Handbuch der experimentellen Pharmakologie
Handbook of Experimental Pharmacology

Heffter-Heubner New Series

XXXVII

Angiotensin

Contributors

D. Allmann · Y. S. Bakhle · E. G. Biglieri · J. R. Blair-West · D. F. Bohr
R. Boucher · G. W. Boyd · F. M. Bumpus · R. D. Buñag · J. P. Coghlan
E. L. Cohen · R. D. Collins · J. W. Conn · H. R. Croxatto · J. O. Davis
D. A. Denton · C. J. Dickinson · F. E. Dorer · C. M. Ferrario · A. Friedman
F. Fyhrquist · J. Genest · T. L. Goodfriend · F. Gross · J. B. Hobbs
J. R. Kahn · P. A. Khairallah · M. C. Khosla · P. Kincaid-Smith
H. G. Langford · W. P. Leary · J. G. Ledingham · K. E. Lentz · M. Levine
J. W. McCubbin · J. C. Melby · L. G. Navar · I. H. Page · M. J. Peach
W. S. Peart · A. L. Robertson · J. W. Ryan · M. Schambelan
B. A. Scoggins · L. Skeggs · R. R. Smeby · J. Stewart · J. R. Stockigt
K. Thurau · R. K. Türker · M. B. Vallotton · J. R. Vane

Editors

Irvine H. Page · F. Merlin Bumpus

With 70 Figures

Springer-Verlag Berlin · Heidelberg · New York 1974

IRVINE H. PAGE, M. D., Emeritus Director of Research, The Cleveland Clinic Foundation, Cleveland, OH 44106/USA

F. MERLIN BUMPUS, Ph. D., Chairman, Division of Research, The Cleveland Clinic Foundation, Cleveland, OH 44106/USA

ISBN-13:978-3-642-65602-6 e-ISBN-13:978-3-642-65600-2
DOI: 10.1007/978-3-642-65600-2

Softcover reprint of the hardcover 1st edition 1974

Angiotensin

Contributors

D. Allmann · Y. S. Bakhle · E. G. Biglieri · J. R. Blair-West · D. F. Bohr
R. Boucher · G. W. Boyd · F. M. Bumpus · R. D. Buñag · J. P. Coghlan
E. L. Cohen · R. D. Collins · J. W. Conn · H. R. Croxatto · J. O. Davis
D. A. Denton · C. J. Dickinson · F. E. Dorer · C. M. Ferrario · A. Friedman
F. Fyhrquist · J. Genest · T. L. Goodfriend · F. Gross · J. B. Hobbs
J. R. Kahn · P. A. Khairallah · M. C. Khosla · P. Kincaid-Smith
H. G. Langford · W. P. Leary · J. G. Ledingham · K. E. Lentz · M. Levine
J. W. McCubbin · J. C. Melby · L. G. Navar · I. H. Page · M. J. Peach
W. S. Peart · A. L. Robertson · J. W. Ryan · M. Schambelan
B. A. Scoggins · L. Skeggs · R. R. Smeby · J. Stewart · J. R. Stockigt
K. Thurau · R. K. Türker · M. B. Vallotton · J. R. Vane

Editors

Irvine H. Page · F. Merlin Bumpus

With 70 Figures

Springer-Verlag New York · Heidelberg · Berlin 1974

IRVINE H. PAGE, M. D., Emeritus Director of Research, The Cleveland Clinic Foundation, Cleveland, OH 44106/USA

F. MERLIN BUMPUS, Ph. D., Chairman, Division of Research, The Cleveland Clinic Foundation, Cleveland, OH 44106/USA

ISBN 0-387-06276-9 Springer-Verlag New York · Heidelberg · Berlin
ISBN 3-540-06276-9 Springer-Verlag Berlin · Heidelberg · New York

Printing: Carl Ritter und Co., Wiesbaden
Binding: Brühlsche Universitätsdruckerei, Gießen

Preface

The history of arterial hypertension is both long and short; long, since BRIGHT (1827) first related hardness of the pulse to hardness of the kidneys and hypertrophy of the heart; short in that modern research began in the late twenties. Most of what we know of these diseases has been discovered in the past fifty years.

The modern story should have begun in 1897 when an extract of kidney was shown to be pressor. But little was done with knowledge until about 1929 when the relationship of this kidney extract called „renin" to hypertension was postulated. The pressor effects were, however, unlike most of those seen with substances such as epinephrine or vasopressin. Plasma was required for action of renin and the active substance appeared to be protein. In 1939, it was shown that renin was not in itself a pressor substance but rather a proteolytic enzyme which produced a powerful pressor substance acting on a substrate synthesized by the liver. Later it was noted that the first definable step after the formation of this peptide was cleaving of the decapeptide which had little or no demonstrable activity, with loss of two amino acids to form the octapeptide called „angiotensin". Within a decade synthesis was achieved which made the substance available for world-wide study. It was not long before attempts were made to measure renin and angiotensin, the latter measurement having been only recently achieved with some degree of elegance. Measurement of renin, while still crude, is serviceable.

Initially, it seemed that the action of angiotensin was relatively simple but this proved grossly misleading. Not only did it have a varied life in the soma but also a seemingly independent one in the nervous system. It gave rise to a number of interesting byplays such as causing the large release of catecholamines from the adrenal medulla and the augmentation of the action of tyramine by way of norepinephrine. Soon it was shown to be the primary stimulant for the release of adrenal cortical aldosterone and hence to have a strong action on salt metabolism. Some evidence implicated it in the production of vascular disease. Even after two decades, the multiplicity of its actions appear not to have been fully uncovered. To call attention to its many functions is one of the purposes of this book.

It has seemed that hypertension is, in principle, a group of diseases differing from the kinds in which a single cause can be found and often eliminated. Since blood pressure is only part of a mechanism the function of which is to perfuse tissues, it seemed appropriate to group hypertension with what might be called "diseases of regulation". To visualize and help conceptualize such disease, a mosaic was proposed in 1948 in which the many elements of the mechanisms controlling tissue perfusion were arranged to indicate their interrelationships. The mosaic showed that equilibria are maintained among these diverse regulatory factors to ensure an orderly distribution of blood. Since the elements are so many and varied, the mosaic provided a structure on which they could be integrated. The earliest form is shown in the accompanying octagon (Figure 1). There is no limit to the amount of knowledge that can be so integrated.

Books today are expensive and time-consuming to read. Much of the material up to 1946 was admirably covered in "Renal Hypertension", by BRAUN-MENENDEZ,

Fasciolo, Leloir, Muñoz and Taquini. This was followed by Page and McCubbin's "Renal Hypertension" in 1968 which aimed at a certain completeness without repetition. The present book was written by a number of highly competent investigators. Editing was minimal in some cases and, as is always the case, to the maximum the author would tolerate in others. The book is not intended for the casual reader but rather for serious students of the problem, hence the differences in points of view and opinions have not been erased in the interest of simplicity. It is not always easy reading but we hope it will always be rewarding.

Cleveland, Winter 1973

Irvine H. Page
F. Merlin Bumpus

Table of Contents

Contributors

Allmann, David, The University of Wisconsin Medical Center, Dept. of Pharmacology, 426 North Charter Street, Madison, WI 53706/USA

Bakhle, Y. S., Dept. of Pharmacology, Institute of Basic Medical Sciences, Royal College of Surgeons of England, Lincoln's Inn Fields, London, WC 2 A 3PN/Great Britain

Biglieri, E. G., Clinical Study Section, Building 100, San Francisco General Hospital, San Francisco, CA 94100/USA

Blair-West, J. R., Howard Florey Institute of Experimental Physiology and Medicine, University of Melbourne, Parkville, Victoria/Australia

Bohr, David F., The University of Michigan, Medical School, Dept. of Physiology, Medical Science Building, Ann Arbor, MI 48104/USA

Boucher, R., Clinical Research Institute of Montreal, 110 Pine Avenue West, Montreal 130/Canada

Boyd, G. W., Senior Lecturer in Medicine, Medical Unit, St. Mary's Hospital Medical School, University of London, Paddington, London W 2/Great Britain

Bumpus, F. M., Research Division, The Cleveland Clinic Foundation, Cleveland, OH 44106/USA

Buñag, Ruben D., Dept. of Pharmacology, Medical Center, University of Kansas, AT 39th Street, Rainbow Boulevard, Kansas City, KS 66103/USA

Coghlan, J. P., Howard Florey Institute of Experimental Physiology and Medicine, University of Melbourne, Parkville, Victoria/Australia

Cohen, E. L., Dept. of Internal Medicine, Division of Endocrinology and Metabolism and the Metabolism Research Unit, The University of Michigan Medical Center, Ann Arbor, MI 48104/USA

Collins, R. D., Clinical Study Section, Building 100, San Francisco General Hospital, San Francisco, CA 94100/USA

Conn, J. W., Dept. of Internal Medicine, Division of Endocrinology and Metabolism and the Metabolism Research Unit, The University of Michigan Medical Center, Ann Arbor, MI 48104/USA

Croxatto, H. R., Dept. of Physiology and Embryology, Catholic University of Chile, Santiago/Chile

Davis, James O., Dept. of Physiology, University of Missouri, School of Medicine, Columbia, MO 65201/USA

Denton, D. A., Howard Florey Institute of Experimental Physiology and Medicine, University of Melbourne, Parkville, Victoria/Australia

Dickinson, C. John, Dept. of Medicine, University College Hospital, Medical School, University Street, London, WC 1 E 6JJ/Great Britain

Dorer, Frederic E., Veterans Administration, 10701 East Boulevard, Cleveland, OH 44106/USA

Ferrario, Carlos M., Research Division, The Cleveland Clinic Foundation, Cleveland, OH 44106/USA

Friedman, A., University of Melbourne, Dept. of Medicine, Royal Melbourne Hospital, P.O. Box 3050, Victoria/Australia

Fyhrquist, Frej, The University of Wisconsin Medical Center, Dept. of Pharmacology, 426 North Charter Street, Madison, WI 53706/USA

Genest, J., Director, Clinical Research Dept., 110 Pine Avenue West, Montreal 130/Canada

Goodfriend, T. L., The University of Wisconsin Medical Center, Dept. of Pharmacology, 426 North Charter Street, Madison, WI53706/USA

Gross, Franz, Director of the Pharmacological Institute, Hauptstraße 47—51, 6900 Heidelberg/Federal Republic of Germany

Hobbs, J. B., University of Melbourne, Dept. of Medicine, Royal Melbourne Hospital, P.O. Box 3050, Victoria/Australia

Kahn, Joseph R., Veterans Administration, 10701 East Boulevard, Cleveland, OH 44106/USA

Khairallah, Philip A., Research Division, The Cleveland Clinic Foundation, Cleveland, OH 44106/USA

Khosla, M. C., Research Division, The Cleveland Clinic Foundation, Cleveland, OH 44106/USA

Kincaid-Smith, P., University of Melbourne, Dept. of Medicine, Royal Melbourne Hospital, P.O. Box 3050, Victoria/Australia

Langford, Herbert G., Dept. of Physiology and Biophysics, University of Mississippi, Medical Center, Jackson, MS 39216/USA

Leary, W. P., University of Natal, Dept. of Physiology, Faculty of Medicine, P.O. Box 39, Congella, Durban/South Africa

Ledingham, J. G., Radcliffe Infirmary, Oxford, OX2 6HE/Great Britain

Lentz, Kenneth E., Veterans Administration, 10701 East Boulevard, Cleveland, OH 44106/USA

Levine, Melvin, Veterans Administration, 10701 East Boulevard, Cleveland, OH 44106/USA

McCubbin, J. W., Research Division, The Cleveland Clinic Foundation, Cleveland, OH 44106/USA

Melby, J. C., Dept. of Medicine, Boston University Medical Center, Boston, MA 02118/USA

Navar, Luis G., Dept. of Physiology and Biophysics, University of Mississippi; Medical Center, Jackson, MS 39216/USA

Page, I. H., 8907 Carnegie Avenue, Cleveland, OH 44106/USA

Peach, M. J., Dept. of Pharmacology, University of Virginia, Charlottesville, VA 22903/USA

Peart, W. S., Director, Medical Unit, St. Mary's Hospital, University of London, London W 2/Great Britain

Robertson, A. Lazzarini, Institute of Pathology, Case Western Reserve University, School of Medicine, Cleveland, OH 44106/USA

Ryan, James W., Box 875, Biscayne Annex, Dept. of Medicine, Miami, FL 33152/USA

Schambelan, M., Clinical Study Section, Building 100, San Francisco General Hospital, San Francisco, CA 94100/USA

Scoggins, B. A., Howard Florey Institute of Physiology and Medicine, University of Melbourne, Parkville, Victoria/ Australia

Skeggs, L., Veterans Administration, 10701 East Boulevard, Cleveland, OH 44106/USA

Smeby, R. R., Research Division, The Cleveland Clinic Foundation, Cleveland, OH 44106/USA

Stewart, John, University of Colorado, School of Medicine, Dept. of Biochemistry, 4200 East Ninth Avenue, Denver, CO 80220/USA

Stockigt, J. R., Clinical Study Section, Building 100, San Francisco General Hospital, San Francisco, CA 94100/USA

Thurau, Klaus, Dept. of Physiology, University of Munich, Pettenkoferstraße 12, 8 München 2/Federal Republic of Germany

Türker, R. K., Dept. of Pharmacology, Faculty of Medicine, University of Ankara, Sihhiye-Ankara/Turkey

Vallotton, M. B., Université de Genève, Laboratoire d'Investigation Clinique, Hôpital Cantonal, Genève/Switzerland

Vane, J. R., Dept. of Pharmacology, Royal College of Surgeons of England, Lincoln's Inn Fields, London WC2 A 3 PN/Great Britain

The Biological Production of Angiotensin

LEONARD T. SKEGGS, FREDERIC E. DORER, JOSEPH R. KAHN
KENNETH E. LENTZ, and MELVIN LEVINE

With 3 Figures

The reaction of kidney renin with its plasma substrate to form angiotensin has been studied for many years using both crude and purified materials derived from many species. Much effort has been expended in the attempt to show the existence or efficacy of inhibitors or activators of the reaction. Many enzymological studies have been carried out to determine optimum pH, Michaelis constants, and maximal velocities. Much of the work prior to 1968 has been reviewed in a publication edited by PAGE and MCCUBBIN (1968).

Renin Substrate

The principal pathway for the generation of angiotensin is represented in Fig. 1. Converting enzyme and the fate of Ang. II are discussed elsewhere in this volume.

Asp-Arg-Val-Tyr-Ile-His-Pro-Phe-His-Leu-Leu-Val-Tyr-Ser-R
(renin substrate, angiotensinogen)
↓ renin
Asp-Arg-Val-Tyr-Ile-His-Pro-Phe-His-Leu + Leu-Val-Tyr-Ser-R
(angiotensin I)
↓ converting enzyme
Asp-Arg-Val-Tyr-Ile-His-Pro-Phe + His-Leu
(angiotensin II)

Fig. 1. Biochemical relationships of the renin-angiotensin system. (After SKEGGS et al., 1968)

The amino-acid sequences of angiotensin shown in Fig. 1 are those of the human (ARAKAWA et al., 1967), the horse (LENTZ et al., 1956; SKEGGS et al., 1956) and the hog (BUMPUS et al., 1957). The bovine form has valine in place of isoleucine in position 5 (ELLIOTT and PEART, 1957).

Assay

Renin substrate (also called angiotensinogen) is measured indirectly by exhaustive incubation with an excess of renin followed by assay of the angiotensin produced. Precautions must be taken to prevent enzymatic and manipulative losses of the product. Substrate concentration is expressed in terms of angiotensin released, preferably in comparison with standard Ang. I.

Distribution

Renin substrate was originally found in the α_2-globulin fraction of plasma (Plentl et al., 1943); more recently it has also been demonstrated in lymph at plasma concentrations (Horky et al., 1971). Levels in normal human serum vary from 600 to 900 ng per ml (as Ang. II) (Gould et al., 1966). Very small amounts have been discovered in dog brain (2.5 to 3 ng per g wet tissue) (Ganten et al., 1972).

Formation

A number of early experiments involving hepatectomy in experimental animals provided indirect evidence that the liver was a principal source of the renin sub-

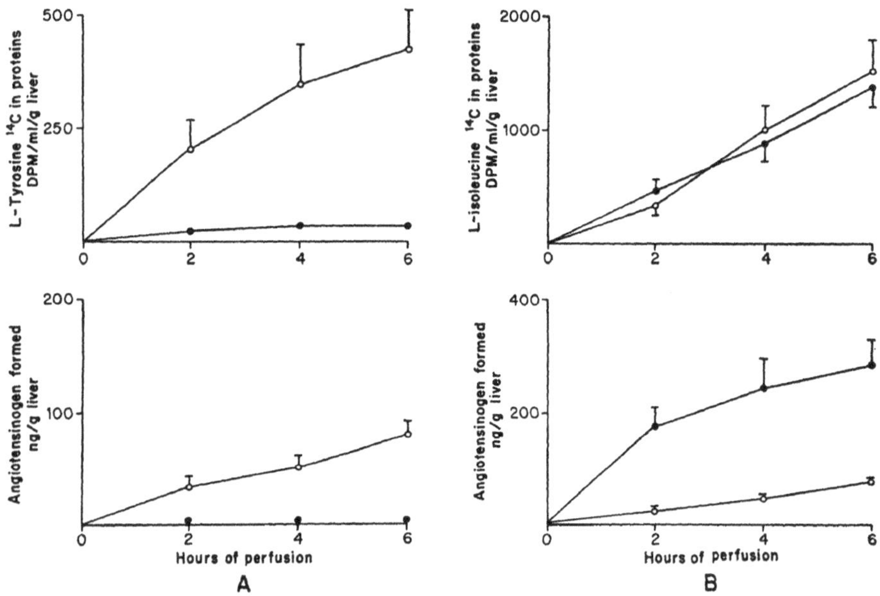

Fig. 2. A.: Angiotensinogen formation and l-tyrosine-^{14}C incorporation into proteins by perfused livers from normal (○) and from puromycin treated rats (●). DPM = Disintegrations per minute. — B.: Angiotensinogen formation and l-isoleucine-^{14}C incorporation into proteins by perfused livers from normal (○) and from 18-h nephrectomized rats (●). DPM = Disintegrations per minute. (After Nasjletti and Masson, 1972)

strate in plasma (Page et al., 1941). Recently Nasjletti and Masson (1972) have demonstrated the synthesis of renin substrate during the perfusion of isolated rat livers for up to 8 h. Inhibition of the synthesis of substrate by puromycin (Fig. 2 A) indicated that most, if not all, of the substrate released into the perfusate was newly synthesized protein. The substrate thus produced in the liver is secreted into the plasma (and probably the lymph) where it may be attacked by renin. Ganten et al. (1972), however, have reported that none of the components of the renin-angiotensin system passed the bloodbrain barrier, and concluded that the small amounts of substrate found in the brain may be synthesized there *de novo*.

Factors Affecting Plasma Levels

The concentration of substrate in the plasma may be decreased by adrenalectomy (BRAUN-MENENDEZ et al., 1946, p. 224). It is increased in pregnancy (GOULD et al., 1966), in malignant hypertension (HELMER and JUDSON, 1963; GOULD et al., 1966), in severe hypoxia (GOULD and GOODMAN, 1970), by nephrectomy (COLLINS and HARAKAL, 1954), and following the administration of ACTH (HELMER and GRIFFITH, 1952; HAYNES et al., 1953), adrenal cortical hormones (HAYNES et al., 1953), and estrogens (HELMER and GRIFFITH, 1952). The most impressive change in substrate level occurs in the rat in the 24-h period following bilateral nephrectomy when the concentration may increase 4 to 15 times (REGOLI et al., 1961; BLAQUIER, 1965). The mechanism controlling the substrate level is not known. It is almost certainly based on the regulation of synthesis by the liver, not by the rate of utilization by circulating renin (TATEISHI et al., 1971). It is interesting that the rate of substrate synthesis observed by NASJLETTI and MASSON (1972) was much greater in perfused livers of bilaterally nephrectomized rats (Fig. 2 B).

Purification and Properties of Hog Substrate

Substrate has been purified from hog plasma by a multistep procedure (SKEGGS et al., 1963) which involved ammonium sulfate fractionation, partial acid denaturation of impurities, ion-exchange chromatography, solvent partitioning, and countercurrent distribution. One major form (A) and two minor forms (B and C) were found by DEAE-cellulose column chromatography. B and C were each further separated into additional forms, 1 and 2, during countercurrent distribution in a polyethylene glycol-Li_2SO_4 system. The final purified products had molecular weights of approximately 58,000 as determined by ultracentrifugation. The several types of substrate were separable by electrophoresis. A migrating between α_2 and β-globulin, both B forms moving as slow α_2-globulins, and the C forms as α_2-globulins. Chemical analysis showed that the substrates were glycoproteins with almost identical amino acid compositions. There were, however, substantial differences in their glucosamine, neutral hexose and sialic acid content (Table 1). The Michaelis constants (K_m) for the different forms of substrate as determined with purified homologous renin are: A, 1.76×10^{-6} *M*; B_1 and B_2, 0.71×10^{-6} *M*; C_1, 1.32×10^{-6} *M*; and C_2, 1.20×10^{-6} *M* (SKEGGS et al., 1967).

Structure of the Tetradecapeptide Substrate

Protein substrate isolated from horse plasma may be degraded with trypsin to yield a tetradecapeptide with full substrate activity (SKEGGS et al., 1957). The structure of the latter compound, shown in Fig. 1, was determined by sequential analysis (SKEGGS et al., 1957) and was confirmed by synthesis (SKEGGS et al., 1958). The Asn^1, Val^5 analog of the equine tetradecapeptide also has been synthesized (MONTAGUE et al., 1966); it was found to be kinetically identical with the synthetic equine tetradecapeptide when incubated with hog renin (SKEGGS et al., 1968). The production of the tetradecapeptide substrate from the natural protein substrate through the action of trypsin has always been puzzling. Trypsin is a highly specific peptidase (with esterase activity) and has not been observed to hydrolyze a peptide bond formed from the carboxyl group of serine. LEE and WILSON (1971) have now prepared the tetradecapeptide substrate from the protein substrate by treatment with alcoholic NaOH. They suggest that the tetradecapeptide may be covalently bonded to the parent protein by an ester linkage between the serine hydroxyl group and the carboxyl group of either arginine or lysine (Fig. 3). Such a structure would imply that the carboxyl group of serine is free and that the protein substrate would have two terminal amino groups. It is of interest to note that both the fluorodinitrobenzene and the phenyl isothiocyanate methods revealed

Table 1. *Comparison of the chemical composition of substrates A, C_1 and C_2 (from* SKEGGS *et al., 1963)*

Constituent	Assumed No. of residues per mole A	C_1	C_2
Aspartic acid	37	36	36
Threonine	36	36	36
Serine	36	39	36
Glutamic acid	45	46	45
Proline	30	28	28
Glycine	34	34	33
Alanine	42	42	43
Cystine	2	2	2
Valine	34	34	33
Methionine	7	7	7
Isoleucine	9	9	9
Leucine	67	67	67
Tyrosine	8	8	7
Phenylalanine	24	23	21
Ammonia	40	44	47
Lysine	18	18	17
Histidine	10	10	9
Arginine	21	20	20
Glucosamine	4	5	7
Sialic acid	2	3	3
Neutral hexose	8	9	12

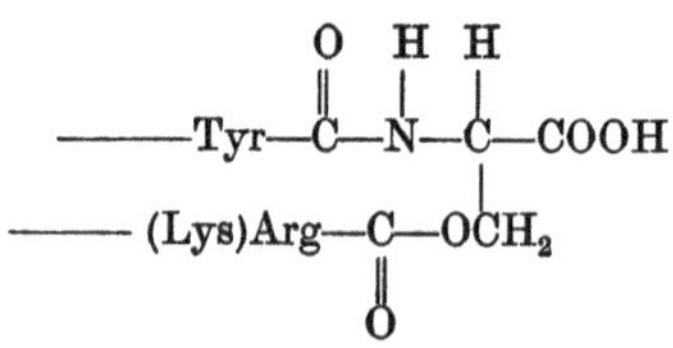

Fig. 3. Proposed ester linkage between C-terminal serine of tetradecapeptide and protein in renin substrate. (After LEE and WILSON, 1971)

aspartic acid as the only N-terminal amino acid in the purified protein substrate (SKEGGS et al., 1963).

A number of peptides have been synthesized which represent portions of the tetradecapeptide substrate and which include the hydrolyzable Leu-Leu bond (SKEGGS et al., 1968). The hydrolysis of these peptides has been studied using purified hog renin (Table 2). A chemical method of determining the rate of hydrolysis was necessary since not all the products were biologically active. The maximum affinity of renin and substrate is obtained when the full tetradecapeptide

Table 2. *Kinetic data describing action of renin on nine peptides (from* SKEGGS *et al., 1968)*

Peptide														Renin concentration	$K_m \times 10^6$ *M*	Average $\times 10^6$ *M*	$V_{max} \times 10^6$ *M*/min	$V_{max} \times 10^6$ *M*/min per Goldblatt units/ml
														Goldblatt units/ml				
1	2	3	4	5	6	7	8	9	10	11	12	13	14					
Asp	Arg	Val	Tyr	Ileu	His	Pro	Phe	His	Leu	Leu	Val	Tyr	Ser	0.0457	3.66	3.68	0.48	10.2
														0.0915	3.70		0.92	
Asn	Arg	Val	Tyr	Val	His	Pro	Phe	His	Leu	Leu	Val	Tyr	Ser	0.0457	3.18	4.06	0.37	9.1
														0.0915	4.95		0.94	
		Val	Tyr	Ileu	His	Pro	Phe	His	Leu	Leu	Val	Tyr	Ser	0.0195	30.1	28.0	0.91	8.9
														0.1830	26.0		1.45	
			Tyr	Ileu	His	Pro	Phe	His	Leu	Leu	Val	Tyr	Ser	0.0457	23.0	26.1	0.51	9.8
														0.0915	29.2		0.78	
				Ileu	His	Pro	Phe	His	Leu	Leu	Val	Tyr	Ser	0.0457	32.2	30.7	0.55	10.9
														0.0915	29.2		0.88	
					His	Pro	Phe	His	Leu	Leu	Val	Tyr	Ser	0.0915	52.4	46.8	1.08	11.7
														0.1830	41.3		2.13	
					His	Pro	Phe	His	Leu	Leu	Val	Tyr		0.0915	55.2	54.9	0.74	7.6
														0.1830	54.6		1.32	
						Pro	Phe	His	Leu	Leu	Val	Tyr	Ser	0.183	50.8	53.6	0.10	0.55
														0.366	56.5		0.21	
					His	Pro	Phe	His	Leu	Leu	Val			0.183	∞	∞		0

is used. Removal of the Asp-Arg from the N-terminal position increases the K_m nearly 10-fold. Further increases in the K_m occur when the molecule is shortened to an octapeptide having Pro^7 as its N-terminal residue. Although the octapeptide has a very low V_{max}, the β-naphthyl amide of its N-benzyloxycarbonyl derivative has been used for assaying renin (REINHARZ and ROTH, 1969). The octapeptide having His^6 as its N-terminal residue and Tyr^{13} as its C-terminal residue has a similar K_m but a much greater V_{max}. Since the peptide terminating in Val^{12} is inactive, Tyr^{13} is apparently essential for the action of hog renin. The nonapeptide His^6 through Ser^{14} has been used successfully as the substrate in an automated chemical method for the assay of renin in kidney extracts (LEVINE et al., 1970).

Human Substrate

Partially purified human substrate has been prepared by ROSENTHAL et al. (1971) by a three-step procedure. After fractionation with ammonium sulfate, the substrate was passed over a column of Sephadex G-75, and the richest fraction was further treated by preparative disc electrophoresis.

The kinetics of the reaction of human renin on homologous substrate have been studied (HAAS and GOLDBLATT, 1967; GOULD and GREEN, 1971; ROSENTHAL et al., 1971). The reported K_m values vary from 0.12×10^{-6} M (ROSENTHAL et al., 1971) to 0.93×10^{-6} M (GOULD and GREEN, 1971). The renin-substrate concentration of human serum varies from an average value of 0.78×10^{-6} M in a normal population to as high as 6×10^{-6} M in patients with malignant hypertension, and may therefore exert as great an influence on the velocity of the renin reaction as the renin concentration itself (GOULD and GREEN, 1971).

Substrate from Other Species

It has long been known that substrates from different species vary markedly in their susceptibility to hydrolysis by heterologous renin. The most extreme example is that of human substrate which is not attacked by other renins except those of primates (BRAUN-MENENDEZ et al., 1946, pp. 134, 135). Conversely, animal substrates are acted upon readily by human renin to produce angiotensin. It has recently been reported by SEN et al. (1971) that the plasmas of rabbit, rat, dog and hog contain a form of substrate (about 40% of the total) which is cleaved only by homologous renin while the remaining portion (60%) may be hydrolyzed by either homologous or heterologous renin. No attempt was made to separate the two types of substrate from any of the species studied. It is not known whether the forms of substrate isolated from hog plasma (SKEGGS et al., 1963) differ in their susceptibility to hydrolysis by homologous and heterologous renins. CARRETERO et al. (1971) have reported the presence of yet another source of Ang. I in dog and rat plasma. This is a previously unknown form of substrate that is not acted upon by hog kidney renin, but is attacked by dog uterine renin. There is some difficulty in reconciling the results of SEN et al. (1971) with those of CARRETERO and co-workers (1971). In the first instance, additional angiotensin could be produced from dog or rat plasma by incubation with homologous renin after the plasma had been treated exhaustively with hog renin. However, in the second instance, no additional angiotensin could be produced in dog or rat plasma by homologous renins if the plasma was first treated with hog renin. The two sets of experiments differed in that the latter workers used plasma from nephrectomized animals.

Other Sources of Angiotensin

It has been reported that Ang. I is present in the kidneys of dogs and humans and is released into the circulation via the renal vein (ITSKOVITZ and ODYA, 1971). The high concentrations which were found were measured by immunoassay and were not confirmed by direct pressor assay. SCHWEIKERT et al. (1972) have claimed that the pressor substance of GROLLMAN and KRISHNAMURTY (1971) ("nephrotensin"), which is said to be found in renal venous blood, is in fact Ang. I complexed with α_2-globulin. In any event, it is reasonable to suppose that Ang. I may be produced by renin fixed within the juxtaglomerular cells acting *in situ* upon the substrate from plasma. The reported production of Ang. I by the incubation of isolated glomeruli in the absence of substrate (FINKIELMAN and NAHMOD, 1969) has not yet been confirmed.

Renin

Distribution

Although renin has now been found in many different tissues of the body, it is predominantly located in the kidney. GOORMAGHTIGH's (1939) conclusion that renin is elaborated and stored in the juxtaglomerular apparatus has been confirmed many times (PAGE and McCUBBIN, 1968, p. 50). A method has recently been developed for the determination of renin activity in a single juxtaglomerular apparatus removed from the kidney by microdissection (DAHLHEIM et al., 1970).

The subcellular localization of renin, as determined by differential centrifugation of homogenized kidney preparations, appears to be lysosomal (OGINO et al., 1967) by its appearance in the isolated lysosomal fraction and subsequent solubilization by freezing and thawing, as well as its shift to the soluble portion upon vigorous homogenization (NUSTAD and RUBIN, 1970).

It has not been possible to find sufficient renin activity in the circulating blood of humans with hypertensive cardiovascular disease to provide a reasonable explanation for the elevation in blood pressure (BROWN et al., 1964). This failure has led to a search for the enzyme in blood vessel walls. There, renin might produce Ang. I from plasma substrate, and tissue converting enzymes would then form Ang. II which could be taken up immediately by vicinal receptor sites. In this manner, peripheral vasoconstriction could be produced without renin or angiotensin ever appearing in the circulation. Renin activity has been found in the large arteries and veins of the hog and the dog (DENGLER, 1956; GOULD et al., 1964). The enzyme appeared to be similar to kidney renin, and it was suggested that it had been transferred to the arterial site from the kidney via the circulation. More recent work has shown that renin activity is present in the mesenteric vessels of 24-h nephrectomized dogs (GANTEN et al., 1970), and that this activity increases during severe hemorrhage. Simultaneously, it was shown that the renin activity in portal vein blood of such animals increases and at a faster rate than in arterial blood. It is thus implied that the splanchnic area has the potentiality for synthesizing and releasing renin into the general circulation.

Significant amounts of renin activity have also been found in the uterus and the placenta (GOULD et al., 1964; GROSS et al., 1964), in the adrenals and the brain (GANTEN et al., 1972), and in the liver (GOULD et al., 1964). The renin of the uterus is similar to kidney renin (ANDERSON et al., 1968; RYAN and JOHNSON, 1969) and has been shown to increase during pregnancy (FERRIS et al., 1967). Dog uterine renin produces Ang. I from homologous plasma, but a hitherto unknown form of substrate appears to be involved (CARRETERO et al., 1971).

The renin-like activity, discovered in brains of rats and dogs (FISCHER-FERRARO et al., 1971; GANTEN et al., 1972), persists after nephrectomy and, since renin was incapable of passing the blood-brain barrier, it appears to be synthesized in the brain itself (GANTEN et al., 1972). The pH optimum for the reaction of dog-brain renin with homologous plasma substrate has been reported to be 5 by GANTEN et al. (1972); but FISCHER-FERRARO et al. (1971) found it to lie between 7 and 7.5. The concentration of renin in the brain was decreased after giving aldosterone and increased by administration of progesterone (GANTEN et al., 1971).

A pressor substance discovered in the submaxillary gland of the mouse (WERLE et al., 1957) was found to be a renin-like enzyme (TURRIAN, 1960). It is present in extremely high concentrations and has been purified (WERLE et al., 1968; TAYLOR et al., 1971). Rat antiserum to the submaxillary gland enzyme of the mouse cross-reacts with kidney renin of dog, pig, or mouse, but not with kidney renin of human (WERLE et al., 1968). The molecular weight of the enzyme from mouse submaxillary gland is reported to be 43,000 (TAYLOR et al., 1971).

Purification and Properties of Animal Renins

Renin has been prepared in crude form from the kidneys of a large number of species (Table 3) (HAAS et al., 1954). There have been several significant attempts

Table 3. *Renin content of the kidneys of various species (from* HAAS *et al., 1954)*

	Renin extracted units renin/ g kidney	Protein extracted mg protein/ g kidney	Specific activity units renin/ mg dry substance
Rabbit	12	19	0.63
Mouse	9	20	0.44
Cat	7.1	14	0.50
Hog	4.3	20	0.22
Rat	2.2	26	0.08
Dog	1.0	18	0.06
Beef	1.0	17	0.06
Guinea pig	0.40	20	0.02
Sheep	0.17	19	0.009
Human	0.11	19	0.006
Horse	0.08	19	0.004
Macaca mulatta monkey	0.02	16	.

at purification of hog and beef renin (Table 4). The first was that of HAAS and co-workers [1953 (1)] who attained a 56,000-fold purification of hog renin using classical methods of organic solvent and salt fractionation. NAIRN et al. (1960), using starch gel electrophoresis as the final step, obtained a small yield of the hog enzyme purified almost 18,000-fold. PEART et al. (1966) purified hog renin 13,500-fold using a series of chromatographic columns followed by starch gel electrophoresis. A 1900-fold purification of renin from an aqueous extract of bovine kidneys has been reported by NEWSOME (1969) using ammonium sulfate fractionation, gel filtration, batch adsorption on CM-Sephadex, DEAE-cellulose chromatography, and preparative disc electrophoresis. Analytical disc electrophoresis of the final product showed that the renin activity was associated with at least four electrophoretic components. WILLARD et al. (1970) also reported obtaining multiple

Table 4. *Compilation of purifications of animal renins obtained by various investigators*

Reference	Purification factor up to columns	Columns used	Purification factor on columns	Over-all for columns	Other methods	Purification factor	Over-all purification
HAAS et al., 1953 (1)	—	None	—	—	salts, pH, organic solvents	56,000	56,000
PASSANANTI, 1959	650	DEAE-cellulose	10	10	1st 5 steps of HAAS et al., 1953 (1)	—	6,500
NAIRN et al., 1960	40	None	—	—	starch gel electrophoresis	16	17,700
KEMP and RUBIN, 1962	—	DEAE-cellulose	10—20	10—20	adsorption on kaolin	10	—
MAIER and MORGAN, 1966	16.4	TEAE-cellulose GE-cellulose Sephadex G-75	10 3.4 6.5	220	—	—	3,500
PEART et al., 1966	16	DEAE-cellulose CM-Sephadex Sephadex G-100	19 3.6 9.0	615	starch gel electrophoresis	—	13,500
NEWSOME, 1969	3.3	Sephadex G-25 Sephadex G-100 DEAE-cellulose	2.4 3.4 5.9	49	CM-Sephadex (batch) preparative disc electrophoresis	3.3 3.6	1,900

forms of beef kidney renin by means of electrofocusing, as did RUBIN (1972) for hog kidney renin.

The existence of hog renin in multiple forms has been demonstrated by SKEGGS et al. (1967). Chromatography on DEAE-cellulose in a descending pH gradient yielded renins I through IV eluting at pH 5.2, 4.7, 4.5, and 4.25, respectively. Only renin I was found when great care was taken to perform the preliminary isolation and dialysis at neutral pH. Dialysis of renin I at pH 5 or treatment under very mild acid conditions converted it to renin II. The Michaelis constants obtained using purified hog substrate were 1.7, 1.0, 1.0, and 1.2×10^{-6} M for renins I through IV respectively, values which do not imply significant differences.

LEVINE and co-workers (1972), using a 3500-fold purified hog kidney renin prepared by batch methods, found a molecular weight of about 40,000 by gel filtration on BioGel P-150. This is close to the earlier value of 42,000 to 49,000 reported by KEMP and RUBIN (1964), and is in agreement with the more recent value of 40,000 found by ultracentrifugation (RUBIN, 1972).

Purification and Properties of Human Renin

The purification of human renin has been attempted by several groups of workers (DEXTER et al., 1945; HAAS et al., 1965; LUBASH and PEART, 1966). The most recent effort was that of LUCAS et al. (1970) who used ammonium sulfate fractionation and chromatography on DEAE-cellulose, CM-Sephadex, and Sephadex G-200, followed by preparative polyacrylamide gel electrophoresis. The final product yielded a single band on analytical disc gel electrophoresis. The maximum specific activity obtained was between 5 and 13 Goldblatt units per mg protein. The molecular weight of human renin is 42,000 as determined by gel filtration, the isoelectric point is 5.25, and the pH optimum of the reaction with homologous substrate is 5.5 (WALDHAUSL et al., 1970).

It has been shown that human kidney renin, like hog kidney renin, exists in several forms (SKEGGS et al., 1972). An aqueous extract of human kidneys was treated with DEAE-cellulose, precipitated with ammonium sulfate, and dialyzed against distilled water. Upon chromatography on DEAE-cellulose at pH 5.5 in an increasing salt gradient, two major forms (A and D) and two minor forms (B and C) were obtained. All four forms were found to have molecular weights of approximately 39,500 as determined by gel filtration on BioGel P-150. Renins A and D were subjected to countercurrent distribution in a solvent system composed of polyethylene glycol-NaH_2PO_4, pH 4. By this means, it was shown that renin A consisted of two components having distribution coefficients of 1.95 and 3.55, while renin D consisted of five components having distribution coefficients of 0.11, 0.39, 0.66, 1.90 and 3.16. That there may be important differences among the forms of human renin is shown by the diversity of their pH-velocity curves with homologous substrate (SKEGGS et al., 1972; SKEGGS, LENTZ, KAHN, LEVINE, DORER, unpublished observations). Furthermore, various preparations of these forms differ enormously in their abilities to hydrolyze the natural homologous substrate as compared with the tetradecapeptide substrate. In view of the latter observation, it would be hazardous to attempt to assay human renin using a simple peptide substrate.

Pseudorenin

Ang. I may also be produced by the recently discovered enzyme, pseudorenin (SKEGGS et al., 1969). This enzyme has been found in every tissue yet studied, including plasma. It is in especially high concentration in salivary gland, spleen, and thymus of the rat. Pseudorenin hydrolyzes both the tetradecapeptide substrate and highly purified hog substrate. The pH optimum for its enzymatic reaction is 4.5 to 5.0. It does not attack the protein substrate in plasma because of the presence of pseudorenin inhibitor. Attempts to purify the inhibitor have shown that it is intimately associated with plasma proteins (SKEGGS, LENTZ, KAHN, DORER, LEVINE, unpublished observations). Although certain protein fractions appear to be more inhibitory than others, it has not yet been possible to achieve significant purification of the inhibitor. Recent studies involving fractionation of human kidneys (SKEGGS et al., 1972) have shown that the pseudorenin from this source may exist in several forms with molecular weights ranging from 43,000 to 158,000 or more, and with pH-activity curves which differ markedly from each other. It would appear that pseudorenin is an intracellular enzyme, possibly located in high concentration within a micro-environment where the plasma inhibitor does not exist. The source of the substrate for the enzyme is not known, nor is the function of the angiotensin that might be produced.

Modified Renin

The effect of chemical modification of renin has received limited attention. Early studies by HAAS et al. [1953 (2)] have shown that renin is relatively unaffected by heavy metal ions with the exception of high concentrations (0.001 *M*) of Fe^{3+}, Au^{+}, Cu^{2+}, Ag^{+}, and Pt^{4+}. However, the test for inactivation was by means of direct pressor assay in the dog, which might have allowed dissociation of the metal-enzyme complex to occur. HAAS et al. (1965) have also made an extensive study of the acetylation of renin, a reaction which both inactivates the enzyme and, at the same time, renders it antigenic in the homologous species. DEODHAR et al. (1964) found that reaction with *p*-chloromercuribenzoate, iodoacetate, iodine, or formaldehyde inactivates renin. More recently, REINHARZ and co-workers (1971) have verified the observation that acetylation inactivates renin, and have tested other chemical agents as well. Reaction with fluorodinitrobenzene, diazobenzene sulfonic acid, or phenyl isocyanate was found to inactivate the enzyme, indicating that amino groups are important to the biological activity of the molecule. Renin activity was unaffected by diisopropyl fluorophosphate or by dialysis against EDTA. These investigators found no inactivation of renin after treatment of the enzyme with *p*-chloromercuribenzoate, as measured by a chemical assay (REINHARZ et al., 1971). It is of interest in this respect that in many cases the biological assay showed a greater inhibition after chemical treatment of the enzyme than did the chemical assay.

An active, water-insoluble derivative of renin has been prepared by the binding of partially purified hog renin to Sepharose 4B (SEKI et al., 1970). Enzyme activity was measured by incubation with hog renin substrate followed by pressor assay in the rat. The bound renin had about one half the hydrolytic activity of the soluble enzyme, and was stable for many months in the refrigerator.

Modifiers of the Renin Reaction

The kidney has long been thought to exert a protective action in experimental hypertension (FASCIOLO et al., 1938). When one normal kidney is present, it is more difficult to establish sustained hypertension in dogs than when both renal arteries are clamped or when one is clamped and the contralateral kidney is removed. Bilaterally nephrectomized animals are much more sensitive to injected renin than are normal animals. For this reason, it was natural for investigators to look to the kidneys as a possible source of antihypertensive substances. Smeby et al. (1967) have succeeded in preparing a phospholipid from kidney tissue which in large amounts prevents an *in vivo* response to injected renin. It is also capable of lowering the blood pressure of rats with acute or chronic renal hypertension (Sen et al., 1968). Recently Rakhit (1971) has determined that the structure of the inhibitor is phosphatidylethanolamine with a large percentage of polyunsaturated fatty acids. The isolated phospholipid is not the active inhibitor, but rather a preinhibitor which is converted to the active lysophospholipid by hydrolysis with phospholipase A or by plasma (Smeby et al., 1967).

The existence of an inhibitor in normal rat plasma has been proposed by Montague (1968) on the basis of kinetic studies. Blaquier (1965) and Poulsen (1971), on the other hand, could find no evidence for the presence of inhibitors of the reaction between renin and its substrate. This was true for normal, salt-depleted, and nephrectomized rats (Poulsen, 1971). A difference in level of renin inhibitor found in rat plasma based on the strain of animal used has been reported (Iwai et al., 1970).

Renin is inhibited by heparin (Sealey et al., 1967), bile (Hiwada et al., 1969) and certain small peptides such as Leu-Leu-Val-Tyr-OEt (Kokubu et al., 1968). The action of renin on highly purified protein substrates can also be inhibited by several peptides whose structures represent portions of the tetradecapeptide substrate molecule (Table 2). Low concentrations of these peptides produce partial inhibition of hog renin but complete inhibition occurs only at very high concentrations of peptide. Although these peptides are inhibitory in aqueous solutions, they are completely ineffective in the presence of plasma (Skeggs, Lentz, Kahn, unpublished observations).

A system capable of the slow inactivation of renin *in vitro* has been described for rat and human plasma (Schaechtelin et al., 1968; Regoli, 1970). The system is destroyed by acidification to pH 3, and is inoperative in the presence of EDTA. Red cells are said to exert a protective action on serum renin (Michelakis and Mizukoshi, 1971). The disappearance of renin from the circulation of rats apparently does not depend upon the plasma-inactivating system, but upon the non-excretory removal of renin by the kidneys (Peters-Haefeli, 1971). This would provide a partial explanation of the increased sensitivity of nephrectomized animals to injected renin.

Conclusion

We have attempted, in this chapter, to present a concise, yet over-all view of angiotensin-forming reactions, particularly that of renin with its substrate. It may be noted that there is considerable disagreement among workers on many aspects of this subject. In part, this disagreement can be traced to technical difficulties. The biological products which are required are difficult to prepare and to characterize. Assays, for the most part, are biological and imprecise. The validity of certain immunoassays is doubtful. Standardizations of assays are not always based on the same form of angiotensin, and frequently the purity of the standard is uncertain. Finally, there is no agreement on a uniform method for the expression of results. All these difficulties must be kept in mind in attempting to evaluate the apparently contradictory results which so frequently appear in this field.

References

ANDERSON, R. C., HERBERT, P. N., MULROW, P. J.: A comparison of properties of renin obtained from the kidney and uterus of the rabbit. Amer. J. Physiol. **215**, 774 (1968).

ARAKAWA, K., NAKAMURA, M.: Studies on human angiotensin. Circulat. Res. **20—21** (Suppl. II), 101 (1967).

BLAQUIER, P.: Kinetic studies of renin-angiotensinogen reaction after nephrectomy. Amer. J. Physiol. **208**, 1083 (1965).

BRAUN-MENENDEZ, E., FASCIOLO, J. C., LELOIR, L. F., MUNOZ, J. M., TAQUINI, A. C.: Renal hypertension. Springfield/Illinois: Charles C. Thomas 1946.

BROWN, J. J., DAVIES, D. L., LEVER, A. F., ROBERTSON, J. I. S.: Variations in plasma renin concentration in several physiological and pathological states. Canad. med. Ass. J. **90**, 201 (1964).

BUMPUS, F. M., SCHWARZ, H., PAGE, I. H.: Synthesis and pharmacology of the octapeptide angiotonin. Science **125**, 886 (1957).

CARRETERO, O. A., BUJAK, B., HOULE, J. A.: Renin isozymes of extrarenal origin. Amer. J. Physiol. **220**, 1468 (1971).

COLLINS, D. A., HARAKAL, C. D.: Changes in hypertensinase and hypertensinogen following nephrectomy. Circulat. Res. **2**, 196 (1954).

DAHLHEIM, H., GRANGER, P., THURAU, K.: A sensitive method for determination of renin activity in the single juxtaglomerular apparatus of the rat kidney. Pflügers Arch. ges. Physiol. **321**, 303 (1970).

DENGLER, H.: Über einen reninartigen Wirkstoff in Arterienextrakten. Naunyn-Schmiedebergs Arch. exp. Path. Pharmak. **227**, 481 (1956).

DEODHAR, S. D., CUPPAGE, F. E., GABLEMAN, E.: Studies on the mechanism of experimental proteinuria induced by renin. J. exp. Med. **120**, 677 (1964).

DEXTER, L., HAYNES, F. W., BRIDGES, W. C.: The renal humoral pressor mechanism in man. I. Preparation and assay of human renin, human hypertensinogen, and hypertensin. J. clin. Invest. **24**, 62 (1945).

ELLIOTT, D. F., PEART, W. S.: The amino acid sequence in a hypertensin. Biochem. J. **65**, 246 (1957).

FASCIOLO, J. C., HOUSSAY, B. A., TAQUINI, A. C.: The blood-pressure raising secretion of the ischaemic kidney. J. Physiol. (Lond.) **94**, 281 (1938).

FERRIS, T. F., GORDEN, P., MULROW, P. J.: Rabbit uterus as a source of renin. Amer. J. Physiol. **212**, 698 (1967).

FINKIELMAN, S., NAHMOD, V. E.: *In vitro* production of angiotensin I by renal glomeruli. Nature (Lond.) **222**, 186 (1969).

FISCHER-FERRARO, C., NAHMOD, V. E., GOLDSTEIN, D. J., FINKIELMAN, S.: Angiotensin and renin in rat and dog brain. J. exp. Med. **133**, 353 (1971).

GANTEN, D., HAYDUK, K., BRECHT, H. M., BOUCHER, R., GENEST, J.: Evidence of renin release or production in splanchnic territory. Nature (Lond.) **226**, 551 (1970).

GANTEN, D., MINNICH, J. L., GRANGER, P., HAYDUK, K., BRECHT, H. M., BARBEAU, A., BOUCHER, R., GENEST, J.: Angiotensin-forming enzyme in brain tissue. Science **173**, 64 (1972).

GANTEN, D., GRANGER, P., GANTEN, U., BOUCHER, R., GENEST, J.: An intrinsic renin-angiotensin system in the brain. In: Hypertension 1972. Berlin-Heidelberg-New York: Springer 1972.

GOORMAGTIGH, N.: La présence de cellules endocrines dans la paroi des artérioles du rein et leur comportement dans l'ischémie renale. C. R. Soc. Biol. (Paris) **132**, 465 (1939).

GOULD, A. B., SKEGGS, L. T., Jr., KAHN, J. R.: The presence of renin activity in blood vessel walls. J. exp. Med. **119**, 389 (1964).

GOULD, A. B., SKEGGS, L. T., KAHN, J. R.: Measurement of renin and substrate concentrations in human serum. Lab. Invest. **15**, 1802 (1966).

GOULD, A. B., GOODMAN, S. A.: The effect of hypoxia on the renin-angiotensinogen system. Lab. Invest. **22**, 443 (1970).

GOULD, A. B., GREEN, D.: Kinetics of the human renin and human substrate reaction. Cardiovasc. Res. **5**, 86 (1971).

GROLLMAN, A., KRISHNAMURTY, V. S. R.: A new pressor agent of renal origin: its differentiation from renin and angiotensin. Amer. J. Physiol. **221**, 1499 (1971).

GROSS, F., SCHAECHTELIN, G., ZIEGLER, M., BERGER, M.: A renin-like substance in the placenta and uterus of the rabbit. Lancet **1964 I**, 914.

HAAS, E., GOLDBLATT, H.: Kinetic constants of the human renin and human angiotensinogen reaction. Circulat. Res. **20**, 45 (1967).

HAAS, E., GOLDBLATT, H., GIPSON, E. C.: Extraction, purification, and acetylation of human renin and the production of antirenin to human renin. Arch. Biochem. Biophys. **110**, 534 (1965).

HAAS, E., LAMFROM, H., GOLDBLATT, H.: (1) Isolation and purification of hog renin. Arch. Biochem. Biophys. **42**, 368 (1953).

HAAS, E., LAMFROM, H., GOLDBLATT, H.: (2) Biochemical and physicochemical studies on renin. Arch. Biochem. Biophys. **44**, 63 (1953).

HAAS, E., LAMFROM, H., GOLDBLATT, H.: A simple method for the extraction and partial purification of renin. Arch. Biochem. Biophys. **48**, 256 (1954).

HAYNES, F. W., FORSHAM, P. H., HUME, D. M.: Effects of ACTH, cortisone, desoxycorticosterone, and epinephrine on the plasma hypertensinogen, and renin concentration of dogs. Amer. J. Physiol. **172**, 265 (1953).

HELMER, O. M., GRIFFITH, R. S.: The effect of the administration of estrogens on the renin-substrate (hypertensinogen) content of rat plasma. Endocrinology **51**, 421 (1952).

HELMER, O. M., JUDSON, W. E.: The quantitative determination of renin in the plasma of patients with arterial hypertension. Circulation **27**, 1050 (1963).

HIWADA, K., KOKUBU, T., YAMAMURA, Y.: Inhibitory effect of rabbit bile on renin angiotensinogen reaction system. Jap. Circulat. J. (En.) **33**, 1231 (1969).

HORKY, K., ROJO-ORTEGA, J. M., RODRIGUEZ, J., BOUCHER, R., GENEST, J.: Renin, renin substrate, and angiotensin I-converting enzyme in the lymph of rats. Amer. J. Physiol. **220**, 307 (1971).

ITSKOVITZ, H. D., ODYA, C.: Intrarenal formation of angiotensin I. Science **174**, 58 (1971).

IWAI, J., KNUDSEN, K. D., DAHL, L. K.: Genetic influence on the renin angiotensin system. Evidence for a renin inhibitor in hypertension prone rats. J. exp. Med. **131**, 543 (1970).

KEMP, E., RUBIN, I.: Renin purification by DEAE cellulose chromatography. Scand. J. clin. Lab. Invest. **14**, 207 (1962).

KEMP, E., RUBIN, I.: Molecular weight of renin determined by Sephadex gel filtration. Acta chem. scand. **18**, 2403 (1964).

KOKUBU, T., UEDA, E., FUJIMOTO, S., HIWADA, K., KATO, A., AKUTSU, H., YAMAMURA, Y.: Peptide inhibitors of the renin-angiotensin system. Nature (Lond.) **217**, 456 (1968).

LEE, H.-J., WILSON, I. B.: On the structure of renin substrate. Biochim. biophys. Acta (Amst.) **243**, 530 (1971).

LENTZ, K. E., SKEGGS, L. T., Jr., WOODS, K. R., KAHN, J. R., SHUMWAY, N. P.: The amino acid composition of hypertensin II and its biochemical relationship to hypertensin I. J. exp. Med. **104**, 183 (1956).

LEVINE, M., DORER, F. E., KAHN, J. R., LENTZ, K. E., SKEGGS, L. T.: Chemical determination of hog kidney renin by an automated method. Analyt. Biochem. **34**, 366 (1970).

LEVINE, M., LENTZ, K. E., SKEGGS, L. T., KAHN, J. R., DORER, F. E.: Preparation of hog renin free of pseudorenin. In: Hypertension—1972. Berlin-Heidelberg-New York: Springer 1972.

LUBASH, G. D., PEART, W. S.: Purification of human renin. Biochim. biophys. Acta (Amst.) **122**, 289 (1966).

LUCAS, C. P., FUKUCHI, S., CONN, J. W., BERLINGER, F. G., WALDHAUSL, W.-K., COHEN, E. L., ROVNER, D. R.: Purification of human renin. J. Lab. clin. Med. **76**, 689 (1970).

MAIER, G. D., MORGAN, W. S.: Purification of hog renin by column chromatography. Biochim. biophys. Acta (Amst.) **128**, 193 (1966).

MICHELAKIS, A. M., MIZUKOSHI, H.: Distribution and disappearance rate of renin in man and dog. J. clin. Endocr. **33**, 27 (1971).

MONTAGUE, D.: Kinetics of renin-angiotensinogen reaction in plasma of normal and nephrectomized rats. Amer. J. Physiol. **215**, 78 (1968).

MONTAGUE, D., RINIKER, B., BRUNNER, H., GROSS, F.: Synthesis and biological activities of a tetradecapeptide renin substrate. Amer. J. Physiol. **210**, 591 (1966).

NAIRN, R. C., CHADWICK, C. S., FRASER, K. B.: Purification of renin by electrophoresis, adsorption and immunological methods. Brit. J. exp. Path. **41**, 214 (1960).

NASJLETTI, A., MASSON, G. M. C.: Studies on renin substrate formation in a liver perfusion system. Circulat. Res. (1972) in press.

NEWSOME, H. H.: Purification of bovine renin. Biochim. biophys. Acta (Amst.) **185**, 247 (1969).

NUSTAD, K., RUBIN, I.: Subcellular localization of renin and kininogenase in the rat kidney. Brit. J. Pharmacol. **40**, 326 (1970).

OGINO, K., MATSUNAGA, M., SAITO, N., KIRA, J., TAKAYASU, M.: Renin and acid adenosine triphosphatase as lysosomal enzymes. Jap. Circulat. J. (En.) **31**, 1 (1967).

PAGE, I. H., MCCUBBIN, J. W.: Renal hypertension. Chicago: Year Book Medical Publishers 1968.

PAGE, I. H., MCSWAIN, B., KNAPP, G. M., ANDRUS, W. D.: The origin of renin-activator. Amer. J. Physiol. **135**, 214 (1941).

PASSANANTI, G. T.: The purification of renin by use of ion-exchange chromatography. Biochim. biophys. Acta (Amst.) **34**, 246 (1959).

PEART, W. S., LLOYD, A. M., THATCHER, G. N., LEVER, A. F., PAYNE, N., STONE, N.: Purification of pig renin. Biochem. J. **99**, 708 (1966).

PETERS-HAEFELI, L.: Rate of inactivation of endogenous or exogenous renin in normal and in renin-depleted rats. Amer. J. Physiol. **221**, 1339 (1971).

PLENTL, A. A., PAGE, I. H., DAVIS, W. W.: The nature of renin activator. J. biol. Chem. **147**, 143 (1943).

POULSEN, K.: No evidence of active renin-inhibitors in plasma. The kinetics of the reaction between renin and substrate in non-pretreated plasma. Scand. J. clin. Lab. Invest. **27**, 37 (1971).

RAKHIT, S.: On the structure of the renin inhibitor from hog kidney. Canad. J. Biochem. **49**, 1012 (1971).

REGOLI, D.: Renin inactivation by human plasma. Canad. J. Physiol. Pharmacol. **48**, 350 (1970).

REGOLI, D., BRUNNER, H., GROSS, F.: Untersuchungen über den Mechanismus der Wirkungsverstärkung von Renin nach Nephrektomie. Helv. physiol. pharmacol. Acta **19**, C 101 (1961).

REINHARZ, A., ROTH, M.: Studies on renin with synthetic substrates. Europ. J. Biochem. **7**, 334 (1969).

REINHARZ, A., ROTH, M., HAEFELI, L., SCHAECHTELIN, G.: Effect of some chemical agents on renin activity *in vitro*. Enzyme **12**, 212 (1971).

ROSENTHAL, J., WOLFF, H. P., WEBER, P., DAHLHEIM, H.: Enzyme kinetic studies on human renin and its purified homologous substrate. Amer. J. Physiol. **221**, 1292 (1971).

RUBIN, I.: Purification of hog renin. Properties of purified hog renin. Scand. J. clin. Lab. Invest. **29**, 51 (1972).

RYAN, J. W., JOHNSON, D. C.: The renin-like enzyme of rabbit uterus. Biochim. biophys. Acta (Amst.) **191**, 386 (1969).

SCHAECHTELIN, G., BAECHTOLD, N., HAEFELI, L., REGOLI, D., GAUDRY-PAREDES, A., PETERS, G.: A renin-inactivating system in rat plasma. Amer. J. Physiol. **215**, 632 (1968).

SCHWEIKERT, J. R., CAREY, R. M., LIDDLE, G. W., ISLAND, D. W.: Characterization of the renal pressor substance of Grollman as angiotensin I. Circulat. Res. (1972) in press.

SEALEY, J. E., GERTEN, J. N., LEDINGHAM, J. G. G., LARAGH, J. H.: Inhibition of renin by heparin. J. clin. Endocr. **27**, 699 (1967).

SEKI, T., JENSSEN, T. A., LEVIN, Y., ERDOS, E. G.: Active waterinsoluble derivative of renin. Nature (Lond.) **225**, 864 (1970).

SEN, S., HIRASAWA, K., SMEBY, R. R., BUMPUS, F. M.: Measurement of plasma renin substrate using homologous and heterologous renin. Amer. J. Physiol. **221**, 1476 (1971).

SEN, S., SMEBY, R. R., BUMPUS, F. M.: Antihypertensive effect of an isolated phospholipid. Amer. J. Physiol. **214**, 337 (1968).

SKEGGS, L. T., Jr., KAHN, J. R., LENTZ, K. E., SHUMWAY, N. P.: The preparation, purification and amino acid sequence of a polypeptide renin substrate. J. exp. Med. **106**, 439 (1957).

SKEGGS, L. T., Jr., KAHN, J. R., SHUMWAY, N. P.: The isolation and assay of hypertensin from blood. J. exp. Med. **95**, 241 (1952).

SKEGGS, L. T., Jr., LENTZ, K. E., HOCHSTRASSER, H., KAHN, J. R.: The purification and partial characterization of several forms of hog renin substrate. J. exp. Med. **118**, 73 (1963).

SKEGGS, L. T., LENTZ, K. E., KAHN, J. R., DORER, F. E., LEVINE, M.: Pseudorenin. A new angiotensin-forming enzyme. Circulat. Res. **25**, 451 (1969).

SKEGGS, L. T., LENTZ, K. E., KAHN, J. R., HOCHSTRASSER, H.: Studies on the preparation and properties of renin. Circulat. Res. **20—21** (Suppl. II), 91 (1967).

SKEGGS, L. T., LENTZ, K. E., KAHN, J. R., HOCHSTRASSER, H.: Kinetics of the reaction of renin with nine synthetic peptide substrates. J. exp. Med. **128**, 13 (1968).

SKEGGS, L. T., LENTZ, K. E., KAHN, J. R., LEVINE, M., DORER, F. E.: Multiple forms of human kidney renin. In: Hypertension 1972. Berlin-Heidelberg-New York: Springer 1972.

SKEGGS, L. T., Jr., LENTZ, K. E., KAHN, J. R., SHUMWAY, N. P., WOODS, K. R.: The amino acid sequence of hypertensin II. J. exp. Med. **104**, 193 (1956).

SKEGGS, L. T., Jr., LENTZ, K. E., KAHN, J. R., SHUMWAY, N. P.: The synthesis of a tetradecapeptide renin substrate. J. exp. Med. **108**, 283 (1958).

SMEBY, R. R., SEN, S., BUMPUS, F. M.: A naturally occurring renin inhibitor. Circulat. Res. **20—21** (Suppl. II), 129 (1967).

TATEISHI, H., NASJLETTI, A., MASSON, G. M. C.: Role of renin in the regulation of angiotensinogen levels in plasma. Proc. Soc. exp. Biol. (N. Y.) **137**, 1424 (1971).

TAYLOR, J., COHEN, S., MICHELAKIS, A., MURAKAMI, K., INAGAMI, T.: Isolation and characterization of a renin-like enzyme from mouse submaxillary glands. Fed. Proc. **30**, 1146 (1971).

TURRIAN, H.: Quelques caractéristiques du principe hypertensif contenu dans les glandes salivaires de la souris. Helv. physiol. pharmacol. Acta **18**, 259 (1960).

WALDHAUSL, W. K., LUCAS, C. P., CONN, J. W., LUTZ, J. H., COHEN, E. L.: Studies on the partial isolation of human renin. Biochim. biophys. Acta (Amst.) **221**, 536 (1970).

WERLE, E., TRAUTSCHOLD, I., KRAMMER, K., SCHMAL, A.: Anreicherung und Immunspezifität des Isorenins der Glandula submaxillaris der Maus. Hoppe-Seylers Z. physiol. Chem. **349**, 1441 (1968).

WERLE, E., VOGEL, R., GOLDEL, L. F.: Über ein blutdrucksteigerndes Prinzip in Extrakten aus der Glandula submaxillaris der weißen Maus. Naunyn-Schmiedebergs Arch. exp. Path. Pharmak. **230**, 236 (1957).

WILLARD, R. F., WILKINSON, J. S., TURNER, M. D., GLASGOW, J. L., BONAR, J. R.: Studies on renin: purification and characterization. Fed. Proc. **29**, 941 (1970).

The Fate of Angiotensin I*

J. R. VANE

With 7 Figures

Introduction

The isolation of two forms of angiotensin by SKEGGS et al. (1954) and of a plasma enzyme which changed one into the other (SKEGGS et al., 1956), led to the belief that conversion of angiotensin I (Ang. I) to angiotensin II (Ang. II) in circulating blood was rapid enough to account for its vaso-active effects *in vivo*. This was because (a) both Ang. I and Ang. II produced the same shaped blood pressure response, so the *in-vivo* conversion must have been rapid and (b), in blood-free tissues, such as the rabbit aorta strip (HELMER, 1957) and saline-perfused rat kidneys (SKEGGS et al., 1956), Ang. I was ineffective, but Ang. II was active.

CARLINI et al. (1958), however, found Ang. I to be strongly active on guinea-pig isolated ileum and in saline-perfused hindquarters of the rat, although it was weakly active on the isolated rat uterus. They concluded that "the responding tissue might have some role in the conversion of hypertensin I into II", but this work was largely ignored and it was not until NG and VANE (1967; 1968) demonstrated conversion of Ang. I to Ang. II in the pulmonary circulation that the importance of the plasma enzyme was questioned. They found that conversion in dog's blood was too slow to account for the rapid pressor effects of Ang. I and concluded that "for the generation of circulating Ang. II the lungs are the most important site. It is possible that other tissues can also generate Ang. II locally but that this is destroyed before reaching the general circulation". At that time NG and VANE failed to demonstrate significant conversion of Ang. I to Ang. II in kidney or hind leg, but it is now apparent that a varying degree of conversion can take place in kidney, hind legs and intestine (see later). Thus, the emphasis accorded to different sites of conversion of Ang. I to Ang. II has changed over the years. In this review, I shall discuss the fate of Ang. I in plasma, in lungs and in other vascular beds. At the same time, I shall attempt to place in perspective the results obtained by extraction of converting-enzyme activity from broken cell preparations of different tissues. The physiological significance of the location of converting enzyme will also be discussed with particular reference to the supposed intra-renal role of the renin-angiotensin system.

Methods for Measuring Conversion

Methods for assessing converting-enzyme activity *in vitro* are reviewed elsewhere in this volume (BAKHLE, 1972). Various methods have been used to study the conversion of Ang. I to Ang. II in tissues. The blood-bathed organ technique developed by VANE (1964; 1969) measures the concentration of Ang. II by its

* Including literature published before March, 1972.

differential effects on the rat colon (REGOLI and VANE, 1964), chick rectum (MANN and WEST, 1950) and rat stomach strip (VANE, 1957) all superfused (GADDUM, 1953) in series with arterial or venous blood. The rat colon contracts to Ang. II, whereas the additional tissues increase the specificity of the assay by detecting the presence of other substances such as prostaglandins [FERREIRA and VANE, 1967 (1)] which might contribute to the response of the rat colon.

A similar bioassay can be used when organs are perfused through their vessels with a physiological salt solution such as Krebs' solution. The effluent from the organ superfuses a series of assay tissues, carefully chosen to augment specificity, and the change in activity of Ang. I or Ang. II is estimated by comparing their effects either infused through the organ or directly over the assay tissues (BAKHLE et al., 1969). Because there is no recirculation of the perfusion fluid, the specificity of this modification of the blood-bathed organ technique can be even further enhanced by the infusion of pharmacological antagonists to render the assay tissues insensitive to substances such as catecholamines, acetylcholine, serotonin and histamine (VANE, 1969).

Another advantage of this modification is that it allows study of the way a substance is affected by the storage or enzymic processes in the tissues during a single passage through the vasculature.

The sensitivity of the method is high with either blood- or saline-superfused assay tissues. This is because the most sensitive assay tissues available are used; thus the method measures concentrations of Ang. II in the "physiological" range, often lower than those required to raise the blood pressure (HODGE et al., 1966; REGOLI and VANE, 1966). The interpretation of results obtained with these bioassay techniques has been challenged by TÜRKER et al. [1971 (1)] who found that Ang. I released a substance from perfused lungs which was different from Ang. II in that it contracted rat aorta made tachyphylactic to Ang. II. They concluded that the release of rat aorta- (and rat colon)-contracting substances other than Ang. II from isolated perfused lungs during Ang. I infusion meant that the degree of conversion of Ang. I to Ang. II was lower than previously thought. Certainly, other smooth muscle-contracting substances can be released by vasoactive substances (usually in high concentrations) from organs such as lung, spleen and kidney, as has now been shown by many workers [FERREIRA and VANE, 1967 (1); DAVIS et al., 1968; PIPER and VANE, 1969; 1971; ALABASTER and BAKHLE, 1970; MCGIFF et al., 1970 (1); 1970 (2); RYAN and STEWART, 1970; AIKEN and VANE, 1971; FERREIRA et al., 1971; TÜRKER et al., 1971 (1)]. In most of these instances the substances released have been identified as prostaglandin or prostaglandin-like. The chick rectum readily distinguishes between angiotensin and prostaglandins, for it does not react to Ang. I or Ang. II, but is strongly contracted by the commonly released prostaglandins such as E_1, E_2 and $F_{2\alpha}$. It is for this reason that we always include a chick rectum in our parallel-bioassay system. TÜRKER et al. [1971 (1)] did not use this preparation in their assay system, so it is not known whether the rat colon contracting substance released from lungs by Ang. I was prostaglandin-like. It did, however, contract the rat aorta, an activity which makes it unlikely to be a known prostaglandin.

It is difficult to interpret the experiments of TÜRKER et al. for other reasons. First, the isolated lung system they used inactivated Ang. II by 40—75%, a result at variance with the experience of others (GOFFINET and MULROW, 1965; NG and VANE, 1967; 1968; 1970; HODGE et al., 1967; LEARY and LEDINGHAM, 1969; BIRON et al., 1969; BAKHLE et al., 1969; AIKEN and VANE, 1970), who find no inactivation either in saline- or blood-perfused lungs, unless the lung preparation deteriorates (BAKHLE et al., 1969).

Secondly, the same authors [Türker et al., 1971 (2)] now suggest that the aortic strips used in their modification of the cascade superfusion technique metabolize Ang. II in the superfusion fluid to such an extent that the response of the next tissue in the series is substantially reduced. This result, which must reflect on their previous conclusions [Türker et al., 1971 (1)] needs comment, for when assay tissues are superfused in series with a medium containing an agonist, any significant removal of the agonist by each tissue would lessen the response of the next one. The contractions would then become smaller and smaller and the size of the response of an assay tissue would depend upon its position in the cascade. We have often looked for such effects on our commonly selected assay tissues by making infusions of Ang. II or other agonists to different parts of the

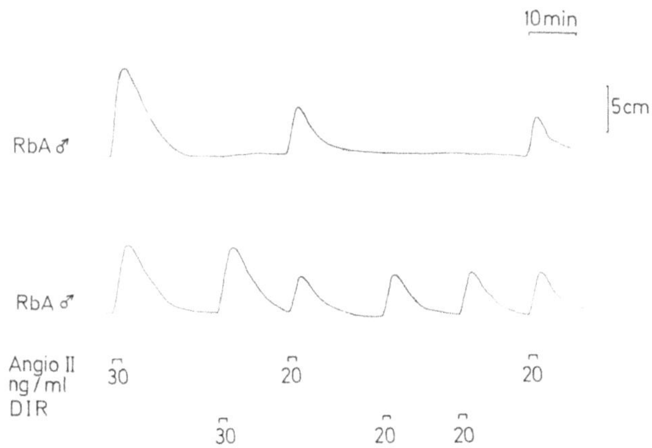

Fig. 1. Two strips of rabbit aorta were superfused in series with Krebs' solution at 5 ml/min. Infusions of Ang. II (20 and 30 ng/ml) were made so that they reached the lower strip alone, or after first superfusing the upper strip. The contractions of the lower strip were the same in both situations, showing that the upper strip had not removed activity from the superfusion fluid. Time 10 min, vertical scale 5 cm

cascade so that they reached some or all of the assay tissues. We were unable to detect either removal of the infused substance by the tissues, or the liberation from the tissues of other active substances. We have also changed the order of the assay tissues without detecting any interaction between them. An example is shown in Fig. 1 in which two strips of rabbit aorta were superfused in series. The second strip gave the same reaction to Ang. II whether the infusion was made to it alone, or to the other strip first. Such negative results are not surprising when the volume of superfusion fluid is compared with the volume of the biophase of an assay tissue weighing 50 to 200 mg. The outside surface of these tissues is irrigated at 5 to 15 ml/min, so that each drop of superfusion fluid is in contact with the biophase for a fraction of a second. It is difficult to envisage a sufficiently great diffusion of Ang. II into the biophase, followed by inactivation therein, for the overall concentration of Ang. II in the superfusion fluid to be significantly reduced.

If some readers feel that bioassay methods, especially those devised and used by the author and his colleagues, have been defended with too much vigour, they should remember that these techniques are relatively easy to use, highly sensitive and, when used properly, specific. What is more, bioassay measures that aspect of a molecule's properties in which the biologist is interested, i.e., the *biological* activity. Thus, even if a metabolic product of a substance such as Ang. II has some biological activity, the bioassay accords that product the weighting it deserves in terms of its physiological action.

Methods based on the superfusion of assay tissues with blood or the effluent from a perfused organ also have the advantage of immediacy and continuity. Intermittent blood sampling procedures may miss a transient change easily detected by the continuous technique; furthermore, the results can be seen as the experiment progresses, thus allowing modifications of the protocol. Many advances have been made in recent years, not only in the field of the renin-angiotensin system, but also in that of prostaglandins, catecholamines and pulmonary pharmacology through the use of these bioassay methods. The method of parallel assay (GADDUM, 1959) coupled with the use of specific antagonists provides strong evidence for identity of a substance. Until recently, specific antagonists for Ang. II had not been discovered but now that they have [KHAIRALLAH et al., 1970; MARSHALL et al., 1970; TÜRKER et al., 1971 (3); PALS et al., 1971 (1); 1971 (2); REGOLI et al., 1971] their use, as well as the use of converting-enzyme inhibitors, should help allay the doubts of those who criticize bioassays.

Conversion of Ang. I to Ang. II has also been estimated by using radioactive Ang. I and separating and measuring labelled histidyl-leucine (OPARIL et al., 1970; 1971) or labelled Ang. II (RYAN et al., 1970) in the outflow from the organ, or by using radio immunoassay based on antibodies capable of distinguishing between Ang. I and Ang. II (OPARIL et al., 1970; 1971). However, radioimmunoassays for Ang. II are no more specific than a single bioassay. CAIN et al. (1969) found that more than 70% of the immunoreactive material in venous blood after Ang. II infusion was due to material other than Ang. II, possibly metabolic fragments. DÜSTERDIECK and MCELWEE (1971) also showed that the nonapeptide des-Leu^{10} Ang. I retained 10% cross-reactivity with Ang. I antibodies. Thus, carboxypeptidase activity in the lung (OPARIL et al., 1970; BARRETT and SAMBHI, 1971) may lead to a product which is detected by radioimmunoassay for Ang. I but has no known physiological activity. PAGE (1970) also described a protein fraction of blood which reacts with Ang. I antibody. In view of these important findings, it is surprising that radioimmunoassays of Ang. I and Ang. II still retain the aura of credibility amongst those who attack the more specific bioassay techniques.

Other methods of estimating conversion of Ang. I to Ang. II in organs depend upon the cardiovascular response, either in the animal as a whole or in the organ itself. For instance, lung activation of Ang. I has been measured by comparing intravenous and intra-aortic injections for their effects on blood pressure. This "systemic blood pressure response" technique has been used extensively by BIRON and his colleagues for estimating both conversion and inactivation of the angiotensins (BIRON and HUGGINS, 1968; BIRON et al., 1968; STANLEY and BIRON, 1969; BIRON et al., 1969; BIRON and CAMPEAU, 1971). It has the advantage of simplicity but the disadvantage of relying on an unspecific response (a rise in blood pressure) complexely controlled by many factors, including nervous reflexes arising from the heart and lungs.

Conversion within an organ has been measured by recording the changes in arterial inflow induced by intra-arterial injections of Ang. I or Ang. II (NG and VANE, 1968; FRANKLIN et al., 1970; GILMORE et al., 1971; OSBORN et al., 1971; TILDESLAY et al., 1971; DISALVO and MONTEFUSCO, 1971; DISALVO et al., 1971; AIKEN and VANE, 1972). By comparing the amounts of peptide required to produce equivalent reductions in flow, and assuming that Ang. I has little or no vasoconstrictor activity in its own right, conversion of Ang. I to Ang. II at sites able to cause a local vasoconstriction can be estimated.

Thus, several types of biological and radiochemical assays have been used to estimate conversion of Ang. I to Ang. II. The credibility of each of them is enhanced in those situations where results obtained with one type are confirmed by those obtained by another.

Some years ago, FERREIRA (1965) isolated a peptide fraction of the venom from *Bothrops jararaca* which potentiated the effects of bradykinin on various isolated organs. This fraction was also found to inhibit converting enzyme (BAKHLE, 1968; BAKHLE et al., 1969; NG and VANE, 1970), as do the individual peptides [FERREIRA et al., 1970 (1)] which were purified [FERREIRA et al., 1970 (2)] from the extract. Peptides corresponding to some of the natural ones have now been synthesized (STEWART et al., 1971; ONDETTI et al., 1971) and these are potent converting-enzyme inhibitors *in vitro* [AIKEN and VANE, 1970; 1971; CUSHMAN and CHEUNG, 1971 (1); 1971 (2); 1972; SANDER et al., 1971; YANG et al., 1971; BAKHLE, 1971] and *in vivo* (ENGEL et al., 1971; KRIEGER et al., 1971; DISALVO et al., 1971; AIKEN and VANE, 1972). Use of these peptide inhibitors of converting enzyme has already helped to clarify the pharmacology of Ang. I. For instance, AIKEN and VANE (1970) showed that the effects of Ang. I on several isolated smooth-muscle preparations were selectively inhibited by the pentapeptide inhibitor (Pca-Lys-Trp-Ala-Pro) whereas those of Ang. II were not. They interpreted their results to mean that there was a variable activity of converting enzyme in smooth muscle and that only a small part (1—5%) of the activity of Ang. I was due to its own intrinsic activity. The discordant results of YAMAMOTO et al. (1971) were due to an inexplicable loss of activity of the sample of pentapeptide inhibitor which they used (TÜRKER, personal communication). OPARIL et al. (1971) have confirmed that most of the activity of Ang. I on strips of rabbit aorta is abolished by a peptide inhibitor of conversion, indicating that intramural conversion accounts for that part of the activity which is abolished. These inhibitors of converting enzyme activity should prove invaluable, not only for dissecting the role that Ang. II plays in the maintenance of different types of hypertension (KRIEGER et al., 1971) but also for distinguishing and delineating the sites of Ang. II generation (see below).

Conversion of Angiotensin I in Plasma and Blood

Converting-enzyme activity was first isolated by SKEGGS et al. (1956) from horse plasma. Since then, it has been found in plasma of all other species investigated, including man [PIQUILLOUD et al., 1970; POULSEN and BING, 1970; POULSEN and POULSEN, 1971; LEE et al., 1971 (1)], rats [LOYKE, 1970; POULSEN and BING, 1970; CUSHMAN and CHEUNG, 1971 (1); POULSEN and POULSEN, 1971), mice (POULSEN and BING, 1970), guinea pigs [LEE et al., 1971 (2); YANG et al., 1971), pigs [DORER et al., 1970; LEE et al., 1971 (2); 1971 (3); YANG et al., 1971), rabbits (UEDA et al., 1971) and cats (PEACH et al., 1971). Guinea-pig blood has higher converting-enzyme activity and higher bradykininase activity than most species. YANG et al. (1971) identify both these actions with the same enzyme.

Most of the papers cited use one or more stages of purification before measuring converting-enzyme activity, and it then becomes difficult to calculate the rate of conversion which takes place in blood in the animal's circulation. This value is important in order to assess the contribution that plasma-converting enzyme makes to the formation of Ang. II *in vivo*. By using the blood-bathed organ technique with blood circulating through an incubating coil, NG and VANE (1967) demonstrated that conversion of Ang. I in dogs' blood was slow, needing at least 3 min to show substantial generation of Ang. II. The experiments were complicated by the fact that there was also angiotensinase activity present in the blood, but even so, there was no doubt that the enzyme in blood worked too slowly to account for the rapid pressor effect of Ang. I after intravenous injection, especially when the amount converted by blood in one circulation time (15—30 sec, SPECTOR, 1956) was calculated to be about 10%. LEE et al. [1971 (1)] have also calculated the half-life of physiological concentrations of Ang. I in pig blood to be 3.3 min. OPARIL et al. (1970) confirmed the relative unimportance of blood-converting enzyme in dogs, using both tritiated Ang. I and radioimmunoassay. They found that Ang. I had a half-life of 3 min and in 15 sec only 8% had been converted. They, too, found angiotensinase activity but their measurements, like those of NG and VANE, did not reveal whether Ang. I as well as Ang. II could be fragmented by the plasma angiotensinase. There was some discrepancy between the percent conversion calculated from the results with tritium-labelled Ang. I (which showed 56% unconverted in 1 min) and that calculated from the results with radioimmunoassay, which showed 90% unconverted in 1 min. A possible explanation of this discrepancy arises from the observation of PAGE (1970), who found that a protein fraction of blood also reacted with the Ang. I antibody.

With human blood, OSBORN et al. (1970) also found slow conversion, a maximum of 20% being achieved in 1 min. POULSEN and POULSEN (1971) estimated simultaneously the converting enzyme and angiotensinase activities of plasma from rat and man. They found the half-life of Ang. I in plasma to be 1 to 2 min.

None of these results on plasma conversion of Ang. I assesses the possible degradation of Ang. I by angiotensinases *before* conversion to Ang. II. DEODHAR (1960) showed that rabbit serum inactivated Ang. I and Ang. II at the same slow rate. If this finding also applies to the blood angiotensinases of other species (and aminopeptidases, at least, may not distinguish between Ang. I and Ang. II) then we can conclude that Ang. I in plasma can be both slowly converted to Ang. II and slowly degraded to substances which would yield relatively inactive products if attacked by converting enzyme. In any event, there is general agreement that the rate of generation of Ang. II by plasma-converting enzyme (except perhaps in the guinea pig) is too slow to account for the rapid activation of Ang. I *in vivo*. Also, there is no evidence that the plasma converting enzyme can be activated, either by oxygenation of the blood, or by passage through an organ. NG and VANE (1967) found the conversion of Ang. I to Ang. II to be similar in venous and arterial blood and conversion in tissues such as the lung can be demonstrated in saline-perfused organs. Thus, there is no need to propose activation of blood enzyme to account for rapid conversion in tissues. Indeed, it may be that blood enzyme simply represents "leakage" of enzyme from its normal tissue-bound sites in, for example, the lungs.

Conversion of Angiotensin I in Tissues

The most comprehensive survey of tissue content of converting-enzyme activity has been that of CUSHMAN and CHEUNG [1971 (1)]. They used a spectrophotometric method [CUSHMAN and CHEUNG, 1971 (2)] to measure hippuric acid, formed by the action of converting enzyme on hippuryl-L-histidyl-L-leucine, a substrate that is not hydrolyzed by most other tissue peptidases. In cell-free homogenates of the twenty-five tissues of rat which they studied (Table 1) they found detectable converting-enzyme activity in all but the gastrocnemius muscle and liver. In those which demonstrated sufficient activity, they characterized the enzyme further by showing that (a) it was inhibited by the pentapeptide inhibitor of converting enzyme, (b) the activity was chloride-dependent and (c) the activity was stimulated by cobalt ions.

Three tissues were outstanding for their converting-enzyme activity; lung, testis and epididymis. The high lung activity fitted well with earlier results *in vivo* in dogs (NG and VANE, 1967; 1968) and other species (BIRON and HUGGINS, 1968)

Table 1. *Activities of angiotensin-converting enzyme in rat tissues [from* CUSHMAN *and* CHEUNG, *1971 (1)]*

Tissue	Specific activity[a]	Percent inhibition		Percent activation
		With pentapeptide[b]	Without NaCl	With $Co(NO\text{-})_2$
Epididymis	122 ± 12	99 ± 0.3	97 ± 0.7	44 ± 15
Testis	85 ± 4.3	99 ± 0.4	99 ± 0.3	36 ± 5
Lung	48 ± 5.0	98 ± 0.4	98 ± 0.7	56 ± 16
Duodenum	8.6 ± 1.0	92 ± 3.7	94 ± 3.4	118 ± 25
Pancreas	7.4 ± 1.2	80 ± 7.7	93 ± 6.1	−21 ± 22
Jejunum	6.0 ± 1.1	97 ± 2.0	95 ± 2.0	152 ± 28
Ovary	3.4 ± 0.5	97 ± 0.9	91 ± 1.5	67 ± 17
Ileum	3.3 ± 0.6	99 ± 0.4	96 ± 3.0	141 ± 38
Aorta	2.9 ± 1.0	97 ± 1.7	85 ± 4.1	93 ± 68
Stomach	2.7 ± 0.4	95 ± 3.7	89 ± 8.8	74 ± 27
Uterus	2.2 ± 0.2	71 ± 5.9	49 ± 12	58 ± 5
Seminal vesicle	2.0 ± 0.1	91 ± 8.0	99 ± 0.2	132 ± 27
Thymus	1.9 ± 0.3	62 ± 7.5	62 ± 3.2	145 ± 22
Thyroid	1.7 ± 0.4	58 ± 13	55 ± 10	107 ± 42
Serum	1.6 ± 0.1	97 ± 1.3	97 ± 1.3	36 ± 18
Brain	1.5 ± 0.2	x	x	x
Colon	1.2 ± 0.1	↓	↓	↓
Submaxillary	1.0 ± 0.1			
Spleen	0.9 ± 0.2			
Kidney	0.6 ± 0.2			
Adrenal	0.5 ± 0.1			
Heart	0.5 ± 0.3			
Diaphragm	0.3 ± 0.2			
Gastrocnemius	<0.2			
Liver	<0.2			

[a] m-units/mg protein (mean ± S.E., n = 5).

[b] Pyrrolidone carboxylyl-Lys-Trp-Ala-Pro. This specific inhibitor of angiotensin-converting enzyme also potentiates the biological activities of bradykinin, and was named BPP5a by STEWART et al. (1971).

x Activities were too low to permit accurate measurement of inhibition.

but the even higher activity in testes and epididymis was a new and intriguing observation. The converting-enzyme activity may have been associated with spermatogenesis, for it was lacking in immature rats. It remains to be seen whether anyone will now propose a role for the renin-angiotensin system in reproduction or fertility.

Where comparisons were possible, CUSHMAN and CHEUNG's estimates of tissue converting-enzyme activity agreed well with those of ROTH et al. (1969), but were mostly in disagreement with those of HUGGINS and THAMPI (1968) who found much lower activities in general and only small differences in activity between lung, liver, diaphragm and heart. CUSHMAN and CHEUNG suggested that the preliminary acidification and ammonium sulphate fractionation used by HUGGINS and THAMPI could have resulted in a low yield of the enzyme. However, there is also variation between the results of CUSHMAN and CHEUNG (1972) and those of DEPIERRE and ROTH (1972). Both groups avoided ammonium sulphate fractionation, both used short synthetic substrates for the enzyme and yet there are considerable differences in the activities found in lung tissues. For instance, CUSHMAN and CHEUNG (1972) found rabbit lung (20 mU/mg protein) and guinea-pig lung (23 mU/mg protein) had similar specific activities whereas DEPIERRE and ROTH (1972) found rabbit lung (109 mU/g tissue) contained three times the activity of guinea-pig lung (30 mU/g tissue). One source of these discrepancies may be the different homogenization and centrifugation procedures used. DEPIERRE and ROTH (1972) centrifuged the homogenized lung tissue at 107,000 × g and measured the converting-enzyme activity in both supernatant and pellet (Table 2). CUSHMAN and CHEUNG [1971 (1); 1972], however, discarded the 5000 × g precipitate and

Table 2. *Comparison of converting enzyme activity in lungs of different species*

	DEPIERRE and ROTH, 1972 m U/g Tissue Total	Pellet	Supernatant	CUSHMAN and CHEUNG, 1972 m U/mg Protein Supernatant from 5000 g
Rat	144	46	98	48
Rabbit	109	106	3.2	20
Dog	62	52	10	10
Guinea Pig	30	26	4	24

measured the activity of the supernatant. It is noticeable that both groups find rat lung to have the highest activity. In this tissue, the enzyme is associated more with the supernatant from centrifugation at 107,000 × g, whereas in the other species, the activity is mainly associated with the pellet. Thus, the discrepancy may be because the 5000 × g precipitate, which CUSHMAN and CHEUNG discarded, contained in some species disproportionately high amounts of converting-enzyme activity. This could happen, perhaps, if the cell structures of the elements of the lungs which contain converting enzyme (vascular tissue?) are less easily broken by homogenization than, say, those of the alveoli.

The results highlight one aspect of the dichotomy associated with the use of macerated tissue as an indication of the possible physiological role of an enzyme in a tissue. On the one hand, the maceration and centrifugation procedure may discard or destroy enzyme activity, yielding artificially low estimates. On the other hand, the process of maceration may liberate peptidase activity which is not normally available to Ang. I, because of cell barriers, thus giving unrealistically high estimates of activity. An illustration of this latter point arises from liberation of angiotensinase activity in lung tissue. Both *in vivo* and in fresh lung perfusions, Ang. II survives passage through the pulmonary circulation (GOFFINET and MULROW, 1965; NG and VANE, 1967; 1968; 1970; HODGE et al., 1967; LEARY and LEDINGHAM, 1969; BIRON et al., 1969; BAKHLE et al., 1969; AIKEN and VANE, 1970) but it is rapidly inactivated by broken-cell preparations of lung tissue (BAKHLE, 1968; HOLLEMANS et al., 1969).

Another approach to measurement of converting-enzyme activity *in vitro* is to use isolated organs, either perfused through their blood vessels or bathed on their external surface with an artificial salt solution. This keeps the cellular architecture of the tissue intact, at least until it becomes distorted by edema. Isolated lungs perfused with saline solution tend to become edematous within 2 h. At this stage, they inactivate Ang. II to an increasing extent (BAKHLE et al., 1969) showing that as the cell integrity is compromised, an angiotensinase becomes available to the perfusion fluid. Damage of this type can be postponed by addition of dextran or some other non-diffusable agent to the perfusion fluid. Results obtained with these techniques in general correspond to those obtained *in vivo*, so they will be presented together.

a) Lung

NG and VANE (1967) showed that *in vivo*, Ang. I was converted to Ang. II in the 3 to 5 sec that it takes for blood to pass through the pulmonary circulation (Fig. 2). Conversion of Ang. I has now been established in the lungs of guinea pig, rat, cat, dog and man (NG and VANE, 1968; 1970; BIRON and HUGGINS, 1968; STANLEY and BIRON, 1969; BIRON et al., 1969; OPARIL et al., 1970; 1971; BARRETT and SAMBHI, 1971) sometimes by perfusing lungs with a saline solution [AIKEN and VANE, 1970; BAKHLE et al., 1969; RYAN et al., 1970; TÜRKER et al., 1971 (1)]. Such an experiment is illustrated in Fig. 3 (from AIKEN and VANE, 1970). Guinea-pig lungs were perfused with Krebs' solution; the lung effluent then superfused a rat-colon preparation which detected Ang. II. The pentapeptide converting-enzyme inhibitor was continuously infused into the lung effluent so that converting-enzyme activity in the rat colon itself was suppressed. Ang. II (0.3 to 3 ng/ml) induced graded contractions of the rat colon but Ang. I (10 ng/ml) was ineffective when applied directly to the assay tissue. However, when Ang. I (3 to 10 ng/ml) was infused through the lungs, the contractions of the rat colon indicated a 50% conversion to Ang. II. Allowing for the impurity of the Ang. I sample, as demonstrated by bioassay [VANE, 1971 (1)] the conversion becomes 73%. The generation of Ang. II from Ang. I was almost completely suppressed when the converting enzyme inhibitor was infused through the isolated lungs, but returned afterwards. This experiment demonstrates well the ability of the pulmonary circulation to convert Ang. I to Ang. II in the absence of blood.

The only failure to demonstrate lung conversion *in vivo* was by KREYE and GROSS (1971) in the rat. Apart from this one discrepancy, the main area of disagreement is around the degree of conversion of Ang. I to Ang. II in one transit through the pulmonary circulation. *In vivo*, estimates are complicated by recirculation of that fraction of Ang. II (10 to 40%) which escapes inactivation in peripheral vascular beds (AKINKUGBE et al., 1966; NG and VANE, 1967; 1968; HODGE et al., 1967; BIRON et al., 1968; HAAS et al., 1968). Allowing for a 30 to 40% recirculation, NG and VANE (1967; 1968) estimated that 80% or more of the Ang. I was converted to Ang. II in one transit through dog lungs. BIRON and HUGGINS (1968) estimated a 40% conversion in rat lungs, but this was probably an underestimate for they made no allowance for the amount of Ang. II recirculating. OPARIL et al. (1970) took blood samples from dogs quickly enough to exclude recirculation. By peptide release and by radioimmunoassay, they estimated a 53% conversion. However, this was with Ang. I at 10,000 times the "physiological" concentration, and they also obtained evidence for carboxypeptidase activity in the lungs, cleaving leucine from Ang. I. Later, using similar techniques but one fifth the concentration of Ang. I, OPARIL et al. (1971) showed an average of 56% conversion in a single passage through dog lung. The complication of recirculation does not apply to

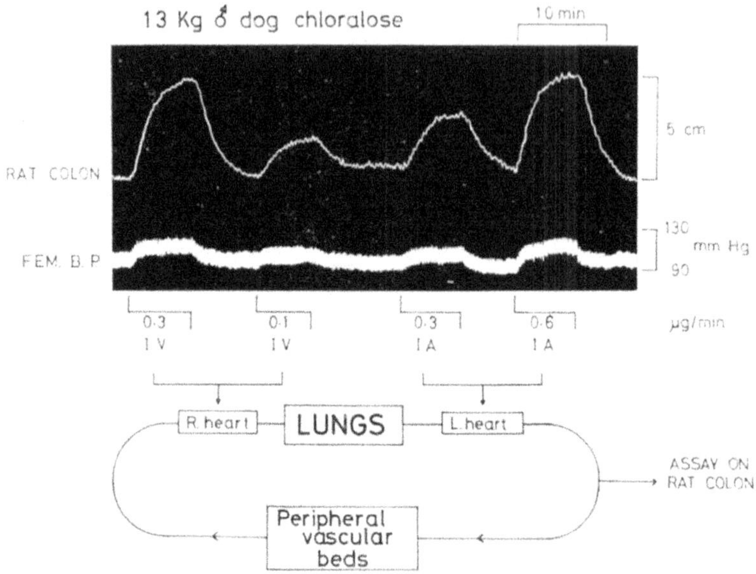

Fig. 2. A rat colon preparation was superfused at 10 ml/min with arterial blood from a 13 kg male dog anaesthetized with chloralose. The lower tracing is of mean blood pressure. Infusion of angiotensin I intravenously had greater effects on blood pressure and on the rat colon than did infusions into the root of the ascending aorta. This shows that activation of Ang. I has taken place in the pulmonary circulation. Time 10 min; Vertical scale 5 cm. (From NG and VANE, 1967)

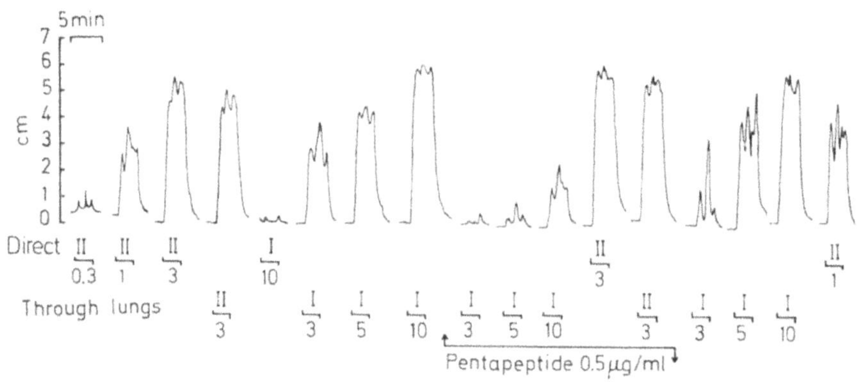

Fig. 3. Isolated lungs from a guinea-pig were perfused through the pulmonary artery with Krebs' solution at 10 ml/min. The effluent superfused a rat colon, the contractions of which are shown. Ang. I (I) or Ang. II (II) was infused for 3 min to give the concentrations shown (ng/ml). Direct infusion of Ang. II (0.3 to 3 ng/ml) into the pulmonary effluent caused graded contractions of the colon. When Ang. II was infused through the lungs it gave a similar effect. Ang. I (10 ng/ml) had no direct effect on the rat colon but when infused through the lungs caused graded contractions representing about 50% conversion to Ang. II. When the pentapeptide inhibitor of converting enzyme (pentapeptide 0.5 ng/ml) was also infused through the lungs, the conversion of Ang. I to Ang. II was greatly reduced but the effects of Ang. II were unchanged. Conversion of Ang. I recovered when the pentapeptide infusion was stopped. Time 5 min; vertical scale in cm. (From AIKEN and VANE, 1970)

isolated lungs perfused with salt solution, and using these from various species, estimates of conversion range from 0 with a fast rate flow in rat lungs (BIRON and CAMPEAU, 1971) to 73% in guinea-pig lungs (AIKEN and VANE, 1970).

An important and clarifying contribution was made by BARRETT and SAMBHI (1971) who studied pulmonary activation of Ang. I in rat lungs *in situ*. At low doses of Ang. I (0.35 μg) they found 80% conversion to Ang. II in the lungs, but as the amounts injected were increased (200 μg) this dropped to 30%, indicating an apparent saturation of the converting process. At the same time, increasing amounts of des-Leu^{10} Ang. I were detected, due to the action of pulmonary carboxypeptidase. They reasoned that this carboxypeptidase activity protected the arterial circulation against formation of excessive amounts of Ang. II and was

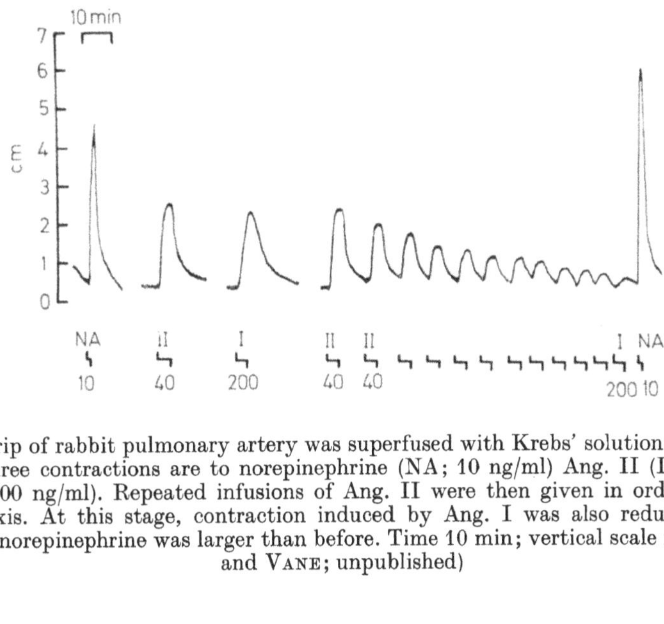

Fig. 4. A strip of rabbit pulmonary artery was superfused with Krebs' solution at 10 ml/min. The first three contractions are to norepinephrine (NA; 10 ng/ml) Ang. II (II; 40/ml) and Ang. I (I 200 ng/ml). Repeated infusions of Ang. II were then given in order to produce tachyphylaxis. At this stage, contraction induced by Ang. I was also reduced, but that induced by norepinephrine was larger than before. Time 10 min; vertical scale in cm. (AIKEN and VANE; unpublished)

only functional when concentrations of Ang. I were high. Their results suggest that at physiological concentrations, there is almost quantitative conversion of Ang. I to Ang. II in the lungs. The carboxypeptidase activity is seen with high "non-physiological" concentration of Ang. I and this is coupled with a lower overall conversion to Ang. II. These findings may well explain some reports [OPARIL et al., 1970; RYAN and STEWART, 1970; TÜRKER et al., 1971 (1)] of formation or release by lungs during Ang. I infusion of substances other than Ang. II and histidyl-leucine, for the concentrations of Ang. I used in these experiments were comparatively high, ranging from 25 ng/ml to 700 μg/ml. Even after severe haemmorhage, Ang. II concentrations in arterial blood are only 1 ng/ml (HODGE et al., 1966).

Where is converting enzyme located in lung tissue? AIKEN and VANE (1970) showed that contractions induced by Ang. I in isolated strips of various arteries from rat, rabbit, cat and dog were slower than those induced by Ang. II. Cross-tachyphylaxis between Ang. I and Ang. II (Fig. 4) indicated that both substances were acting at the same receptor site, a conclusion also reached from work with angiotensin antagonists [TÜRKER et al., 1971 (3)]. Furthermore, a converting-enzyme inhibitor specifically reduced the effects of Ang. I but not those of Ang. II.

They concluded from these results that most of the contractor effects of Ang. I on the isolated vascular smooth muscle were produced after intramural conversion to Ang. II. Calculation of the percentage conversion of Ang. I to Ang. II within the wall of the vascular strip (Fig. 5) showed higher activity for pulmonary arteries (30 to 43%) than for any other artery tested. Aortae of rats and carotid arteries of rabbits, cats and dogs exhibited much lower intramural conversion (5 to 10%) and celiac, renal, femoral and axillary arteries even less (0 and 4%). The high intramural conversion in strips of pulmonary artery is an interesting corollary of the high conversion in blood- or saline-perfused lungs. Converting enzyme might,

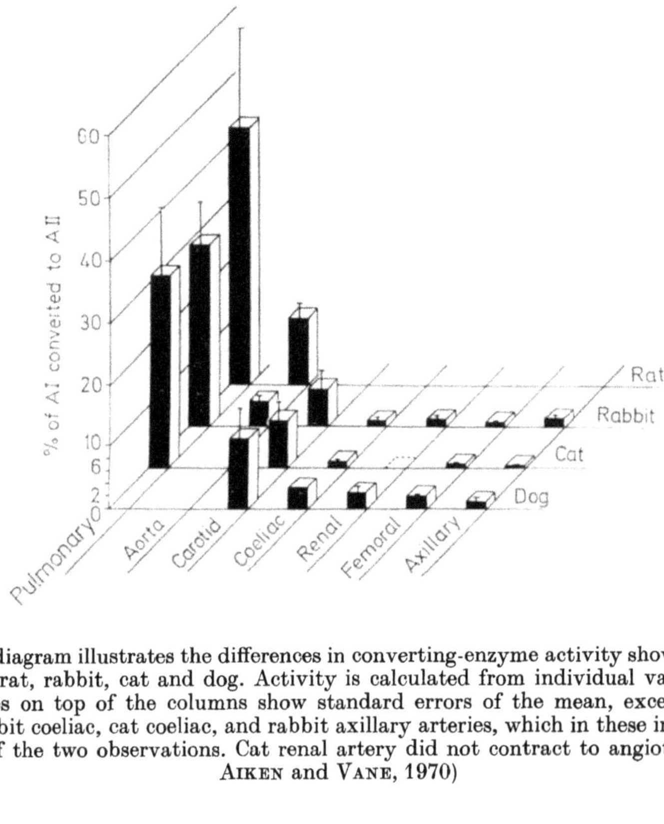

Fig. 5. The diagram illustrates the differences in converting-enzyme activity shown by arterial strips from rat, rabbit, cat and dog. Activity is calculated from individual values, and the vertical lines on top of the columns show standard errors of the mean, except for rabbit carotid, rabbit coeliac, cat coeliac, and rabbit axillary arteries, which in these instances show the range of the two observations. Cat renal artery did not contract to angiotensin. (From AIKEN and VANE, 1970)

therefore, be located in vascular tissue and cell fractionation studies of lung tissue are consistent with this view (BAKHLE, 1968; BAKHLE and REYNARD, 1971; SANDER and HUGGINS, 1971). If converting enzyme were present in the endothelial cells of pulmonary blood vessels, the enormous surface area to which Ang. I was exposed would explain its rapid conversion in the pulmonary circulation.

The metabolic function of the lungs has become increasingly evident over the last few years (VANE, 1968; 1969; HEINEMANN and FISHMAN, 1969) and there is a striking analogy between their respiratory and metabolic functions. As well as removing the waste product, carbon dioxide, they inactivate several vasoactive hormones such as acetylcholine, serotonin, bradykinin, prostaglandin E_1, E_2 and $F_{2\alpha}$ (VANE, 1969). Thus, the arterial circulation is protected from these powerful substances by this strategically placed metabolic organ. Just as the lungs add the vital substance oxygen to the blood passing through them, so they add Ang. II, the most potent vasoconstrictor substance known. There is also evidence (PIPER and VANE, 1969; 1971) that other vasoactive substances may be liberated from the lungs into the blood stream, suggesting that they have an endocrine function. If this seems too immoderate a view, at least the lungs can be regarded as a staging post, where a new life or new form is given to some passing hormones. In this context it is interesting to note that the nonapeptide bradykinin is almost completely inactivated on passage through the pulmonary circulation [FERREIRA and VANE, 1967 (2)]. Following this, NG and VANE (1968) suggested (probably for the wrong reasons) that the same lung enzyme might be responsible for both inactivating bradykinin and activating Ang. I, although this possibility was discounted by SCHOLZ and BIRON (1969). The substrate specificity of an enzyme can only effectively be established on a homogeneous form of the protein. CUSHMAN and CHEUNG (1972) were the first to purify lung converting enzyme to homogeneity, and others have performed similar purifications of plasma enzymes (YANG et al., 1971) and kidney enzymes (ELISSEEVA et al., 1971). In each instance, it is clear that converting enzyme also inactivates bradykinin. Thus, one enzyme can remove from blood the potent vasodilator, bradykinin and add to blood the potent vasoconstrictor, Ang. II. However, no evidence is available as to whether the kininase activity of converting enzymes is physiologically important, for there is at least one other kininase in lung tissue (RYAN et al., 1968).

b) Peripheral Vascular Beds

The fate of Ang. I in peripheral vascular beds is different from that in the lungs, for at "physiological" concentrations it can be both activated and inactivated. Thus, if the arteriovenous blood concentrations of Ang. I across an organ are compared (NG and VANE, 1968) an overall disappearance of activity occurs, amounting to 40 to 50% in the head, 60 to 90% in the hind legs and 80 to 90% in the kidney. This overall inactivation of Ang. I in one passage through the different vascular beds is similar to that found for Ang. II and since tissue angiotensinases include aminopeptidases and/or endopeptidases (LEARY and LEDINGHAM, 1972) it is possible that the same enzymes degrade both Ang. I and Ang. II, which only differ structurally at the carboxy end of the molecule. However, an overall inactivation of Ang. I on passage through an organ, as measured by a change in biological activity, may include and disguise some conversion to Ang. II followed by inactivation of the newly-formed Ang. II before it reaches the venous circulation; indeed, this sequence of events has now been established.

1. Hindquarters

HALVORSEN et al. (1959) were the first to suggest conversion of Ang. I in hindquarters for they found Ang. I was active in perfused preparations, and BARAC (1962) found Ang. I was vasoconstrictive in the hindquarters of dogs. Some conversion of Ang. I also appears to take place in the hind legs of sheep (OSBORN et al., 1971) and toads (CARLINI et al., 1958; HALVORSEN et al., 1959). However, neither NG and VANE (1968) nor OPARIL et al., (1970) were able to detect conversion of Ang. I to Ang. II in the hind legs of dogs. Recently, AIKEN and VANE (1972) using the same techniques as NG and VANE (1968) but with the additional help of a converting enzyme inhibitor, found an average value of 40% conversion of Ang. I to Ang. II when measured by the vasoconstrictor response. They also measured, during Ang. I infusion, the venous output of Ang. II-like activity from the legs by the blood-bathed organ technique; this represented a conversion of only 11%. OPARIL et al. (1970) estimated a similar conversion from the amount of Ang. II in femoral venous blood but attributed it to formation in plasma. It was because of this that they concluded a lack of conversion in the hind legs. The detection of less Ang. II in the venous outflow than the amount calculated from the vasoconstrictor activity of Ang. I suggests that in the hind legs, as in the kidney, conversion of Ang. I to Ang. II takes place at a site which allows vasoconstriction but thereafter there is some 60 to 70% inactivation of the newly-formed Ang. II. This is represented diagramatically in Fig. 6 in which the probable disposition of Ang. I and Ang. II in the hind legs of dogs is compared. In view of this *in-vivo* conversion of Ang. I to Ang. II in hindquarters, it is surprising that CUSHMAN and CHEUNG [1971 (1)] were unable to detect converting-enzyme activity in the gastrocnemius muscle of the rat.

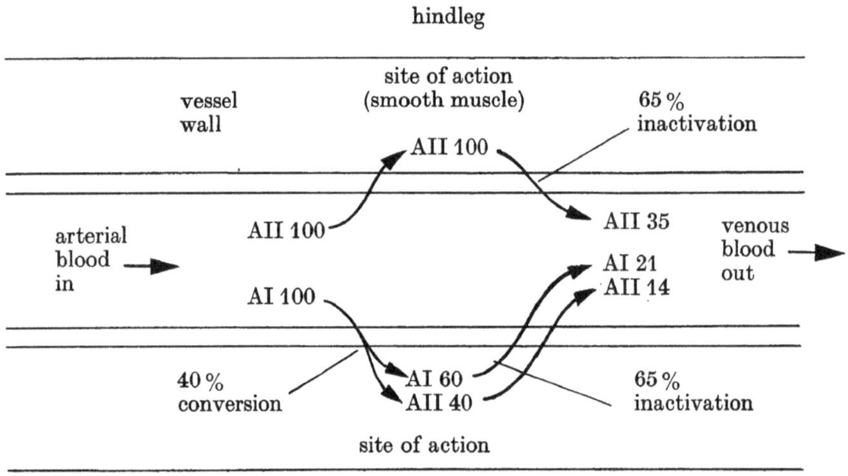

Fig. 6. The diagram shows the possible fate of Ang. I and Ang. II in the hindlegs. Ang. II (100%) produces vascular contraction and is then partially inactivated so that only 35% of the arterial concentration is found in the venous effluent. Ang. I (100%) is partially converted to Ang. II. The 40% Ang. II formed produces vascular contraction and then both Ang. I and Ang. II are inactivated, so that the venous effluent contains, in terms of the arterial concentration of Ang. I, 21% Ang. I and 14% Ang. II. (AIKEN and VANE, unpublished)

2. Intestine

CARLINI et al. (1958) and GROSS and TURRIAN (1960) showed that Ang. I had more than 50% of the potency of Ang. II on guinea-pig isolated ileum; HUGGINS and THAMPI (1968) also noted that the guinea-pig ileum reacted strongly to Ang. I. We have also found a high relative potency of Ang. I on this tissue (AIKEN and VANE, unpublished) and further shown that the activity of Ang. I virtually abolished by the pentapeptide converting-enzyme inhibitor (Fig. 7).

In isolated smooth muscle preparations from the rat, AIKEN and VANE (1970) found much less conversion of Ang. I. The contractions of the rat colon and the rat ileum preparations induced by Ang. I represented 4% conversion, whereas that of the rat uterus represented only 0.8%. DISALVO and MONTEFUSCO (1971) compared the vasoconstrictor effects of Ang. I and Ang. II injected into the superior mesenteric arteries of dogs before and after converting-enzyme inhibition. They calculated that conversion of Ang. I in the intestinal vascular bed averaged 25%. Thus, the evidence so far available indicates considerable variation from species to species in the conversion of Ang. I to Ang. II in the intestine.

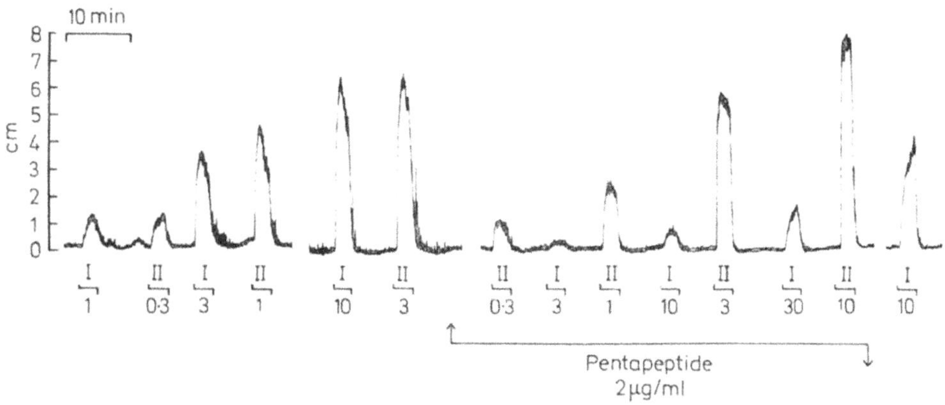

Fig. 7. A piece of guinea pig ileum was superfused with Krebs' solution at 10 ml/min. Infusions of Ang. I (I) or Ang. II (II) for 3 min gave graded contractions; the figures refer to the final concentration in ng/ml. Ang. I had about 30% of the activity of Ang. II. When the pentapeptide inhibitor of converting enzyme (pentapeptide, 2 µg/ml) was infused the contractions induced by Ang. I were selectively reduced, so that the activity now represented only about 1% of that of Ang. II. This experiment illustrates high intramural conversion of Ang. I to Ang. II. Time 10 min; vertical scale in cm. (AIKEN and VANE, unpublished)

3. Adrenal Gland

PEACH et al. (1971) found Ang. I to be a potent stimulant of catecholamine secretion from cat adrenal medulla. The maximum possible conversion to Ang. II within the gland was 15 to 20% and this degree of conversion could not explain the potency of Ang. I as an adrenal medullary stimulant.

4. Kidney

Although SKEGGS et al. (1956) and BAKHLE et al. (1969) using rat perfused kidneys and NG and VANE (1967; 1968) using dog kidneys failed to demonstrate conversion of Ang. I to Ang. II, several workers have since estimated conversion ranging from 2 to 20%. Most of the recent work has been in dogs.

AIKEN and VANE (1972) allowed for a small (1 to 4% relative to Ang. II) inherent activity of Ang. I on Ang. II receptors (AIKEN and VANE, 1970) and this explains the difference between their figures of 2% conversion and the 4% of DISALVO et al. (1971), who assumed Ang. I to be completely inactive before conversion to Ang. II. AIKEN and VANE (1972) also measured the output of newly-formed Ang. II into the renal vein during administration of Ang. I. in the renal artery. This represented less conversion (1%) than that calculated from the renal vasoconstrictor effects. Thus, some of the Ang. II formed in the kidney from bloodborne Ang. I is probably inactivated before reaching the renal vein. The estimate of 7 to 10% conversion, made from radioimmunoassay results by OPARIL et al. (1970) may be high, because of the immuno-reactivity of other substances apart from Ang. II. However, there is a large discrepancy between the low estimates of conversion of NG and VANE (1968), DISALVO et al. (1971) and AIKEN and VANE (1972) and the estimate of 20% by FRANKLIN et al. (1970). There are several possible contributions to this discrepancy. First, implicit in FRANKLIN et al.'s method of calculating the relative potency of Ang. I to Ang. II is the erroneous assumption that the effects of a drug are linearly proportional to the dose, rather than to the $\log_{10}$ dose. Recalculation of their results on a log dose-response basis reduces the estimate of conversion to 14 to 17%. Another contribution to the discrepancy may be differences in potency of the Ang. I and Ang. II used in different laboratories. From the data of FRANKLIN et al. (1970) it appears that their Ang. I was more potent and their Ang. II less potent than that of AIKEN and VANE (1972). These differences in potency would be cumulative in any calculation of conversion based on relative potency of Ang. I and Ang. II. Perhaps the only conclusions that can be sensibly reached at this stage are (a) that a small degree of conversion can be detected in the renal vascular beds (including those of the sheep; TILDESLEY et al., 1971) and (b) that all those working with synthetic peptide hormones should heed the pitfalls associated with their use. Some of these are discussed below.

Differences in potency of peptides between laboratories may be due to several causes [VANE, 1971 (1); BANGHAM et al., 1971). Many workers, knowing that Ang. II adsorbs to glass, are careful to make up, store and use solutions in plastic containers or in siliconized glassware. Nevertheless, dilute solutions of Ang. II sometimes lose their potency, perhaps partly because Ang. II also adsorbs to plastics, such as polyvinyl chloride and polystyrene (BUMPUS, personal communication). Often the inactivation is capricious and, when it occurs, may take 5 min or 5 h. It can also happen within the tubing of an infusion pump. This inactivation is presumably due to bacterial contamination, for it is prevented by an antibacterial procedure based on that of LEARY (1970). It consists of filling the tubing of the infusion pumps and the polyethylene containers with a laboratory detergent such as 'Decon 75' overnight. After washing with distilled water for 5 min they are then washed with 0.01% solution (w/v) of the antiseptic chlorhexidine digluconate ('Hibitane', ICI) for 15 min. This is followed by further washing in distilled water for 5 min and sterile saline for 10 min. This treatment effectively prevents inactivation of dilute Ang. II solutions during the course of a day's experiment.

Even more hazardous and less easy to detect is the activation of Ang. I which can occur while the solution is being used. We have also seen activation in the tubing of infusion pumps so that, even though the reservoir contains Ang. I, a much more active solution is delivered after passing through the pump. This activation, which may represent conversion by bacteria, is also prevented by the procedure outlined above.

Without such antibacterial precautions, there is the strong possibility that, during an acute experiment, solutions of Ang. II will become less active and those of Ang. I will become more active. It is hardly necessary to stress how such changes will affect results in which conversion of Ang. I to Ang. II is being measured by a comparison of their potencies.

Another serious hazard in the use of synthetic peptides is the presence of biologically active or inactive impurities synthesized during manufacture and not excluded later. One manufacturer quotes "95% chemical purity" for the angiotensins and for bradykinin and its analogues. A sample of one of these peptides, methionyl-lysyl bradykinin, contained 25% lysyl bradykinin and about 3% bradykinin (CAMARGO et al., 1972). Such contamination with other biologically active substances, often with widely differing potencies, must substantially affect interpretation of comparative results. Even 5% impurity may be significant. For example, the ratio of potencies of Ang. I and Ang. II on the rat colon preparation is about 1:16. A 5% contamination of the Ang. I sample with Ang. II will double its apparent activity.

These problems would be largely eliminated if biologists working with peptides such as Ang. I and Ang. II would use the following procedure.

a) Prepare, store and use solutions of the peptides in conditions which minimize the possibility of bacterial contamination. We have found the antibacterial procedure described above to be adequate. The use of bacitracin has been suggested by PICKENS et al. (1965), but addition of preservatives to solutions may introduce further biological activity (SOMLYO and SOMLYO, 1970).

b) Check the solutions by bioassay both at the beginning and end of an experiment, until they are sure their precautions are adequate. Results of assays carried out in different laboratories will be more meaningful if the same stable reference standards are used by all. Such standards for many peptide hormones, including Ang. I and Ang. II, are now available from the Division of Biological Standards, National Institute for Medical Research, Mill Hill, London, England (BANGHAM et al., 1972).

c) Perform and publish experiments to check the biological purity of the synthetic peptide. A comparison of the potencies of the angiotensins in a particular tissue or organ is more reliable when their purity is validated by effects (1) on blood pressure after intravenous injection, to show the relative activity of Ang. I after conversion to Ang. II, and (2) on an isolated organ such as the rat uterus or rat colon, as an indication of lack of conversion of Ang. I before use.

d) Insist that the manufacturers of the peptides define clearly and more exactly the constitution and amounts of possible contaminants in their products. These figures, together with the batch numbers, should also be published.

Intra-Renal Role of the Renin-Angiotensin System

It has been suggested (THURAU, 1964; LEYSSAC, 1967; BRITTON, 1968) that the renin-angiotensin system has an important intra-renal role and that the function of renin liberated by the kidney is to generate Ang. II to act locally. Our results throw little light on this hypothesis for the juxtaglomerular apparatus contains converting-enzyme activity (THURAU, 1972) and Ang. II formation may be in the interstitial spaces rather than in blood (BAILIE et al., 1971). However, the overall distribution of converting enzyme in the body suggests an alternative hypothesis. The very small proportion of blood-borne Ang. I converted to Ang. II in kidney, with high conversion in lungs and some conversion in other vascular beds, suggests that the kidneys are exceptional for their low converting-enzyme activity. This may be a protective function; release of renin from the stores in the kidney could then take place without an immediate local generation of Ang. II by the relatively high concentration of renin that must exist in the blood into which it is released. The finding of concentrations of Ang. I in the renal venous blood 45 times higher than those of Ang. II (ITSKOVITZ and ODYA, 1971) fits with this concept.

Thus, without effective converting enzyme, the renal vascular bed, which is highly sensitive to Ang. II, will only receive Ang. II formed by converting enzyme in the lungs, after the renin content of the renal venous blood has been diluted with the rest of the cardiac output. Other results also suggest that the kidney is selectively protected against the actions of Ang. II. McGIFF et al. [1970 (1)] found that infusions of vasoconstrictor amounts of Ang. II into the kidney released into renal venous blood a prostaglandin-like material identified as prostaglandin E_2. We have confirmed this release (AIKEN and VANE, 1973) and further shown that when prostaglandin synthesis and release is prevented by a potent prostaglandin synthetase inhibitor, indomethacin [VANE, 1971 (2)] the vasoconstrictor effects of Ang. II in the kidney (but not those in the hind legs) are substantially enhanced. Thus, the local generation of a vasodilator prostaglandin may be a second mechanism by which the renal circulation is protected against the effects of Ang. II.

Another reason (admittedly teleological) for regarding Ang. II as a circulating hormone rather than a local intra-renal one arises from consideration of the factors which govern release and metabolism of vasoactive substances (VANE, 1969). A local hormone is released by cells near its site of action and is rapidly inactivated before it can have a general action. Possible examples of such hormones are acetylcholine and noradrenaline released from nerve endings, serotonin, bradykinin and some of the prostaglandins. For each of these, there are powerful local, circulatory and/or pulmonary mechanisms for rapid inactivation before they reach the arterial circulation (VANE, 1969), where they would have a general effect. When a circulating hormone, such as adrenal medullary adrenaline, vasopressin, oxytocin, etc. is released, the substance has no vascular effects on the gland itself, but has free access to the systemic circulation through the pulmonary vascular bed. The characteristics of the renin-angiotensin system, including the long half-line of renin in the circulation ($>$ 20 min, NG and VANE, 1968) and the activation of Ang. I in the lungs, all suggest that Ang. II is a circulating rather than a local hormone.

If, then, there are some grounds for doubting the intra-renal role proposed for the renin-angiotensin system, what mechanism can replace it? There are several indications to suggest that a local release of prostaglandin has many of the necessary characteristics. First, it almost certainly falls into the class of a local hormonal mechanism, for locally generated prostaglandins affect nearby cells in spleen (FERREIRA et al., 1971), intestine (FERREIRA et al., 1972) and kidney (AIKEN and VANE, 1971). Furthermore, several tissues including liver and lungs contain powerful inactivating enzymes which remove prostaglandins from the circulation [FERREIRA and VANE, 1967 (1); PIPER et al., 1970; PACE-ASCIAK et al., 1970; NAKANO, 1970; NAKANO and PRANCAN, 1971). Secondly, a review of the mechanisms of prostaglandin release (PIPER and VANE, 1971) shows that tissues do not store prostaglandins but that many types of cell can synthesize them rapidly when stimulated. Types of excitation which initiate prostaglandin production and release include chemical, pathological, physiological and mechanical. Amongst the mechanical stimuli are such mild deformations of cells as are caused by touch [PALMER et al., 1970 (1); 1970 (2)] vibration (GRYGLEWSKI and VANE, 1972) or distention (BERRY et al., 1971). Thirdly, prostaglandin release from the kidney can be induced by vasoconstrictor substances [McGIFF et al., 1970 (1)] or ischaemia [McGIFF et al., 1970 (2)]. The reactive hyperemia which follows renal artery occlusion has also been linked with prostaglandin release (HERBACZYNSKA-CEDRO and VANE, 1972). Lastly indomethacin, which abolishes prostaglandin synthesis, induces vasoconstriction in the dog kidney, reducing normal blood flow by about 15% (AIKEN and VANE, 1971) and at the same time, prevents the autoregulatory fall in resistance associated with a reduction in renal perfusion pressure (HERBACZYNSKA-CEDRO and VANE, 1972). Thus some aspects of renal autoregulation may be accounted for by local generation, not of the vasoconstrictor Ang. II, but of a vasodilator prostaglandin.

There is, however, yet another possibility. A renin-like enzyme has been extracted from vascular tissue (DENGLER, 1956; GOULD et al., 1964). The contiguity of converting enzyme and renin in vascular tissue might allow intramural generation of Ang. II from renin substrate, thereby selectively contributing to the local control of tone in those vessels sensitive to Ang. II. If this were so, the renin-angiotensin system would be somewhat analogous to the sympathetic nervous system: a local mechanism, generating a local hormone (Ang. II or noradrenaline) which would not reach the bloodstream in amounts sufficient to have a general effect; reinforced by an endocrine system (secretion of renin from the kidney or adrenaline from the adrenal medulla) designed to have a more general effect through the systemic circulation.

Summary

1. Bioassay will continue to make significant contributions to our knowledge of the renin-angiotensin system. Now that inhibitors of the formation and activity of Ang. II are available, substances which act like Ang. II in parallel assay systems should be identified as "angiotensin-like" until use of converting-enzyme inhibitors and/or receptor antagonists confirms the identity. In the same way, substances reacting with antibodies for Ang. I or Ang. II should be identified as "immuno-reactive material" rather than as Ang. I or Ang. II until it has been demonstrated that the particular antibody has little or no cross-reactivity with metabolic fragments of the angiotensin or with other plasma constituents.

2. Blood converting-enzyme activity is of little physiological significance for Ang. II formation in most species. The same applies to blood angiotensinase activity, which can slowly degrade both Ang. I and Ang. II.

3. Tissue conversion of Ang. I to Ang. II is much faster than plasma conversion and is, therefore, of greater physiological importance. Tissue conversion varies from organ to organ within a species and probably from species to species.

There are also substantial variations in different laboratories in the measurement of the degree of conversion. Some of the factors responsible for this variation have already been discussed, but activity in different tissues may be influenced by a factor, or factors, as yet unidentified. Many external factors can influence enzyme activity including such chemicals as laboratory insecticides (Conney, 1967). A low-salt diet reduces converting-enzyme activity (Gilmore et al., 1971).

4. Whether measured *in vivo*, by perfusion *in vitro*, or after tissue maceration, lung displays high converting-enzyme activity in all species so far studied. Indeed, with the possible exception of testes, lung shows higher converting-enzyme activity than any other tissue in the body. Most estimates of the degree of *in-vivo* conversion vary between 40 to 100%. At "physiological" concentrations, conversion is substantially complete. When this is considered alongside the fact that the pulmonary circulation handles the total cardiac output a second or so before the blood is pumped to the target organs, it is evident that the lungs must play a predominant role in the formation of blood-borne Ang. II.

5. Because of conversion to Ang. II in the lungs, concentration of Ang. I reaching the arterial circulation will be correspondingly low. Whether converting enzyme-activity in vascular beds such as the hind leg or intestine has an important role in contributing to the total amount of Ang. II available to local receptors depends upon the rate of formation of fresh Ang. I in the arterial circulation between the left ventricle and the vascular bed concerned. Little is known about this, although the finding of relatively high concentrations of Ang. I in arterial blood (Itskovitz and Odya, 1971) suggests that formation may be rapid.

6. As well as a variable degree of conversion of Ang. I to Ang. II in peripheral vascular beds, there is also a direct inactivation of Ang. I, perhaps by the same enzymes that inactivate Ang. II. When converting enzyme is inhibited, peripheral

inactivation of Ang. I should effectively prevent a build-up of Ang. I in the circulation.

7. Consideration of the characteristics of the renin-angiotensin system, including the long half-life of renin and the siting of lung converting-enzyme, lead to the conclusion that release of renin and the consequent formation of Ang. II has a systemic function. The postulated intra-renal role of the renin-angiotensin system has been discussed in the light of the increasing evidence that prostaglandin release may have an important local function in the kidney.

References

AIKEN, J. W., VANE, J. R.: The renin-angiotensin system: inhibition of converting enzyme in isolated tissues. Nature (Lond.) **228**, 30 (1970).

AIKEN, J. W., VANE, J. R.: Blockade of angiotensin-induced prostaglandin release from dog kidney by indomethacin. Pharmacologist **13**, 293 (1971).

AIKEN, J. W., VANE, J. R.: Inhibition of converting enzyme of the renin-angiotensin system in kidneys and hindlegs of dogs. Circulat. Res. **30**, 263 (1972).

AIKEN, J. W., VANE, J. R.: Intrarenal prostaglandin release attenuates the renal vasoconstructor activity of angiotensin. J. Pharmacol. exp. Ther. **184**, 678 (1973).

AKINKUGBE, O. O., BROWN, W. C. B., CRANSTON, W. I.: Pressor effects of angiotensin infusions into different vascular beds in the rabbit. Clin. Sci. **30**, 409 (1966).

ALABASTER, V. A., BAKHLE, Y. S.: The release of biologically active substances from isolated lungs by 5-hydroxytryptamine and tryptamine. Brit. J. Pharmacol. **40**, 582 P (1970).

BAILIE, M. D., RECTOR, F. C., SELDIN, D. W.: Angiotensin II in arterial and renal venous plasma and renal lymph in the dog. J. clin. Invest. **50**, 119 (1971).

BAKHLE, Y. S.: Conversion of angiotensin I to angiotensin II by cell-free extracts of dog lung. Nature (Lond.) **220**, 919 (1968).

BAKHLE, Y. S.: Inhibition of angiotensin I converting enzyme by venom peptides. Brit. J. Pharmacol. **42**, 252 (1971).

BAKHLE, Y. S.: Converting enzyme activity *in vitro*. This volume p. 41 (1973).

BAKHLE, Y. S., REYNARD, A. M.: Characteristics of the angiotensin I converting enzyme from dog lung. Nature (Lond.) New Biology **229**, 187 (1971).

BAKHLE, Y. S., REYNARD, A. M., VANE, J. R.: Metabolism of the angiotensins in isolated perfused tissues. Nature (Lond.) **222**, 956 (1969).

BANGHAM, D. R., CALAM, D. H., COTES, P. M., PARSONS, J. A., ROBINSON, C. J.: Investigation and treatment of endocrinological disorders. Lancet **1972 I**, 315.

BANGHAM, D. R., CALAM, D. H., PARSONS, J. A., ROBINSON, C. J.: Purity of synthetic peptide preparations. Nature (Lond.) **232**, 631 (1971).

BARAC, G.: Angiotensines et circulation sanguine des muscles squélettiques chez le Chien. C. R. Soc. Biol. (Paris) **156**, 1722 (1962).

BARRETT, J. D., SAMBHI, M. P.: Pulmonary activation and degradation of angiotensin I: a dual enzyme system. Res. Comm. Chem. Path. Pharmac. **2**, 128 (1971).

BERRY, E. M., EDMUNDS, J. F., WYLLIE, J. H.: Release of prostaglandin E_2 and unidentified factors from ventilated lung. Brit. J. Surg. **58**, 189 (1971).

BIRON, P., CAMPEAU, L.: Pulmonary and extrapulmonary fate of angiotensin I. Rev. canad. Biol. **30**, 27 (1971).

BIRON, P., CAMPEAU, L., DAVID, P.: Fate of angiotensin I and II in the human pulmonary circulation. Amer. J. Cardiol. **24**, 544 (1969).

BIRON, P., HUGGINS, C. G.: Pulmonary activation of synthetic angiotensin I. Life Sci. **7**, 965 (1968).

BIRON, P., MEYER, P., PANISSET, J. C.: Removal of angiotensins from the systemic circulation. Canad. J. Physiol. Pharmacol. **46**, 175 (1968).

BRITTON, K. E.: Renin and renal autoregulation. Lancet **1968 II**, 329.

CAIN, M. D., CATT, K. J., COGHLAN, J. P.: Immunoreactive fragments of angiotensin II in blood. Nature (Lond.) **223**, 617 (1969).

CAMARGO, A. C., PINTO, J. R., GREENE, L. J.: Brain peptidases; conversion inactivation of kinin hormones. J. Neurochem. **19**, 37 (1972).

CARLINI, E. A., PICARELLI, Z. P., PRADO, J. L.: Pharmacological activity of hypertensin I and its conversion into hypertensin II. Bull. Soc. Chim. biol. (Paris) **40**, 1825 (1958).

CONNEY, A. H.: Pharmacological implications of microsomal enzyme induction. Pharmacol. Rev. **19**, 317 (1967).

CUSHMAN, D. W., CHEUNG, H. S.: (1) Concentrations of angiotensin converting enzyme in tissues of the rat. Biochim. biophys. Acta (Amst.) **250**, 261 (1971).

CUSHMAN, D. W., CHEUNG, H. S.: (2) Spectrophotometric assay and properties of the angiotensin-converting enzyme of rabbit lung. Biochem. Pharmacol. **20**, 1637 (1971).

CUSHMAN, D. W., CHEUNG, H. S.: Studies *in vitro* of angiotensin-converting enzyme of lung and other tissues. (GENEST, J., Ed.). Berlin-Heidelberg-New York: Springer 1972.

DAVIS, B. N., HORTON, E. W., WITHERINGTON, P. G.: The occurence of prostaglandin E_2 in splenic venous blood of the dog following splenic nerve stimulation. Brit. J. Pharmacol. **32**, 127 (1968).

DENGLER, J.: Über ein Reninantigen-Wirkstoff in Arterienextrakten. Naunyn-Schmiedebergs Arch. Pharmak. exp. Path. **227**, 481 (1956).

DEODHAR, S. D.: Immunologic production of anti-angiotensin. J. exp. Med. **1**, 429 (1960).

DEPIERRE, D., ROTH, M.: Activity of a dipeptidyl carboxypeptidase (angiotensin converting enzyme) in lungs of different animal species. Experientia (Basel) **28**, 154 (1972).

DISALVO, J., MENTA, M., MONTEFUSCO, C. B., PETERSON, A.: Intrarenal conversion of angiotensin I to angiotensin II in the dog. Circulat. Res. **29**, 398 (1971).

DISALVO, J., MONTEFUSCO, C. B.: Conversion of angiotensin I to angiotensin II in the canine mesenteric circulation. Amer. J. Physiol. **221**, 1576 (1971).

DORER, F. E., SKEGGS, L. T., KAHN, J. R., LENTZ, K. E., LEVINE, M.: Angiotensin converting enzyme. Method of assay and partial purification. Ann. Biochem. **33**, 102 (1970).

DÜSTERDIECK, G., MCELWEE, G.: Estimation of angiotensin II concentration in human plasma by radio-immunoassay. Some applications to physical and clinical studies. Europ. J. clin. Invest. **2**, 32 (1971).

ELISSEEVA, Y. E., OREKHOVICH, V. N., PAVLIKHINA, L. V., ALEXEENKO, L. P.: Carboxy-cathepsin — a key regulatory component of two physiological systems involved in regulation of blood pressure. Clin. chim. Acta. **31**, 413 (1971).

ENGEL, S. L., SCHAEFFER, T. R., GOLD, B. I., RUBIN, B.: Inhibition of angiotensin converting enzyme *in vivo* by peptides from snake venom. Proc. XXV Intern. Cong. Physiol. Sci. **9**, 163 (1971).

FERREIRA, S. H.: A bradykinin-potentiating factor (BPF) present in the venom of *Bothrops Jararaca*. Brit. J. Pharmacol. **24**, 163 (1965).

FERREIRA, S. H., BARTELT, D. C., GREENE, L. J.: (2) Isolation of bradykinin potentiating peptides from *Bothrops Jararaca* venom. Biochemistry **9**, 2583 (1970).

FERREIRA, S. H., GREENE, L. J., ALABASTER, V. A., BAKHLE, Y. S., VANE, J. R.: (1) Activity of various fractions of bradykinin-potentiating factor against angiotensin converting enzyme. Nature (Lond.) **225**, 379 (1970).

FERREIRA, S. H., HERMAN, A., VANE, J. R.: Prostaglandin generation maintains the smooth muscle tone of the rabbit isolated jejumum. Brit. J. Pharmacol. **44**, 328 P (1972).

FERREIRA, S. H., MONCADA, S., VANE, J. R.: Indomethacin and aspirin abolish prostaglandin release from the spleen. Nature (Lond.) New Biol. **231**, 237 (1971).

FERREIRA, S. H., VANE, J. R.: (1) Prostaglandins: their disappearance from and release into the circulation. Nature (Lond.) **216**, 868 (1967).

FERREIRA, S. H., VANE, J. R.: (2) The disappearance of bradykinin and eledoisin in the circulation and vascular beds of the cat. Brit. J. Pharmacol. Chemother. **30**, 417 (1967).

FRANKLIN, W. G., PEACH, M. J., GILMORE, J. P.: Evidence for the renal conversion of angiotensin I in the dog. Circulat. Res. **27**, 321 (1970).

GADDUM, J. H.: The technique of superfusion. Brit. J. Pharmacol. Chemother. 8, 321 (1953).

GADDUM, J. H.: Bioassay procedures. Pharmacol. Rev. **11**, 241 (1959).

GILMORE, J. P., MERRILL, J., PEACH, M. J.: Further evidence for the renal conversion of angiotensin. Fed. Proc. **30**, 449 Abs. (1971).

GOFFINET, J. A., MULROW, P. J.: Estimation of angiotensin clearance by an *in vivo* assay. Clin. Res. **11**, 408 (1965).

GOULD, A. B., SKEGGS, L. T., KAHN, J. R.: Presence of renin activity in blood vessel walls. J. exp. Med. **119**, 389 (1964).

GROSS, F., TURRIAN, H.: In: Polypeptides which affect smooth muscles and blood vessels (SCHACHTER, M., Ed.). p. 137. Oxford: Pergamon Press 1960.

GRYGLEWSKI, R., VANE, J. R.: The release of prostaglandins and rabbit aorta contracting substance (RCS) from rabbit spleen and its antagonism by anti-inflammatory drugs. Brit. J. Pharmacol. **45** (1972).

HAAS, E. H., GOLDBLATT, H., LEWIS, V., GIBSON, E. C.: Inhibition of angiotensin and its protection by a cofactor in blood. Amer. J. Physiol. **215**, 1420 (1968).

HALVORSEN, K. A., FASCIOLO, J. C., CALVO, R.: Comparaison des activités hypertensives et vasoconstrictrice des angiotensines I et II. C. R. Soc. Biol. (Paris) **153**, 489 (1959).

HEINEMANN, H. O., FISHMAN, A. P.: Non-respiratory functions of mammalian lung. Physiol. Rev. **49**, 1 (1969).

HELMER, O. M.: Differentiation between two forms of angiotonin by means of spirally cut strips of rabbit aorta. Amer. J. Physiol. **188**, 571 (1957).

Herbaczynska-Cedro, K., Vane, J. R.: An intra-renal role for prostaglandin production. V. Int. Congress on Pharmac. (1972).
Hodge, R. L., Lowe, R. D., Vane, J. R.: The effects of alteration of blood volume on the concentration of circulating angiotensin in anaesthetized dogs. J. Physiol. **185**, 613 (1966).
Hodge, R. L., Ng, K. K. F., Vane, J. R.: Disappearance of angiotensin from the circulation of the dog. Nature (Lond.) **215**, 138 (1967).
Hollemans, H. J. G., van der Meer, J., Kloosterziel, W.: Identification of the incubation product of Boucher's renin activity assay, by means of radio-immunoassays for angiotensin I and angiotensin II, and a converting enzyme preparation from lung tissue. Clin. chim. Acta **23**, 7 (1969).
Huggins, C. G., Thampi, N. S.: A simple method for the determination of angiotensin converting enzyme. Life Sci. **7**, 633 (1968).
Itskovitz, H. D., Odya, C.: Intra-renal formation of angiotensin I. Science **174**, 58 (1971).
Khairallah, P. A., Toth, A., Bumpus, F. M.: Analogs of angiotensin II. Mechanism of receptor interaction. J. Med. Chem. **13**, 181 (1970).
Kreye, V. A. W., Gross, F.: Conversion of angiotensin I to angiotensin II in peripheral vascular beds of the rat. Amer. J. Physiol. **220**, 1294 (1971).
Krieger, E. M., Salgado, H. C., Assan, C. J., Greene, L. J., Ferreira, S. H.: Potential screening test for detection of overactivity of renin-angiotensin system. Lancet **1971 I**, **269**.
Leary, W. P. P.: Aspects of the renin-angiotensin system. D. Phil. Thesis Univ. of Oxford (1970).
Leary, W. P. P., Ledingham, J. G.: Removal of angiotensin by isolated perfused organs of the rat. Nature (Lond.) **222**, 959 (1969).
Leary, W. P. P., Ledingham, J. G.: Catabolism of angiotensin II. This volume, p. 111 (1973).
Lee, H. J., Larue, J. N., Wilson, I. B.: (1) Human plasma converting enzyme. Arch. Biochem. **142**, 548 (1971).
Lee, H. J., Larue, J. N., Wilson, I. B.: (2) Angiotensin-converting enzyme from guinea pig and hog lung. Biochim. biophys. Acta (Amst.) **250**, 549 (1971).
Lee, H. J., Larue, J. N., Wilson, I. B.: (3) Angiotensin-converting enzyme from porcine plasma. Biochim. biophys. Acta (Amst.) **235**, 521 (1971).
Leyssac, P. P.: Intrarenal function of angiotensin. Fed. Proc. **26**, 55 (1967).
Loyke, H. F.: Converting enzyme in rat serum. Proc. Soc. exp. Biol. (N. Y.) **134**, 248 (1970).
Mann, M., West, G. B.: The nature of hepatic and splenic sympathin. Brit. J. Pharmacol. Chemother. **5**, 173 (1950).
Marshall, G. R., Vine, W., Needleman, P.: A specific competitive inhibitor of angiotensin II. Proc. nat. Acad. Sci. (Wash.) **67**, 1624 (1970).
McGiff, J. C., Crowshaw, K., Terragno, N. A., Lonigro, A. J.: (1) Release of a prostaglandin like substance into the renal venous blood in response to angiotensin II. Circulat. Res. **27**, Suppl. I, I—121 (1970).
McGiff, J. C., Crowshaw, K., Terragno, N. A., Lonigro, A. J., Strand, J. C., Williamson, M. A., Lee, J. B., Ng, K. K. F.: (2) Prostaglandin like substances appearing in canine renal venous blood during renal ischaemia. Circulat. Res. **27**, 765 (1970).
Nakano, J.: Metabolism of prostaglandin E_1 in dog kidneys. Brit. J. Pharmacol. **40**, 317 (1970).
Nakano, J., Prancan, A. V.: Metabolic degradation of prostaglandin E_1 in the rat plasma and in rat brain, heart, lung, kidney and testicle homogenates. J. Pharm. Pharmacol. **23**, 231 (1971).
Ng, K. K. F., Vane, J. R.: Conversion of angiotensin I to angiotensin II. Nature (Lond.) **216**, 762 (1967).
Ng, K. K. F., Vane, J. R.: Fate of angiotensin I in the circulation. Nature (Lond.) **218**, 144 (1968).
Ng, K. K. F., Vane, J. R.: Some properties of angiotensin converting enzyme in the lung *in vivo*. Nature (Lond.) **225**, 1142 (1970).
Ondetti, M. A., Williams, N. J., Sabo, E. F., Pluščec, J., Weaver, E. R., Kocy, O.: Angiotensin-converting enzyme inhibitor from the venom of *Bothrops Jararaca*. Isolation, elucidation of structure and synthesis. Biochemistry **10**, 4033 (1971).
Oparil, S., Sander, C. A., Haber, E.: *In vivo* and *in vitro* conversion of angiotensin I to angiotensin II in dog blood. Circulat. Res. **26**, 591 (1970).
Oparil, S., Tregear, G. W., Koerner, T., Barnes, B. A., Haber, E.: Mechanism of pulmonary conversion of angiotensin I to angiotensin II in the dog. Circulat. Res. **29**, 682 (1971).
Osborn, E. C., Pickens, P. T., Willicombe, P. R., Pirie, A. T., Mahler, R. F.: Studies with angiotensins I and II; the use of phenylthiocarbamyl derivatives. Clin. Sci. **38**, 211 (1970).
Osborn, E. C., Tildesley, G., O'Gorman, L. P., Mahler, R. F.: The effect of angiotensin I and II on hind-limb blood flow in sheep. J. Pharm. Pharmacol. **23**, 466 (1971).

PACE-ASCIAK, C., MORAWSKA, K., WOLFE, L. S.: Metabolism of prostaglandin $F_{1\alpha}$ by the rat stomach. Biochim. biophys. Acta (Amst.) **218**, 288 (1970).

PAGE, L. B.: Discussion contribution. Circulat. Res. **26** and **27**, 1—103 (1970).

PALMER, M. A., PIPER, P. J., VANE, J. R.: (1) The release of rabbit aorta contracting substance (RCS) from chopped lung and its antagonism by anti-inflammatory drugs. Brit. J. Pharmacol. **40**, 581 P (1970).

PALMER, M. A., PIPER, P. J., VANE, J. R.: (2) Release of vasoactive substances from lungs by injection of particles. Brit. J. Pharmacol. **40**, 547 P (1970).

PALS, D. T., MASUCCI, F. D., DENNING, G. S., SIPOS, F., FESSLER, D. R.: (2) Role of the pressor action of angiotensin II in experimental hypertension. Circulat. Res. **29**, 673 (1971).

PALS, D. T., MASUCCI, F. D., SIPOS, F., DENNING, G. S.: (1) A specific competitive antagonist of the vascular action of angiotensin II. Circulat. Res. **29**, 664 (1971).

PEACH, M. J., BUMPUS, F. M., KHAIRALLAH, P. A.: Release of adrenal catecholamines by angiotensin I. J. Pharmacol. exp. Ther. **176**, 366 (1971).

PICKENS, P. T., BUMPUS, F. M., LLOYD, A. M., SMEBY, R. R., PAGE, I. H.: Measurement of renin activity in human plasma. Circulat. Res. **17**, 438 (1965).

PIPER, P. J., VANE, J. R.: Release of additional factors in anaphylaxis and its antagonism, by anti-inflammatory drugs. Nature (Lond.) **223**, 29 (1969).

PIPER, P. J., VANE, J. R.: The release of prostaglandins from lung and other tissues. Ann. N. Y. Acad. Sci. **180**, 363 (1971).

PIPER, P. J., VANE, J. R., WYLLIE, J. H.: Inactivation of prostaglandins by the lungs. Nature (Lond.) **225**, 600 (1970).

PIQUILLOUD, Y., REINHARZ, A., ROTH, M.: Studies on the angiotensin converting enzyme with different substrates. Biochim. biophys. Acta (Amst.) **206**, 136 (1970).

POULSEN, K., BING, J.: Species specific differences in converting enzyme and in angiotensin I. Acta. path. microbiol. scand. Section A **78**, 665 (1970).

POULSEN, K., POULSEN, L. L.: Simultaneous determination of converting enzyme and angiotensinase activity by radio-immunoassay. Clin. Sci. **40**, 443 (1971).

REGOLI, D., PARK, W. K., RIOUX, F., CHAN, C. S.: Antagonists of angiotensin. Substitution of an aliphatic chain to phenyl ring in position 8. Rev. canad. Biol. **30**, 319 (1971).

REGOLI, D., VANE, J. R.: A sensitive method for the assay of angiotensin. Brit. J. Pharmacol. Chemother. **23**, 351 (1964).

REGOLI, D., VANE, J. R.: The continuous estimation of angiotensin formed in the circulation of the dog. J. Physiol. (Lond.) **183**, 513 (1966).

ROTH, M., WEITZMAN, A. F., PIQUILLOUD, Y.: Converting enzyme content of different tissues of the rat. Experientia (Basel) **25**, 1247 (1969).

RYAN, J. W., ROBLERO, J., STEWART, J. M.: Inactivation of bradykinin in the pulmonary circulation. Biochem. J. **110**, 795 (1968).

RYAN, J. W., STEWART, J. M., LEARY, W. P. P., LEDINGHAM, J. G.: Metabolism of angiotensin I in the pulmonary circulation. Biochem. J. **120**, 221 (1970).

SANDER, G. E., HUGGINS, C. G.: Subcellular distribution of angiotensin I converting enzyme. Nature (Lond.) **230**, 27 (1971).

SANDER, G. E., WEST, D. W., HUGGINS, C. G.: Peptide inhibitors of pulmonary angiotensin I converting enzyme. Biochim. biophys. Acta (Amst.) **242**, 662 (1971).

SCHOLZ, H. W., BIRON, P.: Non identity between pulmonary bradykininase and converting-enzyme activity. Rec. canad. Biol. **28**, 197 (1969).

SKEGGS, L. T., KAHN, J. R., SHUMWAY, N. P.: Preparation and function of the hypertensin converting enzyme. J. exp. Med. **103**, 295 (1956).

SKEGGS, L. T., MARSH, W. H., KAHN, J. R., SHUMWAY, N. P.: The existence of two forms of hypertensin. J. exp. Med. **99**, 275 (1954).

SOMLYO, A. P., SOMLYO, A. V.: Vascular smooth muscle. II. Pharmacology of normal and hypertensive vessels. Pharmacol. Rev. **22**, 257 (1970).

SPECTOR, W. G.: Handbook of biological data, p. 285. Philadelphia: Saunders 1956.

STANLEY, P., BIRON, P.: Renal response to angiotensin I during cardiopulmonary by-pass. Experientia (Basel) **25**, 46 (1969).

STEWART, J. M., FERREIRA, S. H., GREENE, L. J.: Bradykinin potentiating peptide PCA-LYS-TRP-ALA-PRO: an inhibitor of the pulmonary inactivation of bradykinin and conversion of angiotensin I to II. Biochem. Pharmacol. **20**, 1557 (1971).

THURAU, K.: Renal haemodynamics. Amer. J. Med. **36**, 698 (1964).

THURAU, K.: Functional and enzymatic analysis of the juxta-glomerular apparatuses. Hypertension 1972 (GENEST, J., Ed.). Berlin-Heidelberg-New York: Springer 1972.

TILDESLEY, G., OSBORN, E. C., WILLICOMBE, P. R., MAHLER, R. F.: The effect of angiotensin I on renal blood flow in sheep. J. Pharm. Pharmacol. **23**, 547 (1971).

TÜRKER, R. K., YAMAMOTO, M., BUMPUS, F. M., KHAIRALLAH, P. A.: (1) Lung perfusion with angiotensins I and II. Evidence of release of myotropic and inhibitory substances. Circulat. Res. **28**, 559 (1971).

TÜRKER, R. K., YAMAMOTO, M., BUMPUS, F. M., KHAIRALLAH, P. A.: (2) Loss of activity of angiotensin I and II by superfusion over rabbit aorta and rat colon. Pharmacologist **13**, 214 (1971).

TÜRKER, R. K., YAMAMOTO, M., KHAIRALLAH, P. A., BUMPUS, F. M.: (3) Competitive antagonism of 8-ala-angiotensin II to angiotensins I and II on isolated rabbit aorta and rat ascending colon. Europ. J. Pharmacol. **15**, 285 (1971).

UEDA, E., AKUTSU, H., KOKUBU, T., YAMAMURA, Y.: Partial purification and properties of angiotensin I converting enzyme from rabbit plasma. Jap. Circulat. (En.) J. **35**, 801 (1971).

VANE, J. R.: A sensitive method for the assay of 5-hydroxytryptamine. Brit. J. Pharmacol. **12**, 344 (1957).

VANE, J. R.: The use of isolated organs for detecting active substances in the circulating blood. Brit. J. Pharmacol. **23**, 360 (1964).

VANE, J. R.: The alteration or removal of vaso-active substance in the pulmonary circulation. In: Importance of fundamental principles in drug evaluation (TEDESCHI, D. H., TEDESCHI, R. E., Eds.), p. 217. New York: Raven Press 1968.

VANE, J. R.: The release and fate of vaso-active substances in the circulation. Brit. J. Pharmacol. **35**, 209 (1969).

VANE, J. R.: (1) Purity and stability of synthetic peptides such as angiotensin and kinins. Nature (Lond.) **230**, 382 (1971).

VANE, J. R.: (2) Inhibition of prostaglandin synthesis as a mechanism of action for aspirin-like drugs. Nature (Lond.) New Biology **231**, 232 (1971).

YANG, H. Y. T., ERDOS, E. G., LEVIN, Y.: Characterization of a dipeptide hydrolase (kininase II: angiotensin I converting enzyme). J. Pharmacol. exp. Ther. **177**, 291 (1971).

YAMAMOTO, M., TÜRKER, R. K., LEWIS, L. A.: Studies on the conversion of angiotensin I to angiotensin II. Fed. Proc. **30**, 432 (1971).

Converting Enzyme *in Vitro* Measurement and Properties

Y. S. BAKHLE

Introduction

In 1954 SKEGGS, MARSH, KAHN and SHUMWAY reported that angiotensin, the pressor product of renin's incubation with its substrate, was actually a mixture of two forms, Ang. I and Ang. II, separable by counter-current distribution. Ang. I, the initial product of renin's action, was itself transformed into Ang. II by an enzyme present in plasma and requiring chloride ion for its activity. This enzymic activity was called "converting enzyme". Since Ang. I and Ang. II were equally pressor (when injected intravenously into rats), they suggested that the action of converting enzyme was the removal of some groups from Ang. I "leaving that portion of the molecule responsible for its pressor activity unchanged". The following year HELMER (1955) showed that there was a pharmacological difference between the two forms, Ang. I being inactive and Ang. II active in contracting the rabbit aortic strip. He also showed that plasma would convert the inactive Ang. I to the active Ang. II *in vitro*, although both forms were equipressor *in vivo*. Following this suggestion that Ang. II was the true vasoconstrictor and pressor agent, SKEGGS et al. (1956) showed that in isolated kidneys perfused with an artificial salt solution, only Ang. II increased perfusion pressure and not Ang. I. From these experiments, they concluded that there was enough converting enzyme (CE) in plasma to transform Ang. I to Ang. II so that, *in vivo*, the two forms were equipressor, and that the rate-limiting step in the overall formation of Ang. II was the rate of reaction of renin with its substrate.

During the next twelve years, little work was reported on CE. In a review on the renin-angiotensin system in 1965, PEART was able to cover the subject of CE fully in three lines of print. In 1968, two papers from different sources reopened the study of CE (BAKHLE; HUGGINS and THAMPI) and the eighty to ninety papers published on CE in the next three years mean it is no longer possible to review the subject with PEART's enviable brevity.

One crucial factor in this reawakening of interest in CE was an advance in chemistry — the development of the solid-phase method of peptide synthesis (MERRIFIELD, 1964) to a stage where the synthesis of oligopeptides about 10 residues long could be successfully undertaken. This meant that the substrate of CE, the decapeptide Ang. I, was available in milligram quantities, without isolating it from the reaction of purified renin with purified renin substrate as SKEGGS and his colleagues had to. Another factor was the recognition of the pulmonary circulation as an important locus of CE (NG and VANE, 1967). The combination of these factors raised the problems of whether the plasma or the lung were the physiologically important locus of CE and whether it was the same enzyme in both places. At the same time it provided a source of enzyme and a convenient supply of substrate, so that closer study of these problems was possible.

This section is confined to a discussion of the properties of CE activity studied *in vitro*. The properties of CE *in vivo* and in isolated organs perfused with blood or physiological salt solutions are dealt with elsewhere in this volume (VANE, 1972).

The original definition of Ang. I-converting enzyme activity was in terms of its function — to convert the decapeptide Ang. I to the octapeptide Ang. II (SKEGGS et al., 1954) — and it remains the essential criterion for this activity. These authors also established other properties of this peptidase activity, which have served as additional criteria for the identification of converting-enzyme activity.

The more important of these are:

1. The removal of the two C-terminal amino acids as a dipeptide unit (LENTZ et al., 1956).

2. The absence of any point of hydrolysis in the substrate apart from the Phe^8-His^9 bond. This means that Ang. II is a limit peptide for CE and that there is no angiotensin inactivation reaction catalyzed by this enzyme (LENTZ et al., 1956).

3. The requirement for halide ions, usually expressed as dependence on chloride ion (SKEGGS et al., 1954).

4. Inhibition by EDTA (SKEGGS et al., 1956).

The majority of preparations catalyzing the conversion of Ang. I to Ang. II satisfy the four additional criteria as well, but there are now several notable exceptions (see below). Thus, a carboxypeptidase acting on Ang. I could be classified as a converting enzyme if it produced Ang. II but it would not satisfy all the other four criteria. I shall, therefore, discuss together those peptidases that convert Ang. I to Ang. II and also satisfy all four additional criteria, and then discuss those peptidases which although capable of converting Ang. I to Ang. II have failed to satisfy one or more of the additional criteria.

Assay Methods

The various assay methods that have been used (almost a different one for each preparation) will be discussed first as the reliability of the assay reflects on the validity of the results obtained with it. The assays are most conveniently grouped into those that use Ang. I as substrate and those that use another synthetic peptide as substrate (see Table 1).

1. Methods Using Angiotensin I as Substrate

These methods may be further subdivided into those utilizing the biological activity of the Ang. II produced and those in which chemical and physical methods are used to measure either of the products, Ang. II or His-Leu.

a) Biological Methods

The bioassay of Ang. II is reviewed thoroughly elsewhere in this volume but some comments can properly be made here. There are various isolated organs, e.g. rat uterus, rat colon, rabbit aorta, on which Ang. II is so much more potent than Ang. I that the biological activity of a mixture of substrate Ang. I and product Ang. II is essentially due to the Ang. II for a wide range of concentrations.

This differential sensitivity was demonstrated with spiral strips of rabbit aorta, in one of the first papers on CE (HELMER, 1957), and more recently, HUGGINS et al. (1970) have used this tissue in their studies on lung and plasma CE. The rat uterus is 10 to 40 times more sensitive to Ang. II than to Ang. I and has been used

Table 1. *Assay methods for converting enzyme*

The details are taken from the descriptions of the method in the references. The limit of sensitivity values have been estimated (except for ref. 17) by the writer

Amount of substrate per ml of standard assay	Product measured	Method of measurement	Approximate limit of sensitivity	Reference
		A. *With Ang. I as substrate*		
20—40 µg	Ang. I	Rabbit aorta	2.5 ng/ml	15
200 ng	Ang. I	Rat uterus	0.5—1 ng/ml	1
2 µg	Ang. I	Rat uterus	0.5—1 ng/ml	6
200 ng	Ang. I	Rat uterus	0.5—1 ng/ml	23
5—10 µg	Ang. I	Rat colon	2.5 ng	2—5
33 ng	Ang. I	Rat blood pressure	0.5—1 ng	18
125 ng	Ang. I	Rat blood pressure	0.5—1 ng	19
1 µg[a]	Ang. I	Rat blood pressure	0.5—1 ng	7
17.5 µg 1260 cpm ^{14}C	His-Leu	Radiometric		14
250—375 ng 80,000 cpm ^{3}H	His-Leu	Radiometric		20
0.25—6.25 µg 4,000 cpm ^{14}C	His-Leu	Radiometric	400 cpm	17
No data given ^{3}H	His-Leu	Radiometric		13
0.5 µg[b] ^{35}S	PTC-Ang. II	Radiometric		21
67 µg	His-Leu	Spectrofluorimetric	~ 1 nmole	8
75 µg	His-Leu	Spectrofluorimetric	~12 nmoles	10
100 µg	His-Leu	Photometric (ninhydrin)	~ 2 nmoles	11
		B. *With short substrates*		
75 µg Z-Phe-His-Leu Z-Pro-Phe-His-Leu	His-Leu	Spectrofluorimetric	~ 1 nmole/ml	22
5 µmoles Hippuryl-His-Leu	Hippuric acid	Photometric	~ 5 nmoles/ml	9
300 nmoles *t*-BOC-Phe(NO_2)-Phe-Gly	*t*-BOC-Phe(NO_2)	Photometric	~50 nmoles/ml	24
No data given Hippuryl-Phe-Pro	Phe-Pro	Photometric (ninhydrin)	?	12
3.6 nmoles Dansyl-Gly-Gly-Gly[c] ^{14}C	Dansyl-Gly	Radiometric	?	16

[a] In this assay 1 µg of Ang. I is adsorbed on a standard amount of ion exchange resin.
[b] The substrate here is PTC-Ang. I labelled with ^{35}S, of unstated specific activity.
[c] The hydrolysis of this substrate has not been shown to be dependent on chloride ion.

1. Andersen (1967); 2. Bakhle (1968); 3. Bakhle (1971); 4. Bakhle (1972); 5. Bakhle and Reynard (1971); 6. Barrett and Sambhi (1969); 7. Boucher et al. (1970); 8. Boucher et al. (1970); 9. Cushman and Cheung, (1971a); 10. Cushman and Cheung, (1972); 11. Dorer et al, (1970); 12. Elisseeva and Orekhovich (1963); 13. Fitz and Overturf (1972); 14. Huggins and Thampi (1968); 15. Huggins et al. (1970); 16. Igic et al. (1972); 17. Lee et al [1971 (1—4)]; 18. Loyke (1968); 19. Loyke (1970); 20. Oparil et al. (1970); 21. Osborn et al. [1970 (2)]; 22. Piquilloud et al. (1970); 23. Ueda et al. (1971); 24. Yang et al. (1971).

by Bumpus et al. (1956), Andersen (1967), Barrett and Sambhi (1969) and Ueda et al. [1971 (1, 2)]. The rat colon with a sensitivity to Ang. II 15 to 20 times that to Ang. I (Ng and Vane, 1967) has been used in the work of Bakhle and his colleagues.

The advantage of this type of assay is that small amounts of Ang. II may be measured, as are produced from correspondingly small (nearly physiological) amounts of Ang. I. High concentrations of Ang. I are metabolized by carboxypeptidases as well as by CE in the pulmonary circulation of the rat (BARRETT and SAMBHI, 1971). Furthermore, it is not necessary to separate product Ang. II from residual substrate Ang. I before assay. The disadvantages are chiefly those inherent in any bioassay, with the further point that since we are only following biological activity, *any* peptide fragment of Ang. I with greater activity than Ang. I will be represented to some extent as Ang. II. There is no identification of the biologically active material as Ang. II beyond that afforded by parallel bioassay techniques.

The traditional method of bioassay is to make use of the pressor activity of Ang. II but since Ang. I given i.v. is equipressor to Ang. II, assay of Ang. II produced from Ang. I is possible only after separation of the peptides. The first separation was achieved by SKEGGS et al. (1954), using counter-current distribution in 49 transfers, although fewer transfers have been used (DORER et al., 1970).

This method was superseded by a number of chromatographic techniques. WISENBAUGH et al. (1964) used Whatman no. 1 paper with a solvent system of 1 M NaCl and 0.02 HCl to give separation of Ang. I (R_F 0.3 to 4) from Ang. II (R_F 0.7 to 0.8) after 8 to 10 h. The Ang. II was eluted from the paper with distilled water (18 to 20 h) and assayed by its pressor effect. LOYKE (1964, 1968, 1970) has used the separation procedure of WISENBAUGH et al. coupled with the pressor assay in rats in his studies on serum CE in hypertensive rats.

ELISSEEVA et al. (1971) separated Ang. II, formed by "carboxycathepsin", from Ang. I by thin layer chromatography on silica gel. Two solvent systems were used in succession (*sec.*-BuOH: 3% NH_3 25:11, v/v; *n*-BuOH: NH_3: H_2O-120:7:7:, v/v) to give adequate but not striking separation of Ang. I and Ang. II. The octapeptide was then assayed by its pressor effect in rats.

BOUCHER et al. (1970) have modified their earlier procedure (BOUCHER et al., 1964) so that Ang. I, adsorbed on Dowex 50W-X2, is now treated with CE at pH 7.4 and both substrate Ang. I and product Ang. II are retained on this resin. The reaction is stopped with EDTA, and after washing, both peptides are eluted from the first ion-exchange resin with 4 M pyridine and passed into a column of Dowex 50W-X8 which retains only the unreacted Ang. I, allowing Ang. II to pass through and be collected. The Ang. II is then measured by its pressor effect in nephrectomized rats. The separation of Ang. I and Ang. II on the second column is good, only 2 to 3% of Ang. I being eluted by 4 M pyridine (compared with 90 to 100% of the Ang. II), and the reproducibility of the assay is within 15%. The effect of carboxypeptidases, which will generate Ang. II from Ang. I in this system, is eliminated by preincubation of plasma, resin and adsorbed substrate at 0 to 5 °C. One disadvantage is that there is a basal conversion during the preincubation of 25 ng/1000 ng Ang. I, compared with the total conversion of 100 ng/1000 ng Ang. I after the additional 20 min incubation at 37 °C. This rather high blank: sample ratio could perhaps be improved by increasing the level of substrate. Another inconvenience is that the Ang. II is finally eluted in pyridine and an evaporation step is therefore essential before bioassay is undertaken.

b) Physicochemical Methods for Assay of CE

The methods which do not rely on bioassay of Ang. II produced from Ang. I may be divided into those measuring Ang. II and those measuring His-Leu.

The former group consists almost entirely of radio-immunoassays of Ang. II as described in the work of several groups in different countries and reviewed elsewhere in this volume. An interesting variation in which *E. coli* and T_4 phage coupled to Ang. II is used as the indicator system has been described by HURWITZ et al. (1971). The immunoassay of Ang. II is fully discussed in this volume, but here attention must be drawn to the admittedly (CAIN et al., 1969; DUSTERDIECK and MCELWEE, 1971) high degree of cross reaction of Ang. II antibodies with the hepta- and hexapeptides, des-[Asp^1]- and des-[Asp^1-Arg^2]-Ang II. Thus both Ang. II *and* two of its metabolites (with less biological activity) would all react as Ang. II.

The other common radiometric assay for CE uses Ang. I with radioactively labelled Leu^{10} and measures the radioactive His-Leu formed after separation from substrate. Both ^{3}H- and ^{14}C-labelled substrates have been synthesized and used. The method was first described by HUGGINS and THAMPI (1968) who synthesized [5-Ile-10-^{14}C(U) Leu]-Ang. I of relatively low specific activity (90 cpm/nmole). This was split by CE to give Ang. II and His-Leu and all three components of the reaction mixture, Ang. I, Ang. II and His-Leu, were most conveniently separated by chromatography on glass fibre papers impregnated with silica gel (SG-Gelman) developed with n-BuOH:NH_3:H_2O (120:7:7, v/v) giving R_F values of 0.7 (His-Leu), 0.45 (Ang. I) and 0.25 (Ang. II). The papers were dried and cut into strips and radioactivity was measured by scintillation counting. The amount of conversion was calculated from the radioactivity travelling with marker His-Leu. Only the area of the chromatogram corresponding to the marker Ang. II showed activity on the rabbit aorta and the amount of conversion measured as Ang. II produced (on the aorta) correlated well with that measured as labelled His-Leu formed. They were able to identify the products of acid hydrolysis of the His-Leu-like material as histidine and leucine only.

A crucial requirement in this type of assay is the ability to separate labelled Leu from the other two radioactive species. Leucine could be liberated by carboxypeptidases from Ang. I giving a nonapeptide which is not a substrate for CE and which is only slowly hydrolyzed to Ang. II (LENTZ et al., 1956) by carboxypeptidase itself. Leucine could also be formed by dipeptidase attack on the His-Leu produced by CE. In either circumstance, overlap of ^{14}C-Leu with either radioactive His-Leu or Ang. I would lead to false estimates of CE activity. HUGGINS and THAMPI (1968) did not mention the R_F of Leu in their chromatographic system, so we cannot judge how well their method fulfils this requirement, although they did state that there was no carboxypeptidase activity in their CE preparation.

Another radioactive form of Ang. I, [^{3}H-Leu^{10}]-Ang. I, is commercially available and was used by OPARIL et al. (1970). They were able to separate Leu, His-Leu and Ang. I by electrophoresis (2000 volts, 3 h) in pyridine-acetate buffer (at pH 3.5) on Whatman 3 MM paper. The products of incubating [^{3}H]-Ang. I with their CE preparations were subjected to electrophoresis and identified by comparison with markers of [^{3}H]-Ang. I, His-Leu and Leu. The paper was dried, cut into strips and the radioactivity measured by scintillation counting. They do not quote values for the mobilities in their system, but from their diagrams Leu moves about 5 cm, angiotensin 15 cm and His-Leu 24 cm from the origin, with good resolution between radioactive peaks. When these authors needed to handle larger numbers of samples they preferred columns of ion-exchange resins for the separation. All the peptides from an incubation mixture were absorbed on Dowex 50-X2 (H^+) at acid pH, then eluted with 0.2 N NH_4OH and 0.1 N diethylamine. Half this sample was chromatographed on SE-Sephadex G-25 columns to separate Ang. I from Leu and His-Leu, and the other half chromatographed on the short column of an amino-acid analyzer to separate Leu from His-Leu. The materials from this column chromatography were subjected to electrophoresis as before, as a check, and there was good correlation between the two separation procedures.

Their column-chromatographic procedure was found to be more rapid than their electrophoretic method, and may thus be expected to take less than 3 h. Although they do not say so, the efficiency of radioactive counting is probably greater with aqueous solutions of isotope as obtained from the column chromatography than with isotope absorbed on paper.

The electrophoretic separation of Ang. I, His-Leu and Leu has, however, been used to handle large numbers of samples arising from the chromatographic separation of CE on Sephadex columns. LEE et al. [1971 (1—4)] used [^{14}C-Leu^{10}]-Ang. I as substrate and separated labelled His-Leu from substrate by electrophoresis in pyridine-acetate buffer at pH 3.6 (2500 volts, 30 to 60 min). These authors were monitoring the purification of plasma and lung CE. FITZ and OVERTURF [1972 (1)] used [^{3}H-Leu^{10}]-Ang. I with the electrophoretic separation method of OPARIL et al. (1970), to follow CE extracted from human lung during its chromatography on Sephadex columns.

A different radiometric assay for CE has been developed by OSBORN et al. [1970 (2)]. These authors have synthesized Ang. I and Ang. II labelled at Asp^{1} by allowing the natural peptides to react with ^{35}S-phenylisothiocyanate to give the ^{35}S-phenylthiocarbamyl derivatives, [PTC]-Ang. I and [PTC]-Ang. II [1966, 1970 (1)]. On paper chromatography (developed with *sec*-BuOH: 30% ammonia-100:44, v/v), the R_F values are 0.85 (PTC-Ang. I) and 0.79 (PTC-Ang. II) but resolution is not complete [OSBORN et al., 1970 (2)] and the measurement of the amount of conversion of PTC-Ang. I to PTC-Ang. II is consequently less precise that it is in methods where substrate and product may be completely separated. Although the biological activity of the PTC derivatives parallels that of the natural peptides at a quarter of their potency (OSBORN et al., 1966), it is not yet known whether CE accepts [PTC]-Ang. I as though it were the natural substrate or as an alternative substrate like those to be discussed later.

Another method of separating His-Leu from substrate Ang. I, which may be the most convenient method described so far, is to filter the reaction mixture through a Diaflo membrane that retains molecules with molecular weights greater than 550 (PEACH, 1971; PEACH et al., 1971). Ang. I and Ang. II are retained while His-Leu (and presumably Leu) pass through the filter. When [^{14}C]-Ang. I in Locke's solution is filtered ,only 10% of the original radioactivity appears in the filtrate, but when [^{14}C]-Ang. I. that has been incubated with cat plasma is filtered, 90% of the radioactivity appears in the filtrate. There was no further identification of the radioactivity in the filtrate which could be any Leu-containing peptide up to a molecular weight of 550. Although this method was not adequate to differentiate between CE and carboxypeptidase activity, it deserves to be investigated further because of the simplicity of the separation procedure.

There are only two photometric assays for CE using Ang. I as substrate, the fluorimetric method developed by PIQUILLOUD et al. (1970) and the ninhydrin method used by DORER et al. (1970). PIQUILLOUD et al. modified an existing method (GREGERMANN, 1967) for measuring histidine in which it is allowed to react with *o*-phthaldialdehyde in the presence of alkali after which the fluorescence of the resulting adduct in acid solution is measured. They carried out most of their experiments with two synthetic substrates, Z-Pro-Phe-His-Leu or Z-Phe-His-Leu, which will be discussed later. This fluorimetric assay has been used more recently by BOUCHER et al. (1972), who found a good correlation between fluorimetric and biological assays of CE activity only when Ang. I was used as substrate for both assays. When they used one of the synthetic peptides used by PIQUILLOUD et al., Z-Phe-His-Leu, in the fluorimetric assay, the correlation between bioassay and fluorimetric assays was "not as expected". The authors did not say whether the synthetic substrate gave higher or lower values than the natural substrate. Ang. I, Ang. II and leucine do not give rise to fluorescence under the conditions employed, and the contribution to the total fluorescence due to the adduct with histidine is negligible. The sensitivity of this method, in which the production of 10 nmoles His-Leu and thus of 10 nmoles, (approx. 10 μg) Ang. II is easily detectable, is comparable to that of the ninhydrin method used by DORER et al. (1970) in their purification of pig plasma CE (see Table 1).

The latter authors allow the incubation mixture to react with ninhydrin, without separating the peptides, and measure the total optical density, to which Ang. I, Ang. II, His-Leu, His and Leu will all contribute. As a control, they incubate the same mixture in the absence of chloride ion, and again measure the total ninhydrin colour. The difference in optical density between these values (chloride-chloride free) is a measure of the peptides produced in the presence of chloride ion, and assuming that the only chloride-activated peptidase acting on Ang. I which produces His-Leu is CE, this difference can be converted with a calibration curve for standard His-Leu to units of CE activity. A further essential control was to show that His-Leu itself was not split by the enzyme preparation.

c) *Discussion*

All these assay methods using the natural substrate can be grouped into two other groups, those in which Ang. II is measured and those in which His-Leu is measured. There are several reasons why it is preferable to measure Ang. II. Since we are interested in CE primarily because of its role in a biological system, it is most relevant to measure the biologically important product. Even though the biological assays (blood pressure, smooth muscle contraction, and immunoreaction) will also measure two of the metabolites of Ang. II, the hepta- and hexa-peptides to some extent, they have the virtue of being *bio*assays. We cannot entirely discount the possible contribution of the hepta- and hexa-peptides to the overall biological effects of the renin-angiotensin system. Another reason for measuring Ang. II concentrations is that many degradation products of Ang. I would, on present evidence (see below), be substrates for CE. ARAKAWA et al. (1968) have shown that leucine aminopeptidase will cleave successive N-terminal residues from human Ang. I up to a limit tripeptide, Phe^{8}-His^{9}-Leu^{10}, trypsin will produce the octapeptide [des-Asp^{1}-Arg^{2}]-Ang. I and α-chymotrypsin the pentapeptide His^{6}-Pro^{7}-Phe^{8}-His^{9}-Leu^{10}. All these peptides, on treatment with CE, could liberate His-Leu but none would yield biologically active fragments of Ang. II. Thus the rate of His-Leu formation would be unrepresentative of the rate of Ang. II formation, and the presence of amino- or endopeptidases in extracts with CE activity could significantly depress the amount of biological activity produced without necessarily affecting the amount of His-Leu produced.

Bioassay of Ang. II allows the measurement of low concentrations (100 pg/ml to 100 ng/ml, approximately 10^{-10} M to 10^{-7} M), which are close to the normal and pathological concentrations of Ang. II found in plasma. In rat lung, Ang. I, in amounts exceeding 25 μg, is hydrolyzed mainly by a carboxypeptidase and not by CE (BARRETT and SAMBHI, 1971). If this phenomenon is found to be generally applicable, investigations of CE activity must be carried out with substrate levels nearest to those existing *in vivo*.

The chemical assay in which Ang. II is measured by a radiometric method using ^{35}S PTC-Ang. [OSBORN et al., 1970 (2)] has a crucial disadvantage in that the chromatographic system used separates the substrate (PTC-Ang. I) only partially from product (PTC-Ang. II). Moreover the PTC-angiotensins are not substrates for aminopeptidases (OSBORN et al., 1966) so that there will be no inactivation of PTC-Ang. II in extracts containing both CE and aminopeptidases and the CE activity measured will be correspondingly higher.

The disadvantage of the biological assay methods is that they are not suitable for large numbers of samples such as would be produced, for instance, by column chromatography, and in none of the preparations of CE that have been purified has a bioassay or immunoassay been used to monitor the various purification steps.

The His-Leu concentrations must be measured by chemical or physical methods, and the advantage of these is that they are more capable of handling large numbers of samples with the minimum of labour. The photometric methods devised by DORER et al. (1970) and by PIQUILLOUD et al. (1970) are particularly valuable in monitoring column chromatography of CE, although the more cumbersome electrophoretic method using radioactive substrates had been used by LEE et al. [1971 (1—3)] and by FITZ and OVERTURF [1972 (1)] in their purification procedures. The main source of interference in the photometric assays is dipeptidase activity, liberating Leu from the His-Leu formed by CE. Thus His and Leu will appear only in the presence of chloride ion and this would cause either a reduction in activity, as measured by the fluorimetric method (PIQUILLOUD et al., 1970), or an increase in activity, as measured by the ninhydrin method of DORER et al. (1970). The amount of such dipeptidase activity must therefore be established using synthetic His-Leu as substrate.

In the radiometric assays again His-Leu is measured and again the presence of dipeptidases could lead to a falsely low estimation of CE activity. However, since in this assay Leu is separated from His-Leu and has a radioactive label, it can easily be measured separately and the amount of Leu due to carboxypeptidase activity, or to dipeptidase activity, or to both, may be estimated from the results of incubations carried out with and without chloride ion. The lack of separation of Leu from His-Leu and the absence of tests showing the level of carboxypeptidase activity are two serious disadvantages in the otherwise attractive radiometric method of PEACH (1971).

Measurements of the amount of labelled His-Leu produced by CE from Ang. I provide no information about angiotensinase attack on Ang. II as the tracer has been lost from the Ang. II produced and further hydrolysis of Ang. II can only be monitored by bioassay. An alternative is to use angiotensins radioactively-labelled in Phe^8 (RYAN et al., 1971) which allows a number of hydrolysis products to be followed.

This insensitivity to contaminating angiotensinases is sometimes an advantage, allowing measurements of CE against a high background of angiotensinases in a crude tissue extract, as would be required if extracts of a number of tissues were scanned to find the richest source of CE preparatory to further purification.

2. Methods Using Short Substrates

a) Physicochemical Methods

None of the short substrates have significant biological activity and their hydrolysis must therefore be followed by a physicochemical assay. The short substrates are all short peptides, some designed as analogues of the carboxyterminal of Ang. I e.g. Hippuryl-His-Leu (HHL), [CUSHMAN and CHEUNG, 1971 (1)], Z-Pro-Phe-His-Leu and Z-Phe-His-Leu (PIQUILLOUD et al., 1970). ERDOS and his colleagues (YANG et al., 1971; IGIC et al., 1972) have synthesized a number of short substrates, many of which have little structural analogy with Ang. I, to estimate "dipeptide hydrolase" which also converts Ang. I to Ang. II.

The method of PIQUILLOUD et al. (1970) has already been referred to in the previous section and depends on the fluorimetric estimation of His-Leu released from the substrates Z-Pro-Phe-His-Leu and Z-Phe-His-Leu. They favour the use of the tripeptide Z-Phe-His-Leu as it is hydrolyzed about ten times faster than either Ang. I or the tetrapeptide by the CE activity in human or horse plasma. A similar situation was reported by CUSHMAN and CHEUNG [1971 (1)], in that their short substrate HHL is hydrolyzed far faster then Ang. I by their preparation of CE from rabbit lungs. In their assay, the hippuric acid released is estimated by its UV absorption at 228 nm, after separation from product and unreacted substrate by extraction into ethyl acetate. Endopeptidases and aminopeptidases do not hydrolyze HHL and in their preparation of CE, there was no carboxypeptidase activity, although this may not be the case in other preparations.

Of the numerous short peptides used by ERDÖS and his colleagues, the substrate which is perhaps most versatile and convenient is ^{14}C-Dansyl-Gly-Gly-Gly which is hydrolyzed to DNS-Gly and Gly-Gly (IGIC et al., 1972). The product and unreacted substrate may be separated by thin-layer chromatography, detected by the fluorescence of the dansyl group, and measured in terms of the radioactivity. Carboxypeptidase activity would form DNS-Gly-Gly and since all three dansyl peptides are well separated, the presence of such activity would be easily detected. However, we do not know if the hydrolysis of this substrate is chloride-dependent. The hydrolysis of another substrate, *t*-BOC-Phe(NO_2)-Phe-Gly (BPPG) by "dipeptide hydrolase" an enzyme described by YANG et al. (1971), is chloride-dependent and this substrate could therefore serve as a substrate for CE estimation. The basis of the assay is an increase in UV absorption at 310 nm as the terminal dipeptide is released from BPPG. The method is described only briefly, so possible interference by other products of the substrate cannot be adequately assessed.

b) Discussion

These assays are well suited to handle large numbers of samples and have been used by each group to follow the purification of enzyme activity during extensive purification procedures. The short substrates are not attacked by angiotensinases, either endo- or aminopeptidases, so that CE activity may be measured accurately in the less purified extracts as well. These substrates are more easily synthesized and more stable than the natural substrate. Nevertheless all these advantages may be negated as the parameters measured with a short substrate will not necessarily correlate with those obtained using a natural substrate. Several examples of this discrepancy have already been reported.

The order of potency of three peptide inhibitors of CE obtained from an assay using Ang. I differs from that obtained when HHL is used as the substrate (BAKHLE, 1971; CUSHMAN and CHEUNG, 1972). BOUCHER et al. (1972) found that correlation between their bioassay method and the fluorimetric method of PIQUILLOUD et al. (1970) was adequate only when Ang. I was the substrate in the fluorimetric assay and not when the short substrate was used. Furthermore, the same authors described an enzyme catalyzing the conversion of Ang. I to Ang. II which did not hydrolyze the short substrate Z-Phe-His-Leu. Thus this CE activity, which might be physiologically significant, was missed when the short substrate HHL was used [CUSHMAN and CHEUNG ,1971 (2)]. Recently CUSHMAN and CHEUNG (1972) have prepared CE from rabbit lung and followed the purification with the HHL assay, checking each stage with a fluorimetric assay using Ang. I as substrate. This enzyme has different pH optima, different optimal concentrations of chloride ion and different Km and Vmax values for the two substrates. If further examples of this discrepancy are found it will cast serious doubts on the relevance of results obtained with only the short substrates to the behaviour of the enzyme with the natural substrate and *in vivo.*

3. Summary of Assay Methods

When all these methods for measuring CE activity are considered, the final choice may depend as much on the facilities available as on any definite scientific advantage. Thus the bioassays require ready access to animals, not always easy in biochemistry departments, and the electrophoretic methods require access to a high voltage electrophoresis apparatus, which may be a problem in physiology and pharmacology departments. Whichever method is used there are good reasons, outlined above, for using Ang. I as the substrate in preference to the artifical substrates. Radiometric assay has been used to follow purification procedures but it is less convenient than the photometric assays, although the sensitivity of the radiometric method is higher than that of the fluorimetric assays and close to that of bioassay. For this reason, a combination of bioassay of Ang. II produced and fluorimetric assay of the His-Leu produced (PIQUILLOUD et al., 1970) would seem to be the best method of measuring CE activity. The bioassay facilitates measurement of the angiotensinase content of the preparation and the fluorimetric assay is capable of handling the large number of samples involved in monitoring the purification procedures.

Sources of Converting Enzyme

CE-activity is present in many tissues from a variety of animals. Three groups of workers, each using a different assay, have surveyed the CE content of several rat tissues [HUGGINS and THAMPI, 1968; ROTH et al., 1969; CUSHMAN and CHEUNG, 1971 (2)]. CUSHMAN and CHEUNG (1972) have compared the CE content of a selection of tissues from 5 species of common laboratory animals and DEPIERRE and ROTH (1972) have measured CE in the lungs of eleven species. Table 2 lists the sources of CE with selected references. The criterion for inclusion in the table is that some properties of the enzyme extracted from that tissue have been measured and not merely that its presence has been demonstrated. Furthermore, where there are several references to the same work, often as abstracts, preliminary papers, etc., only the reference with the fullest details is quoted, unless there are significant differences in the results.

1. Blood

There is CE in the blood of animals and man and the first studies on CE were carried out with a preparation derived from horse plasma (SKEGGS et al., 1954). The plasma enzyme has been the most frequently studied perhaps because of the ready supply of blood and because it is easier to purify an initially soluble enzyme. Thus three purifications of pig plasma CE [DORER et al., 1970; YANG et al., 1971; LEE et al., 1971 (1)] and two of human plasma CE [PIQUILLOUD et al., 1970; LEE et al., 1971 (2)] have been described. The preparation of rabbit plasma CE reported by UEDA et al. (1970) has two important differences from other preparations. Firstly, CE was not separated from dipeptidase activity in spite of a sixty three-fold purification and secondly, the enzyme was inhibited by 10^{-3} M DFP. In their paper (UEDA et al., 1971) on this enzyme there is no mention of the DFP effect, and the degree of dipeptidase contamination is very small — 70 nmoles hydrolyzed out of 1 mole added, over 20 h incubation.

Table 2. *Sources of converting enzyme activity*

Animal	Tissue: Blood, plasma or serum	Lung	Kidney
Mouse	POULSEN and BING, 1970		
Rat	ANDERSEN, 1967 BOUCHER et al., 1972 POULSEN and BING, 1970 LOYKE, 1964; 1968; 1970	BOUCHER et al., 1972	GRANGER et al., 1971
Guinea pig	YANG et al., 1971 LEE et al., 1971 (3)	LEE et al., 1971 (3)	
Rabbit	UEDA et al., 1970; 1971	SANDER and HUGGINS, 1971 CUSHMAN and CHEUNG, 1971 (1); 1972	
Pig	DORER et al., 1970 HUGGINS et al., 1970 LEE et al., 1971 (2) YANG et al., 1971	LEE et al., 1971 (3) YANG et al., 1971 IGIC et al., 1972	
Dog	OPARIL et al., 1970; 1971	BAKHLE, 1968 BAKHLE and REYNARD, 1971 HUGGINS et al., 1970	
Horse	SKEGGS et al., 1956 PIQUILLOUD et al., 1970 HUGGINS et al., 1970		
Man	BOUCHER et al., 1970 FITZ et al., 1971 LEE et al., 1971 (1) PIQUILLOUD et al., 1970 POULSEN and POULSEN, 1971	FITZ and OVERTURF, 1970; 1972 (1)	
Ox			ELISSEEVA et al., 1971

2. Lung

The physiological importance of plasma CE was challenged by the high level of CE activity exhibited *in vivo* by the pulmonary circulation (NG and VANE, 1967; BIRON, 1968; OPARIL et al., 1970). This concentration of activity in lung was confirmed by all the surveys of CE *in vitro* from rat tissues [HUGGINS and THAMPI, 1968; ROTH et al., 1969; CUSHMAN and CHEUNG, 1971 (2)] and was also shown to be true for 4 other species of laboratory animals (CUSHMAN and CHEUNG, 1972). In homogenates of lung, CE is both soluble and particulate. The particulate form may be readily "solubilized", (IGIC et al., 1972) though this "solubilized" CE has a different sedimentation velocity from that of the CE already in the supernatant [LEE et al., 1971 (3)]. A highly purified CE has been prepared from acetone powders of rabbit lung (CUSHMAN and CHEUNG, 1972). Two other purified preparations from pig (IGIC et al., 1972) and human lung [FITZ and OVERTURF, 1972 (1)] may not fulfil all the criteria for CE activity.

The type of pulmonary cell that contains CE is not known nor are all the subcellular localizations of the enzyme clearly established, although it seems that CE is associated with the plasma membranes, probably of the vascular endothelial cells. This hypothesis was advanced when the CE activity of dog lung was found to be concentrated in a light particulate fraction (BAKHLE, 1968) and more refined studies on rabbit lung (SANDER and HUGGINS, 1971) have confirmed that CE is concentrated in a particulate fraction with enzymic activities and morphology compatible with plasma membranes. In describing a plasma-membrane fraction from rat lung, RYAN and SMITH (1971) mention that it has CE activity (0.1 nmole/min/mg protein) and will hydrolyze bradykinin. Thus it is clear that some CE activity is associated with cell membranes but what proportion of the total CE activity is membrane-bound seems to vary from species to species. A recent survey of CE in the lungs of eleven species showed that the activity in the 107,000 g pellet was greater (2.5- to 30-fold) than that in the supernatant fraction, except in rat and mouse lung (DEPIERRE and ROTH, 1972). In these experiments CE was measured by the chloride-dependent hydrolysis of Z-Phe-His-Leu. The soluble CE obtained in homogenates may be an artefact of homogenization.

The involvement of the vascular endothelial cells was deduced from the rapidity of conversion *in vivo* or in perfused isolated lungs. In support of this, RYAN et al. (1971) found that isolated lungs perfused with radioactive Ang. I for 2 to 3 min retained less that 0.5% of the total radioactivity. Furthermore, since CE and bradykininase activity in the lung are closely linked (ALABASTER and BAKHLE, 1972; IGIC et al., 1972) and bradykinin is metabolized in the pulmonary circulation without leaving the vascular bed, then CE may be located in a cell type with similarly free access to the vascular perfusion fluid. The pinocytotic vesicles in the vascular endothelial cells of the lung described by SMITH and RYAN (1969) may also be important in pulmonary CE activity.

3. Other Tissues

The only tissues so far shown to contain more CE than the lung are testicular tissue of rat, guinea pig and rabbit (Table 3); human seminal plasma contains as much CE as rat lung [CUSHMAN and CHEUNG, 1971 (2); 1972; see also BOUCHER et al., 1972). The CE content of rat testicular tissue increases from the ages of 23 days to 40 to 50 days when full sexual maturation has taken place. The presence of CE in this tissue, which is not usually associated with the regulation of blood pressure or of electrolyte balance, gives rise to the suspicion that in this case, Ang. I is not its natural substrate. The involvement of this peptidase in reproductive processes is being investigated.

The three surveys of CE in rat tissues are in fair qualitative agreement (Table 4), all showing lung to be one of the richest sources, but whereas the results of ROTH et al. (1969) correspond quantitatively with those of CUSHMAN and CHEUNG [1971 (2)], HUGGINS and THAMPI (1968) found generally lower values in all the tissues they examined (allowing for the difference between grams wet weight and mg protein) and less difference between lung and the other tissues. This discrepancy may be due to the initial homogenization of the tissues in 10^{-3} M EDTA, a procedure used by the last authors, which could have inactivated much of the CE present. Another contributing factor to the low levels of activity reported by HUGGINS and THAMPI (1968) is their use of Ang. I as substrate whereas ROTH et al. (1969) and CUSHMAN and CHEUNG [1971 (2)] used short substrates which are both hydrolyzed faster than Ang. I by CE.

CE has also been reported in the juxtaglomerular apparatus of rat kidney (GRANGER et al., 1971) and in rat (HORKY et al., 1971) and dog (BAILIE et al., 1971) lymph, and CE activity is one of the properties of a peptidase ("carboxycathepsin") isolated from bovine kidney (ELISSEEVA et al., 1971). A peptidase from porcine kidney cortex ("kininase II") (ERDÖS and YANG, 1967) is identical to the "dipeptide hydrolase" purified from porcine plasma (YANG et al., 1971) and lung (IGIC et al., 1972).

Table 3. *Converting enzyme activity in tissues from five species (from* Cushman *and* Cheung, *1972)*

Animal	Specific activity of converting enzyme (milliunits/mg protein)[a]			
	Lung	Testis	Kidney	Serum
Dog	10.5	8.5	2.5	0.3
Cat	14.5	6.5	5.1	0.3
Rabbit	20.5	39.5	33.0	0.9
Guinea pig	23.5	55.0	3.2	15.5
Rat	48.0	85.0	0.6	1.6

[a] One unit of enzyme activity catalyzes the formation of 1 μmole of hippuric acid per minute from Hippuryl-His-Leu.

Table 4. *Converting enzyme in tissues of the rat*

The values from Huggins and Thampi are expressed as μmoles His-Leu produced/min/g wet weight of tissues, and those from the other two references as μmoles product/min/mg protein

Tissue	Substrate		
	Ang. I Huggins and Thampi (1968)	Z-Phe-His-Leu Roth et al. (1969)	HHL Cushman and Cheung [1971(2)][a]
Serum or plasma	3.7	1.03	1.6
Heart	6.8	0.15	0.5
Brain	3.7	1.47	1.5
Liver	10.4	0.23	<0.2
Diaphragm	13.8	0.71[b]	0.3
Kidney	5.9	0.63	0.6
Lung	12.5	37.0	48.0
Ileum	13.5	4.67	3.3
Aorta	0	—	2.9
Uterus	0.3	—	2.2[c]

[a] Cushman and Cheung have also assayed several other rat tissues for CE, see their paper for the full table.

[b] Roth et al's value here refers to muscle (probably striated) and not specifically to diaphragm.

[c] This value may include some atypical converting enzyme activity (vid. infra).

Although there is some correlation between the CE activity shown by a tissue or its vascular bed *in vivo* and that shown in homogenates of the tissue in some cases, the absolute or relative amounts of CE in tissue homogenates should not be assumed to reflect the CE content of those tissues *in vivo*. The relation between *in vivo* and *in vitro* CE is dealt with elsewhere in this volume (Vane, 1972).

Methods of Preparation

1. Blood

CE in blood has been studied in many states of purity. Ng and Vane (1967), Oparil et al. (1970) and Osborn et al. [1970 (1)] used whole blood, though the

Table 5. *Purification of converting enzyme*

Tissue	Animal (reference)	Steps in purification	Purification (fold)	Yield %	Specific activity milliunits/mg protein[a]
Plasma	Pig [2]	i $(NH_4)_2SO_4$ ii CM-cellulose iii Alumina gel	74	25	8.5
	Pig [10]	i $(NH_4)_2SO_4$ ii DEAE-Sephadex iii Sephadex G-200	200	20	200 (with HGG)[b]
	Pig [7]	i $(NH_4)_2SO_4$ ii Sephadex G-200 iii DEAE-cellulose	165	14	50
	Man [6]	i $(NH_4)_2SO_4$ ii Sephadex G-200	67	70	6
	Rabbit [9]	i $(NH_4)_2SO_4$ ii DEAE Sephadex iii Sephadex G-200	63	9.3	0.143
	Guinea pig [8]	i $(NH_4)_2SO_4$ ii Sephadex G-200 iii DEAE cellulose			15.6
Lung	Pig [8]	i 80,000 g supernatant ii $(NH_4)_2SO_4$ iii Sephadex G-200			3.8
	Guinea pig [8]	i 80,000 g supernatant ii $(NH_4)_2SO_4$ iii Sephadex G-200	230	117[c]	10.5
	Rabbit [1] [8]	i Acetone powder ii "$CaPO_4$" gel iii DEAE-cellulose iv Biogel-P300	285	25	1,200
	Pig [5]	i 105,000 g supernatant ii Sephadex G-200 iii DEAE-Sephadex iv Biogel-P300			28,000 (with HGG)[b]
	Man [4]	i Homogenate supernatant ii $(NH_4)_2SO_4$ iii Sephadex G-200			
Kidney	Ox [3]	i Homogenate supernatant ii $(NH_4)_2SO_4$ iii Sephadex G-75, 200 iv DEAE-cellulose	1,500		

[a] One unit of activity catalyzes the formation of 1 μmole product/min from Ang. I as substrate, unless otherwise stated.

[b] HGG = Hippuryl-Gly-Gly.

[c] Yield exceeds 100% as there are enzymes interfering with the CE assay, in the crude homogenate.

References

1. CUSHMAN and CHEUNG (1972); 2. DORER et al. (1970); 3. ELISSEEVA et al. (1971); 4. FITZ and OVERTURF [1972 (1)]; 5. IGIC et al. (1972); 6. LEE et al. [1971 (1)]; 7. LEE et al. [1971 (2)]; 8. LEE et al. [1971 (3)]; 9. UEDA et al. (1971); 10. YANG et al. (1971).

majority of workers have at least prepared plasma or serum from blood. Untreated (apart from anticoagulants other than EDTA) plasma has been used to measure the net conversion of Ang. I (ANDERSEN, 1967; OPARIL et al., 1970; FITZ et al., 1971; PEACH, 1971) with allowance for the angiotensinase activity, although the absolute rates of Ang. II formation may be calculated in untreated plasma under certain circumstances (POULSEN and POULSEN, 1971). The next stage of purification is generally the removal of angiotensinase activity by the transient acidification (pH 3.5 to 4, room temperature, 25 min) of plasma (SKEGGS et al., 1954; HELMER, 1957; LOYKE, 1964; POULSEN and BING, 1970). It should now be possible to measure how much CE activity is also lost by this step. Further stages of purification require ammonium sulphate fractionation and subsequent chromatographic procedures, although PIQUILLOUD et al. (1970) produced, from human plasma, CE of reasonably high activity by a single passage through a column of Sephadex G-200.

The preparation and purity data of more highly purified CE are outlined in Table 5. It is of particular interest that LEE et al. include dialysis against 5 mM EDTA in their procedure [1971, (1, 2)] and still retain CE activity, the purified enzyme being inhibited by 0.5 mM EDTA. DORER et al. (1970) and LEE et al. [1971 (2)] have used the same source, porcine plasma, and the same substrate, Ang. I, and thus the activity may be directly compared. CE activity purified by YANG et al. (1971) from porcine plasma was assayed with a short substrate (Hippuryl-Gly-Gly, HGG). Assuming a 1:20 ratio between the hydrolysis rates of Ang. I and HGG, (see CUSHMAN and CHEUNG, 1972), the purified enzyme would have a specific activity of about 1.4 units/mg protein with Ang. I as substrate.

2. Lung

A similar progression in purity is seen with the preparation of CE from lung. HOLLEMANS et al. (1969) homogenized lungs for 20 min, allowing the temperature to rise to 60°, centrifuged the suspension and used the supernatant as a source of CE. This somewhat vigorous homogenization inactivated angiotensinases present in homogenates of lung prepared at lower temperatures, although they did not measure the specific activity of CE in the extracts. The next state of purification is represented by the preparations of BAKHLE (1968) and BAKHLE and REYNARD (1971) in which low temperature homogenization was followed by differential centrifugation to concentrate CE in the high speed pellet, and angiotensinases in the final supernatant. Vmax values were not reported; however, 20 to 25% conversion of Ang. I was obtained with a substrate range of 2 to 100 μg of Ang. I/ml, using the CE derived from the high-speed pellet. SANDER and HUGGINS (1971) elaborated the procedure further by homogenizing rabbit lung in isotonic sucrose in the presence of Mg ions, following this by differential centrifugation to concentrate CE in the 25,000 × g pellet and further centrifugation of this pellet on a discontinuous density gradient to give a material capable of forming 2.5 μg Ang. II/min/mg protein (equivalent to about 2.5 nmoles/min/mg). Another preparation of CE, from canine lungs by HUGGINS et al. (1970), involved ammonium sulphate fractionation of lung homogenates to yield a preparation "almost free of angiotensinase", capable of converting 6.7 nmoles of Ang. I to Ang. II/min/mg protein. It is not clear whether the human-lung CE purified by FITZ and OVERTURF [1972 (1)] is a particulate or a soluble enzyme. They derived their enzyme from lung homogenates by ammonium sulphate fractionation followed by chromatography on Sephadex G-200. It was free from angiotensinase and dipeptidase activity. However this CE is not inhibited by EDTA and does not therefore fulfil all the criteria for CE activity.

The more highly purified preparations described in the literature are two from porcine lung [LEE et al., 1971 (3); IGIC et al., 1972], one from guinea-pig lung [LEE et al., 1971 (3)] and one from rabbit lung (CUSHMAN and CHEUNG, 1972). In all these preparations, CE was present in a soluble form and in three also in a particulate form which it was possible to solubilize [LEE et al., 1971 (3); IGIC et al., 1972). IGIC et al. found the solubilized enzyme had the same relative activities towards a series of substrates as did the soluble enzyme. LEE et al. [1971 (3)], however, found the solubilized enzyme had a different sedimentation velocity from the soluble enzyme.

A high degree of purification is possible with chromatographic procedures and the final product obtained from rabbit lung by CUSHMAN and CHEUNG (1972) consists of a single component (disc-gel electrophoresis) and represents a 285-fold purification over the starting material. A similar degree of purification is reported by LEE et al. [1971 (3)] for guinea-pig lung CE, though no values are quoted for their porcine lung enzyme, perhaps because the crude porcine lung homogenate contained too much His-Leu hydrolyzing activity for the authors' assay method. LEE et al. [1971 (3)] concentrated activity in a high speed supernatant by differential centrifugation before starting chromatographic procedures, and the same approach is used by IGIC et al. (1972) in their preparation of CE from pig lung ("dipeptide hydrolase"). The porcine lung enzyme showed four bands on gel electrophoresis but the CE activity was concentrated in only one band. When the material in this band was resubjected to gel electrophoresis it moved as a single component. The best preparations of IGIC et al. had a specific activity of 28 units/mg with HGG as substrate. This value is equivalent to about 1.4 units/mg with Ang. I as substrate, assuming the 1:20 ratio between Ang. I and HGG reaction rates as before.

The lung enzyme obtained by IGIC et al. (1972) in a partially purified form was coupled to Sepharose 4B and the enzyme-Sepharose complex was shown to hydrolyze bradykinin and convert Ang. I to Ang. II. The efficiency of the coupling procedure or the activity of the coupled enzyme relative to that of the free enzyme has not been reported. It would be particularly interesting to measure kinetic and substrate parameters for the coupled enzyme.

Properties of Converting Enzymes

1. Molecular Weight

LEE et al. [1971 (1, 2, 3)] have estimated the MW of CE from porcine and human plasma and porcine and guinea-pig lung. The molecular weights of the plasma converting enzymes [LEE et al., 1971 (1, 2)] were derived from their sedimentation velocity in sucrose gradients with catalase, cytochrome C and *E. coli* alkaline phosphatase. In the later paper [LEE et al., 1971 (3)], this method and gel filtration on Sephadex G-150 were used with the same three standard proteins as markers, and gave the same values. All four samples of CE have a MW of about 150,000 daltons. It is noticeable that the MW does not change with the degree of purification from 63-fold (human plasma) to 230-fold (guinea-pig lung).

FITZ and OVERTURF [1972 (1)] used gel filtration on Sephadex G-200 with apo-ferritin, γ-globulin, ovalbumin and chymotrypsinogen as marker proteins to estimate the MW of CE from human lung as 480,000 daltons. However this is the same as the MW of apo-ferritin and represents the high MW end of the range of markers used. Only 75% of the CE activity elutes at this volume, immediately after the void volume of the column, and about 25% elutes later at a volume corresponding to a MW of around 175,000. It is thus possible that the molecular weights of the guinea pig- and the porcine-lung CE and the human lung CE are comparable for the monomer and the 480,000-dalton material represents a polymeric species of CE. However, as the human-lung CE is atypical in its resistance to inhibition by EDTA, it is perhaps not to be expected that it will correspond with the other typical forms of CE in other respects.

2. Temperature and pH Stability

There are three reports on the temperature stability of CE activity, each from a different organ and species. HOLLEMANS et al. (1969) found that CE activity from human lung survived a temperature of 60° while the angiotensinases present in the extract were inactivated. They did not determine whether the CE activity was reduced by this procedure. The "carboxycathepsin" from bovine kidney is more thermolabile, losing 80 to 90% of its activity (towards Hip-Phe-Pro) within 5 min at 60°, whereas at 50° inactivation takes 80 min (OREKHOVICH, 1968). CE from rabbit plasma is stable at 56° for 30 min, partially inactivated at 60° for 30 min and totally inactivated after 30 min at 65° [UEDA et al., 1971 (1)]. From these two latter examples it would seem likely that HOLLEMANS et al. did inactivate a significant proportion of the CE originally present in their lung extract.

Only UEDA et al. [1971 (1)] and OREKHOVICH (1968) have reported on the pH-stability of CE activity. The former authors find their rabbit-plasma enzyme fully active after 2 h at pH 5.5, 6.5 or 7.5 but partially inactivated after 2 h at pH 4.5 or 8.5. "Carboxycathepsin" is described as having maximum stability over the pH range 6.0 to 8.0. These results suggest that the transient-acidification method of inactivating angiotensinases (BRAUN-MENENDEZ et al., 1946), in which the pH is brought down to about 4 for 30 min and then restored to about 7, which has been frequently used (SKEGGS et al., 1954; HELMER, 1957; LOYKE, 1970; POULSEN and BING, 1970) will also inactivate a small proportion of the CE activity present.

3. pH-Dependence of Activity

There is general agreement that CE has maximal activity between pH 6.5 and 8, with most estimates of the pH optimum falling between pH 7 and 8 (see Table 6). ELISSEEVA et al. (1971) also describe their "carboxycathepsin" as a neutral peptidase but have not determined the pH optimum with Ang. I as substrate, and the same reservation must be applied to the values given by YANG et al. (1971), who used a tripeptide chromogenic substrate (BPPG). The reason for this reservation is that the pH optimum for Ang. I differs from that of shorter substrates by up to 1 pH unit in the two cases examined [PIQUILLOUD et al., 1970; CUSHMAN and CHEUNG, 1971 (1)] and it may differ in all cases.

There are only two reports of the pH optimum varying with the buffer, SKEGGS et al. (1954) reporting a value of pH 6.5 in phosphate and 8.0 in tris buffers, and YANG et al. (1971) reporting 7.7 in phosphate and 7.4 in tris. These latter authors also find that the rate of BPPG hydrolysis was 60% lower in phosphate buffers than in tris. There are no other reports of the inhibitory effects of phosphate on CE activity.

4. Substrate Specificity

It is clear that CE will cleave a wide variety of peptides by removing dipeptide fragments starting from the C-terminal. One consequence of this mode of hydrolysis is that the undecapeptide Ang. II-His-His-Leu is not hydrolyzed to Ang. II by CE *in vivo* (NG and VANE, 1970). Similarly the nonapeptide, [des Leu[10]]-Ang. I,

Table 6. *Properties of converting enzyme prepared from different sources*

Tissue	Animal	pH Optimum (buffer)	Substrate	Km.	(Cl^-) max.	Activity ratio without Cl/with Cl	References
Plasma	Guinea pig		Ang. I	0.048 mM		*	[9]
	Horse	6.5 (phosphate)	Ang. I			*	[13]
		8.0 (tris)					
		7.25 (phosphate)	Ang. I	0.048 mM	17 mM	*	[6]
	Man	7.5 (barbital-Na/acetate)	Ang. I				[5]
	Man	7.2—7.8 (phosphate)	Ang. I	0.04 mM		*	[7]
		7.5	Ang. I			*	[10]
	Man	7.5—8.5	Z-Pro-Phe-His-Leu .	0.06, 0.04 mM		1/100	[10]
			Z-Phe-His-Leu .				[10]
	Pig	7.8 (phosphate)	Ang. I		100 mM	5/90	[4]
	Pig	7.4 (tris)	BPPG[a]			*	[14]
	Pig	7.2—7.8 (phosphate)	Ang. I	0.04 mM		*	[8]
	Rat	7—8 (borax-phosphate)	Ang. I			*	[2]
Lung	Dog	7.25 (phosphate)	Ang. I	0.0052 mM		3.5/8.2	[6]
	Dog	7.0 (phosphate)	Ang. I		170 mM	2/100	[1]
	Guinea pig	7.2—7.8	Ang. I	0.02 mM		*	[9]
	Pig	7.2—7.8	Ang. I	0.026 mM		*	[9]
	Rabbit					0/2.9	[12]
	Rabbit	7.5	Ang. I	0.05 mM	30 mM	1/100	[3]
		8.3 (phosphate)	Hip-His-Leu	2.1 mM	300 mM	1/7.5	[3]
Kidney	Ox	7.0—7.3	Hip-Phe-Pro			*	[11]

* Denotes that dependence on chloride ions has been demonstrated.

[a] BPPG = *t*-BOC-Phe(NO_2)-Phe-Gly.

References

1. Bakhle and Reynard (1971); 2. Boucher et al. (1972); 3. Cushman and Cheung (1972); 4. Dorer et al. (1970); 5. Fitz et al. (1971); 6. Huggins et al. (1971); 7. Lee et al. [1971 (1)]; 8. Lee et al. [1971 (2)]; 9. Lee et al. [1971 (3)]; 10. Piquilloud et al. (1970); 11. Orekhovich (1968); 12. Sander et al. (1971); 13. Skeggs et al. (1954); 14. Yang et al. (1971).

in vivo (LENTZ et al., 1956) or *in vitro* (OPARIL et al., 1971) does not produce Ang. II. Presumably a dodecapeptide could give rise to Ang. II in two stages and the tetradecapeptide renin substrate, Ang. II-Leu-Val-Tyr-Ser, gives a slight pressor response on injection in rats (SKEGGS et al., 1969). There are some limitations on possible substrates. The C-terminal residue must be present as the free carboxylic acid, because amides or esters are not substrates *in vivo* (SCHWYZER, 1961) or *in vitro*, and this terminal aminoacid must be of the L-configuration (OPARIL et al., 1971). [D-Phe^8]-Ang. I (GUTTMANN, 1961) may be a substrate for CE. Although this peptide is inactive (i.e. non-pressor) *in vivo*, so is [D-Phe^8]-Ang. II itself and an assay for any His-Leu liberated would be necessary to settle this point. A further limitation at the C-terminal is that although positively-charged amino acids e.g. Arg, are acceptable (thus bradykinin may be, and in most cases, is a substrate for CE), the presence of an acidic C-terminal e.g. Glu, makes the peptide resistant to attack by CE (OREKHOVICH, 1968).

Peptide bonds involving the imino group of proline are not hydrolyzed. Thus R_1-Pro^{7}Phe-OH would not be hydrolyzed but R_1-Phe-Pro-OH would be a substrate. Thus Ang. II is the limit peptide produced by CE from Ang. I as the next dipeptide that could be removed from Ang. II would require cleavage of the His--Pro- bond in which the imino group of proline is involved. For the same reason, [Pro^9-Phe^{10}]-Ang. I is non-pressor *in vivo* (SCHWYZER and TURRIAN, 1960). There is a lower limit to the size of peptide substrate, although at present no upper limit has been described. Thus dipeptides, either with blocked N-terminals e.g. Z-Phe-Pro, Hippuryl-Phe (OREKHOVICH, 1968) or with free N-terminals, e.g. His-Leu, are not substrates, but tripeptides and higher peptides of suitable structure are substrates. Apart from these major limitations, CE will hydrolyze a variety of peptides ranging from Hippuryl-Gly-Gly (HGG) to the B-chain of insulin (IGIC et al., 1972).

One group of peptides that have not yet been examined as possible substrates are those derived from Ang. I by the loss of successive amino acids from the N-terminal. In this way, the C-terminal grouping, which seems to determine acceptability as a substrate, is kept intact and the hydrolysis of the C-terminal His-Leu dipeptide could be followed by a suitable method (see above). The action of CE on such peptides could not be followed by bioassay as only the heptapeptide, [des-Asp^1]-Ang. II has significant biological activity. This point has already been discussed in the comparison of assay methods using Ang. I as substrate.

Another analogue of Ang. I that is a substrate for CE is the PTC-derivative described by OSBORN and his colleagues [OSBORN et al., 1970 (1)]. The PTC-group is attached to the N-terminal and though this group reduces biological activity of [PTC]-Ang. II to a quarter of that of Ang. II (OSBORN et al., 1966) ,it does not prevent [PTC]-Ang. I being converted to [PTC]-Ang. II by blood, plasma and *in vivo*. The *in-vitro* conversion of [PTC]-Ang. I by plasma is lower than that of Ang. I, but *in vivo* (rats, guinea-pigs and rabbits) the shape of the pressor response-time curve was very similar [OSBORN et al., 1970 (1)]. Perhaps the lung CE is less affected than plasma CE by the change at the N-terminal of Ang. I.

A wide range of other substrates for CE are given in the lists provided by ELLISEEVA et al. (1971), YANG et al. (1971) and IGIC et al. (1972) (Table 7). It is interesting that neither of the enzymes described by these two groups of workers was originally characterized as CE. "Carboxycathepsin" was purified by ELISSEEVA and her colleagues (ELISSEEVA and OREKHOVICH, 1963; OREKHOVICH, 1968) as a proteinase from bovine kidney cortex, active at neutral pH, dependent on chloride ion and capable of cleaving dipeptides from the C-terminal of a number of short peptides, particularly Hippuryl-Phe-Pro (Hip-Phe-Pro). The action of this enzyme on Ang. I and bradykinin had not been investigated nor had its CE activity been established until recently (ELISSEEVA et al., 1971). ERDOS and his colleagues isolated and purified an enzyme ("kininase II") from plasma and kidney which hydrolyzed the C-terminal dipeptide from bradykinin (ERDÖS and YANG, 1966, 1967; YANG and ERDÖS, 1967). This enzyme was then shown to hydrolyze His-Leu from Ang. I and to liberate dipeptides from other substrates, (YANG et al., 1971) and, as a consequence, renamed "dipeptide hydrolase" (DH). Although this porcine

Table 7. *Substrate specificity of peptidases with converting-enzyme activity*
"Carboxycathepsin" from bovine kidney (ELISSEEVA and OREKHOVICH; ELISSEEVA et al.)
"Dipeptide hydrolase" from porcine plasma (YANG et al.) or from porcine lung (IGIC et al.)

YANG et al., 1971 IGIC et al., 1972	ELISSEEVA and OREKHOVICH, 1963 ELISSEEVA et al., 1971
	Substrates
Hip-Gly-Gly	Hip-Phe-Pro
Hip-His-Leu	Hip-Lys-Gly
Cbo-Pro-Leu-Gly	Hip-Phe-Phe
t-BOC-Phe(NO_2)-Phe-Gly[a]	Hip-Gly-Pro
Dansyl-Gly-Gly-Gly[b]	
Ac-Ser-Pro-Phe-Arg	Cbz-Gly-Phe-Phe-Tyr
Bradykinin	Cbz-Pro-Phe-His-Leu
Angiotensin I	Hip-Phe-Glu-γ-benzylester
Insulin (B chain)[b]	Cbz-Phe-Gly-Pro-Phe-Arg
	Cbz-Val-His-Pro-Phe-His-Leu
	Bradykinin
	Angiotensin I
	Not Substrates
Hip-Gly	Hip-Phe
Hip-Phe NH_2	Cbz-Phe-Pro
Cbo-Gly-Gly	Cbz-Glu-Tyr
t-BOC-Phe(NO_2)-Phe	Hip-Phe-Glu
Angiotensin II	Hip-Phe-Phe-NH_2
	Hip-Gly-Phe-NH_2
	Hip-Gly-Pro-NH_2
	Gly-Pro-Ala-Gly-Pro-Ala
	Insulin (B chain)
	Human serum albumin
	Ovalbumin

[a] Only tested by YANG et al.
[b] Only tested by IGIC et al.

plasma DH preparation shows a chloride-dependent hydrolysis of a tripeptide chromogenic substrate (BPPG), no similar chloride requirement for the hydrolysis of any substrate has been demonstrated in the lung DH preparation (IGIC et al., 1972). This note of caution must be sounded as at least one example of CE activity from lung [FITZ and OVERTURF, 1972 (1)] is atypical in its response to EDTA, and there is a chloride-independent CE in rat submaxillary gland (BOUCHER et al., 1972) (see below).

An important difference between the short peptide substrates and Ang. I is reflected in a generally higher hydrolysis rate for the short substrates, viz. HHL-22 µmoles/min; Ang. I 1.2 µmoles/min [CUSHMAN and CHEUNG, 1971 (1)]. PIQUIL-

LOUD et al. (1970) also report that Z-Phe-His-Leu is hydrolyzed about 10 times faster than Ang. I. However, Ang. I has a lower Km (40 µM) than HHL (2 mM) [CUSHMAN and CHEUNG, 1971 (1)]. The activation of CE by chloride ion also varies with the substrate. Thus HHL needs 300 mM NaCl for maximal activation compared with 30 mM NaCl for Ang. I on the same enzyme [CUSHMAN and CHEUNG, 1971 (1)]. The chloride ion may help binding of substrates and it is interesting that as the Km falls from 2.1 mM (HHL) to about 40 µm (Ang. I) and then to about 1 µM (bradykinin), the requirement for chloride activation falls from 300 mM to less than 30 mM and then to zero. This relation between chloride requirement and Km should be extended to other shorter substrates and perhaps the substrates derived from bradykinin may need less chloride than those resembling Ang. I. This may give some clue as to the mechanism of chloride activation of this enzyme.

One general point must be made about synthetic peptides used as substrates. The purity of chemically synthesized, biologically active peptides may be checked by bioassay but the purity of biologically inactive peptides may only be based on physicochemical data. Unfortunately some samples of synthetic Ang. I and bradykinin with adequate physiochemical purity have lacked full biological activity, suggesting that the physicochemical parameters measured cannot differentiate between peptides chemically similar but biologically dissimilar. Since close analogues of substrates are often good inhibitors, particular care must be exercised in the use of peptide analogues and in the interpretation of results obtained with them (BANGHAM et al., 1971; VANE, 1971).

Naturally occurring peptide hormones other than those mentioned may be substrates for CE, though several e.g. oxytocin, vasopressin, gastrin, cholecystokinin, are C-terminal amides and are thus resistant to attack by CE. The extent to which hydrolysis of insulin by CE (IGIC et al., 1972) contributes to the overall biological inactivation of this blood-borne hormone has yet to be determined. Moreover, ELISSEEVA and OREKHOVICH (1963) find insulin to be resistant to hydrolysis by carboxycathepsin.

The wide substrate specificity of CE that has been only recently recognized has given rise to a number of different names for this enzyme, both systematic and trivial; "α-carboxypeptide dipeptidohydrolase", "dipeptidyl carboxypeptidase", "dipeptide hydrolase", "carboxycathepsin". It is true that "Ang. I-converting enzyme" is not a good example of a trivial name — for which brevity is essential — and since there are kinin converting enzymes (catalysing the hydrolysis of Met-Lys-bradykinin to bradykinin) merely to call it "converting enzyme" will only cause confusion. Another suggestion ,"convertase" has a definitely carbohydrate implication. Furthermore, CE is probably the same as a bradykininase and this function must be accommodated in the trivial designation.

Another source of confusion is the unit used to quantitate the activity of preparations of CE. The most popular method [ROTH et al., 1969; PIQUILLOUD et al., 1970; DORER et al., 1970; LEE et al., 1971 (1—4); CUSHMAN and CHEUNG, 1971 (1, 2); BOUCHER et al., 1972] is to measure the amount of product formed from either Ang. I or a short substrate, but PIQUILLOUD et al. and CUSHMAN and CHEUNG then express their rate as µmoles product/min, and DORER et al. and BOUCHER et al. choose µmoles/h. Perhaps the most convenient rate unit would be µmoles product formed/min and one unit of activity would form one µmole product/min/mg protein. Milliunits of CE activity representing nmoles product/min/mg protein could be used to describe lower activities (ROTH et al., 1969) and these have been used in Table 5, so that as far as possible comparisons can be easily made.

5. Effect of Anions

A characteristic property of CE is its dependence on chloride ions. In their first paper dealing with the two forms of angiotensin, SKEGGS et al. (1954), showed that in the absence of chloride only Ang. I could be found and that as the chloride concentration was increased to 0.1 M only Ang. II was present. Fluoride, bromide and nitrate could substitute to some extent for chloride but other anions such as bicarbonate, sulphate and phosphate all failed to activate plasma CE. Most subsequent work with CE has confirmed the chloride dependence (see Table 6) and there are only a few peptidases known to convert Ang. I to Ang. II which do not require chloride ion (see below).

The quantitative aspects of the chloride dependence are less uniform, both in the degree of activation produced, which varies from 100-fold (PIQUILLOUD et al., 1970) to 2.3-fold (HUGGINS et al., 1970), and in the optimal chloride concentration, which varies from 17 mM to 170 mM (Table 6). Chloride ion is also necessary for the hydrolysis of the shorter peptide substrates of CE [PIQUILLOUD et al., 1970; CUSHMAN and CHEUNG, 1971 (1); YANG et al., 1971] although the optimal chloride concentration may be different from that for Ang. I conversion [see Table 6, CUSHMAN and CHEUNG, 1971 (1)]. There is agreement that other halide ions can partially activate CE and other monovalent anions with the exception of nitrate are ineffective (SKEGGS et al., 1967; PIQUILLOUD et al., 1970; BAKHLE and REYNARD, 1971). Multivalent anions are unable to activate CE. No inhibitory anions have been found, apart from cyanide, (HUGGINS et al., 1970) which may, at 100 mM, have been acting more as a chelating agent.

Ionic stimulation of enzymes offers a control mechanism for the activity of the enzyme and, bearing in mind the effects of varying sodium chloride intake on blood pressure both in man and in animals, the chloride ion activation of CE might provide a method of controlling the renin-angiotensin system. Unfortunately for this hypothesis, the chloride ion concentration at half maximal CE activity varies from 1 meq/litre to 50 meq/litre (for the different preparations) and these levels have to be contrasted with the normal blood concentration of 80 to 100 meq/litre. Since the CE is either in blood (plasma) or in close proximity to it (lung), it is unlikely that the concentrations of chloride at the enzyme can fall to levels low enough to limit the activity of CE. In kidney, where local chloride concentrations may vary widely, CE activity may be controlled in this way but there is at present no evidence to support this possibility.

Attention has already been drawn to the variation of chloride ion requirements with different substrates (see above), but the mechanism by which chloride activation takes place is unknown. Anion stimulation of activity occurs with other enzymes (JOHNSON, 1941; WEBB and MORROW, 1959; KAIKUCHI and TOMIZAWA, 1964), notably the chloride-activated aminopeptidase described by MCDONALD et al. (1966, 1969) which also splits dipeptide units from its substrates. However, substrates not requiring chloride have not yet been described for this aminopeptidase, in analogy with bradykinin and CE.

Some possible mechanisms of chloride activation are:

1. Direct involvement of Cl′ in the binding of substrates, perhaps by masking of some electrophilic centre in the active site.

2. Allosteric effects causing a rearrangement of the same active site.

3. Allosteric effects causing *another* active site to be formed. In this case there must be sufficient interaction between the two sites to allow for the inhibition of Ang. I conversion by bradykinin.

Now that highly purified preparations of CE are available, the question of what physical changes, if any, arise in the presence of chloride ion could be examined. The alteration of substrate specificity by chloride ion should provide enough problems to occupy enzymologists for several years.

6. Effect of Cations

The effect of cations has been studied both on normal enzymic activity and on CE inhibited by chelating agents.

With Ang. I as substrate none of the cations studied stimulates the activity of normal CE (see Table 8), although the hydrolysis of HHL (or HGG, YANG et al., 1971) is stimulated by Co to about 150% of normal activity [CUSHMAN and CHEUNG, 1971 (1)]. Several cations depress the hydrolysis of either type of substrate, the most consistently inhibitory being Ni and Zn.

Table 8. *Effects of cations (up to 1 meq/litre) on converting enzyme activity (references in brackets)*

Cations added	Substrate[a]		
	Ang. I [1, 3, 4]	HHL [2, 5]	HGG [5]
Ca	0 [3, 4]		
Ba	0 [4]		
Mg	0 [1, 3, 4]		
Zn	– [1, 3, 4]	– [2]	
Cd		– [2]	
Hg	– [4]	– [2]	
Mn	0 [1, 4]	0 [2]	
Co	0 [1, 3, 4]	+ [2, 5]	+ [5]
Ni	– [1, 4]	– [2]	
Fe	– [4]	– [2]	
Cu	– [4]	– [2]	
Sn	0 [4]		
Pb	– [4]		

[a] HHL = Hippuryl-His-Leu; HGG = Hippuryl-Gly-Gly.
0 = no effect; + = stimulation; – = inhibition.

References

1. BAKHLE and REYNARD (1971); 2. CUSHMAN and CHEUNG [1971 (1)]; 3. DORER et al. (1970); 4. HUGGINS et al. (1970); 5. YANG et al. (1971).

The effect of cations on EDTA-inhibited CE has been studied with enzyme that had been dialyzed against EDTA, and with normal enzyme in the presence of added EDTA. Again, there is general agreement on the ability of Co and Mn to restore activity to either form of inhibited enzyme (see Table 9). The hydrolysis of HHL is not only restored but increased by Co under these conditions. There is disagreement, however, about the effectiveness of Zn and of Ca. In two examples, Zn restored activity to EDTA-inhibited CE, although this cation inhibited normal activity of the same enzyme (DORER et al., 1970; CUSHMAN and CHEUNG, 1971).

No clear conclusions can be drawn from these effects of cations on CE, if only because the concentrations of cations and EDTA used vary widely. Thus DORER et al.

(1969) find Zn at 30 μM reactivates CE dialyzed against EDTA (500 μM) but at 100 μM Zn the activity is almost back to the fully inhibited level. HUGGINS et al. (1970) used either 100 μM or 1 mM Zn to look for reactivation of EDTA (1 mM)-dialyzed enzyme; FITZ et al. (1971) used 4 mM Zn for reactivation after dialysis against 3 mM EDTA.

Inhibition by Cd, Hg and Cu might suggest the inactivation of a sulphydryl group involved in the peptidase function but this suggestion is not supported by the results obtained with sulphydryl reagents (see below). Only two examples of stimulation of normal CE have been reported and the short substrate was used in both cases. In general the enzyme does not require added cations for activity, which implies that its native cation is tightly bound as all the preparations will

Table 9. *Ability of divalent cations to restore activity to converting enzyme inhibited by EDTA*

Cations added	Method of inhibition by EDTA						
	Dialysed against EDTA				Added EDTA		Not specified
	Substrate[a]						
	-Ang. I [3, 5, 6]		-HHL [2, 7]		-Ang. I [1, 5, 6]		-HPP [4]
Ca	+ [6]	0 [3, 5]		0 [2]	+ [6]	0 [5]	+ 0
Ba				0 [2]			
Mg		0 [3, 5, 6]		0 [2, 7]	+ [6]	0 [1, 5]	
Zn	+ [3]	0 [5, 6]	+ [2, 7]		+ [5, 6]	0 [1]	+
Cd			+ 0 [7]				+ 0
Mn	+ [3, 6]	0 [5]	+ [2, 7]		+ [1, 6]	0 [5]	+
Co	+ [3, 5]	+ 0 [6]	+ + [2, 7]		+ [1, 5, 6]		+
Ni		0 [6]		0 [7]		0 [1, 5]	+ 0
Fe							+ 0
Cu				0 [2]			

[a] HHL = Hippuryl-His-Leu; HPP = Hippuryl-Phe-Pro
0 = no activity restored, + = most of activity restored, + + = activity stimulated.

References

1. BAKHLE and REYNARD (1971); 2. CUSHMAN and CHEUNG [1971 (1)]; 3. DORER et al. (1970); 4. ELISSEEVA et al. (1971); 5. FITZ et al. (1971); 6. HUGGINS et al. (1970); 7. YANG et al. (1971).

have been dialyzed against buffer or water at some stage in their preparation. From the results of the reactivation experiments, it would seem that either Co or Mn is the closest substitute for the cation in the native enzyme, with Zn only sometimes effective. This combination of efficacy of Co and Mn and non-efficacy of Zn is an unusual characteristic of this peptidase.

7. Inhibitors

The inhibitors of CE may be conveniently divided into non-peptide inhibitors and peptide inhibitors.

a) Non-Peptide Inhibitors

Table 10 summarizes the results given in several papers for the more commonly used inhibitors. The first section deals with chelating agents. The inhibition of CE by EDTA, first reported by SKEGGS et al. (1956), has been confirmed by every report. Other chelating agents such as BAL, *o*-phenanthroline, and EGTA (FITZ et al., 1971) are also effective at less than 1 mM, but the effects quoted for 2:2′-dipyridyl and 8-hydroxyquinoline vary from paper to paper. Inhibition obtained by dialysis of CE against 1 mM EDTA is not reversed by dialysis against buffer, but when more dilute EDTA (0.1 mM) is used, the inhibition is reversible by dialysis against buffer [Cushman and Cheung, 1971 (1)]. This is a further indication of the firmness with which the native metal is held by the enzyme.

Table 10. *Effect of various compounds on converting enzyme activity*
Results obtained with the compounds in concentrations up to 1 mM only have been included

Compound	Effect			
	Inhibitory		Non-inhibitory	
	Reference	Substrate	Reference	Substrate
	a) Chelating agents			
EDTA	All references			
2:3-Dimercaptopropanol (BAL)	Bakhle and Reynard, 1971	Ang. I		
	Cushman and Cheung, 1971	HHL[a]		
o-Phenanthroline	Cushman and Cheung, 1971	HHL		
	Yang et al., 1971	BPPG[b]		
2:2′-Dipyridyl	Boucher et al., 1972	Ang. I	Cushman and Cheung, 1971	HHL
			Fitz et al., 1971	Ang. I
8-Hydroxyquinoline	Fitz et al., 1971	Ang. I	Bakhle, 1968	Ang. I
	b) Sulphydryl compounds and reagents			
N-Ethylmaleimide	Huggins et al., 1970	Ang. I	Bakhle and Reynard, 1971	Ang. I
			Cushman and Cheung, 1971	HHL
p-Chloromercuribenzoate	Huggins et al., 1970	Ang. I	Cushman and Cheung, 1971	HHL
2-Mercaptoethanol			Bakhle, 1968	Ang. I
			Cushman and Cheung, 1971	HHL
Dithiothreitol	Cushman and Cheung, 1971	HHL	Huggins et al., 1970	Ang. I
Gluthathione	Igic et al., 1972	Ang. I		

[a] HHL = Hippuryl-His-Leu.
[b] BPPG = t-BOC-Phe(NO_2)-Phe-Gly.

Two points of interest arise from this susceptibility to inhibition by EDTA. The first is that two groups of workers use EDTA in their purification procedures for CE and retain both activity and inhibition by subsequent treatment with EDTA. Thus Huggins and Thampi (1968) homogenized tissue in saline containing 1 mM EDTA at pH 4.7. Both this concentration of EDTA and the low pH (see above) would be enough to inactivate a considerable portion of the CE activity. Perhaps they were measuring in those tissue extracts another His-Leu-liberating peptidase resistant to EDTA as is present in rat (BOUCHER et al., 1972) and man [FITZ and OVERTURF, 1972 (1)]. It is interesting that EDTA has not been used in subsequent preparations of CE from HUGGINS' laboratory (HUGGINS et al., 1970; SANDER and HUGGINS, 1971).

The other group is LEE et al.; in their purifications of CE from porcine [1971 (1)] and human plasma [1971 (2)] they dialyzed the extracts against 1 mM EDTA for an unspecified time and then against buffer before chromatography. The purified material liberated His-Leu from Ang. I, required NaCl for enzyme activity and was inhibited by EDTA. The authors do not comment on the fact that EDTA at a lower concentration than that used during purification inhibits the purified enzyme. They, too, have omitted to use this method in subsequent [1971 (3)] preparations.

The second point has been made by several authors (HOLLEMANS et al., 1969; BARRETT and SAMBHI, 1969; UEDA et al., 1971) and is that in the assay for renin described by BOUCHER et al. (1964), in which renin and renin substrate are incubated at pH 5.5 in the presence of EDTA, the angiotensin formed is Ang. I and not Ang. II, as both the low pH and the EDTA prevent the formation of Ang. II. As long as the angiotensin was assayed by its pressor effect in rats, this did not matter, as the Ang. I would be equipotent to Ang. II *in vivo*, but for radio-immunoassay the nature of the angiotensin is crucial, since the antibodies distinguish between Ang. I and Ang. II. The realization that the product of the method of BOUCHER et al. and of many other methods was Ang. I, because either inhibitors or low pH were involved, led to the development of the radio-immunoassay of Ang. I.

There is less agreement about the effects of sulphydryl compounds (see Table 10). Although 2-mercaptoethanol, β-mercaptoethylamine (YANG et al., 1971) and sulphide ions (CUSHMAN and CHEUNG, 1971) are not inhibitors (up to 1 mM), both glutathione and dithiothreitol may be inhibitory. Cysteine and thioglycolic acid are also inhibitors of HHL hydrolysis [CUSHMAN and CHEUNG, 1971 (1)]. As far as reagents for sulphydryl groups are concerned, opinion is equally divided on whether N-ethylmaleimide and *p*-chloromercuribenzoate are inhibitors or not. YANG et al. found *p*-chloromercuriphenyl sulphonic acid did not inhibit hydrolysis of BPPG. Neither iodoacetic acid nor its amide are inhibitors of HHL hydrolysis [CUSHMAN and CHEUNG, 1971 (1)].

The esterase inhibitor DFP is generally not an inhibitor of CE (BOUCHER et al., 1970), though HUGGINS et al. (1970) reported that phenylmethylsulphonyl fluoride (PMSF), a related inhibitor, did inhibit conversion of Ang. I by plasma CE but not by dog-lung CE. The chloroketones TLCK (chlorotosylamidoaminoheptanone) and TPCK (tosylamidophenylethylchloromethyl ketone) do not inhibit HHL hydrolysis and nor do aminooxyacetic acid or hydroxylamine [CUSHMAN and CHEUNG, 1971 (1)].

b) Peptide Inhibitors

The peptide inhibitors of CE are as diverse as its substrates. Some inhibit the conversion of Ang. I to Ang. II because they are alternative substrates e.g. bradykinin, Met-Lys-bradykinin, HHL; others, like Ang. II and His-Leu, may inhibit through product inhibition but there is some disagreement as to their action (see Table 11); the peptide inhibitors from snake venom can behave as competitive or non-competitive inhibitors, and one, the pentapeptide from *Bothrops jararaca* venom, is slowly degraded by the purified enzyme (CUSHMAN and CHEUNG, 1972).

The alternative peptide substrates of CE will inhibit the conversion of Ang. I (see Table 11) to a variable degree, the longer substrates like bradykinin and insulin being the more potent inhibitors. SANDER et al. (1971) showed that inhibition by bradykinin and Met-Lys-bradykinin follows competitive kinetics. However other large peptides e.g. soybean-trypsin inhibitor (BOUCHER et al., 1972) aprotinin (Trasylol) (BAKHLE, 1968) and human fibrinopeptides A and B [CUSHMAN and CHEUNG, 1971 (1)] do not inhibit CE.

Amino-acids (phenylalanine, YANG et al., 1971; ε-aminocaproic acid, BAKHLE, 1968) and dipeptides unrelated to angiotensin (or bradykinin) also fail to inhibit CE (YANG et al., 1971). The C-terminal dipeptides of Ang. I or bradykinin inhibit Ang. I conversion, though there is disagreement about this as there is over the inhibitory effect of Ang. II, the other product of CE (see Table 11).

The first group of venom peptides to be studied as inhibitors of CE (see Table 12) were derived from the venom of *Bothrops jararaca* and originally characterized as potentiators of the effects of bradykinin (BPF, FERREIRA, 1965). BPF

Table 11. *Peptide inhibitors of converting enzyme*

Inhibitor peptide	Substrate peptide			
	Angiotensin I			Hip-His-Leu
	I_{50} (M)		I_{100} (M)	I_{50} (M)
	SANDER et al. 1971	LEE et al. 1971 (2)	YANG et al. 1971	CUSHMAN and CHEUNG, 1971 (1)
His-Leu	1—5 × 10^{-3}	<10^{-3}	10^{-3}	
Phe-Arg	~ 10^{-3}		10^{-3}	
Hip-His-Leu	10^{-3}		10^{-3}	
Hip-Gly-Gly	<5 × 10^{-3}			
Bradykinin	~8 × 10^{-6}			10^{-6}—10^{-5}
Met-Lys-bradykinin	~3 × 10^{-5}			
Angiotensin II		~10^{-4}		10^{-5}—10^{-4}
Insulin (pig)			10^{-6}	
Insulin (bovine)	<5 × 10^{-5}			

inhibits bradykininases in tissues and in blood and in 1968 BAKHLE showed that BPF was also a potent inhibitor of CE from canine lung. BPF was separated into its component peptides and one of these, a pentapeptide Pca-Lys-Trp-Ala-Pro, was synthesized by FERREIRA et al., 1970. ONDETTI et al. (1971) also separated and synthesized several other peptides from BPF. Most of the peptides isolated from BPF by the two groups were identical in composition. Many of the peptides isolated by FERREIRA et al. [1970 (1)] which were potentiators of the action of bradykinin (on the guinea-pig ileum) were also tested as inhibitors of canine-lung CE [FERREIRA et al., 1970 (2)], and there was no clear distinction between the two levels of activity. However, several peptides were very potent as CE inhibitors, especially a nonapeptide referred to as IV-1-D. The structure of this nonapeptide was shown by ONDETTI et al. (1970) to be Pca-Trp-Pro-Arg-Pro-Glu-Ile-Pro-Pro, and the synthetic nonapeptide has been designated SQ 20881 in their papers.

The inhibition of CE by some of the synthetic *Bothrops* peptides has been studied by BAKHLE (1971, 1972) and in more detail by CUSHMAN and CHEUNG (1972). The studies agree that the nonapeptide is the most potent inhibitor among the longer peptides (9 to 13 residues), but the latter authors find the pentapeptide

Table 12. *Venom peptide inhibitors of converting-enzyme activity*

Venom peptides	Inhibitory potency (expressed as I_{50}, μM)				
	Form of venom peptide				
	Natural	Synthetic			
	Substrate	Angiotensin I		HHL[b]	HGG[b]
	FERREIRA et al., 1970 (2)	BAKHLE, 1972	CUSHMAN and CHEUNG, 1972		IGIC et al., 1972
Bothrops jararaca					
Pca-Lys-Trp-Ala-Pro (V—3—A, SQ 20,475)[a]	1.4	0.9	0.7	0.07	
Pca-Trp-Pro-Arg-Pro-Gln-Ile-Pro-Pro (IV—1—D, SQ 20,881)	0.019	0.024	3.6	0.56	0.03
Pca-Asn-Trp-Pro-Arg-Pro-Gln-Ile-Pro-Pro (SQ 20,861)		0.02	10	2.5	
Pca-Trp-Pro-Arg-Pro-Thr-Pro-Gln-Ile-Pro-Pro (IV—1—Bα, SQ 20,661)			18	5.0	
Pca-Asn-Trp-Pro-His-Pro-Gln-Ile-Pro-Pro-Pro (IV—1—Bβ, SQ 20,858)			21	5.8	
Pca-Gly-Gly-Trp-Pro-Arg-Pro-Gly-Pro-Pro-Gln-Ile-Pro-Pro (III—1—A, SQ 20,718)			36	15	
Pca-Ser-Trp-Pro-Gly-Pro-Asn-Ile-Pro-Pro (IV—1—A, SQ 20,859)	0.87	3.2	76	34	
Agkistrodon halys blomhoffii					
Pca-Gly-Leu-Pro-Pro-Arg-Pro-Lys-Ile-Pro-Pro (potentiator B)	0.12	0.12			
Pca-Gly-Leu-Pro-Pro-Gly-Pro-Pro-Ile-Pro-Pro (potentiator C)	3.0	3.0, 2.5[c]			0.03
Pca-Lys-Trp-Asp-Pro-Pro-Pro-Val-Ser-Pro-Pro (potentiator E)		—[d]			

[a] The designation V—3—A etc. is that used by FERREIRA et al. [1970 (1)]. SQ 20,475 etc. is that used by CUSHMAN and CHEUNG (1972) to denote the synthetic peptides prepared by ONDETTI et al. (1971).

[b] HHL = Hippuryl-His-Leu; HGG = Hippuryl-Gly-Gly.

[c] The second value is that from SANDER et al. (1971).

[d] This peptide was non-inhibitory at concentrations up to 300 μM.

more potent as an inhibitor of the hydrolysis of Ang. I (or HHL) than the nonapeptide. This discrepancy is probably due to the different concentrations of Ang. I used. CUSHMAN and CHEUNG used their optimal concentration of Ang. I, 0.3 mM, whereas BAKHLE used a much lower concentration, 5 μg/ml (about 5 μM) of Ang. I.

The type of inhibition caused by the pentapeptide also varies with the substrate, being competitive with Ang. I but non-competitive with HHL. The longer *Bothrops* peptides are also competitive inhibitors of Ang. I conversion.

Another group of peptide inhibitors has been isolated from the venom of *Agkistrodon halys blomhoffii*. These peptides were also isolated as potentiators of bradykinin and three of the most potent, referred to as potentiators B, C and E have been purified, their structure established and their synthesis accomplished (KATO and SUZUKI, 1971). They are all undecapeptides and have been tested as inhibitors of Ang.-I conversion by BAKHLE (1972; also quoted in KIMURA et al., 1970; and in KATO and SUZUKI, 1971) and by SANDER and HUGGINS (1971) and UEDA et al. [1971 (2)]. The natural and synthetic forms of these peptides have identical potency (cf. *Bothrops* peptides), and although potentiator B is only twice as potent as C in potentiating bradykinin on the guinea-pig ileum, B is 20 to 25 times as potent as C in inhibiting CE. Peptide E, which is 75 times less potent than C in potentiating bradykinin, has no inhibitory effect on CE at 0.3 mM, i.e. 100 times the I_{50} of peptide C (BAKHLE, 1972). Inhibition of Ang. I conversion by potentiator C is competitive (SANDER and HUGGINS, 1971). Potentiator C is also an inhibitor of the hydrolysis of HGG and other short substrates catalyzed by lung or plasma "dipeptide hydrolase" (YANG et al., 1971; IGIC et al., 1972) with an I_{50} value 100 times lower than those obtained with CE and Ang. I. The *Bothrops* peptides are also better inhibitors with the shorter substrates (see Table 12). The venom peptides also inhibit CE in perfused isolated lungs (BAKHLE, REYNARD and VANE, 1969; AIKEN and VANE, 1970; BAKHLE, 1971, 1972; IGIC et al., 1972) and *in vivo* (NG and VANE, 1970; ENGEL et al., 1971).

The action does appear to be related to the structure. All the inhibitory peptides except the *Bothrops* pentapeptide have a C-terminal dipeptide Pro-Pro which would make them resistant to hydrolysis by CE; the *Bothrops* pentapeptide has the C-terminal Ala-Pro and is a substrate for CE (CUSHMAN and CHEUNG, 1972). *In vivo*, the pentapeptide has a transitory effect whereas the action of the longer peptides persist for hours (ENGEL et al., 1971; BAKHLE and FERREIRA, unpublished experiments). Secondly, the presence of a basic amino-acid residue e.g. Arg, Lys, His, seems to be required for high activity and where they are absent, as in the last *Bothrops* peptide in Table 12 or in potentiator C, the inhibitory potency is low. Potentiator E has a Lys residue but its effect may be neutralized by the Asp residue, two residues away. The Tyr residue in Ang. II is an essential requirement for vasoconstrictor activity, and although all the *Bothrops* peptides have aromatic residues (Trp and not Tyr), such residues are not essential for high inhibitory potency — see potentiator B. However, both the enzymic site in CE and the receptor site for Ang. II require a free carboxylic acid group at the C-terminal.

So far only peptides from the venoms of *B. jararaca* and *A. halys blomhoffii* have been purified and studied as CE inhibitors, but it is very likely that other venoms, not necessarily from *Viperidae*, will contain peptides of similar activity. Peptide inhibitors of CE may be of clinical value, for instance, in the diagnosis of hyperactivity of the renin-angiotensin system (KRIEGER et al., 1971), but the concomitant inhibition of bradykininase is a serious disadvantage. They have, however, immediate significance for fundamental research both in the renin-angiotensin system and in peptidase biochemistry.

8. General Comparison of CE Activities

Reasonably detailed descriptions of CE from several species (as summarized in Table 6) have now been published, and it seems that these enzymes are all closely related. However, one species-specific parameter has been described by POULSEN and BING (1970) for plasma converting enzymes from man, rat and mouse. Mouse Ang. I (from the reaction of mouse renin with mouse plasma) is converted rapidly by mouse plasma CE, but only slowly by rat or human plasma CE, whereas rat and human Ang. I are rapidly converted by all three plasma enzymes. The rates of reaction of the three Ang. I preparations with homologous plasma converting enzymes are identical. However, *in vivo*, mouse Ang. I is equipressor in rats and mice.

Since the pressor activity of Ang. I *in vivo* is mainly due to conversion in the lungs (NG and VANE, 1967; BIRON, 1968), this result would imply that rat-lung CE is able to convert mouse Ang. I rapidly and it is thus different from rat-plasma CE. Although no direct efforts have been made to differentiate between tissue converting enzymes, support for the presence of such differences *in vivo* may be drawn from isolated findings by several authors. The findings of POULSEN and BING quoted above suggest a difference between rat-lung and rat-plasma CE. A similar difference is implied in the results of CARRETERO et al. (1969) and LOYKE (1964). Whereas LOYKE finds a low level of CE in serum from CCl_4-treated rats, CARRETERO et al. find that the *in-vivo* pressor response to Ang. II, Ang. I and renin is unaffected by CCl_4 treatment. These results are compatible if CCl_4 treatment selectively reduces serum CE without affecting lung CE.

Examples of differences between lung and plasma converting enzymes *in vitro* are more difficult to find. The properties, summarized in Table 6, of lung converting enzymes overlap to a great extent with those of the plasma enzymes. In particular, the Km values for plasma CE are all about 40 to 50 μM, and those for lung CE are between 20 and 50 μM, except for one value of 5 μm (HUGGINS et al., 1970). These values all refer to Ang. I as substrate. The similarity of Km between the lung and plasma enzyme is surprising in view of the great difference in conversion rates in blood and in the pulmonary circulation *in vivo* (NG and VANE, 1967; OPARIL et al., 1970), which might reasonably have been expected to show itself as a difference in Km values for the enzymes *in vitro*. This is because the different *in-vivo* conversion rates cannot be explained merely by the greater specific activity of lung tissue. The ratio activity/g lung: activity/ml plasma, is only 3:4 for the rat (HUGGINS and THAMPI, 1968), 3:2 for guinea pig and 1:1 for pig [LEE et al., 1971 (3)]. Higher values of this ratio are obtained if the activities/mg protein are compared (Table 4), but this is not a direct estimate of *tissue* content. The possibility of different Km values is supported by the report of a comparatively crude and particulate preparation of lung CE (HUGGINS et al., 1970) which has a Km ten times lower than that of the highly purified but soluble preparations (Table 6).

A possible explanation of this situation is that the Km of lung CE *in situ* is probably one tenth or less that of plasma CE and that this difference accounts for the different conversion rates *in vivo*. In extracts of lung, the lower Km is retained as long as the enzyme is particulate, i.e. membrane bound. Solubilization of the enzymes may cause a conformational change leading to a higher value for Km, and in a soluble form lung CE may indeed be identical with plasma CE. It is, then, the fact that CE is soluble that determines its higher Km, whether this is due to a natural process such as the formation of the plasma enzyme, or to homogenization or the use of detergents.

In those species where both lung and plasma enzymes have been studied *in vitro*, only one qualitative difference has emerged. This is in the human-lung CE, which is not inhibited by EDTA [FITZ and OVERTURF, 1972 (1)] and is therefore clearly different from human-plasma CE. This lung enzyme may have other atypical properties — its chloride dependence for instance, has not been measured.

9. Converting Enzyme and Bradykininase

Enzymes inactivating bradykinin are present in many preparations of CE. The work of ELISSEEVA et al. (1971) and YANG et al. (1971) shows clearly that even highly purified enzymes will both convert Ang. I to Ang. II and hydrolyze, and thus inactivate, bradykinin. It is therefore highly probable that converting enzyme and bradykininase are two functions of the same protein, modified in the former case by chloride ions. Whether this bradykininase is the rate-limiting enzyme in the inactivation of bradykinin in blood or in lung is a question that still has to be settled.

Atypical Converting Enzyme

This section deals with those enzymes capable of catalyzing the conversion of Ang. I to Ang. II but which, as shown in Table 13, fail to satisfy one or more of the four additional criteria laid down for inclusion in the group of typical converting enzymes. The terms "typical" and "atypical" are preferred to other terms like "true" [LEE et al., 1971 (3)], because the two classes of CE are distinguished by biochemical criteria which may or may not have physiological significance. Any peptidase that generates Ang. II from Ang. I faster than the Ang. II is inactivated may be a physiologically significant CE, regardless of its mechanism of action or requirements for activation. The β-CE activity in rat plasma (BOUCHER et al., 1972) may in certain circumstances prove to be of greater importance to the overall activity of the renin-angiotensin system than the typical plasma CE activity.

Table 13. *Atypical converting enzymes*

Enzyme	Criteria for "typical" CE				
	His-Leu dipeptide	Ang. II-Limit peptide	Chloride dependence	EDTA inhibition	References
Subtilisin BPN′	Yes	No	?	?	[3]
α-Amylase	?	No	?	?	[1]
Dipeptidyl carboxypeptidase *Corynebacterium equi*	Yes	Yes	No	Yes	[6]
CE from rat uterus, thymus, thyroid	?	?	No	?	[4]
β-CE (rat)	Yes	Yes	No	No	[2]
Human lung CE	Yes	Yes	?	No	[5]

References

1. BARRETT and SAMBHI (1969); 2. BOUCHER et al. (1972); 3. CARLINI and HUGGINS (1968); 4. CUSHMAN and CHEUNG [1971 (2)]; 5. FITZ and OVERTURF [1972 (1)]; LEE et al. [1971 (4)].

1. Bacterial Enzymes

HUGGINS and his colleagues have been investigating the production of oxytocic materials from plasma by a variety of enzymes (Ang. II is oxytocic while Ang. I is not). The earlier papers (HUGGINS and WALASZEK, 1959; WALASZEK and HUGGINS, 1960) described an oxytocic principle arising from the reaction of crude α-amylase on human plasma fraction IV—4. This was followed in 1962 (CARLINI and HUGGINS) by the report of the formation of an oxytocic material from Ang. I by crude α-amylase. There was an increase in oxytocic activity for the first 10 min of incubation followed by a decrease, all activity disappearing after 30 min. No oxytocic activity was generated by purified crystalline α-amylase. In two papers (PAVESI and HUGGINS, 1968; BUTT and HUGGINS, 1968), the proteinase subtilisin BPN′ or subtilisin Carlsberg), a likely contaminant of α-amylase, was shown to liberate a "vasopressor polypeptide A" from plasma fraction IV—4 and also to catalyze its inactivation. The biological activity (WALASZEK et al., 1962) and amino-acid content (ARIAS, 1965) of the vasopressor polypeptide resembled that of Ang. II, and subtilisin BPN′ formed Ang. II from [^{14}C-Leu^{10}]-Ang. I with the liberation of His-Leu (^{14}C), and subsequent degradation of Ang. II (THAMPI and HUGGINS, 1968). The conversion was maximal at pH 6 with no formation below pH 4 to 5, although there was considerable conversion at pH 8. Formation of polypeptide A from fraction IV—4 by subtilisin BPN′ is inhibited by DFP and PMSF but not by EDTA, and has a similar pH optimum (PAVESI and HUGGINS). No mention is made of chloride or any other anion dependence.

The CE activity of crude α-amylase was confirmed by BARRETT and SAMBHI (1969) who achieved complete conversion of small amounts of Ang. I before significant degradation took place. They suggested its use in the renin assay of BOUCHER et al. (1964) to convert the Ang. I produced in this assay quantitatively to Ang. II so that the final measurement of renin activity could be made by immunoassay of Ang. II.

Recently another bacterial peptidase has been extracted from *Corynebacterium equi* which is more like typical CE [LEE et al., 1971 (4)]. Thus it hydrolyzes dipeptide fragments from the C-terminal of peptides where the terminal amino acid is present as the carboxylic acid and will not hydrolyze the imino-peptide bond of proline peptides. It is inhibited by EDTA and not by DFP, but it does not require chloride ion for its activity.

2. Mammalian Enzymes

The other atypical CE preparations are from mammalian sources. The most fully investigated is the peptidase from rat submaxillary glands, "β-converting enzyme" (BOUCHER et al., 1972). Only a crude extract (homogenization, followed by centrifugation, to give a clear supernatant as the enzyme preparation) was studied and compared with typical CE (from rat lung or plasma) using Ang. I as substrate. Conversion of Ang. I was measured by the method of PIQUILLOUD et al. (1969), assaying His-Leu liberated. Preliminary experiments had been carried out using the rat pressor bioassay method of BOUCHER et al. (1970) which gave similar results to those obtained with the fluorimetric assay. Although the authors do not state it specifically, it must be assumed that Ang. II was the limit peptide. There was approximately 20 times as much activity in the submaxillary glands as in the lungs per gram of tissue and the velocity of conversion catalyzed by β-CE was greater than that of lung or plasma CE. The pH optima are different: 6.5 to 7.2 for β-CE, 7 to 8 for typical CE, and the substrate specificity also differs, Z-Phe-His-Leu being almost totally resistant to β-CE. Furthermore, chloride ion is not required for β-CE conversion, and the inhibitors of typical CE, EDTA, dipyridyl and the pentapeptide Pca-Lys-Trp-Ala-Pro have no effect on β-CE. However, soybean trypsin inhibitor and a component of rat plasma are potent inhibitors of β-CE. Fractionation of plasma proteins has allowed the authors to separate the inhibitor and disclose β-CE activity in plasma.

This β-CE is therefore a dipeptidyl carboxypeptidase; it liberates His-Leu from Ang. I and does not form Ang. II from the nonapeptide, [des-Leu[10]]-Ang. I (LENTZ et al., 1956), and is capable of converting Ang. I in the absence of chloride, as is the enzyme from *C. equi*. It would be interesting to see whether or not bradykinin is a substrate for these enzymes. The function of β-CE in the submaxillary glands is not known. It may be secreted into saliva, or act as a kininase involved with salivary kallikrein or with the postulated function of bradykinin in reactive hyperaemia in these glands. The presence of a potent inhibitor in normal rat plasma clearly implies that β-CE is not meant to act on blood-borne Ang. I in normal circumstances.

The investigations into human lung CE by FITZ and OVERTURF [1972 (1)] have not been completed, but one atypical parameter has been established. This is its lack of inhibition by EDTA in concentrations up to 100 mM. Otherwise, this CE liberates His-Leu from Ang. I and can be separated from the angiotensinases present in the lung homogenate. All the incubations were carried out in the presence of chloride, so that the relation of activity to chloride-ion concentration is not known. The situation is further complicated by the multiple forms of CE in the human lung extract, which are separable by gel filtration on Sephadex G-200 [FITZ and OVERTURF, 1972 (2)]. Although the majority of the activity elutes as though it had a MW of 480,000, about 25% of the CE activity elutes later. Assay of this lesser CE peak showed the presence of Leu as well as His-Leu after incubation, suggesting contamination with carboxypeptidase or dipeptidase activities. LEE et al. [1971 (3)] found a high level of dipeptidase activity capable of hydrolyzing His-Leu in extracts of porcine lung.

It is interesting to note that when FITZ and OVERTURF first described human-lung CE in 1970, they prepared it by a different method; homogenization in 1 mM EDTA, acetone powder, ammonium sulphate fractionation, gel filtration; and reported that its conversion of Ang. I was inhibited by EDTA (30 mM), as was their preparation of human plasma CE. The two enzymes also eluted from the gel filtration column in similar volumes and the authors concluded at that time that the two enzymes were similar and perhaps identical. The later papers make no reference to this earlier work, so the reasons for changing the preparative methods have not been given and the relation of this change to the change in properties of the enzymes cannot be assessed.

The last examples of atypical CE are also from rat tissues. In their survey of rat tissues for CE activity, CUSHMAN and CHEUNG [1971 (2)] used four criteria for CE activity; the liberation of His-Leu from the tripeptide HHL, stimulation of hydrolysis by added Co, inhibition by the pentapeptide Pca-Lys-Trp-Ala-Pro and dependence on chloride ion. The activity from four tissues, uterus, thymus, thyroid and pancreas was less dependent on chloride ion than the activity from the other tissues. Furthermore, the activity from uterus, thymus and thyroid were resistant to inhibition by the pentapeptide.

Thus, at least part of the HHL-hydrolyzing activity from these rat tissues is not due to a typical CE. In the light of the study by BOUCHER et al. (1972), it would be more valuable to perform these surveys with Ang. I as substrate rather than with short peptide substrates. This point is emphasized by the low activity found by CUSHMAN and CHEUNG [1971 (2)] in the rat submaxillary gland using HHL as substrate (1 nmole His-Leu/mg/min), and the high activity found by BOUCHER et al. using Ang. I as substrate (13 nmole His-Leu/mg/min). It appears that this "β-CE" will hydrolyze neither Z-Phe-His-Leu *nor* HHL. BOUCHER et al.

were not, however, able to find "β-CE" in submaxillary-gland extract until the rats weighed at least 250 g, and they routinely used 400 g rats for preparation of "β-CE". CUSHMAN and CHEUNG used "mature" Sprague-Dawley rats which may have weighed only just 250 g or perhaps less.

Pathological Factors Affecting Converting-Enzyme Activity *in Vitro*

1. Liver Damage

RAASCHOU (1949) and LOYKE (1960) showed that hypertension rarely co-existed with impaired hepatic function. The latter author extended this to the treatment of hypertensive rats with CCl_4 to induce liver damage. Hypertension caused by renal artery clips or by desoxycorticosterone acetate was ıeversible by a series of injections of CCl_4. The serum CE activity in the rats was measured by incubating Ang. I with serum (10 min, 37°), separating Ang. I and Ang. II in the incubation mixture by the chromatographic method of WISENBAUGH et al. (1964), and assaying the peptides by their pressor effect in rats. The serum fıom normal or hypertensive untreated rats converted nearly all the Ang. I to Ang. II, whereas that from CCl_4-treated rats converted less of the Ang. I (28% conversion as against 94% conversion, LOYKE, 1968). Furthermore, rats resistant to CCl_4 treatment had serum CE activity in the normal range. Addition of CCl_4 to normal serum inhibited conversion (LOYKE, 1968) and addition of serum from CCl_4-treated rats to normal serum inhibited the CE activity of normal serum (LOYKE, 1964). In a later paper LOYKE (1970) uses longer incubation times (up to 120 min) and at 60 mın the noımal serum has converted all, and the CCl_4-treated hypertensive serum has converted none of the Ang. I to Ang. II. The untreated hypertensive serum samples contain both peptides, thus exhibiting a level of CE activity between those of normal and of treated serum. Therefore, a small decrease in CE activity may be compatible with hypertension, though a more pronounced fall makes CE the rate-limiting step and produces an overall lowering of blood pressure. LOYKE (1968) suggested that CCl_4 either inhibits serum CE directly or else causes the production of an inhibitory substance from the damaged liver.

However, hepatic damage does not influence plasma CE activity in the blood from patients with cirrhosis or from rats with ligated common bile ducts as compared with the normal values (ANDERSEN, 1967). Two points must be noted about this work. Firstly, all the plasma samples are dialyzed for 24 h so that if there were a low-MW substance inhibitory to CE, it could have been lost, and secondly, as ANDERSEN himself points out, CCl_4 may produce its effect through a reaction specific to this substance and not through hepatic damage.

The results of CARRETERO et al. (1969) may make investigations of plasma CE irrelevant to the situation *in vivo*. They compared the pressor potency of Ang. I and Ang. II in normal rats and in rats given CCl_4 over eleven weeks in a manner and quantitity comparable to that used by LOYKE. No only were the relative potencies of Ang. I and Ang. II the same in treated and untreated rats, but the size of the responses to standard doses and the responses to renin were all unchanged by CCl_4 treatment. These results suggest that, even if changes in plasma CE do occur, the lung CE and hence the total *in-vivo* conversion is unchanged. The work of DAUDA et al. (1969) is more relevant to that of CARRETERO et al. than to LOYKE's, although they conclude that their results are not consistent with those of the latter author. The design of these experiments was as follows. Ang. I was generated *in vitro* by the reaction of renin and renin substrate and then converted to Ang. II, not *in vitro*, but *in vivo* in normal oı CCl_4-treated rats. The Ang. I generated was equivalent in pressor potency to 64 to 68 ng Ang. II/ml in normal rats, but to only 38 to 40 ng/ml in CCl_4-treated rats. These results conflict more with those of CARRETERO et al. on total *in-vivo* CE levels and give no information about the level of blood CE. The reduced effect of the Ang. I samples in treated rats is due, according to DAUDA et al., to increased angiotensinase activity. Experiments by CARRETERO et al. showed no sign of increased angiotensinase activity. Well designed and clearly executed experiments are needed to decide the relevance of blood CE levels to the efficacy of the renin-angiotensin system in rats with hepatic damage caused by CCl_4 or other treatments.

2. Hypertension

OSBORN et al. [1970 (2)] measured the conversion of [PTC]-Ang. I to [PTC]-Ang. II by plasma of normotensive and hypertensive subjects but were unable to correlate conversion rates with blood pressure. Plasma CE in other states has been examined by KURIHARA et al. (quoted by BOUCHER et al., 1972) in rabbits. Increases or decreases in sodium content, or hypertension caused by clipping of renal arteries had no effect on plasma CE. In patients with essential hypertension, plasma CE was also unchanged, though renal failure and severe respiratory insufficiency caused the activity to decline (DEWAILLY et al., quoted by BOUCHER et al., 1972). Following a report that oral contraceptives increased the pressor potency of exogenous renin in rats, (DOUGLAS et al., 1970) the conversion of Ang. I to Ang. II in rats treated with oral contraceptives was studied by BELL and BAKHLE (1971). Both low (1.5% mestranol) and high (4% mestranol) oestrogen formulations of norethynodrel (Enavid, Enavid E) given over three weeks caused an increased pressor response to renin and to Ang. I as against controls. However, neither CE in plasma nor the CE activity in the pulmonary circulation of isolated lungs perfused with Krebs solution from treated animals was different from that in untreated littermates.

No reports have yet appeared of variations in lung or other tissue converting enzymes *in vitro* due to physiological or pathological changes in the animal.

There has been an enormous increase in the work carried out and published on CE in the last three years (Nov. 1968—Jan. 1972). In this time, CE has developed from a semi-purified enzyme of interest to only a few, to a highly purified homogenous protein with enzymic properties relevant to both clinical medicine and enzyme biochemistry.

In concluding this review, I would like to mention the properties of CE that seem to provide best areas for further progress. In clinical medicine, the relevance of CE to the overall functioning of the renin-angiotensin system has been recognized, although no useful correlations between CE activity and blood pressure have emerged. This may be because CE activity in blood has been investigated most often whereas the CE activity in pulmonary and perhaps in peripheral vascular beds is a more effective determinant of circulating Ang. II levels. The venom-peptide inhibitors will be important tools in such investigations both *in vivo* and *in vitro*. The difference between lung and blood CE demonstrated in the results of some workers (LOYKE, 1968; CARRETERO et al., 1969; POULSEN and BING, 1970; FITZ and OVERTURF, 1972) needs further investigation *in vitro* and the inquiry could be extended to CE from those peripheral vascular beds showing significant CE activity *in vivo*. Peripheral CE activity and localized Ang. II generation become additionally significant if the interaction between Ang. II and sympathetic nerve function is a physiologically important way of modulating sympathetic activity *in vivo*.

More fundamental questions arise from the enzymic properties of CE. Although this enzyme is a carboxypeptidase, it is set apart from other carboxypeptidases by three intriguing properties: the cleavage of dipeptide units, the dependence on chloride ion, and the inability to hydrolyze peptide bonds involving proline. The most closely related enzymes are a group of aminopeptidases. This group includes Cathepsin C from liver and spleen (McDONALD et al., 1969), dipeptidyl aminopeptidase I from pituitary gland (McDONALD et al., 1968) and a glucagon-degrading enzyme from liver (KAIKUCHI and TOMIZAWA, 1964). McDONALD et al. (1969) have suggested that they are all examples of Cathepsin C. These enzymes cleave dipeptide units from the free N-terminal, have an absolute dependence on chloride and do not cleave dipeptides from proline. A further similarity to CE is that several biologically active peptides are substrates for these aminopeptidases, although in each case studied (glucagon, Ang. II, gastrin tetrapeptide, oxidized insulin, synthetic β-corticotropin and purified ACTH) enzymic attack results in biological inactivation (McDONALD et al., 1969). Though there are diffeıences between these two groups of dipeptidyl peptidases, the similarities are sufficiently striking to encourage speculation on many questions. Why are many peptide hormones metabolized by dipeptidyl peptidases? Is there significance in the removal of *two* amino-acid residues? Is the association between chloride activatıon and cleavage of dipeptides fortuitous? How does chloride ion interact with the protein and substrate?

Since both Cathepsin C and CE have now been prepared as highly purified, homogenous proteins from readily accessible sources, it should be possible to test many of the possible answers to such questions.

References

AIKEN, J. W., VANE, J. R.: The renin-angiotensin system: inhibition of converting enzyme in isolated tissues. Nature (Lond.) **228**, 30 (1970).

ALABASTER, V. A., BAKHLE, Y. S.: Converting enzyme and bradykinase in the lung. Suppl. II to Circulat. Res. **31**, II-72 (1972).

ANDERSEN, J. B.: Converting enzyme activity in liver damage. Acta path. microbiol. scand. **71**, 1 (1967).

ARAKAWA, K., MINOHARA, A., YAMADA, J., NAKAMURA, M.: Enzymatic degradation and electrophoresis of human angiotensin I. Biochim. biophys. Acta (Amst.) **168**, 96 (1968).

ARIAS, F.: Studies on the structure of the vasopressor polypeptide A. Dissertation, Tulane Univ. 1965.

BAILIE, M. D., RECTOR, Jr., F. C., SELDIN, D. W.: Angiotensin II in arterial and renal venous plasma and renal lymph in the dog. J. clin. Invest. **50**, 119 (1971).

BAKHLE, Y. S.: Conversion of angiotensin I to angiotensin II by cell-free extracts of dog lung. Nature (Lond.) **220**, 919 (1968).

BAKHLE, Y. S.: Inhibition of angiotensin I converting enzyme by venom peptides. Brit. J. Pharmacol. **43**, 252 (1971).

BAKHLE, Y. S.: Inhibition of converting enzyme by venom peptides. Hypertension 1972 541 (GENEST, J., Ed.). Berlin-Heidelberg-New York: Springer 1972.

BAKHLE, Y. S., REYNARD, A. M.: Characteristics of the angiotensin I converting enzyme from dog lung. Nature (Lond.) New Biol. **229**, 187 (1971).

BAKHLE, Y. S., REYNARD, A. M., VANE, J. R.: Metabolism of the angiotensins in isolated perfused tissues. Nature (Lond.) **222**, 956 (1969).

BANGHAM, D. R., CALAM, D. H., PARSONS, J. A., ROBINSON, C. J.: Purity of synthetic peptide preparations. Nature (Lond.) **232**, 631 (1971).

BARRETT, J. D., SAMBHI, M. P.: Simultaneous assay of angiotensin I and II and determination of converting enzyme activity. J. Pharmacol. exp. Ther. **170**, 326 (1969).

BARRETT, J. D., SAMBHI, M. P.: Pulmonary activation and degradation of angiotensin I; a dual enzyme system. Res. Commun. Chem. Path. Pharmac. **2**, 128 (1971).

BELL, C., BAKHLE, Y. S.: Increased systemic conversion of angiotensin I following oral contraceptive treatment of female rats. Proc. Aust. Soc. Clin. Exp. Pharmac. (1971).

BIRON, P.: Renal and pulmonary activation of angiotensin I. Clin. Res. **16**, 511 (1968).

BIRON, P., CAMPEAU, L.: Pulmonary and extrapulmonary fate of angiotensin I. Rev. canad. Biol. **30**, 27 (1971).
BIRON, P., HUGGINS, C. G.: Pulmonary activation of synthetic angiotensin I. Life Sci. **7**, 965 (1968).
BOUCHER, R., KURIHARA, H., GRISE, C., GENEST, J.: Measurement of plasma angiotensin I converting enzyme activity. Suppl. to Circulat. Res. **26** and **27**, 1 (1970).
BOUCHER, R., SAIDI, M., GENEST, J.: A new angiotensin I converting enzyme system. Hypertension 1972, 512 (GENEST, J., Ed.). Berlin-Heidelberg-New York: Springer 1972.
BOUCHER, R., VEYRAT, R., DE CHAMPLAIN, J., GENEST, J.: New procedures for measurement of human plasma angiotensin and renin activity levels. Canad. med. Ass. J. **90**, 194 (1964).
BRAUN-MENENDEZ, E., FASCIOLO, J. C., LELOIR, S. F., MÜNOZ, J. M., TAQUINI, A. C.: Renal hypertension. Springfield/Illinois: Thomas 1946.
BUMPUS, F. M., SCHWARZ, H., PAGE, I. H.: Partial separation of an oxytocic principle from preparations of angiotonin. Circulat. Res. **4**, 448 (1956).
BUMPUS, F. M., SMEBY, R. R., PAGE, I. H.: Angiotensin, the renal pressor hormone. Circulat. Res. **9**, 762 (1961).
BUTT, C. Y. K., HUGGINS, C. G.: Formation of vasopressor polypeptide by subtilisin Carlsberg, a proteolytic enzyme of *Bacillus subtilis*. Biochem. Pharmacol. **17**, 1709 (1968).
CAIN, M. D., CATT, K. J., COGHLAN, J. P.: Immuno-reactive fragments of angiotensin II in blood. Nature (Lond.) **223**, 617 (1969).
CARLINI, E. A., HUGGINS, C. G.: Enzymic conversion of Val^5-angiotensin I into an oxytocic principle by impure preparations of α-amylase. Biochem. Pharmacol. **II**, 171 (1962).
CARLINI, E. A., PICARELLI, Z. P., PRADO, J. L.: Pharmacological activity of hypertensin I and its conversion into hypertensin II. Bull. Chim. Biol. **40**, 1825 (1958).
CARRETERO, O. A., BUMPUS, F. M., SMEBY, R. R.: Pressor response to angiotensin I and II in rats treated with carbon tetrachloride. Nature (Lond.) **221**, 1067 (1969).
CUSHMAN, D. W., CHEUNG, H. S.: (1) Spectrophotometric assay and properties of the angiotensin converting enzyme of rabbit lung. Biochem. Pharmacol. **20**, 1673 (1971).
CUSHMAN, D. W., CHEUNG, H. S.: (2) Concentrations of angiotensin converting enzyme in tissues of the rat. Biochim. biophys. Acta (Amst.) **250**, 261 (1971).
CUSHMAN, D. W., CHEUNG, H. S.: Studies *in vitro* of angiotensin converting enzyme of lung and other tissues. Hypertension 1972, 532 (GENEST, J., Ed.). Berlin-Heidelberg-New York: Springer 1972.
DAUDA, G. Y., DEVENYI, I., SZOKOLY, V.: Converting enzyme in experimental cirrhosis. Acta physiol. Acad. Sci. hung. **35**, 365 (1969).
DEPIERRE, D., ROTH, M.: Activity of a dipeptidyl carboxypeptidase (angiotensin converting enzyme) in lungs of different animal species. Experientia (Basel) **28**, 154 (1972).
DORER, F. E., SKEGGS, L. T., KAHN, J. R., LENTZ, K. E., LEVINE, M.: Angiotensin converting enzyme. Method of assay and partial purification. Analyt. Biochem. **33**, 102 (1970).
DOUGLAS, B. H., HULL, R. P., LANGFORD, H. G.: Effect of an oral contraceptive agent on blood pressure response to renin. Proc. exp. Biol. (N. Y.) **133**, 1142 (1970).
DUSTERDIECK, G., MCELWEE, G.: Estimation of angiotensin concentration in human plasma by radio-immunoassay. Some applications to physiological and clinical studies. Europ. J. clin. Invest. **2**, 32 (1971).
ELISSEEVA, Y. E., OREKHOVICH, V. N.: Isolation of carboxycathepsin and examination of its specificity. Dokl. Akad. Nauk SSSR. **153**, 954 (1963).
ELISSEEVA, Y. E., OREKHOVICH, V. N., PAVLIKHINA, L. V., ALEXEENKO, L. P.: Carboxycathepsin — a key regulatory component of two physiological systems involved in regulation of blood pressure. Clin. chim. Acta **31**, 413 (1971).
ENGEL, S. L., SCHAEFFER, T. R., GOLD, B. I., RUBIN, B.: Inhibition of angiotensin converting enzyme *in vivo* by peptides from snake venom. Proc. 25th. Int. Cong. Physiol. Sci. **2**, 163 (1971).
ERDÖS, E. G., YANG, H. Y. T.: Inactivation and potentiation of the effects of bradykinin. In: "Hypotensive Peptides", ed. by ERDÖS, E. G., BACK, N., SICUTERI, F., WILDE, A. F., S. 235. Berlin-Heidelberg-New York: Springer 1966.
ERDÖS, E. G., YANG, H. Y. T.: An enzyme in the microsomal fraction of kidney that inactivates bradykinin. Life Sci. **6**, 569 (1967).
FERREIRA, S. H.: A bradykinin potentiating factor (BPF) in the venom of *Bothrops jararaca*. Brit. J. Pharmacol. **24**, 163 (1965).
FERREIRA, S. H., BARTELT, DIANA C., GREENE, L. J.: (1) Isolation of bradykinin potentiating peptides from *Bothrops jararaca* venom. Biochemistry **9**, 2583 (1970).
FERREIRA, S. H., GREENE, L. J., ALABASTER, VALERIE A., BAKHLE, Y. S., VANE, J. R.: (2) Activity of various fractions of Bradykinin Potentiating Factor against angiotensin I converting enzyme. Nature (Lond.) **225**, 379 (1970).

Fitz, Annette, Boyd, G. W., Peart, W. S.: Converting enzyme activity in human plasma. Circulat. Res. **28**, 246 (1971).
Fitz, Annette, Overturf, M.: Human lung converting enzyme. J. Lab. clin. Med. **76**, 1035 (1970).
Fitz, Annette, Overturf, M.: (1) Human lung converting enzyme. Hypertension 1972, 507 (Genest, J., Ed.). Berlin-Heidelberg-New York: Springer 1972.
Fitz, Annette, Overturf, M.: (2) Molecular weight of human angiotensin I converting enzyme. J. biol. Chem. **247**, 581 (1972).
Granger, P., Dahlheim, H., Thurau, K.: Contenu en rénine ,angiotensinases et "converting enzyme", de l'appareil juxtaglomérulaire (AJG) du rat. Un. méd. Can. **100**, 786 (1971).
Gregermann, R. I.: Identification of histidylleucine and other histidyl peptides as normal constituents of human urine. Biochem. Med. **1**, 151 (1967).
Guttmann, S.: Synthèse de la Val[5]-D-Phe[8]-angiotensine I et nouvelle synthèse de la Val[5]-angiotensine I. Helv. chim. Acta **44**, 721 (1961).
Helmer, O. M.: A factor in plasma that enhances contraction produced by angiotonin on rabbit aortic strips. Fed. Proc. **14**, 728 (1955).
Helmer, O. M.: Differentiation between two forms of angiotonin by means of spirally cut strips of rabbit aorta. Amer. J. Physiol. **188**, 571 (1957).
Hollemans, H. J. G., van der Meer, J., Kloosterziel, W.: Identification of the incubation product of Boucher's renin activity assay by means of radio-immunoassays for angiotensin I and angiotensin II, and a converting enzyme preparation from lung tissue. Clin. chim. Acta **23**, 7 (1969).
Horky, K., Rojo-Ortega, J. M., Rodriguez, J., Boucher, R., Genest, J.: Renin, renin substrate and angiotensin I converting enzyme in the lymph of rats. Amer. J. Physiol. **220**, 307 (1971).
Huggins, C. G., Corcoran, R. J., Gordon, J. S., Henry, H. W., John, J. P.: Kinetics of the plasma and lung angiotensin I converting enzymes. Suppl. to Circulat. Res. **26** and **27**, I—93 (1970).
Huggins, C. G., Thampi, N. S.: A simple method for the determination of angiotensin I converting enzyme. Life Sci. **7**, 633 (1968).
Huggins, C. G., Walaszek, E. J.: Formation of a pharmacologically active substance from plasma protein. Proc. Soc. exp. Biol. (N. Y.) **100**, 100 (1959).
Hurwitz, E., Dietrich, F. M., Sela, M.: A sensitive technique for detecting and estimating the peptide hormone angiotensin II-beta-amide and its antibodies by using chemically modified bacteriophage and activated sepharose. Europ. J. Biochem. **17**, 273 (1970).
Igic, R., Erdös, E. G., Yeh, H. S. J., Sorrells, K., Nakajima, T.: The angiotensin I converting enzyme of the lung. Suppl. II to Circulat. Res. **31**, II-51 (1972).
Johnson, M. J.: Isolation and properties of a pure yeast polypeptidase. J. biol. Chem. **137**, 575 (1941).
Kaikuchi, S., Tomizawa, H. H.: Properties of a glucagon-degrading enzyme of beef liver. J. biol. Chem. **239**, 2160 (1964).
Kato, H., Suzuki, T.: Bradykinin-potentiating peptides from venom of *A. halys blomhoffii*. Isolation of five bradykinin potentiators and the amino acid sequence of two of them, potentiators B and C. Biochemistry **10**, 972 (1971).
Kimura, T., Kato, H., Sakakibara, S., Suzuki, T.: Synthesis of bradykinin-potentiating peptides isolated from the venom of *Agkistrodon halys blomhoffii*. In Press. Proc. 2nd. Amer. Peptide Symp. Cleveland (1970).
Krieger, E. M., Salgado, H. C., Assan, C. J., Greene, L. J., Ferreira, S. H.: Potential screening test for detection of overactivity of renin-angiotensin system. Lancet **1971**, 269.
Lee, H. J., Larue, J. N., Wilson, I. B.: (1) Human plasma converting enzyme. Arch. Biochem. Biophys. **142**, 548 (1971).
Lee, H. J., Larue, J. N., Wilson, I. B.: (2) Angiotensin converting enzyme from porcine plasma. Biochim. biophys. Acta (Amst.) **35**, 521 (1971).
Lee, H. J., Larue, J. N., Wilson, I. B.: Angiotensin converting enzyme from guinea pig and hog lung. Biochim. biophys. Acta (Amst.) **250**, 549 (1971).
Lee, H. J., Larue, J. N., Wilson, I. B.: (4) Dipeptidyl carboxypeptidase from *Corynebacterium equi*. Biochim. biophys. Acta (Amst.) **250**, 608 (1971).
Lentz, K. E., Skeggs, L. T., Woods, K. R., Kahn, J. R., Shumway, N. P.: The amino acid composition of hypertension II and its biochemical relationship to hypertensin I. J. exp. Med. **104**, 183 (1956).
Loyke, H. F.: Experimental hypertension treated with CCl_4: measurements of adrenal function, vascular responsiveness, angiotensinase and converting enzyme. Proc. Soc. exp. Biol. (N. Y.) **115**, 1035 (1964).
Loyke, H. F.: Converting enzyme in CCl_4-treated renal hypertension. Amer. J. Physiol. **215**, 1334 (1968).

LOYKE, H. F.: Converting enzyme in rat serum. Proc. Soc. exp. Biol. (N. Y.) **134**, 248 (1970).
MCDONALD, J. K., ELLIS, S., REILLY, T. J.: Properties of dipeptidyl arylamidase I of the pituitary. J. biol. Chem. **241**, 1494 (1966).
MCDONALD, J. K., ZEITMAN, B. B., REILLY, T. J., ELLIS, S.: New observations of the substrate specificity of Cathepsin C (Dipeptidyl aminopeptidase I). J. biol. Chem. **244**, 2693 (1969).
MERRIFIELD, R. B.: Solid phase peptide synthesis I. The synthesis of a tetrapeptide. J. Amer. chem. Soc. **85**, 2149 (1963).
NG, K. K. F., VANE, J. R.: Conversion of angiotensin I to angiotensin II. Nature (Lond.) **216**, 762 (1967).
NG, K. K. F., VANE, J. R.: Some properties of angiotensin converting enzyme *in vivo*. Nature (Lond.) **225**, 1142 (1970).
ONDETTI, E. C., WILLIAMS, N. J., SABO, E. F., PLUSCEC, J., WEAVER, E. R., KOCY, O.: Angiotensin converting enzyme inhibitors from the venom of *Bothrops jararaca*. Isolation, elucidation of structure and synthesis. Biochemistry **19**, 4033 (1971).
OPARIL, S., SANDERS, C. A., HABER, E.: *In vivo* and *in vitro* conversion of angiotensin I to angiotensin II in dog blood. Circulat. Res. **26**, 591 (1970).
OPARIL, S., TREGEAR, G. W., KOERNER, T., BARNES, B. A., HABER, E.: Mechanism of pulmonary conversion of angiotensin I to angiotensin II in the dog. Circulat. Res. **29**, 682 (1971).
OREKHOVICH, V. N.: The proteolytic enzymes. Ital. J. Biochem. **17**, 241 (1968).
OSBORN, E. C., HODGES, N. G., PICKENS, P. T., WILLICOMBE, P. R., MAHLER, R. F.: (2) Conversion of [^{35}S] PTC-angiotensin I to PTC-angiotensin II in plasma of normotensive and hypertensive subjects. Clin. Sci. **38**, 217 (1970).
OSBORN, E. C., LOUIS, W. J., DOYLE, A. E.: Preparation, isolation and properties of phenylthiocarbamyl angiotensin. J. exp. Biol. Med. Sci. **44**, 475 (1966).
OSBORN, E. C., PICKENS, P. T., WILLICOMBE, P. R., PIRIE, A. T., MAHLER, R. F.: (1) Studies with angiotensin I and II; the use of phenylthiocarbamyl — derivatives. Clin. Sci. **38**, 211 (1970).
PAVESI, L., HUGGINS, C. G.: Kinetic studies on the formation and destruction of the vasopressor polypeptide Substance A. Biochem. Pharmacol. **17**, 1699 (1968).
PEACH, M. J.: Adrenal medullary stimulation induced by angiotensin I, angiotensin II and analogues. Suppl. to Circulat. Res. **28**, II—107 (1971).
PEACH, M. J., BUMPUS, F. M., KHAIRALLAH, P. A.: Release of adrenal catecholamines by angiotensin I. J. Pharmacol. exp. Ther. **176**, 366 (1971).
PEART, W. S.: Isolation of hypertensin. Biochem. J. **62**, 520 (1955).
PEART, W. S.: The renin-angiotensin system. Pharmacol. Rev. **17**, 143 (1965).
PIQUILLOUD, Y., REINHARZ, A., ROTH, M.: Studies on the angiotensin converting enzyme with different substrates. Biochem. biophys. Acta (Amst.) **206**, 136 (1970).
POULSEN, J., BING, J.: Species specific differences in converting enzyme and angiotensin I. Acta path. microbiol. scand. A **78**, 665 (1970).
POULSEN, J., POULSEN, L. L.: Simultaneous determination of plasma converting enzyme and angiotensinase activity by radio-immunoassay. Clin. Sci. **40**, 443 (1970).
RAASCHOU, F.: Blood pressure and heart weight in chronic hepatitis. Nord. Med. **42**, 1791 (1949).
ROTH, M., WEITZMANN, A. F., PIQUILLOUD, Y.: Converting enzyme content of different tissues of the rat. Experientia (Basel) **25**, 1247 (1969).
RYAN, J. W., NIEMEYER, R. S., GOODWIN, D. W., SMITH, U., STEWART, J. M.: Metabolism of [8-L(C^{14})] Phenylalanine — angiotensin I in the pulmonary circulation. Biochem. J. **125**, 921 (1971).
RYAN, J. W., SMITH, U.: A rapid simple method for isolating pinocytotic vesicles and plasma membrane of lung. Biochim. biophys. Acta (Amst.) **249**, 177 (1971).
SANDER, G. E., HUGGINS, C. G.: Subcellular localisation of angiotensin I converting enzyme in rabbit lung. Nature (Lond.) New Biol. **230**, 27 (1971).
SANDER, G. E., HUGGINS, C. G.: Vasoactive peptides. Ann. Rev. Pharmacol. in Press (1972).
SANDER, G. E., WEST, D. W., HUGGINS, C. G.: Peptide inhibitors of pulmonary angiotensin I converting enzyme. Biochim. biophys. Acta (Amst.) **242**, 662 (1971).
SCHWYZER, R.: Synthetische analogs des hypertensins. Helv. chim. Acta **44**, 667 (1961).
SCHWYZER, R., TURRIAN, H.: The chemistry and pharmacology of angiotensin. Vitam. and Horm. (N. Y.) **18**, 237 (1960).
SKEGGS, L. T., KAHN, J. R., SHUMWAY, N. P.: Purification of hypertensin II. J. exp. Med. **103**, 301 (1956).
SKEGGS, L. T., LENTZ, K. E., GOULD, A. B., HOCHSTRASSER, H., KAHN, J. R.: Biochemistry and kinetics of the renin-angiotensin system. Fed. Proc. **26**, 42 (1967).

SKEGGS, L. T., LENTZ, K. E., KAHN, J. R., DORER, F. E., LEVINE, M.: Pseudorenin. A new angiotensin-forming enzyme. Circulat. Res. **25**, 451 (1969).
SKEGGS, L. T., MARSH, W. H., KAHN, J. R., SHUMWAY, N. P.: The existence of two forms of hypertensin. J. exp. Med. **99**, 275 (1954).
SKEGGS, L. T., MARSH, W. H., KAHN, J. R., SHUMWAY, N. P.: Amino acid composition and electrophoretic properties of hypertensin I. J. exp. Med. **102**, 435 (1955).
SMITH, U., RYAN, J. W.: An electron microscope study of the vascular endothelium as a site for bradykinin and adenosine-5-triphosphate inactivation in rat lungs. Pharmac. Res. Commun. **I**, 197 (1969).
THAMPI, N. S., HUGGINS, C. G.: The angiotensin I converting enzyme activity of subtilisin BPN′ (Nagarse), a crystalline enzyme of *Bacillus subtilis*. Biochem. Pharmacol. **17**, 2018 (1968).
UEDA, E., AKUTSU, H., KOKUBU, T., YAMAMURA, Y.: (1) Partial purification and properties of angiotensin I converting enzyme from rabbit plasma. Jap. Circulat. J. **35**, 801 (1971).
UEDA, E., KOKUBU, T., AKUTSU, H., HIWADA, K., YAMAMURA, Y.: The purification and properties of angiotensin I converting enzyme. Jap. Circulat. J. **34**, 849 (1970).
UEDA, E., KOKUBU, T., AKUTSU, H., YAMAMURA, Y.: (2) Inhibition of angiotensin I converting enzyme and kininase in rabbit plasma by bradykinin potentiating peptide B (Pyr-Gly-Leu-Pro-Arg-Lys-Ile-Pro-Pro). Experientia (Basel) **27**, 1020 (1971).
VANE, J. R.: Purity and stability of synthetic peptides such as angiotensins and kinins. Nature (Lond.) **230**, (1971).
VANE, J. R.: The fate of angiotensin I. This volume (1972).
WALASZEK, E. J., BUNAG, R. D., HUGGINS, C. G.: The characterisation of the hypertensive polypeptide Substance A. J. Pharmacol. exp. Ther. **138**, 139 (1962).
WALASZEK, E. J., HUGGINS, C. G.: Further studies on the vasopressor polypeptide Substance A. Fed. Proc. **19**, 124 (1960).
WEBB, E. C., MORROW, P. F.: The inactivation of an arysulphatase from ox liver by chloride and other ions. Biochem. J. **73**, 7 (1959).
WISENBAUGH, P. E., WILLIS, E. N., HILL, R. W.: Paper chromatographic identifications of angiotensins. Amer. J. Physiol. **207**, 759 (1964).
YANG, H. Y. T., ERDÖS, E. G.: Second kininase in human blood plasma. Nature (Lond.) **215**, 1402 (1967).
YANG, H. Y. T., ERDÖS, E. G., LEVIN, Y.: Characterisation of a dipeptide hydrolase (Kininase II: angiotensin I converting enzyme). J. Pharmacol. exp. Ther. **177**, 291 (1971).

Papers published up to January 1972 and the proceedings of two meetings held in 1971 (published later in 1972) have been included in this review.

The Fate of Angiotensin II

J. W. RYAN

With 3 Figures

I. Introduction

Virtually all existing evidence on the fate of Ang. II *in vivo* bears on the more restricted question of what happens to Ang. II once it enters the circulation. At present, there is little or no evidence on the fate of angiotensin within cells or in body fluids other than blood. For reasons to be discussed, the question of what happens to angiotensin in the circulation is by no means simple as its fate depends to a large degree on where it enters the circulation and on the concentrations achieved. Angiotensin entering portal venous blood has a much shorter half-life than that formed in systemic venous blood (CHAMBERLAIN et al., 1964; METHOT et al., 1964; HODGE et al., 1967). Similarly, angiotensin entering the pulmonary artery has a longer half-life than that formed subsequently within the pulmonary circulation or in the systemic arterial circulation.

In the discussion that follows, the term angiotensin is used to mean

1 2 3 4 5 6 7 8
H-Asp-Arg-Val-Tyr-Ile-His-Pro-Phe-OH

or its Val[5] analog. [Val[5]]-Ang. II has never been isolated from natural sources but is presumed to occur. CAIN et al. (1970) have reported indirect evidence of its occurrence in sheep. At present, there is little reason to believe that the fate of [Val[5]]-Ang. II differs from that of [Ile[5]]-Ang. II. [Ile[5]]-Ang. II occurs in horse (LENTZ et al., 1956; SKEGGS et al., 1956), pig (BUMPUS et al., 1957, 1958) and man (ARAKAWA et al., 1967, 1968). Whether it is the natural form in lower animals is not known, and this may be a problem as most of the studies of the fate of Ang. II have been performed using cats, dogs, rabbits and rats.

In many respects, the techniques and reagents required for definitive studies of the fate of angiotensin are just becoming available. The introduction of two new histidine derivatives, N^{im}-DNP-histidine (R. N. PIASIO, M. LOMBARDO and J. M. STEWART, unpublished, cited by STEWART and YOUNG, 1969) and N^{im}-tosyl-histidine (SAKAKIBARA and FUJII, 1969) has vastly simplified the synthesis of angiotensin, which can now be made in quantity. Simpler synthetic techniques have, in turn, made the production of intrinsically-labelled analogs more economical. Concurrently, there have been improvements in techniques for the purification and identification of peptides which occur in biological extracts in less than picamole quantities [RYAN et al., 1968 (2), 1970 (1, 2), 1971 (2)]. As well, there have been improvements of methods of preparing homogeneous subcellular fractions (SCHNEIDER and KUFF, 1964) and of localizing specific enzymes and radioactive hormones by electron microscopy (SHNITKA and SELIGMAN, 1971; CARO, 1966; SALPETER et al., 1969). Thus, in a technical sense, studies of the fate of Ang. II are just coming of age.

Therefore, this section has been written with two purposes in mind: 1) to review the current status of the field, and 2) to attempt to provide technical guidelines for future studies.

II. Technical Aspects

Present evidence indicates that the greatest proportion of Ang. II is removed from the circulation by enzymic mechanisms, primarily hydrolytic. None of the hydrolase enzymes described so far are known to be specific for Ang. II but are, nonetheless, commonly referred to as angiotensinase enzymes. The term angiotensinase is used here as a general classification of peptidase and protease enzymes capable of catalyzing the hydrolysis of any of the seven peptide bonds of Ang. II.

Historically, the term angiotensinase had a much broader meaning and included oxidase enzymes (see BRAUN-MENENDEZ et al., 1946 for review). In fact, enzymes other than hydrolases have not been considered since the primary structure of Ang. II was established, a point that may merit reinvestigation. Judging from results of studies using synthetic analogs, enzymic side-chain and end-group modifications could markedly reduce biological activity (see Chapter 5, Section A: *Analogues and their Activity*, F. M. BUMPUS, this volume).

Still, the dominant consideration in understanding the means by which Ang. II is inactivated is that it is a linear octapeptide, the complete, unmodified structure of which is required for full biological activity (see Chapter 5, this volume). Only one of its lower homologs (the C-terminal heptapeptide) retains much biological activity. Therefore hydrolysis of any of the other six peptide bonds yields products having no intrinsic angiotensin-like activity. Whether any of the lower homologs can potentiate or antagonize the action of angiotensin is a question of possible importance, as the effects of another polypeptide, bradykinin, are potentiated by its C-terminal pentapeptide (GARBE, 1967).

A. The Problem of Lower Homologs

A point that has been frequently overlooked in studies of hydrolytic degradation of angiotensin (and other polypeptide hormones) is that a linear octapeptide having no repeating amino acids has 35 possible lower homologs (see Table 1), all of which must be accounted for in any attempt to determine the exact mechanisms of hydrolysis. The problem of lower homologs becomes more complicated as the size of the parent polypeptide increases, Ang. I having 54 lower homologs. Even the relatively simple question of conversion of Ang. I to Ang. II becomes complicated if any bond other than Phe^8-His^9 is hydrolyzed in a concurrent or sequential reaction [RYAN et al., 1970 (2), 1971 (2), 1972 (2)].

As one begins to consider side-chain and end-group modifications of Ang. II as well as hydrolytic reactions, the numbers of possible metabolites increase enormously; there being eight additional homologs to consider for each end-group modification and twenty more homologs should there be modifications of the tyrosyl residue.

B. The Problem of Labelled Analogs

Most of the existing evidence on the fate of angiotensin in the circulation is based on bioassay results. The merit of this approach is that a biological assessment is needed to evaluate the appearance or disappearance of a hormonal substance. There is the further point that results of dynamic bioassay systems, such as those used by CHAMBERLAIN et al. (1964) and VANE and his colleagues (VANE, 1964, 1969), have brought out the point that the appearance and disappearance of Ang. II occur very rapidly indeed. However, studies using bioassays as their only means of detection and measurement suffer from several disadvantages. Firstly, through the nature of the approach, only relatively large changes of angiotensin-like

Table 1. *Ile*[5]*-Ang. II and its lower homologs*

Residue No.	1	2	3	4	5	6	7	8
8	Asp-	Arg-	Val-	Tyr-	Ile-	His-	Pro-	Phe
7	Asp-	Arg-	Val-	Tyr-	Ile-	His-	Pro	
7		Arg-	Val-	Tyr-	Ile-	His-	Pro-	Phe
6			Val-	Tyr-	Ile-	His-	Pro-	Phe
6	Asp-	Arg-	Val-	Tyr-	Ile-	His		
6		Arg-	Val-	Tyr-	Ile-	His-	Pro	
5				Tyr-	Ile-	His-	Pro-	Phe
5	Asp-	Arg-	Val-	Tyr-	Ile			
5			Val-	Tyr-	Ile-	His-	Pro	
5		Arg-	Val-	Tyr-	Ile-	His		
4					Ile-	His-	Pro-	Phe
4	Asp-	Arg-	Val-	Tyr				
4				Tyr-	Ile-	His-	Pro	
4		Arg-	Val-	Tyr-	Ile			
4			Val-	Tyr-	Ile-	His		
3						His-	Pro-	Phe
3	Asp-	Arg-	Val					
3					Ile-	His-	Pro	
3		Arg-	Val-	Tyr				
3				Tyr-	Ile-	His		
3			Val-	Tyr-	Ile			
2							Pro-	Phe
2	Asp-	Arg						
2						His-	Pro	
2		Arg-	Val					
2					Ile-	His		
2			Val-	Tyr				
2				Tyr-	Ile			
1	Asp							
1		Arg						
1			Val					
1				Tyr				
1					Ile			
1						His		
1							Pro	
1								Phe
Homolog No.	8	14	18	20	20	18	14	8

activity can be detected. Secondly, the term "angiotensin-like" becomes operative. Even in studies following the fate of pure angiotensin administered intravenously or intra-arterially there is the uncertainty that not all of the biological activity subsequently measured in blood is owing to angiotensin. The problem is not much simplified in studies of the fate of angiotensin during passage through isolated organs perfused with artificial salt solutions, as it is evident that angiotensin can stimulate the release of endogenous substances that have angiotensin-like effects on a given bioassay preparation [RYAN et al., 1970 (2); TÜRKER et al., 1971].

Thirdly, there are problems of sensitivity and specificity. Under physiologic conditions, Ang. II occurs in blood in concentrations of 10^{-10} to 10^{-12} g/ml. Bioassay preparations such as the rat colon and rat blood pressure cannot be relied upon to measure angiotensin at concentrations much lower than 10^{-9} g/ml. BEAULNES and BEEBE (1970) have reported that rabbit atria are much more sensitive, inotropic effects of angiotensin being detectable at 10^{-17} g/ml. This finding needs confirmation. No single bioassay preparation is specific for Ang. II. Selectivity can be increased by using two or more bioassay preparations and by the use of inhibitors to reduce effects of other known biologically active substances (VANE, 1964, 1969). Still there is the problem of unknown excitatory substances. The problem of specificity of response may possibly be solved by the use of specific antagonists of angiotensin itself, and five such compounds are under evaluation [MARSHALL et al., 1970; BUMPUS et al., 1971; STEWART et al., 1971 (2); PALS et al., 1971 (1, 2)] but are not yet widely available.

Should all the above-listed disadvantages of bioassay be corrected, one problem would remain: studies relying only on bioassay results provide little or no evidence on the precise mechanisms by which angiotensin appears in or disappears from the circulation.

For reasons such as these, it has been pointed out repeatedly that definitive studies of the distribution and fate of Ang. II require a suitably-labelled Ang. II (BARBOUR and BARTTER, 1963; BUMPUS et al., 1964).

Finding means of labelling Ang. II (or any other polypeptide hormone) has not been easy. For the purpose of the following discussion, it may be useful to consider minimum requirements. The labelled compound should 1) retain full biological activity, 2) have the same physicochemical properties as the natural compound, and 3) have a specific activity high enough to allow its quantitative measurement at the low concentrations at which the compound occurs normally *in vivo*. As well, it would be a great technical advantage if the labelled compound were reasonably stable.

Angiotensins labelled extrinsically, e.g. with ^{131}I or ^{125}I, are eliminated by the first two criteria. Using mild iodination procedures, the monoiodo-analog retains much of its biological activity and can be made at very high specific activities (LIN et al., 1970; KURCBART et al., 1971). However, iodinated Ang. II is not Ang. II, and those who use an iodo-analog find themselves in the position of having to prove that its fate is the same as that of Ang. II. Whether naturally occurring iodinase enzymes (NAKAGAWA and RUEGAMER, 1967) confuse the study of fate has not been investigated.

It has been suggested that Ang. II should be labelled intrinsically such that each amino acid residue is labelled at the same specific activity as any other residue (BUMPUS et al., 1964). It is probably technically feasible to prepare such a compound using ^{3}H- or ^{14}C-labelled amino acid derivatives during synthesis. However, because of the small concentrations to be used and other reasons to be discussed below, each residue should be labelled at a specific activity allowing its measurement as a free amino acid. Using ^{14}C, each residue should have a specific activity of about 10 Ci/mmole. ^{3}H-tagged residues would run to 40 or 50 Ci/mmole, with angiotensin having a specific activity of $\sim$400 Ci/mmole. The expense of synthesis would be prohibitive, and one can only guess at the seriousness of radiolysis and the consequent purification and repurification problems.

Following the fate of a uniformly-labelled angiotensin raises serious problems of isolation and identification of homologs. As shown in Table 1, restricting metabolic considerations to hydrolytic reactions, Ang. II has 35 possible metabolites. Whereas it is unlikely that all 35 homologs are formed during degradation, those formed must be distinguished from all possible metabolites. All of the eight free amino acids can be identified readily using an amino acid analyzer with a scintillation flow cell attachment. Conceivably, the seven dipeptides could be identified similarly (MANNING and MOORE, 1968). The six tripeptides, five tetrapeptides, etc., could be very difficult to separate, as there is a wide overlap of size, charge and solubility properties.

1. Specific Activity

There is some disagreement about the concentrations of Ang. II in blood under physiologic conditions. Methods of assay of Ang. II and their results is the concern of another chapter (Chapter 6, this volume). Suffice it to say here that few of the recent studies indicate that the concentration of angiotensin in blood exceeds 300 pg ($\sim$0.3 pmole)/ml, and this high level is achieved only under the stimulus of salt depletion (GOCKE et al., 1968, 1969). BOYD et al. (1967), CATT et al. (1967) and CAIN et al. (1970) reckon concentrations to be more commonly about 10 to 50 pg/ml. Therefore, if we assume the lower figures to be correct, a ^{3}H-labelled Ang. II, for use in studies of distribution and fate, should have a specific activity of about 50 Ci/mmole. Using carbon-14, a specific activity of 10 Ci/mmole would be acceptable for measuring angiotensin itself. Radioactive Ang. II currently available from commercial sources does not approach the necessary specific activity. Recently FROMAGEOT's group (MORGAT et al., 1970) described a labelling method in which [diiodo-Tyr^{4}]-Ang. II is dehalogenated in tritium gas. The resulting [^{3}H]-angiotensin can be obtained at activities >50 Ci/mmole.

2. Random Tritiation

Angiotensin II has been tritiated using a modified Wilzbach technique (KHAIRALLAH et al., 1962) yielding a biologically-active, radiochemically homogeneous peptide having a specific activity of 300 μCi/mg ($\sim$300 μCi/μmole). The specific activity of the whole molecule approaches that needed to detect Ang. II at the concentrations likely to occur *in vivo*. However, through the nature of the labelling process, each of the amino acid residues has a much lower specific activity, and single amino acids may be well out of the range of detection by usual scintillation techniques. Using Wilzbach techniques, there is also the well-recognized problem of tritium exchange.

3. Labelling During Synthesis

At present, the radioactive angiotensins available from commercial sources are labelled in one residue during synthesis. The major advantage of the technique is that angiotensin can be labelled in any residue. As indicated above, the radioactive compounds available at present are of low specific activity. The problem of low specific activity should not persist as radioactive amino acids of much higher specific activity are already available.

Radioactive angiotensins labelled in a single residue have the disadvantage that their unlabelled metabolites cannot be traced. As a consequence, it is difficult or impossible to be certain of the sites of primary hydrolysis. Single-step reactions by an aminopeptidase or carboxypeptidase enzyme can be established. However, the theoretical metabolite, H-Ile-His-Pro-Phe-OH, could be formed by the action of an aminopeptidase, endopeptidase or both. Nonetheless, there is a mathematical advantage for isolating and identifying radioactive metabolites. For example, Ang. II labelled in residues 1 or 8 has only seven possible radioactive lower homologs. When the label is in residue 2 or 7 there are 13 possibilities. Labels in residue 4 or 5 (Tyr or Ile) give the least practical advantage as each has 19 possible radioactive lower homologs.

Although angiotensin labelled in a single residue can seldom be used to determine primary sites of hydrolysis, it can be useful for distinguishing between mechanisms of disappearance, e.g. enzymic degradation vs. transfer to other extracellular spaces, cellular uptake, etc. Furthermore the feasibility of using such compounds for some types of autoradiography has been demonstrated (ROBERTSON and KHAIRALLAH, 1971).

Radioactive angiotensin prepared by peptide synthesis is subject to the same problems as any other synthetic polypeptide. Error peptides formed during synthesis may be difficult to separate and may not be biologically inactive. The error peptides, especially those formed by racemization, may be more resistant to enzymic degradation and thereby confuse attempts to establish elimination mechanisms *in vivo*.

As well, both natural and synthetic Ang. II are subject to $\alpha \rightarrow \beta$ shifts of the peptide linkage of aspartic acid. The β-Asp^1-Ang. II is formed on exposure to mineral acids (MARSHALL and MERRIFIELD, 1965) and may also be formed during prolonged storage at pH values near neutrality (RINIKER and SCHWYZER, 1964). This analog is resistant to degradation by aminopeptidase enzymes (KHAIRALLAH et al., 1963).

Some of the technical problems of working with synthetic polypeptide hormones have been reviewed by VANE (1971) and BANGHAM et al. (1971).

4. Labelling by Catalytic Hydrogenation

As mentioned above, MORGAT et al. (1970) have described a method of producing [^{3}H-Tyr^4]-Ang. II by dehalogenating [diiodo-Tyr^4]-Ang. II during catalytic hydrogenation in a tritium atmosphere. The specific activity of the [^{3}H]-Ang. II (56.3 Ci/mmole) approaches the theoretical maximum expected for the addition of two ^{3}H atoms (30 Ci/atom). This radioactive angiotensin would appear to meet the three minimum requirements, namely full biological activity, identical physicochemical properties, and high specific activity. As well, the [^{3}H]-angiotensin is reasonably stable, losing only 10% of its biological activity when stored in 1 mM acetic acid-acetate buffer, pH 4.6, at $-60°$ for three months.

The MORGAT procedure should be applicable to the tritiation of angiotensin I and the tetradecapeptide renin substrate. The latter compound, having two tyrosines, could be used as an exquisitely sensitive substrate for the assay of renin (SKEGGS et al., 1957, 1958), its isoenzymes [RYAN, 1967 (1), 1970; RYAN and JOHNSON, 1969; CARRETERO et al., 1971 (1)] and pseudorenin (SKEGGS et al., 1969).

[^{3}H-Tyr^4]-angiotensin has the technical disadvantages of any other angiotensin labelled in a single residue. It can seldom be used to establish precise cleavage sites, and since the label is near the center of the molecule, there are 19 possible radioactive lower homologs.

There is the further point that the MORGAT procedure may label residues other than tyrosine. Although MORGAT et al. showed that their iodination technique produced the bathochromic shift characteristic of diiodinated tyrosine, they did not rule out the concurrent iodination of histidine. Similarly, it was not shown that all of the radioactivity conferred by subsequent catalytic tritiation was restricted to tyrosine. Histidine is readily iodinated and iodinated histidine, like iodotyrosine, is reduced by catalytic tritiation (PRADELLES et al., 1972). Clearly, the use of [^{3}H-Tyr^4,His^6]-Ang. II, assumed to be [^{3}H-Tyr^4]-Ang. II, could yield misleading results in metabolic studies.

The procedure of MORGAT et al. is reminiscent of the catalytic tritiation of [8-(Br)phenylalanine]-Ang. II (RINIKER and SCHWYZER, unpublished, cited by BUMPUS and SMEBY, 1968). Apparently the product was unstable but this should be reinvestigated.

C. Strategies for Identifying Metabolites

In principle, the problem of isolating and identifying angiotensin II and its metabolites is the same as for any other polypeptide or protein and should yield to the same approaches (see HIRS, 1967; HARTLEY, 1970). In following the fate of angiotensin, one starts with the advantage of knowing the primary structure, therefore end-group determinations should suffice for identification. The difficulty comes in terms of concentrations and relative abundance in biological fluids and tissue extracts.

As one is dealing with an exquisitely potent hormonal substance, the concentrations of angiotensin used for infusion should not greatly exceed that achieved in blood under physiologic conditions (0.001 to 0.1 picamoles/ml). At present there is no reason to believe that angiotensin occurs in higher concentrations in tissues or other body fluids except possibly in renal lymph (BAILIE et al., 1971). Established methods of isolation cannot deal with these quantities. Methods of identifying end-group residues are near the required sensitivity but require homogeneous peptides (see NARITA, 1970 for review).

Starting with blood, Ang. II and its metabolites may represent less than 10^{-12} of the wet weight. Furthermore, both blood and tissues contain peptidase enzymes that must be prevented from causing artifactual degradation during and following sample collection. In general, Ang. II is not very soluble in organic solvents and partitions poorly even in partially-miscible two-phase solvent systems. Some possible metabolites, e.g. the neutral homologs, Asp-Arg-Val-Tyr-Ile, Val-Tyr-Ile and Tyr-Ile, are much more soluble in organic solvents (J. M. STEWART and J. W. RYAN, unpublished), a point that must be taken into account in any attempt at "blind" group purifications. As well, because of the low concentrations and the tendency of angiotensin in dilute solution to adsorb to glass and similar materials, recoveries through separation procedures may be poor.

Problems of contaminants may persist or become more severe during purification because impurities of reagent grade solvents and buffers may exceed the concentrations of angiotensin and its metabolites. Electrophoresis or chromatography on paper can be hazardous, as paper, even after extensive washing, contains amino acids or amino acid polymers. Conversely, elution of small quantities of angiotensin from paper is seldom quantitative (WISENBAUGH et al., 1964).

There are numerous established methods for partial purification of angiotensin from biological extracts (SKEGGS et al., 1952; BOUCHER et al., 1964; BOYD et al.. 1967). Whether these methods are applicable to the parallel purification of all possible metabolites produced by hydrolysis requires investigation. Unfortunately, the surest methods that have been used for the isolation of milligram quantities of angiotensin (e.g. a 700-transfer countercurrent distribution, SKEGGS et al., 1956) cannot be applied to picagram quantities without finding ways of reducing volumes of solvents and exposure to glass. In this regard, the new microcountercurrent techniques of ITO may prove of value (ITO and BOWMAN, 1971).

Judging from previous studies of the fates of radioactive bradykinin [RYAN et al., 1968 (2), 1970 (1)], Ang. I [RYAN et al., 1970 (2), 1971 (2); BARRETT and SAMBHI, 1971; SANDER and HUGGINS, 1971], and one study of Ang. II (OSBORNE et al., 1970), it may not be necessary to isolate angiotensin and its metabolites in order to make identifications. By combining simple desalting and deproteinizing steps with group-purification procedures and selective detection methods, metabolites can be identified tentatively and, sometimes unequivocally, by excluding other possible homologs.

Procedures for removing salt and protein have included selective extractions [RYAN et al., 1970 (2), 1971 (2)], adsorption (PEART, 1955; BOYD, 1967) and gel chromatography (OSBORNE et al., 1970). Gel chromatography offers the further advantage of separation of metabolites by size but effects poor separations of the parent polypeptide and its large homologs from protein and small homologs from salt. Adsorption techniques work well for separating angiotensin from protein and salt but the efficacy of the technique for separating lower homologs has not been tested.

Angiotensin II has a moderately favorable distribution of charged amino acid residues, and group separations can be accomplished by electrophoresis and by ion exchange chromatography [KHAIRALLAH et al., 1962; BUMPUS et al., 1964; RYAN et al., 1970 (2), 1971 (2)]. Except for the free amino acids (which in any event are easily identified) all lower homologs can be classified into three groups: neutral (8 homologs), one positive charge (16 homologs) and two positive charges (3 homologs).

Major problems arise in attempts to separate a given metabolite from all other homologs of the same charge and of similar size. Identifications have been attempted using an Ang. II antibody known to cross-react with some lower homologs (CAIN et al., 1969; OSBORNE et al., 1970; GIESE et al., 1971). However cross-reactions with other homologs of interest were not reported. It may be that immunoadsorption of large homologs will prove useful, but as a single or primary technique of identification it leaves much to be desired. One would need either several highly specific antibodies or a few whose cross-reactions with all possible homologs are known precisely. In any event, immunoadsorption is unlikely to be of value for identifying small, non-antigenic metabolites.

None of the published studies on the fate of Ang. II has solved the problem of separating homologs closely related in size and charge. At present, no single purification procedure nor detection method appears to be sufficiently selective to allow unequivocal identification of a given homolog by exclusion of all others. However, the approaches used to investigate the mechanisms of degradation of bradykinin and the conversion of Ang. I to Ang. II in the lungs [RYAN et al., 1968 (2), 1970 (1, 2), 1971 (2)] should be applicable to studies of Ang. II.

Starting with the parent polypeptide labelled in a single residue, the number of detectable metabolites (and therefore possible homologs) is reduced. The number of possible homologs is reduced further by preliminary classification of metabolites by charge and size. On the basis of this information, likely homologs can be synthesized in quantity and used to find means of separating one from another. The metabolites can be identified by exclusion and by co-electrophoresis and co-chromatography with a synthetic standard. Relatively few laboratories are equipped for peptide synthesis, thus the preparation of homologs appears to be a rate-limiting step. Possibly the collaboration of several laboratories will be necessary to synthesize homologs and find means of distinguishing one from another. Table 2 summarizes the experience of this laboratory in the electrophoretic separation of 9 peptide homologs (synthesized by J. M. STEWART). Each of the first six are separable. These peptides cover the range necessary for studies of the degradation of angiotensin labelled in the phenylalanyl residue. The last three are the neutral homologs that contain isoleucine. Each of the free amino acids can be identified by electrophoresis at pH 1.9 (DREYER and BYNUM, 1967).

When a given metabolite is small, e.g. a free amino acid or a dipeptide, its identification can be confirmed by co-chromatography on an amino acid analyzer with a flow-cell attachment [RYAN et al., 1968 (2), 1970 (1)]. Some dipeptides are prone to diketopiperazine formation and this feature can be used to confirm identifications. Possibly, the use of enzymes such as arginase (DU VIGNEAUD et al., 1953) and tyrosinase (BISSET, 1962) as well as trypsin, chymotrypsin and specific exopeptidases can be used to support identifications. Selective reactants, such as

Table 2. *Electrophoretic behavior of Ang. II and some of its lower homologs*

	Relative migration System			
	I	II	III	IV
Pro-Phe		0.10		
His-Pro-Phe	0.85	0.65	0.50	0.56
Ile-His-Pro-Phe	0.72	0.62	0.53	0.53
Tyr-Ile-His-Pro-Phe	0.60	0.52	0.36	0.39
Val-Tyr-Ile-His-Pro-Phe	0.53	0.51	0.40	0.39
Arg-Val-Tyr-Ile-His-Pro-Phe	0.68	0.65	0.13	0.22
Asp-Arg-Val-Tyr-Ile-His-Pro-Phe	0.62	0.24		0.27
Asp-Arg-Val-Tyr-Ile	0.45	0.10		0.62
Val-Tyr-Ile	0.59	0.12		0.41
Tyr-Ile		0.12		0.75
Arginine (standard)	1.00	1.00	1.00	
Picric acid (standard)				1.00

Electrophoretic systems I, II and IV used Whatman no. 1 paper at pH 1.9, 5.0 and 9.0 respectively. Electrophoresis was performed at 22 v/cm at 10 to 20 mA for 1 h. System III used Whatman CM-82 paper at pH 5.0 at 15 v/cm at 5 to 10 mA for 1.5 h (see RYAN et al., 1972, for further details).

fluorodinitrobenzene, may be useful for confirming identifications of histidine-containing homologs (see GREGERMAN and KOWATCH, 1971), but neither of the latter two approaches has been exploited. Bioassay could be useful for identifying metabolites which retain biological activity, but care must be taken to rule out potentiating or antagonizing effects of inert metabolites and to rule out the presence of biologically-active contaminants that are not structurally related to angiotensin [GARBE, 1967; RYAN et al., 1970 (2); TÜRKER et al., 1971]. For these reasons, it is likely that identifications by bioassay or immunoadsorption are most informative when used after highly-selective chemical separations.

The use of an angiotensin labelled in a single residue has the advantage of reducing the numbers of detectable metabolites and therefore simplifies identifications. However there is a limit to the kinds of information that can be obtained. An angiotensin labelled in two distant residues would facilitate the firm identification of primary sites of hydrolysis but at the cost of producing more detectable metabolites. If one residue were labelled with ^{14}C and another with ^{3}H, for differential counting, some of the practical advantages of angiotensin labelled in a single residue would be preserved. For that matter, a judicious mixture of a ^{3}H-labelled angiotensin with angiotensin labelled with ^{14}C in another residue could do as well.

III. Mechanisms by Which Angiotensin II is Removed from the Circulation

A. Binding at Sites of Action

The reactions of Ang. II with its receptors is the concern of another chapter. Suffice it to say that some portion of Ang. II in the circulation is taken up at sites of action. Current evidence indicates that the quantity so used is probably small and depends upon the amount that is available (KHAIRALLAH et al., 1966, 1970 BAUDOUIN et al., 1971). Whether, having exerted its effects, Ang. II is released again into the circulation is unkown. The effects of angiotensin may be terminated by degradation at sites of action.

Possibly the binding sites associated with pressor responses are not far from the vascular space, as soluble angiotensinase enzymes will reverse angiotensin tachyphylaxis (KHAIRALLAH et al., 1966). Similarly, KLAUS et al. (1965) have shown that the pressor response can be reduced in proportion to the amounts of leucine aminopeptidase or carboxypeptidase A added to the circulation. LUBASH et al. (1971) have reported that during infusion of [Asn^{1}]-Ang. II, plasma enzyme activity is associated inversely with plasma angiotensin and directly with change of blood pressure, findings consistent with the concept that sites of action are accessible to angiotensinase as well as to angiotensin itself. RICHARDSON and BEAULNES (1971) have reported that angiotensin bound to peroxidase exerts a pressor response and that the peroxidase is localized along the plasma membrane of endothelial cells. Assuming that angiotensin is not removed from peroxidase *in vivo*, these results may be significant. Localization of sites of action along the luminal surface of endothelial cells has some appeal as many endothelial cells contain myofibril-like material (MAJNO et al., 1969; PIETRA et al., 1971; SMITH et al., 1971) and have close, possibly low-resistance, junctions with smooth muscle cells (RHODIN, 1967).

B. Enzymic Degradation

Since the discovery of angiotensin, it has been known that blood and tissues contain angiotensinase activity (BRAUN-MENENDEZ et al., 1939; PAGE and HELMER, 1940; FASCIOLO et al., 1940). Initially it was thought that the angiotensinase activity was specific for angiotensin and was, although extractable from a large number of tissues, probably a single enzyme (for review see BRAUN-MENENDEZ et al., 1946). HELMER et al. [1942 (2)] reported that angiotensinase activity of kidney had pH optima at pH 4 and 7, raising the possibility of two or more enzymes. When the primary structure of Ang. II was established (SKEGGS et al., 1956), it became apparent that enzymes having specificities like that of trypsin, chymotrypsin, pepsin, leucine aminopeptidase and carboxypeptidase could reduce or eliminate biological activity (SKEGGS et al., 1956; ELLIOTT and PEART, 1957; RINIKER and SCHWYZER, 1964). It is now evident that most tissues contain a multiplicity of enzymes which are capable of reducing angiotensin to its component amino acids. Which of these enzymes has access to angiotensin *in vivo* has been (SAPIRSTEIN et al., 1946) and still is a central question in studies of the fates of Ang. I and II (JOHNSON and RYAN, 1968).

1. Enzymes of Blood

Plasma and serum. In the first attempts to produce angiotensin *in vitro*, it was evident that prolonged incubations of crude renin-renin substrate preparations resulted in a loss of angiotensin (BRAUN-MENENDEZ et al., 1939; PAGE and HELMER, 1940). Loss of product became less of a problem as purer renin and renin substrate became available (LELOIR et al., 1940) and as bacterial contamination was eliminated. Both kidney extracts and plasma were found subsequently to be capable of inactivating angiotensin, kidney enzymes being at least 800 times more active than plasma or serum (FASCIOLO et al., 1940).

Because of the need of plasma as a source of renin substrate and because of the ease of collecting samples for study, the great preponderance of angiotensinase studies have focussed on plasma enzymes. As well, the large numbers of studies requiring measurement of renin and angiotensin in plasma have been bedeviled by plasma angiotensinase enzymes. The sheer nuisance of these enzymes in plasma renin assays has provoked studies for over 30 years to find ways of eliminating their activities [see BRAUN-MENENDEZ et al., 1946; BROWN et al., 1964; PICKENS et al., 1965; RYAN et al., 1966; RYAN, 1967 (2); RYAN et al., 1968 (1) for review].

Yet taken in the context of the fate of angiotensin *in vivo*, it has been recognized since the 1940's that plasma enzymes may have no more than a minor role in eliminating biological activity (FASCIOLO et al., 1940). The vasopressor response to angiotensin is abrupt and brief, disappearing at rates faster than can be accounted for by plasma enzymes (CAIN et al., 1970).

Through the nature of the experiment, plasma angiotensinase activity is studied *in vitro*, usually with the reaction mixture fortified with a neutral buffer. Virtually all neutral buffers have a greater or lesser capacity of binding divalent cations, and the studies reviewed below should be interpreted with this in mind. Edetic acid is known to inhibit plasma peptidase enzymes (HELMER and JUDSON, 1963; KHAIRALLAH, 1963; KHAIRALLAH and PAGE, 1967) and it has been shown that the plasma enzymes capable of degrading angiotensin may be inhibited completely by combinations of chelating agents [RYAN et al., 1966, 1968 (1); RYAN, 1967 (1, 2); BOYD et al., 1967). In fact, it is difficult to find a study of plasma or serum angiotensinase enzymes in which a buffer has not been employed, and in this sense it may be claimed that we do not know the full potency of plasma angiotensinase activity.

Nonetheless, a significant role for these enzymes in degrading angiotensin *in vivo* is in doubt, as the half-life of angiotensin in whole blood without exogenous buffers greatly exceeds its half-life during circulation through various vascular beds (CHAMBERLAIN et al., 1964; HODGE et al., 1967; LEARY and LEDINGHAM, 1969).

Four plasma angiotensinase enzymes have been described. KHAIRALLAH et al. (1963) found that at neutral or slightly alkaline pH, most angiotensin is degraded by an aminopeptidase, which they named angiotensinase A. Subsequently, KHAIRALLAH and PAGE (1967) showed that angiotensinase A could be separated into two enzymes: A_1, which hydrolyzes [Asn^1]-angiotensin, and A_2, which degrades [Asp^1]-angiotensin. The pH optimum of A_1 is 7.4 and the pH optimum of A_2 is 6.8. Both require Ca^{++} and are inhibited by EDTA. KURTZ and WACHSMUTH (1969) have reported that plasma angiotensinase activity is inhibited by antibodies raised against a renal aminopeptidase. NIGAWARA et al. (1971) have reported that most angiotensinase active at neutral pH is inactivated by prior acidification. REGOLI et al. (1963) claimed to have found an endopeptidase, active at acid pH, in serum, plasma and kidney homogenates. The enzyme was said to hydrolyze [β-L-Asp^1]-Ang. II into two tetrapeptides. However, only the N-terminal tetrapeptide was identified, the remainder of the molecule occurring as free amino acids. KHAIRALLAH and PAGE (1967) found a plasma enzyme capable of hydrolyzing [succinic acid[1]]- and [β-aspartic acid[1]]-angiotensins, substrates resistant to aminopeptidase activities. This enzyme is inhibited by diisopropylfluorophosphate (DFP, 0.5 mg/ml of enzyme) and phenylmethylsulfonyl fluoride (1 mg/ml). It migrates on paper electrophoresis as a β-globulin and may be the enzyme studied by REGOLI et al. (1963). ZWANZIG and OELKERS (1968) using pH-dependence techniques, have confirmed that plasma contains at least three enzymes capable of degrading angiotensin.

Because of the uncertainties of the experiments by REGOLI et al., a search was made for a carboxypeptidase enzyme. When other angiotensinase activity is masked by EDTA, plasma releases the C-terminal phenylalanine without releasing the penultimate proline (JOHNSON, 1967). At neutral pH the plasma carboxypeptidase activity is sluggish in comparison with the activity inhibited by EDTA. MATSUNAGA (1971) recently has presented further evidence of carboxypeptidase activity in plasma.

RIPA and DEGLI ATTI (1969) have postulated the existence of an inhibitor in plasma of angiotensinase activity, but no clear data on this point has been forthcoming.

The origin of the angiotensinase enzymes that occur in plasma under physiologic conditions is not known.

Species variations, the effects of disease and tissue destruction and the effects of drugs on angiotensinase enzymes are discussed in the chapter on *Measurement of Angiotensinase Enzymes* (LEARY and LEDINGHAM, this volume).

Angiotensinase enzymes of blood cells. Red blood cells contain at least two enzymes capable of degrading angiotensin. The best characterized is an aminopeptidase that corresponds in terms of utilization of substrates and response to inhibitors to angiotensinase A (KHAIRALLAH et al., 1963). ITSKOVITZ and MILLER (1967) have reported that ε-aminocaproic acid (EACA) and Hg^{++} inhibit plasma and red cell angiotensinase activities, EACA being more effective against plasma enzymes and Hg^{++} being more effective on red cell enzymes. DAHLHEIM et al. (1969) have confirmed effects of Hg^{++} on angiotensinase enzymes of red cells and have shown that Cd^{++} inhibits as well. KOKUBU et al. (1969) have purified an endopeptidase of rabbit red cells to a specific activity 8,000-fold greater than that of the original hemolysate. The enzyme(s) hydrolyzed the Arg^2-Val^3, Tyr^4-Ile^5 and Ile^5-His^6 bonds, isoleucine being the only free amino acid. KOKUBU et al. reported that hydrolysis of the Tyr^4-Ile^5 bond was primary but the evidence was not conclusive.

Whether the enzymes within red blood cells have access to angiotensin *in vivo* seems doubtful. FASCIOLO et al. (1940) found that washed erythrocytes inactivate angiotensin at rates no faster than do plasma enzymes. Slight hemolysis may increase substantially the rates of inactivation (DEXTER, 1942), a point seldom taken into account in studies of changes of plasma angiotensinase activity in various pathologic states.

Angiotensinase enzymes of white blood cells have not been studied with any depth. Polymorphonuclear cells have been reported to have peptidase enzymes on the exterior of their plasma membranes (GREENBAUM and KIM, 1967), but under physiologic conditions these enzymes are unlikely to have a major role in degrading angiotensin in blood (HODGE et al., 1967). Possibly in conditions characterized by extreme leucocytosis, angiotensinase enzymes of white blood cells could influence the concentrations of angiotensin achieved in blood.

Other body fluids. FRIEDMAN et al. (1943) found that lymph has even less angiotensinase than plasma. Here again, ion-binding buffers may obscure the true activity of peptidase enzymes. Renin, renin substrate, converting enzyme and Ang. II are known to occur in lymph (FRIEDMAN et al., 1943; HORKY et al., 1971; BAILIE et al., 1971), but it is not known whether lymph contributes to angiotensin in blood. Although angiotensinase activity of lymph is slight, it may be sufficient considering the slow, meandering flow.

YANG et al. (1968) have reported that urine contains a carboxypeptidase enzyme capable of reacting with angiotensin. The molecular size of angiotensin is such that it may be filtered by glomeruli. However, whether angiotensin reaches the level of the urinary bladder or even the level of the proximal tubules is an open question. BUMPUS et al. (1964) found little evidence of angiotensin in the urine of rats infused with large quantities of randomly tritiated angiotensin, and LEARY and LEDINGHAM (1969) were unable to find angiotensin-like biological activity in the urine of kidneys perfused *in vitro*. WACHSMUTH (1968) has shown that ground substance of kidney contains an aminopeptidase enzyme. In principle, the filtered angiotensin could be degraded efficiently in transit across the basement membrane of the glomerulus. A basis for hydrolytic reactions of this type has been developed by KATCHALSKI and colleagues (GOLDMAN et al., 1965) from experiences with enzymes attached to artificial membranes.

GREGERMAN (1967) found microgram quantities of the dipeptide, His-Leu, in normal human urine. Whether any proportion of the His-Leu arises from the metabolism of Ang. I is not known.

MAEBASHI and YOSHINAGA (1968) have reported that angiotensin is not degraded in amniotic fluid. Whether cerebrospinal fluid contains angiotensinase activity is not known. Nor is it known whether bile contains angiotensinase enzymes. The latter question may be of little consequence as rat liver perfused with radioactive Ang. II does not secrete angiotensin nor its radioactive metabolites (W. P. LEARY and J. W. RYAN, unpublished).

2. Angiotensinase Enzymes of Disrupted Solid Tissues

Homogenates of every tissue that has been surveyed contain an abundance of enzymes capable of inactivating Ang. II. Characteristically, whole homogenates or the supernatants obtained after low speed centrifugation are capable of reducing milligram quantities of angiotensin to its component amino acids. Recently, however, it has become evident that many of these tissue enzymes do not have access to angiotensin in the circulation. To take the most prominent example, homogenates of lung rapidly degrade angiotensin (JOHNSON, 1967; ITSKOVITZ and MILLER, 1967) yet indirect evidence indicates that only a small proportion of the Ang. II entering the pulmonary artery fails to emerge in the pulmonary vein (HODGE et al., 1967; BIRON et al., 1968, 1969; LEARY and LEDINGHAM, 1969). Therefore, the studies of angiotensinase activities of disrupted tissues and subcellular fractions must be interpreted in terms of the question of access of enzyme to substrate. As well, the technical maneuvers used to facilitate *in vitro* studies, namely the means of tissue disruption, preparation of subcellular fractions, dialysis, protein precipitation, addition of buffers, etc., probably have a strong influence on the observations obtained.

Kidney. As the primary source of renin and as a major target organ of angiotensin, the kidney has been studied extensively. HELMER et al. [1942 (2)] reported that angiotensinase activity of kidney has pH optima at pH 4 and 7. ITSKOVITZ and MILLER (1966) found that most angiotensinase is in the cortex. Destruction of proximal tubules by sodium potassium tartrate may effect a 90% reduction in angiotensinase activity. Destruction of proximal tubules by mercuric chloride reduces activity by 40%. High doses of meralluride also reduce renal angiotensinase activity *in vivo* and *in vitro*. Ammonium (180 mM) reduces the activity of cortical homogenates and has an additive effect with meralluride. GRANGER et al. (1969) found angiotensinase activity in the proximal tubule and in microdissected juxtaglomerular apparatus.

Using early methods of preparing subcellular fractions, DENGLER and REICHEL (1960) found that mitochondrial and microsomal fractions of rat and swine kidneys contained 10 times as much angiotensinase activity as did the cytosol fraction. HESS (1965) confirmed that angiotensinase occurs in its highest specific activity in microsomes. The microsomal enzymes require Ca^{++} and are inhibited by EDTA. Using more selective methods of preparing subcellular fractions, MATSUNAGA et al. (1968, 1969) and SAITO et al. (1969) found large quantities of angiotensinase activity in lysosomal as well as microsomal fractions. The enzymic activity associated with the lysosomal fraction is active at acid pH and is inhibited by diisopropylfluorophosphate. The microsomal fraction is most active at neutral pH. The lysosomal enzyme may correspond to the acid angiotensinase discovered by HELMER et al. [1942 (1)].

Most of the lysosomal enzyme activity is accounted for by a carboxypeptidase. However the lysosomes apparently contain several enzymes capable of hydrolyzing angiotensin as SAITO et al. (1969) have reported that the release of phenylalanine is followed by the release of proline. Histidine and isoleucine are also liberated, presumably in subsequent reactions. Recently MATSUNAGA (1971) has reported a separation of enzymic activities associated with lysosomes. One enzyme releases phenylalanine only and is inhibited by DFP. The specificity of the remainder of the enzymic activity was not determined.

YANG et al. (1968) have described the preparation of a soluble carboxypeptidase from swine kidney cortex. A remarkable feature of the enzyme is that it withstands heating at 62 °C for 10 min. The enzyme releases phenylalanine from [Asn^1]-Ang. II and from a variety of synthetic substrates, including Cbo- and dansyl-derivatives of Pro-Phe and Gly-Pro-Phe. It is inhibited by DFP but not by EDTA, phenanthroline nor p-chloromercuriphenylsulfonic acid (PCMS). YANG et al. named the enzyme angiotensinase C. MATSUNAGA (1971) has claimed that angiotensinase C is identical with the major lysosomal angiotensinase. The heat-resistant carboxypeptidase does not appear to represent a major proportion of the total angiotensinase of kidney, as over 90% of the total angiotensinase activity is inactivated by heating at 56 °C at pH 6.0 for 30 min (RYAN and JOHNSON, 1969).

Starting with the studies of BLAQUIER et al. (1961) and BING (1962), there have been a number of reports on the effect of diet, drugs and various surgical procedures on the angiotensinase content of the kidneys. These studies are reviewed in the accompanying section by LEARY and LEDINGHAM (this volume).

Liver. Like kidney, liver is a rich source of enzymes capable of degrading angiotensin, and many of the investigations of the subcellular location of angiotensinase enzymes have studied these two organs in parallel. An intracellular carboxypeptidase active on angiotensin was first extracted from liver and was described by JOHNSON (1967) and JOHNSON and RYAN (1968). The carboxypeptidase withstands mild heating (56 °C for 30 min) and is not inhibited by EDTA. It accounts for about 30% of the total angiotensinase activity of rabbit liver homogenates. At present, it appears that the lysosomal angiotensinase activity of liver is largely accounted for by the carboxypeptidase (MATSUNAGA, 1971). Like the renal enzyme, the carboxypeptidase is active at acid pH and is inhibited by DFP.

Most of the angiotensinase activity of liver homogenate is active at neutral pH and is inhibited by EDTA (JOHNSON, 1967; JOHNSON and RYAN, 1968). This angiotensinase activity is inactivated by heating at 56 °C. Possibly, as in the kidney, the neutral angiotensinase activity is associated with microsomes, but attempts to separate hepatic microsomes have not been successful (MATSUNAGA and MASSON, 1970).

The carboxypeptidase and EDTA-sensitive angiotensinase enzymes account for most but not all of the soluble angiotensinase activity of liver homogenates. The low-speed supernatant previously dialyzed against EDTA (3 mM) releases

Table 3. *Angiotensinase activity of dog tissues*
Fasciolo units/gm of fresh tissue

Intestinal mucosa	1,200—1,600
Kidney	800
Intestine	400—800
Pancreas	240
Spleen	160—200
Hemolyzed erythrocytes	80—120
Liver	80
Adrenal	40—50
Brain	4—8
Heart	4
Intact erythrocytes	4
Plasma or serum	1—4

Table. 4. *Angiotensinase activity of rabbit tissues*
(Activity at pH 7.4, expressed in mμg of Asn[1], Val[5]-Ang. II inactivated/min/ml of undiluted tissue extract)

Spleen	4,400
Liver	2,300
Salivary gland	2,200
Thymus	2,000
Kidney	700
Lung	600
Adrenal	540
Plasma	500

phenylalanine from Asn[1]-Ang. II at a rate slightly slower than that of the disappearance of biological activity. The residual "third" enzyme is inhibited by N-ethylmaleimide (JOHNSON and RYAN, 1968).

Enzymes of other tissues. Table 3 is modified from that of FASCIOLO et al. (1940) and summarizes the results of a survey of dog tissues.

These results are not invariable and depend on species, buffers, methods of tissue disruption, centrifugation and the type, purity and starting concentrations of angiotensin and probably other factors. Table 4 shows results of a survey of rabbit tissues (JOHNSON, 1967). Species variation is emphasized by the point that sheep kidney contains almost 10 times as much angiotensinase activity per gram of tissue as does rabbit kidney.

As mentioned previously, every tissue that has been studied contains enzymes capable of inactivating angiotensin. BUMPUS et al. (1964) found angiotensinase enzymes in skeletal muscle and aortic tissue as well as adrenals, brain, heart, lung, liver, spleen and kidney. A survey of rat tissues by ITSKOVITZ and MILLER (1967) was in substantial agreement with the results of BUMPUS et al.

At present, virtually nothing is known of the specificities of the enzymes in tissues other than kidney and liver. Nor is anything known of which of the various tissue enzymes have access to angiotensin in the circulation.

3. Angiotensinase Enzymes in Various Vascular Beds

Depending on the value used for the half-life of intravenously-administered angiotensin, it has been concluded that the plasma enzymes account entirely for the disappearance of biological activity, or, quite the opposite, that the plasma enzymes play little or no role. Using crude preparations of angiotensin, CORCORAN et al. (1941) estimated that the disappearance time of the blood pressure response approached 20 to 25 min. Assuming from these data that the half-life of angiotensin is about 10 min, SAPIRSTEIN et al. (1946) calculated that the angiotensinase activity of plasma could account for this rate of disappearance. They went on to show that neither nephrectomy nor evisceration increased or extended pressor responses to angiotensin and concluded that angiotensinase enzymes of solid tissues contribute little to the degradation of circulating angiotensin.

As pure angiotensin and better means of detection became available, estimates of the half-life of angiotensin became very much shorter, recent estimates by radioimmunoassay being of the order of one minute (BOYD et al., 1969; CAIN et al., 1970). Many of the radioimmunoassays in common use cross-react with some lower homologs known to occur in blood (CAIN et et al., 1969; GIESE et al., 1971) and do not distinguish between endogenous and injected angiotensin, thus it is possible that the half-life of angiotensin is considerably less than one minute. Using bioassay techniques, HODGE et al. (1967) estimated that the half-life of angiotensin in dogs is about one circulation time or about 15 sec (SPECTOR, 1956). Similarly, DOYLE et al. (1968) found the half-life of [PTC-^{35}S]-Ang. II to be about one circulation time. Now that an intrinsically-labelled angiotensin of high specific activity is available (MORGAT, 1970), it may be possible to measure the half-life and clearance rate with greater accuracy.

Beginning with studies in 1964, understanding of the immediate fate of Ang. II has been transformed. CHAMBERLAIN et al. (1964), studying the efficacy of renoportal anastomosis for the treatment of renal hypertension, found that angiotensin disappears almost completely during a single circulation through the liver. METHOT et al. (1964), using rats, provided simultaneous confirmation. Subsequently, ABRAMS (1966) showed substantial disappearance of angiotensin during circulation through the liver of the dog. In 1967, HODGE et al. extended these findings to show that angiotensin also disappears during circulation through the head, kidney and hindquarter of the dog. The apparent half-life of Ang. II in blood alone was found to be on the order of $3^1/_2$ min. In striking contrast, they reported indirect evidence indicating that angiotensin II is not lost during circulation through the lungs. These findings have been confirmed by BIRON et al. (1968, 1969) and LEARY and LEDINGHAM (1969).

The bioassay results are clear on the point of disappearance of Ang. II in various vascular beds but provide no evidence on the mechanisms of disappearance. METHOT et al. (1964) assumed that disappearance was accounted for by enzymic degradation. HODGE et al. (1967) took a broader view and considered removal from the vascular space with either degradation or subsequent release back into the bloodstream.

OSBORNE et al. (1970) provided the first direct evidence on the mechanisms of disappearance of angiotensin. Using [4-(^{3}H)Tyr]-Ang. II, these investigators found that 30 to 80% of the biological activity of angiotensin disappears during a single passage through the coronary or renal circulation. However, greater than 80% of the radioactivity was recovered in the venous effluent coincident in time with the emergence of biological activity. Less than 2% of the radioactivity was retained by the heart and less than 3% was retained by the kidneys; the remainder of the radioactivity was not found. On gel chromatography, most of the radioactivity was retarded in elution in comparison with angiotensin, occurring as a complex mixture of lower homologs. Some of the lower homologs were identified tentatively as Arg^2-Phe^8, Val^3-Phe^8 and Asp^1-Tyr^4. For reasons discussed under TECHNICAL ASPECTS, none of the identifications are firm. Nonetheless, the evidence supports the concept that the disappearance of angiotensin in the coronary and renal vascular beds is owing to enzymic hydrolysis.

Although there was no specific comment on this point, the data presented by OSBORNE et al. (1970) shows an apparent discrepancy between degradation as estimated by bioassay and as estimated by the disappearance of radioactive angiotensin. When angiotensin was infused at 10 ng/ml, they found mean values for biological inactivation of $43.5 \pm 3.2\%$ for the heart and $67.0 \pm 5.4\%$ for kidney. However, by integration of the peaks of radioactivity obtained on gel chromatography, it appears that less than 10% of the radioactivity of the renal venous effluent and less than 20% of that of the coronary effluent occurred as Ang. II. This apparent discrepancy is brought out to illustrate the need of measuring metabolism by more than one technique. In studies of the metabolism of Ang. I in the pulmonary circulation, it has been shown that a large proportion of rat colon-stimulating activity is not owing to the expected product, Ang. II, but to another substance which may not be structurally related to Ang. I [RYAN et al., 1970 (2); TÜRKER et al., 1971). Recently, W. P. LEARY and J. W. RYAN (in preparation) used [5-(^{14}C)isoleucine]-Ang. II to obtain direct evidence for the free passage of Ang. II through isolated rat lungs. Bioassay results (blood pressure response) indicated that no loss occurred, but up to 10% of the radioactivity of the pulmonary venous effluent occurred as lower homologs.

The results of OSBORNE et al. (1970) and the relatively free passage of angiotensin through the lungs raise again the important question of the access of enzymes to circulating polypeptide substrates. The lungs, as well as the liver, kidney, spleen and other tissues, are known to contain enzymes capable of hydrolyzing Ang. II (JOHNSON, 1967; ITSKOVITZ and MILLER, 1967). Although angiotensin disappears rapidly during circulation through other vascular beds, there is no evidence that it is exposed to peptidase or protease enzymes as they occur in cytoplasm, lysosomes or internal membrane systems. ROBERTSON and KHAIRALLAH (1971) have presented autoradiographic evidence of the uptake of radioactivity by heart following intraventricular injections of [4-(^{3}H)tyrosine]-Ang. II. However the proportion of radioactivity taken up was small and the radioactivity was not shown to be in the form of angiotensin.

Using large quantities (4.6 μg/min) of randomly tritiated [Asn^1, Val^5]-Ang. II in intravenous infusions (20 min), KHAIRALLAH et al. (1962) and BUMPUS et al. (1964) obtained evidence of uptake in tissues of rats. Immediately after infusions in normal rats, most of the radioactivity was found in the adrenal glands, kidneys, uterus and blood. The radioactivity extracted from these tissues migrated in a single electrophoresis system like authentic [Asn^1, Val^5]-Ang. II. Thirty minutes after ending the infusions, most of the radioactivity was found in kidney and urine. There was a twelve-fold increase in brain. With the exception of a small amount of radioactivity in blood, none of the radioactivity behaved on electrophoresis like angiotensin. BUMPUS et al. pointed out that none of the radioactivity recovered at any stage could definitely be said to occur as angiotensin.

When tritiated Asn^1, Val^5-Ang. II was infused in rats after bilateral nephrectomy, most of the radioactivity was found in liver, spleen, lung and blood. Thirty minutes after infusion, there were substantial decreases of radioactivity in all tissues, raising questions about the method of elimination. Possibly some isotope was lost as water vapor in expired air. The major proportion of the radioactivity of [2-(^{14}C)proline]-bradykinin is ultimately eliminated as $^{14}CO_2$ (J. J. PISANO, personal communication).

OSBORNE et al. (1971) carried out a similar study in which a small dose (25 or 100 ng) of [^{3}H-Tyr^4]-Ang. II (56 Ci/mmole) was administered as a bolus injection into the jugular vein of the rat. Blood and tissues were taken at timed intervals and were extracted for Ang. II, its immunoreactive lower homologs, and other forms of radioactivity. They found that the radioactivity disappears quickly from blood, the major proportion disappearing within the first 5 min. The radioactivity of the larger dose disappeared more rapidly than did that of the lower dose. Disappearance of radioactivity from the blood of bilaterally nephrectomized rats was slower than in controls but was still largely completed within 5 min. Twenty min after injection, plasma radioactivity was found to rise, although the molecular relationship of this radioactivity to the original [^{3}H-Tyr-]-Ang. II was not clear and may have represented new protein synthesis. One min after injection, some of the radioactivity of plasma was found to be associated with large molecular components (as indicated by elution from Sephadex G-25). This association possibly could represent protein binding of angiotensin.

As in the previous study by BUMPUS and colleagues (1964), OSBORNE et al. (1971) found most radioactivity in the kidneys, adrenals, liver and spleen. However, in comparison with the uptake of ^{3}H-inulin, only the adrenals and the liver had proportionately more radioactivity after [^{3}H]-Ang. administration than after that of ^{3}H-inulin. However, they pointed out that while ^{3}H-inulin was excreted rapidly, the radioactivity following injection of [^{3}H]-Ang. II was not excreted rapidly. On this basis, it would appear that the kidney concentrates radioactivity following the intravenous injection of [^{3}H-Tyr^4]-Ang. II. Of the brain regions studied by OSBORNE et al., only the pituitary contained more radioactivity than plasma.

In light of other data on the immediate fate of angiotensin and on the rapidity of metabolism of peptides and free amino acids, it is possible that the data of BUMPUS et al. and OSBORNE et al. show late results of a very extensive series of reactions. Degradation of angiotensin occurs within seconds. Furthermore an organ such as liver can take up free amino acids, incorporate them into proteins and release the proteins back into the circulation within 1 h [RYAN et al., 1971 (1); BRYAN et al., 1972].

At present, there is no clear evidence of how rapidly Ang. II can be taken up from the circulation, but the rate is unlikely to be great. Free amino acids do not readily pass out of the lumen of vessels lined with a continuous endothelium (CHINARD et al., 1962; CHINARD, 1966). The liver is exceptional because of its need of amino acids for the synthesis of plasma proteins. But even in the liver, the proportion of amino acids removed from blood in one circulation time may not be great (GORESKY, 1963, 1964) (see, however, ROBERTSON and KHAIRALLAH, Chapter 27).

Bradykinin and Ang. I are metabolized extensively during one circulation through the lungs, but little or none of either peptide appears to be removed from the vascular space [RYAN et al., 1968 (2), 1970 (2, 2), 1971 (1), 1972 (1, 2)]. Possibly Ang. II is processed similarly in the renal and coronary circulations. OSBORNE et al. (1970) have reported that radioactivity and biological activity emerge simultaneously in the venous effluents of heart and kidney perfused with [4-(^{3}H)tyrosine]-Ang. II and that less than 3% of the radioactivity is retained. Secretion of angiotensinase enzymes into the vascular space appears to be ruled out, as LEARY (1969) has reported that degradation of angiotensin by the effluents of isolated, perfused organs is negligible.

It could be argued that angiotensin passes rapidly from the vascular space, is metabolized and then its metabolites are rapidly returned to the circulation. However it is also possible that the relevant angiotensinase enzymes, at least in some tissues, are on or near the luminal surface of endothelial cells. In this regard, it is of interest that angiotensinase enzymes of rat kidney occur in highest specific activity in the microsomal fraction (DENGLER and REICHEL, 1960; HESS, 1965), a fraction composed of plasma membrane as well as internal membrane systems (THINES-SEMPOUX et al., 1970; ALLAN and CRUMPTON, 1970; TOUSTER et al., 1970).

The plasma membranes of some endothelial cells are known to contain hydrolase enzymes. 5'-Nucleotidase is regarded generally as a plasma membrane "marker" enzyme (EMMELOT et al., 1964). ATPase occurs as well (MARCHESI and BARRNETT, 1963; SMITH and RYAN, 1970, 1971), and VATTER et al. (1968) have reported evidence of esterases capable of hydrolyzing acetate, propionate and butyrate esters of p-nitrothiophenol. These substrates also can be hydrolyzed by enzymes like chymotrypsin. The esterase enzymes, like some angiotensinase activity (PICKENS et al., 1965; KHAIRALLAH and PAGE, 1967), are inhibited by DFP and phenylmethylsulfonyl fluoride. Recently RYAN and SMITH [1971 (1, 2)] and RYAN et al. [1972 (2)] have shown that plasma membrane of lung converts Ang. I to Ang. II (Fig. 1). The Ang. II thus formed is not degraded, a point consistent with the relatively free passage of Ang. II through the pulmonary circulation. The plasma membrane preparation also hydrolyzes [2-(^{14}C)proline]-bradykinin to radioactive Pro^2-Pro^3, a major metabolite produced by intact lungs perfused with bradykinin [RYAN et al., 1968 (2), 1970 (1)].

Little is known of how the various hydrolase enzymes are situated along the plasma membrane of endothelial cells. Cytochemical studies have shown that 5'-nucleotidase and ATPase activities are located predominantly within caveolae intracellulares (Fig. 2) [SMITH and RYAN, 1970, 1971; RYAN and SMITH, 1971 (1, 2)]. The enzymes capable of hydrolyzing p-nitrothiophenyl esters have been studied cytochemically, but the electron-dense deposits were not sufficiently discrete to allow conclusions (VATTER et al., 1968). Recent studies of the fine structure of endothelial cells indicate that the concave surface of caveolae has globular subunits not found on undifferentiated areas of plasma membrane (Fig. 3). It has been suggested that the subunits are enzyme clusters [SMITH and RYAN, 1972 (2)]. At present, there is no direct evidence of the positions of kininase and converting enzyme activities along the plasma membrane. The kinetics of disappearance of Ang. I and bradykinin are similar to that of adenine nucleotides and on this basis it has been postulated that kininase and converting enzyme may have a distribution like 5'-nucleotidase and ATPase [SMITH and RYAN, 1970, 1971, 1972 (1); RYAN et al., 1971 (2), 1972 (2)].

Until more evidence is forthcoming on the immediate fate of Ang. II, it may be premature to speculate on the precise subcellular or even cellular location of relevant angiotensinase enzymes. The structures of various vascular beds differ, and the locations of relevant enzymes may differ. The endothelium of some organs of interest is not continuous: the adrenal cortex and renal glomeruli have fenestrat-

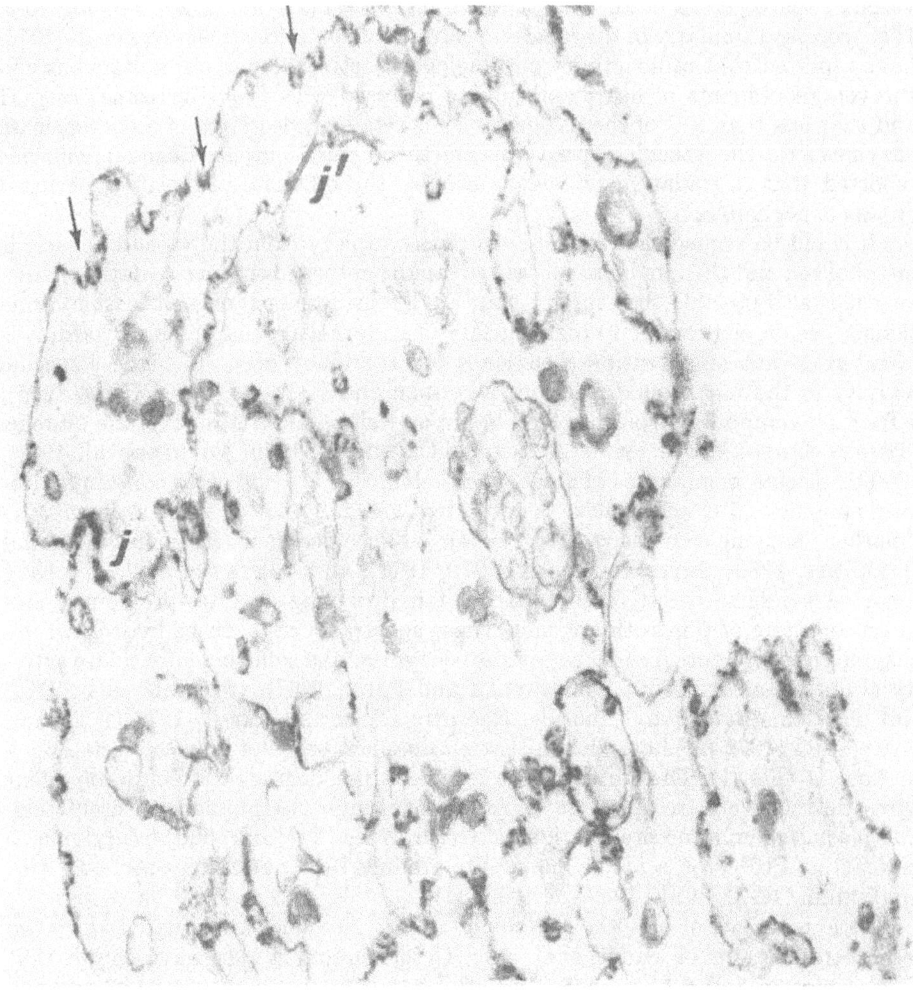

Fig. 1. Pellet obtained on incubation of lung homogenate with 5'-AMP and lead nitrate. The discrete deposition of lead phosphate within caveolae (arrows) allows the collection of long strands of plasma membrane. Cell junctions (j) are preserved, including a tight junction (j[1]). ×54,000. (Reproduced from RYAN and SMITH, 1971, Trans. Assoc. Amer. Physcns., by permission of the publishers)

Fig. 2. a) Section through the capillary endothelium of lungs perfused with AMP and $Pb(NO_3)_2$. Caveolae facing the lumen (L) of the vessel contain an electron-dense reaction product (arrows), presumably insoluble lead phosphate. × 84,000. (Reproduced from SMITH and RYAN, 1971, Chest **59,** 12 S, by permission of the publishers, the American College of Chest Physicians). b) Micrograph showing electron-dense reaction product specifically localized within endothelial caveolae (arrows). This material was briefly pre-fixed in glutaraldehyde and incubated with ATP in the presence of $Pb(NO_3)_2$, NaCl and KCl. × 117,000. (Reproduced from SMITH and RYAN, 1970, Adv. Med. Biol. 8, 249, by permission of the publishers, Plenum Publishing Corp.)

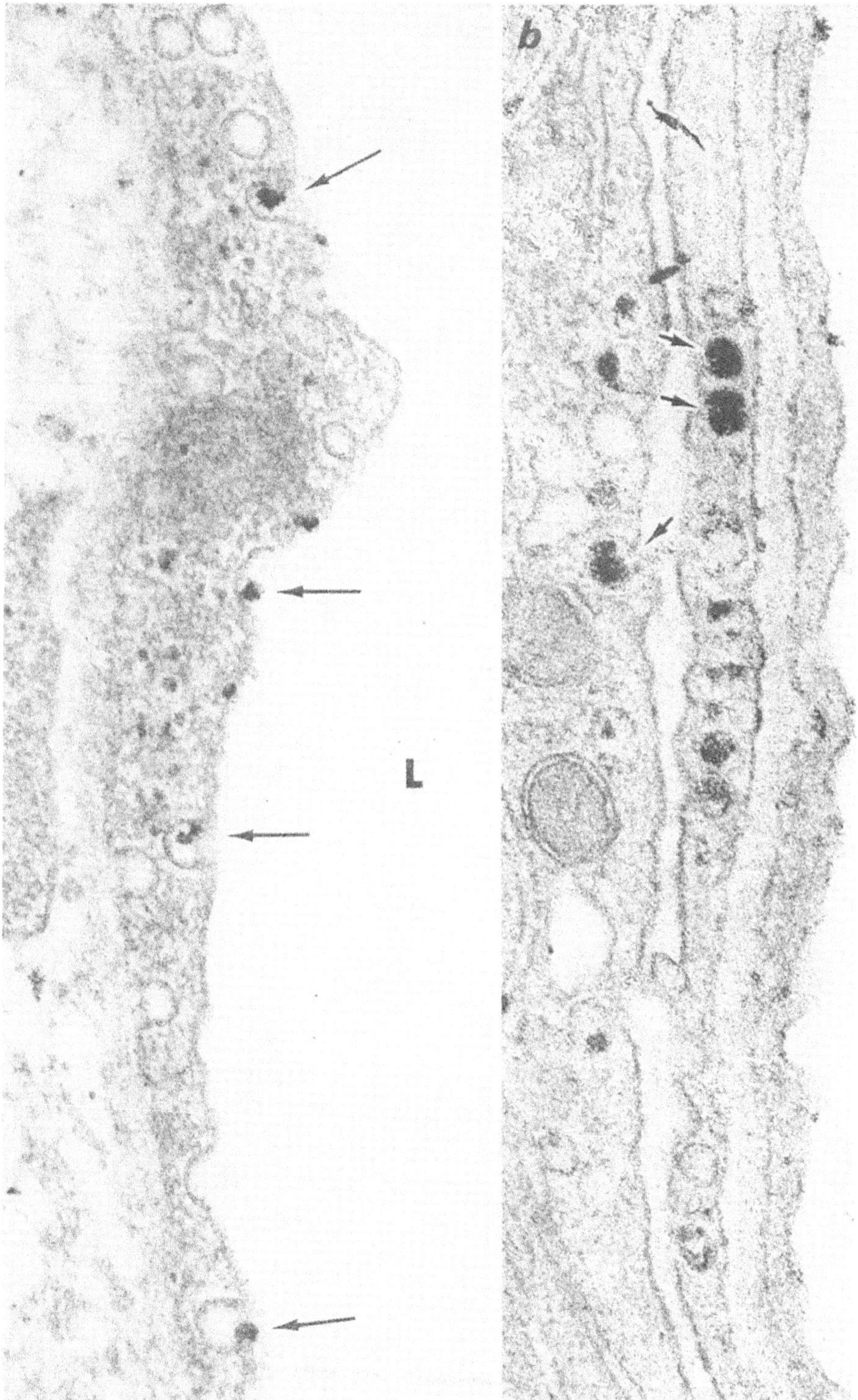

a b

Fig. 2

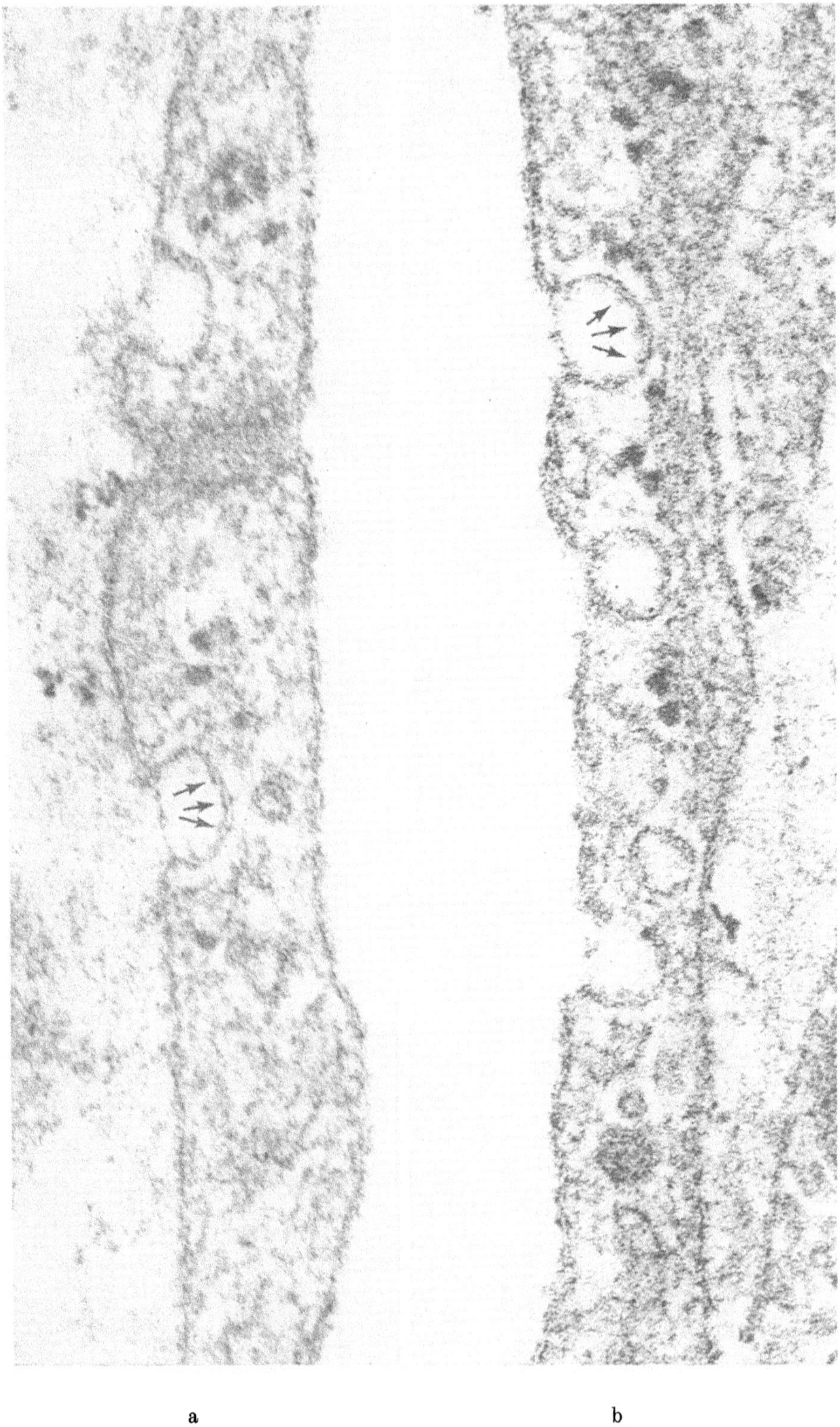

a b

Fig. 3

ed areas, and the lining of the hepatic sinusoids is composed of endothelial cells and Kupffer cells in approximately equal proportions (WIDMANN et al., 1972). With the exception of the study of the coronary and renal circulations (OSBORNE et al., 1970), there is no direct evidence that Ang. II is eliminated by hydrolytic degradation. As well, there are no data on the access of intracellular enzymes to angiotensin. LEARY (1969), using isolated organs perfused *in situ*, has found no evidence of the secretion of soluble angiotensinase enzymes into the vascular space. The slow rate of inactivation of angiotensin by intact red cells as opposed to the vigorous metabolism by hemolysates suggests that the plasma membrane is not very permeable to angiotensin. Estimates of the volumes of distribution and mean transit times of angiotensin and its metabolites in various vascular beds could be instructive [CHINARD et al., 1962; GORESKY, 1963; CHINARD, 1966; RYAN and SMITH, 1971 (1); RYAN et al., 1972 (1, 2)]. If the volume of distribution of angiotensin were found to exceed that of the vascular space, a role for intracellular angiotensinase enzymes would become more tenable. At present, there is no evidence of facilitated uptake of angiotensin.

C. Elimination by Binding

The physicochemical form of angiotensin in the circulation is not known. HAAS et al. (1968) have presented evidence of a co-factor in blood which appears to increase the duration of pressor effects. Possibly angiotensin is bound to the co-factor, the two being difficult to separate *in vitro*. However, formation of an angiotensin co-factor complex *in vivo* is sluggish at best as the pressor response of highly purified angiotensin is much briefer than that of crude angiotensin which contains co-factor. Direct evidence of a complex is lacking, and the possibility must be considered that angiotensin and the co-factor are not linked but relate to each other much like bradykinin and its potentiating factors [FERREIRA, 1965; HAMBERG et al., 1969; STEWART et al., 1971 (1)]. The bradykinin potentiating factors act, at least in part, to extend the duration of bradykinin responses by inhibiting tissue kininase enzymes [RYAN et al., 1970 (1)].

Experience with antibodies to angiotensin proves the point that angiotensin could be eliminated by specific binding [WEISER et al., 1969; BRUNNER et al., 1971; CARRETERO et al., 1971 (2)]. However, angiotensin is not very antigenic unless coupled to macromolecules (GOCKE et al., 1968, 1969; VALLOTTON et al., 1967) or adsorbed on charcoral (BOYD et al., 1967), and the occurrence of natural antibodies to angiotensin has not been shown. Similarly there is, at present, little evidence of the binding of angiotensin to plasma proteins or to small molecular carriers or to inhibitors.

D. Elimination by Synthetic Reactions

LEE et al. (1970) has presented chemical evidence indicating that Ang. II can be condensed with histidyl-leucine to form Ang. I. The product was not isolated nor tested biologically, thus it is questionable that condensation occurred.

Fig. 3. a) and b). High power micrographs showing endothelial caveolae, each of which is covered by a diaphragm composed of a single lamella. The caveolae membrane appears to have a unit membrane construction similar to the plasma membrane, but the inner concave surface of the caveola membrane is studded with regularly spaced subunits (arrows) which give the impression of beading. a) × 223,000; b) × 176,000. (Reproduced from SMITH and RYAN, 1972, Tissue and Cell **4**, by permission of the publishers, The Longman Group Ltd.)

E. Cellular Uptake and Transfer to Extracellular Spaces

Recent studies, using intrinsically labelled angiotensin, have provided little evidence of the uptake of angiotensin by cells or of transfer from the vascular lumen to other extracellular spaces. Although lymph may contain angiotensin, BAILIE et al. (1971) were unable to find evidence of the transfer of [5-(^{14}C)isoleucine]-angiotensin from the vascular space to the renal lymphatic effluent.

Similarly OSBORNE et al. (1970) found that less than 3% of the radioactivity of [4-(^{3}H)tyrosine]-Ang. II was retained during passage through the isolated coronary or renal circulations. Whether any of the retained radioactivity remained in the form of angiotensin was not reported. However, a note of caution seems appropriate because of the relatively high concentrations of angiotensin that have been used. The studies by OSBORNE et al. used angiotensin at 10 ng/ml, almost 1,000 times greater than the concentrations reported to occur physiologically (CAIN et al., 1970). Thus retention of 2 to 3% of the total radioactivity could be significant.

In a subsequent study using anesthetized rats, OSBORNE et al. (1971) found that the kidneys, adrenals, liver and spleen contained more radioactivity 1 min after the intravenous injection of [^{3}H-Tyr^{4}]-Ang. II than could be accounted for as trapped blood. As much as 50% of the radioactivity found in tissues 2 min after injection migrated on paper chromatography like Ang. II or its C-terminal heptapeptide. Through the nature of the experiment, it was not possible to conclude whether the Ang. II-like material was derived primarily from trapped blood or from organ parenchyma.

Acknowledgements

This work was supported in part by grants from the U.S. Public Health Service (HL-14360) and the John A. Hartford Foundation. I thank Dr. UNA SMITH for providing the electron micrographs and for helpful discussion and criticism. I also thank Miss SUEHANNA RICHMOND for typing the manuscript and for checking the bibliography.

References

ABRAMS, J. S.: Blood pressure response to the portal infusion of angiotensin II. Surg. Forum **XVII**, 133 (1966).

ALLAN, D., CRUMPTON, M. J.: Preparation and characterization of the plasma membrane of pig lymphocytes. Biochem. J. **120**, 133 (1970).

ARAKAWA, K., NAKATANI, M., MINOHARA, A., NAKAMURA, M.: Isolation and amino acid composition of human angiotensin I. Biochem. J. **104**, 900 (1967).

ARAKAWA, K., MINOHARA, A., YAMADA, J., NAKAMURA, M.: Enzymatic degradation and electrophoresis of human angiotensin I. Biochim. biophys. Acta (Amst.) **168**, 106 (1968).

BAILIE, M. D., RECTOR, F. C., SELDIN, D. W.: Angiotensin II in arterial and renal venous plasma and renal lymph in the dog. J. clin. Invest. **50**, 119 (1971).

BANGHAM, D. R., CALAM, D. H., PARSONS, J. A., ROBINSON, C. J.: Purity of synthetic peptide preparations. Nature (Lond.) **232**, 631 (1971).

BARBOUR, B. H., BARTTER, F. C.: Angiotensin labeled with I^{131} and with tritium. J. clin. Endocr. **23**, 313 (1963).

BARRETT, J. D., SAMBHI, M. P.: Pulmonary activation and degradation of angiotensin I: A dual enzyme system. Res. Commun. Chem. Path. Pharmacol. **2**, 128 (1971).

BAUDOUIN, M., MEYER, P., WORCEL, M.: Specific binding of ^{3}H-angiotensin II in rabbit aorta. Biochem. biophys. Res. Commun. **42**, 434 (1971).

BEAULNES, A., BEEBE, C.: Comparative cardiac effects of angiotensin, eledoisin and physalaemin. Adv. Exp. Med. Biol. **8**, 149 (1970).

BING, J.: Angiotensinase content of kidneys of normal and hypertensive rats. Acta path. microbiol. scand. **56**, 385 (1962).

BIRON, P., CAMPEAU, L., DAVID, P.: Fate of angiotensin I and II in the human pulmonary circulation. Amer. J. Cardiol. **24**, 544 (1969).

BIRON, P., MEYER, P., PANISSET, J. C.: Removal of angiotensins from the systemic circulation. Canad. J. Physiol. Pharmacol. **46**, 175 (1968).

BISSET, G. W.: Effect of tyrosinase preparations on oxytocin, vasopressin and bradykinin. Brit. J. Pharmacol. **18**, 405 (1962).

BLAQUIER, P., BOHR, D. F., TAQUINI, A. C., HOOBLER, S. W.: Renin and angiotensinase content of the kidney of normal and renal hypertensive rats. Proc. Soc. exp. Biol. (N. Y.) **108**, 711 (1961).

BOUCHER, R., VEYRAT, R., CHAMPLAIN, DE, J., GENEST, J.: New procedures for measurement of human plasma angiotensin and renin activity levels. Canad. med. Ass. J. **90**, 194 (1964).

BOYD, G. W., LANDON, J., PEART, W. S.: Radioimmunoassay for determining plasma-levels of angiotensin II in man. Lancet **1967 II**, 1002.

BOYD, G. W., LANDON, J., PEART, W. S.: The radioimmunoassay of angiotensin II. Proc. Roy. Soc. B. **173**, 327 (1969).

BRAUN-MENENDEZ, E., FASCIOLO, J. C., LELOIR, L. F., MUÑOZ, J. M.: La substancia hipertensora de la sangre del riñon isquemiado. Rev. Soc. argent. Biol. **15**, 420 (1939).

BRAUN-MENENDEZ, E., FASCIOLO, J. C., LELOIR, L. F., MUÑOZ, J. M., TAQUINI, A. C.: Renal Hypertension. 1st ed. Springfield/Illinois: Charles C. Thomas 1946.

BROWN, J. J., DAVIES, D. L., LEVER, A. F., ROBERTSON, J. I. S.: The estimation of renin activity in human plasma. Biochem. J. **93**, 594 (1964).

BRUNNER, H. R., KIRSHMAN, J. D., SEALEY, J. E., LARAGH, J. H.: Hypertension of renal origin: Evidence for two different mechanisms. Science **174**, 1344 (1971).

BRYAN, F. T., RYAN, J. W., NIEMEYER, R. S.: Bradykinin synthesis by liver. Adv. exp. Med. Biol. **21**, 43 (1972).

BUMPUS, F. M., SCHWARZ, H., PAGE, I. H.: Synthesis and pharmacology of the octapeptide angiotonin. Science **125**, 886 (1957).

BUMPUS, F. M., SCHWARZ, H., PAGE, I. H.: Synthesis and properties of angiotonin. Circulation **XVII**, 664 (1958).

BUMPUS, F. M., SMEBY, R. R.: Angiotensin. In: Renal Hypertension. 1st ed. Chicago: Year Book Medical Publishers Inc. 1968.

BUMPUS, F. M., SMEBY, R. R., PAGE, I. H., KHAIRALLAH, P. A.: Distribution and metabolic fate of angiotensin II and various derivatives. Canad. med. Ass. J. **90**, 190 (1964).

BUMPUS, F. M., TÜRKER, R. K., YAMAMOTO, M.: A new potent antagonist of angiotensin II. In: Abstracts of the 2nd International Symposium on Protein and Polypeptide Hormones. Liege, Sept. 28—Oct. 1, 1971.

CAIN, M. D., CATT, K. J., COGHLAN, J. P.: Immunoreactive fragments of angiotensin II in blood. Nature (Lond.) **223**, 617 (1969).

CAIN, M. D., CATT, K. J., COGHLAN, J. P., BLAIR-WEST, J. R.: Evaluation of angiotensin II metabolism in sheep by radioimmunoassay. Endocrinology **86**, 955 (1970).

CARO, L. G.: High resolution autoradiography. In: Methods in Cell Physiology, 1st ed. Vol. II. New York: Academic Press 1966.

CARRETERO, O. A., BUJAK, B., HOULE, J. A.: (1) Renin isozymes of extrarenal origin. Amer. J. Physiol. **220**, 1468 (1971).

CARRETERO, O. A., KUK, P., PIWONSKA, S., HOULE, J. A., MARIN-GREZ, M.: (2) Role of the renin-angiotensin system in the pathogenesis of severe hypertension in rats. Circulat. Res. **XXIX**, 654 (1971).

CATT, K. J., CAIN, M. C., COGHLAN, J. P.: Measurement of angiotensin II in blood. Lancet **1967 II**, 1005.

CHAMBERLAIN, M. J., BROWSE, N. L., GIBSON, D. G., GLEESON, J. A.: Angiotensin and renoportal anastomosis. Brit. Med. J. **1964 II**, 1507.

CHINARD, F. P.: The permeability characteristics of the pulmonary blood-gas barrier. In: Advances in Respiratory Physiology. 1st ed. Baltimore: The Williams and Wilkins Co. 1966.

CHINARD, F. P., ENNS, T., NOLAN, M. F.: The permeability characteristics of the alveolar capillary barrier. Trans. Assoc. Amer. Phycns. **75**, 253 (1962).

CORCORAN, A. C., KOHLSTAEDT, K. G., PAGE, I. H.: Changes of arterial blood pressure and renal hemodynamics by injection of angiotonin in human beings. Proc. Soc. exp. Biol. (N. Y.) **46**, 244 (1941).

DAHLHEIM, H., PETSCHAUER, K., THURAU, K.: Anreicherung und Charakterisierung der Erythrocytenangiotensinase. Pflügers Arch. ges. Physiol. **305**, 105 (1969).

DENGLER, H., REICHEL, G.: Untersuchungen zur intrazellulären Lokalisation der Renin- und Hypertensinase-Aktivität. Experientia (Basel) **16**, 36 (1960).

DEXTER, L.: The hypertensinase content of plasma of normal, hypertensive and nephrectomized dogs. Ann. intern. Med. **17**, **447** (1942).

DOYLE, A. E., LOUIS, W. J., JERUMS, G., OSBORN, E. C.: Metabolism and blood levels following infusion of a radioactive analog of angiotensin. Amer. J. Physiol. **215**, 164 (1968).

DREYER, W. J., BYNUM, E.: High-voltage paper electrophoresis. In: Methods in Enzymology, 1st ed., Vol. XI, New York: Academic Press 1967.
ELLIOTT, D. F., PEART, W. S.: The amino acid sequence in a hypertensin. Biochem. J. **65**, 246 (1957).
EMMELOT, P., BOS, C. J., BENEDETTI, E. L., RÜMKE, P.: Studies of plasma membranes. I. Chemical composition and enzyme content of plasma membranes isolated from rat liver. Biochim. biophys. Acta (Amst.) **90**, 126 (1964).
FASCIOLO, J. C., LELOIR, L. F., MUÑOZ, J. M., BRAUN-MENENDEZ, E.: La hipertensinasa, su dosaje y distribución. Rev. Soc. argent. Biol. **16**, 643 (1940).
FERREIRA, S. H.: A bradykinin-potentiating factor (BPF) present in the venom of Bothrops jararaca. Brit. J. Pharmacol. **24**, 163 (1965).
FRIEDMAN, M., MARX, W., LINDNER, E.: Renin substrate and angiotenase in dogs' lymph and plasma. Proc. Soc. exp. Biol. (N. Y.) **54**, 221 (1943).
GARBE, G.: Quantitative Kininogenbestimmung in menschlichem Plasma. Naunyn-Schmiedebergs Arch. Pharmak. exp. Path. **256**, 112 (1967).
GIESE, J., NIELSEN, M. D., JORGENSEN, M.: New view of cross-reaction in anti-angiotensin sera. Nature (Lond.) New Biol. **229**, 189 (1971).
GOCKE, D. J., GERTEN, J., SHERWOOD, L. M., LARAGH, J. H.: Physiological and pathological variations of plasma angiotensin II in man. Circulat. Res. Suppl. I, **XXIV**, I—131 (1969).
GOCKE, D. J., SHERWOOD, L. M., OPPENHOFF, I., GERTEN, J., LARAGH, J. H.: Measurement of plasma angiotensin II and correlation with renin activity. J. clin. Endocr. **28**, 1675 (1968).
GOLDMAN, R., SILIMAN, H. I., CAPLAN, S. R., KEDEM, O., KATCHALSKI, E.: Papain membrane on a collodion matrix: Preparation and enzymic behavior. Science **150**, 758 (1965).
GORESKY, C. A.: A linear method for determining liver sinusoidal and extravascular volumes. Amer. J. Physiol. **204**, 626 (1963).
GORESKY, C. A.: Initial distribution and rate of uptake of sulfobromophthalein in the liver. Amer. J. Physiol. **207**, 13 (1964).
GRANGER, P., DAHLHEIM, H., THURAU, K.: Renin-, Angiotensinase- und Converting Enzym-Bestimmungen an einzelnen mikrodissezierten juxtaglomerulären Apparaten und Teilen des Nephrons. Pflügers Arch. ges. Physiol. **312**, R 87 (1969).
GREENBAUM, L. M., KIM, K. S.: The kinin forming and kininase activities of rabbit polymorphonuclear leucocytes. Brit. J. Pharmacol. **27**, 230 (1967).
GREGERMAN, R. I.: Identification of histidylleucine and other histidyl peptides as normal constituents of human urine. Biochem. Med. **1**, 151 (1967).
GREGERMAN, R. I., KOWATCH, M. A.: Double isotope derivative assay for angiotensin I: Use for renin measurement. J. clin. Endocr. **32**, 110 (1971).
HAAS, E., GOLDBLATT, H., LEWIS, L., GIPSON, E. C.: Inhibition of angiotensin and its protection by a cofactor in blood. Amer. J. Physiol. **215**, 1420 (1968).
HAMBERG, U., ELG, P., STELWAGEN, P.: Tryptic and plasmic peptide fragments increasing the effect of bradykinin on isolated smooth muscle. Scand. J. clin. Lab. Invest. Suppl. 107, **24**, 9 (1969).
HARTLEY, B. S.: Strategy and tactics in protein chemistry. Biochem. J. **119**, 805 (1970).
HELMER, O. M., JUDSON, W. E.: The quantitative determination of renin in the plasma of patients with arterial hypertension. Circulation **XXVII**, 1050 (1963).
HELMER, O. M., KOHLSTAEDT, K. G., KEMPF, G. F., PAGE, I. H.: (1) The assay of anti-pressor extracts of kidney by in vitro destruction of angiotonin. Fed. Proc. **1**, 114 (1942).
HELMER, O. M., KOHLSTAEDT, K. G., PAGE, I. H.: (2) Destruction of angiotonin by extracts of various tissues. Fed. Proc. **1**, 114 (1942).
HESS, R.: Arylamidase activity related to angiotensinase. Biochim. biophys. Acta (Amst.) **99**, 316 (1965).
HIRS, C. H. W.: Enzyme structure. In: Methods in Enzymology, 1st ed., Vol. XI, New York: Academic Press 1967.
HODGE, R. L., NG, K. K. F., VANE, J. R.: Disappearance of angiotensin from the circulation of the dog. Nature (Lond.) **215**, 138 (1967).
HORKY, K., ROJO-ORTEGA, J. M., RODRIGUEZ, J., BOUCHER, R., GENEST, J.: Renin, renin substrate, and angiotensin I-converting enzyme in the lymph of rats. Amer. J. Physiol. **220**, 307 (1971).
ITO, Y., BOWMAN, R. L.: Development of support-free liquid-liquid partition techniques holds promise for preparative and analytical chromatographic separation of compounds without complications arising from solid supports. Analyt. Chem. **43**, 69 A (1971).
ITSKOVITZ, H. D., MILLER, L.: Differential studies of angiotensinase activities from several tissue sources. Amer. J. Med. Sci. **254**, 659 (1967).
ITSKOVITZ, H. D., MILLER, L. D.: Renal angiotensinase activity. Its localization and the effects of mercury. Circulat. Res. **XIX**, 507 (1966).

JOHNSON, D. C.: The selective inactivation of angiotensinase activity. Thesis, University of Oxford, 1967.
JOHNSON, D. C., RYAN, J. W.: Degradation of angiotensin II by a carboxypeptidase of rabbit liver. Biochim. biophys. Acta (Amst.) **160**, 196 (1968).
KHAIRALLAH, P. A., BUMPUS, F. M., PAGE, I. H., SMEBY, R. R.: Angiotensinase with a high degree of specificity in plasma and red cells. Science **140**, 672 (1963).
KHAIRALLAH, P. A., PAGE, I. H.: Plasma angiotensinases. Biochem. Med. **1**, 1 (1967).
KHAIRALLAH, P. A., PAGE, I. H., BUMPUS, F. M., SMEBY, R. R.: Angiotensin II. Its metabolic fate. Science **138**, 523 (1962).
KHAIRALLAH, P. A., PAGE, I. H., BUMPUS, F. M., TÜRKER, R. K.: Angiotensin tachyphylaxis and its reversal. Circulat. Res. **XIX**, 247 (1966).
KHAIRALLAH, P. A., TOTH, A., BUMPUS, F. M.: Analogs of angiotensin II. II. Mechanism of receptor interaction. J. med. Chem. **13**, 181 (1970).
KLAUS, D., HEIZMANN, A., UEHLEKE, H.: Beeinflussung der Blutdruckwirkung von Angiotensin durch Aminopeptidasen und Carboxypeptidase. Naunyn-Schmiedebergs Arch. exp. Pharmakol. **251**, 28 (1965).
KOKUBU, T., AKUTSU, H., FUJIMOTO, S., UEDA, E., HIWADA, K., YAMAMURA, Y.: Purification and properties of endopeptidase from rabbit red cells and its process of degradation of angiotensin. Biochim. biophys. Acta (Amst.) **191**, 668 (1969).
KURCBART, H., COLI, A., VANCHERI, L., ROSA, U.: Chemical and biological effects associated with the iodination of angiotensin II. Biochim. biophys. Acta (Amst.) **230**, 160 (1971).
KURTZ, A. B., WACHSMUTH, E. D.: Identification of plasma angiotensinase as aminopeptidase. Nature (Lond.) **221**, 92 (1969).
LEARY, W. P.: The inactivation of angiotensin II by isolated perfused organs in the rat. Thesis, University of Oxford, 1969.
LEARY, W. P., LEDINGHAM, J. G.: Removal of angiotensin by isolated perfused organs of the rat. Nature (Lond.) **222**, 959 (1969).
LEE, H.-J., LARUE, J. N., WILSON, I. B.: A possible new component of the renin angiotensin system. Abst. 1141, Fed. Proc. **29**, 448 (1970).
LELOIR, L. F., MUÑOZ, J. M., BRAUN-MENENDEZ, E., FASCIOLO, J. C.: La secreción de renina y la formación de hipertensina. Rev. Soc. argent. Biol. **16**, 75 (1940).
LENTZ, K. E., SKEGGS, L. T., WOODS, K. R., KAHN, J. R., SHUMWAY, N. P.: The amino acid composition of hypertensin II and its biochemical relationship to hypertensin I. J. exp. Med. **104**, 183 (1956).
LIN, S.-Y., ELLIS, H., WEISBLUM, B., GOODFRIEND, T. L.: Preparation and properties of iodinated angiotensins. Biochem. Pharmacol. **19**, 651 (1970).
LUBASH, G. D., MUIESAN, G. E., ALICANDRI, C. L., GARFINKEL, D. J., SIEKIERSKI, E. C., MCCONNAUGHEY, C. K.: Plasma angiotensin, serum 'angiotensinase activity', and blood pressure response during angiotensin II amide infusions in normal volunteers. Experientia (Basel) **27**, 68 (1971).
MAEBASHI, M., YOSHINAGA, K.: Estimation of renin activity in human aminotic fluid of normal and toxemic pregnant women. Tohoku J. exp. Med. **96**, 393 (1968).
MAJNO, G., SHEA, S. M., LEVENTHAL, M.: Endothelial contraction induced by histamine-type mediators. J. Cell. Biol. **42**, 647 (1969).
MANNING, J. M., MOORE, S.: Determination of D- and L-amino acids by ion exchange chromatography as L-D and L-L dipeptides. J. biol. Chem. **243**, 5591 (1968).
MARCHESI, V. T., BARRNETT, R. J.: The demonstration of enzymatic activity in pinocytic vesicles of blood capillaries with the electron microscope. J. Cell. Biol. **17**, 547 (1963).
MARSHALL, G. R., MERRIFIELD, R. B.: Synthesis of angiotensins by the solid-phase method. Biochemistry **4**, 2394 (1965).
MARSHALL, G. R., VINE, W., NEEDLEMAN, P.: A specific competitive inhibitors of angiotensin II. Proc. Natl. Acad. Sci. (Wash.) **67**, 1624 (1970).
MATSUNAGA, M.: Nature of lysosomal angiotensinase activity. Jap. Circulat. J. (En.) **35**, 333 (1971).
MATSUNAGA, M., KIRA, J., SAITO, N., OGINO, K., TAKAYASU, M.: Acid angiotensinase, renin and acid adenosine triphosphatase in rat kidney lysosomes. Jap. Circulat. J. (En.) **32**, 137 (1968).
MATSUNAGA, M., MASSON, G. M. C.: Hepatic and renal neutral angiotensinases. Experientia (Basel) **26**, 1297 (1970).
MATSUNAGA, M., SAITO, N., KIRA, J., OGINO, K., TAKAYASU, M.: Acid angiotensinase as a lysosomal enzyme. Jap. Circulat. J. (En.) **33**, 545 (1969).
METHOT, A. L., MEYER, P., BIRON, P., LORAIN, M. F., LAGRUE, G., MILLIEZ, P.: Hepatic inactivation of angiotensin. Nature (Lond.) **203**, 531 (1964).
MORGAT, J. L., HUNG, L. T., FROMAGEOT, P.: Preparation of highly labelled [^{3}H]-angiotensin II. Biochim. biophys. Acta (Amst.) **207**, 374 (1970).

NAKAGAWA, S., RUEGAMER, W. R.: Properties of a rat tissue iodothyronine deiodinase and its natural inhibitor. Biochemistry **6**, 1249 (1967).

NARITA, K.: End group determination. In: Protein Sequence Determination, 1st ed. Berlin-Heidelberg-New York: Springer 1970.

NIGAWARA, K., TERAYAMA, Y., TATEYAMA, M., SENO, T., SHIRAIWA, Y., FUNYM, T.: A method for the measurement of plasma renin activity. Jap. J. Urol. **62**, 131 (1971).

OSBORNE, M. J., D'AURIAC, A., MEYER, P., WORCEL, M.: Mechanism of extraction of angiotensin II in coronary and renal circulations. Life Sci., **9**, 859 (1970).

OSBORNE, M. J., POOTERS, N., D'AURIAC, G. A., EPSTEIN, A. N., WORCEL, M., MEYER, P.: Metabolism of tritiated angiotensin II in anaesthetized rats. Pflügers Arch. ges. Physiol. **326**, 101 (1971).

PAGE, I. H., HELMER, O. M.: A crystalline pressor substance (angiotonin) resulting from the reaction between renin and renin-activator. J. exp. Med. **71**, 29 (1940).

PALS, D. T., MASUCCI, F. D., DENNING, G. S., SIPOS, F., FESSLER, D. C.: (1) Role of the pressor action of angiotensin II in experimental hypertension. Circulat. Res. **XXIX**, 673 (1971).

PALS, D. T., MASUCCI, F. D., SIPOS, F., DENNING, G. S.: (2) A specific competitive antagonist of the vascular action of angiotensin II. Circulat. Res. **XXIX**, 664 (1971).

PEART, W. S.: A new method of large scale preparation of hypertensin, with a note on its assay. Biochem. J. **59**, 300 (1955).

PICKENS, P. T., BUMPUS, F. M., LLOYD, A. M., SMEBY, R. R., PAGE, I. H.: Measurement of renin activity in human plasma. Circulat. Res. **XVII**, 437 (1965).

PIETRA, G. G., SZIDON, J. P., LEVENTHAL, M. M., FISHMAN, A. P.: Histamine and interstitial pulmonary edema in the dog. Circulat. Res. **XXIX**, 323 (1971).

PRADELLES, P., MORGAT, J. L., FROMAGEOT, P., OLIVER, C., JAQUET, P., GOURDJI, D., TIXIER-VIDAL, A.: Preparation of highly labelled ^{3}H-thyreotropin releasing hormone (PGA-HIS-PRO[NH_2]) by catalytic hydrogenolysis. FEBS Letters **22**, 19 (1972).

REGOLI, D., RINIKER, B., BRUNNER, H.: The enzymatic degradation of various angiotensin II derivatives by serum, plasma or kidney homogenate. Biochem. Pharmacol. **12**, 637 (1963).

RHODIN, J. A. G.: The ultrastructure of mammalian arterioles and precapillary sphincters. J. Ultrastruct. Res. **18**, 181 (1967).

RICHARDSON, J. B., BEAULNES, A.: The cellular site of action of angiotensin. J. Cell Biol. **51**, 419 (1971).

RINIKER, B., SCHWYZER, R.: Synthetische Analoge des Hypertensins. V. α-L, β-L, α-D- und β-D-Asp^1-Val^5-Hypertensin II; desamino-Val^5-Hypertensin II. Helv. chim. Acta **47**, 2357 (1964).

RIPA, R., DEGLI ATTI, B.: Plasmatic and erythrocytic angiotensinase activity in subjects with arterial hypertension. Mal. cardiovasc. **X**, 537 (1969).

ROBERTSON, A. L., KHAIRALLAH, P. A.: Angiotensin II: Rapid localization in nuclei of smooth and cardiac muscle. Science **172**, 1138 (1971).

RYAN, J. W.: (1) Renin-like enzyme in the adrenal gland. Science **158**, 1589 (1967).

RYAN, J. W.: (2) A rapid simple method for the assay of renin in rabbit plasma. Thesis, University of Oxford, 1967.

RYAN, J. W.: Specificity of the renin-like enzyme of rabbit uterus. Biochem. J. **116**, 159 (1970).

RYAN, J. W., BRYAN, F. T., NIEMEYER, R. S.: (1) Kininogen is synthesized in the liver. Cien. Cult. **23**, 515 (1971).

RYAN, J. W., JOHNSON, D. C.: The renin-like enzyme of rabbit uterus. Biochim. biophys. Acta (Amst.) **191**, 386 (1969).

RYAN, J. W., MCKENZIE, J. K., LEE, M. R.: A rapid simple method for the estimation of plasma renin activity in the rabbit. Proc. III International Congr. of Nephrology, Abstract 1966.

RYAN, J. W., MCKENZIE, J. K., LEE, M. R.: (1) A rapid, simple method for the assay of renin in rabbit plasma. Biochem. J. **108**, 679 (1968).

RYAN, J. W., NIEMEYER, R. S., GOODWIN, D. W.: (1) Metabolic fates of bradykinin, angiotensin I, adenine nucleotides and prostaglandins E_1 and $F_1\alpha$ in the pulmonary circulation. Adv. Exp. Med. Biol. **21**, 259 (1972).

RYAN, J. W., NIEMEYER, R. S., GOODWIN, D. W., SMITH, U., STEWART, J. M.: (2) Metabolism of [8-L-(^{14}C)phenylalanine]-angiotensin I in the pulmonary circulation. Biochem. J. **125**, 921 (1971).

RYAN, J. W., ROBLERO, J., STEWART, J. M.: (2) Inactivation of bradykinin in the pulmonary circulation. Biochem. J. **110**, 795 (1968).

RYAN, J. W., ROBLERO, J., STEWART, J. M.: (1) Inactivation of bradykinin in rat lung. Adv. Exp. Med. Biol. **8**, 263 (1970).

RYAN, J. W., SMITH, U.: (1) A rapid, simple method for isolating pinocytotic vesicles and plasma membrane of lung. Biochim. biophys. Acta (Amst.) **249**, 177 (1971).

RYAN, J. W., SMITH, U.: (2) Metabolism of adenosine-5'-monophosphate during circulation through the lungs. Trans. Ass. Amer. Phycns. **84**, 297 (1971).
RYAN, J. W., SMITH, U., NIEMEYER, R. S.: Angiotensin I: Metabolism by plasma membrane of lung. Science **176**, 64 (1972).
RYAN, J. W., STEWART, J. M., LEARY, W. P., LEDINGHAM, J. G.: (2) Metabolism of angiotensin I in the pulmonary circulation. Biochem. J. **120**, 221 (1970).
SAITO, N., SANADA, K., MATSUNAGA, M., MUKAINO, S., KIRA, J., OGINO, K., TAKAYASU, M.: Amino acid analysis after degradation of angiotensin II by rat kidney lysosomes. Jap. Circulat. J. (En.) **33**, 87 (1969).
SAKAKIBARA, S., FUJII, T.: Synthesis and use of N^{im}-Tosyl-L-histidine. Bull. chem. Soc. Jap. **42**, 1466 (1969).
SALPETER, M. M., BACHMANN, L., SALPETER, E. E.: Resolution in electron microscope radioautography. J. cell. Biol. **41**, 1 (1969).
SANDER, G. E., HUGGINS, C. G.: Subcellular localization of angiotensin I converting enzyme in rabbit lung. Nature (Lond.) New Biol. **230**, 27 (1971).
SAPIRSTEIN, L. A., REED, R. K., PAGE, E. W.: The site of angiotonin destruction. J. exp. Med. **83**, 425 (1946).
SCHNEIDER, W. C., KUFF, E. L.: Centrifugal isolation of subcellular components. In: Cytology and Cell Physiology. 3rd ed. New York: Academic Press 1964.
SHNITKA, T. K., SELIGMAN, A. M.: Ultrastructural localization of enzyme. Ann. Rev. Biochem. **40**, 375 (1971).
SKEGGS, L. T., KAHN, J. R., LENTZ, K., SHUMWAY, N. P.: The preparation, purification and amino acid sequence of a polypeptide renin substrate. J. exp. Med. **106**, 439 (1957).
SKEGGS, L. T., KAHN, J. R., SHUMWAY, N. P.: The isolation and assay of hypertensin from blood. J. exp. Med. **95**, 241 (1952).
SKEGGS, L. T., LENTZ, K. E., KAHN, J. R., DORER, F. E., LEVINE, M.: Pseudorenin, a new angiotensin-forming enzyme. Circulat. Res. **XXV**, 451 (1969).
SKEGGS, L. T., LENTZ, K. E., KAHN, J. R., SHUMWAY, N. P.: The synthesis of a tetradecapeptide renin substrate. J. exp. Med. **108**, 283 (1958).
SKEGGS, L. T., LENTZ, K. E., KAHN, J. R., SHUMWAY, N. P., WOODS, K. R.: The amino acid sequence of hypertensin II. J. exp. Med. **104**, 193 (1956).
SMITH, U., RYAN, J. W.: An electron microscopic study of the vascular endothelium as a site for bradykinin and ATP inactivation in rat lung. Adv. Exp. Med. Biol. **8**, 249 (1970).
SMITH, U., RYAN, J. W.: Pinocytocic vesicles of the pulmonary endothelial cell. Chest **59**, 12 S (1971).
SMITH, U., RYAN, J. W.: (1) Pulmonary endothelial cells and metabolism of adenine nucleotides, kinins and angiotensin I. Adv. Exp. Med. Biol. **21**, 267 (1972).
SMITH, U., RYAN, J. W.: (2) Substructural features of pulmonary endothelial caveolae. Tissue and Cell **4**, 49 (1972).
SMITH, U., RYAN, J. W., MICHIE, D. D., SMITH, D. S.: Endothelial projections as revealed by scanning electron microscopy. Science **173**, 927 (1971).
SPECTOR, W. S.: Handbook of Biological Data. 1st ed. Philadelphia: W. B. Saunders Co. 1956.
STEWART, J. M., FERREIRA, S. H., GREENE, L. J.: (1) Bradykinin potentiating peptide PCA-LYS-TRP-ALA-PRO. An inhibitor of the pulmonary inactivation of bradykinin and conversion of angiotensin I to II. Biochem. Pharmacol. **20**, 1557 (1971).
STEWART, J. M., FREER, R. J., PAIVA, T. B., PAIVA, A. C. M.: (2) Alkylating derivatives of angiotensin II and bradykinin. In: Abstracts of the 2nd International Symposium on Protein and Polypeptide Hormones. Liege, Sept. 28—Oct. 1, 1971.
STEWART, J. M., YOUNG, J. D.: Solid Phase Peptide Synthesis. 1st ed. San Francisco: W. H. Freeman and Co. 1969.
THINES-SEMPOUX, D., AMAR-COSTESEC, A., BEAUFAY, H., BERTHET, J.: The association of cholesterol, 5'-nucleotidase and alkaline phosphodiesterase with a distinct group of microsomal particles. J. Cell Biol. **43**, 604 (1970).
TOUSTER, O., ARONSON, N. N., DULANEY, J. T., HENDRICKSON, H.: Isolation of rat liver plasma membranes. J. Cell Biol. **47**, 604 (1970).
TÜRKER, R. K., YAMAMOTO, M., BUMPUS, F. M., KHAIRALLAH, P. A.: Lung perfusion with angiotensin I and II. Evidence of release of myotropic and inhibitory substances. Circulat. Res. **XXVIII**, 559 (1971).
VALLOTTON, M. B., PAGE, L. B., HABER, E.: Radioimmunoassay of angiotensin in human plasma. Nature (Lond.) **215**, 714 (1967).
VANE, J. R.: The use of isolated organs for detecting active substances in the circulating blood. Brit. J. Pharmacol. **23**, 360 (1964).
VANE, J. R.: The release and fate of vaso-active hormones in the circulation. Brit. J. Pharmacol. **35**, 209 (1969).

VANE, J. R.: Purity and stability of synthetic peptides such as angiotensins and kinins. Nature (Lond.) **230**, 382 (1971).

VATTER, A. E., REISS, O. K., NEWMAN, J. K., LINDQUIST, K., GROENEBOER, E.: Enzymes of the lung. 1. Detection of esterase with a new cytochemical method. J. Cell Biol. **38**, 80 (1968).

VIGNEAUD, DU, V., LAWLER, H. C., POPENOE, E. A.: Enzymatic cleavage of glycinamide from vasopressin and a proposed structure for this pressor antidiuretic hormone of the posterior pituitary. J. Amer. chem. Soc. **75**, 4880 (1953).

WACHSMUTH, E. D.: Lokalisation von Aminopeptidase in Gewebeschnitten mit einer neuen Immunofluoreszenztechnik. Histochemie **14**, 282 (1968).

WEISER, R. A., JOHNSON, A. G., HOOBLER, S. W.: The effect of antirenin on the blood pressure of the rat with experimental renal hypertension. Lab. Invest. **20**, 326 (1969).

WIDMANN, J.-J., COTRAN, R. S., FAHIMI, H. D.: Mononuclear phagocytes (Kupffer cells) and endothelial cells. Identification of two functional cell types in rat liver sinusoids by endogenous peroxidase activity. J. Cell Biol. **52**, 159 (1972).

WISENBAUGH, P. E., WILLS, N. E., HILL, R. W.: Paper chromatographic identification of angiotensins. Amer. J. Physiol. **207**, 759 (1964).

YANG, H. Y. T., ERDOS, E. G., CHIANG, T. S.: New enzymatic route for the inactivation of angiotensin. Nature (Lond.) **218**, 1224 (1968).

ZWANZIG, M., VON, OELKERS, W.: Vergleichende Untersuchungen über den Abbau von Angiotensin II und Angiotensin II-Amid durch Peptidasen des menschlichen Plasmas. Verh. Deutsche Ges. inn. Med. **74**, 426 (1968).

Catabolism of Angiotensin II

J. G. LEDINGHAM and W. P. LEARY

Catabolism of Angiotensin II

It has long been evident that there are substances in blood and tissues which are capable of destroying angiotensin. The effects of temperature, pH changes and dialysis on angiotensin survival in renin assay systems indicated that enzymes were probably involved (BRAUN-MENENDEZ and FASCIOLO, 1939; PAGE and HELMER, 1940). The generic term "angiotensinase" is used to describe these enzymes, although their specificity is unproven.

The study of angiotensinases in tissue homogenates, lysed red cells, plasma and serum *in vitro* has provided good data about the biological pathways by which angiotensin may be destroyed. This approach probably has no value in the evaluation of the contribution of specific organs or tissues to the metabolism of angiotensin in health and disease. The presence of these enzymes in blood and in tissue extracts of kidney, liver, lung, uterus, intestinal mucosa, adrenal, pancreas, spleen, brain, skeletal and cardiac muscle (FASCIOLO et al., 1940; ITSKOVITZ and MILLER, 1967; MATSUNAGA et al., 1969) does not imply that they are in any way specific for angiotensin or necessarily play any part in the metabolism of Ang. II *in vivo*. For instance homogenates of lung contain angiotensinases in amounts comparable to those in other organs (ITSKOVITZ and MILLER, 1967; MATSUNAGA et al., 1969) but studies of intact lungs indicate that this peptide is not detectably metabolized in the pulmonary circulation in man or other animals (HODGE et al., 1967; LEARY and LEDINGHAM, 1969; BIRON et al., 1969; BIRON and CAMPEAU, 1971; OSBORN et al., 1969).

Nature of Angiotensinases

Yeast aminopeptidase, pepsin, trypsin, chymotrypsin, carboxypeptidases and papain have been shown to destroy angiotensin by CROXATTO and CROXATTO (1942), CROXATTO et al. (1943), and PLENTL and PAGE (1943). The availability of synthetic angiotensin in 1958 led to further studies into the nature and source of angiotensinases in plasma, serum, red cells and tissue slices or homogenates. Enzymes capable of hydrolyzing the N-terminal bond (aminopeptidases), the middle of the peptide (endopeptidases) and the C-terminal bond (carboxypeptidases) of Ang. II have been described (Table 1).

Aminopeptidases (Angiotensinase "A"). GLENNER et al. (1962) found an enzyme specific for N terminal α-L-glutamyl and α-L-aspartyl residues in rat kidney microsomes. KHAIRALLAH et al. (1963) later described a peptidase of very similar properties, in human plasma and lysed washed red cells. Both enzymes were calcium-dependent, pH optima were similar and neither would destroy β-Asp^1-Ang. II. These enzymes, which had much in common, were named Aminopeptidase A by GLENNER et al. and Angiotensinase A by KHAIRALLAH et al. (1963). NAGATSU et al. [1965 (1 and 2) and 1970] then produced evidence that separate aminopeptidases were responsible for hydrolyzing the Asn^1 and Asp^1 analogues of Ang. II. KHAIRALLAH and PAGE (1967) suggested the enzyme active at pH 7.4, which hydrolyzed the Asn^1 peptide, be called Angiotensinase A_1 and the peptidase specific to [Asp^1]-Ang. II Angiotensinase A_2. MATSUNAGA et al. (1969) have found similar neutral

Table 1. *Identified angiotensinases*

Angiotensinase	Authors	pH Optimum	Inhibitors	Source	Site of Action
Aminopeptidase A	GLENNER et al., 1962	7.0	EDTA	Kidney Microsomes	Asp^1-Arg^2
Angiotensinase A_1	KHAIRALLAH and PAGE, 1967	7.4	Sodium pyrophosphate EDTA	Human plasma Human serum	Asn^1-Arg^2
Aminopeptidase	NAGATSU et al., 1965, 1970			Human red cells Kidney extracts	
Angiotensinase A_2 Aminopeptidase	NAGATSU et al., 1965 KHAIRALLAH and PAGE, 1967; NAGATSU et al., 1970	7.4	EDTA	Human serum Red cell and kidney extracts	Asp^1-Arg^2
Microsomal Aminopeptidase	MATSUNAGA and MASSON, 1970	7.4	EDTA	Kidney Microsomes (SH group independent)	Asn^1-Arg^2
		7.4	EDTA and Thiol reagent	Liver microsomes (SH group dependent)	Asp^1-Arg^2 Asn^1-Arg^2
Angiotensinase B (Endopeptidase)	REGOLI et al., 1963; KHAIRALLAH and PAGE, 1967	7.4	? EDTA	Rat serum Human plasma Rat kidney	Tyr^4-Val^5
Lysosomal Endopeptidase	MATSUNAGA, 1971	5.5	SH group dependent	Kidney and liver lysosomes	Tyr^4-Val^5
Carboxypeptidase	JOHNSON and RYAN, 1968	7.4	N.E.M.	EDTA dialyzed Rabbit-liver extract	Pro^7-Phe^8
Angiotensinase C Carboxypeptidase	YANG et al., 1968	5.6 to 5.7	D.F.P.	Hog kidney Human urine	Pro^7-Phe^8
Lysosomal Carboxypeptidase	MATSUNAGA, 1971	5.5	D.F.P.	Kidney and liver lysosomes	Pro^7-Phe^8

amino-peptidases in the microsomal fragments of many organs, most concentrated in kidney and liver (Table 2). Liver cell sap aminopeptidase may be dependent on sulphhydryl (SH) groups in contrast to the renal microsomal enzyme.

Endopeptidases (Angiotensinase "B"). The effects of rat serum, human plasma and rat kidney homogenate on six analogues of Ang. II were observed by REGOLI et al. (1963). Analogues stable to aminopeptidases were destroyed by all three media, and chromatography of the peptide fragments showed individual amino acids and the tetrapeptide Asp^1-Arg^2-Val^3-Tyr^4. The C-terminal tetrapeptide was not found intact, but the evidence was taken to suggest the presence of an endopeptidase, hydrolyzing the tyrosine--valine linkage. A similar plasma endopeptidase, active at pH 7.4 and inhibited by diisopropyl-fluorophosphate (D.F.P.) was described by KHAIRALLAH and PAGE (1967) and labelled Angiotensinase B. MATSUNAGA (1971) has recently shown chymotrypsin-like activity in the presence of dithiothreitol (D.T.T.) and inhibited by D.F.P. in the lysosomal fraction of rat kidney and liver. This SH group-dependent lysosomal enzyme may be identical to that described by REGOLI et al. (1963) but differs from the Angiotensinase B of KHAIRALLAH and PAGE in that it is not inhibited by D.F.P.

Carboxypeptidases (Angiotensinase "C"). Pancreatic Carboxypeptidase A was shown to release phenylalanine from Ang. II by LENTZ et al. (1956) and JOHNSON and RYAN (1968) have found evidence of carboxypeptidase activity in aqueous extracts of rabbit liver. Another enzyme with the capacity to hydrolyze the terminal peptide bond when proline is the penultimate amino-acid has recently been described by YANG et al. (1968). This enzyme, isolated from porcine kidney cortex or human urine has been called Angiotensinase C. It can be distinguished from Carboxypeptidase A, Cathepsins and other known enzymes; it is inhibited by D.F.P., though not by chelating agents, and has a pH optimum of 5.6 to 5.7.

Table 2. *Neutral aminopeptidases in extracts of various tissues*
(Adapted from MATSUNAGA et al., 1969)

Tissue	Activity per 10 ng of tissue	Protein mg
Kidney	343	0.55
Liver	309	0.76
Spleen	175	0.70
Adrenal	—	0.35
Lung	137	0.30
Heart	28	0.24
Brain	35	0.16
Muscle	17	0.17

[a] Activity is expressed in nanograms of angiotensin inactivated by 0.46 ng of protein at 37 °C for 15 min.

MATSUNAGA and his colleagues (SAITO et al., 1969; MATSUNAGA et al., 1969; MATSUNAGA, 1971) have shown interest in the angiotensinases found in the lysosomal fraction of various tissues, particularly kidney. The evidence now suggests that the main enzyme of this fraction is a carboxypeptidase, inhibited by D.F.P., active at acid pH, and independent of SH groups.

Angiotensinases in Plasma, Serum, and Blood

Peptidases in plasma, serum or whole blood have been the subject of intensive investigation. *In-vitro* methods have suggested the presence of both aminopeptidases and endopeptidases in plasma and serum [REGOLI et al., 1963; KHAIRALLAH and PAGE, 1967; PICKENS et al., 1965; NAGATSU et al., 1965 (1 and 2), 1970]. Studies of the metabolism of (^{35}S) Phenyl thiocarbamyl-Ang. II in human plasma confirm the presence of both types of enzymes, but suggest a dominant role for amino peptidases (DOYLE et al., 1967). Degradation of Ang. II in blood, once thought all-important, is now known to be a slow process of minor significance compared with the rapid catabolism of the peptide in tissue vascular beds (HODGE et al., 1967; NG and VANE, 1968; BAKHLE et al., 1969).

Kidney Angiotensinases

Tissue Extracts. Renal angiotensinases have been measured in homogenates of dog, rat and rabbit kidney by FASCIOLO et al. (1940), REGOLI et al. (1963), LEE (1965), ITSKOVITZ and MILLER (1967) and JOHNSON (1967). YANG et al. (1968) reported the presence of a carboxypeptidase in extracts of hog kidney cortex while other workers have fractionated kidney homogenates and demonstrated that most angiotensinase is present in microsomal and lysosomal fractions (DENGLER and REICHEL, 1960; GLENNER et al., 1962; MATSUNAGA et al., 1968). The nature of these peptidases has been investigated by incubation of [Asn^1-Val^5]-Ang. II or its analogues with kidney homogenates under standard conditions with subsequent bioassay of residual pressor activity. In some experiments, peptide fragments have

Table 3.

Species	Fraction	Angiotensinase identified	Authors
Rat	Microsomes	Aminopeptidase	GLENNER et al. (1962)
Rat	Homogenate	Aminopeptidase and Endopeptidase	REGOLI et al. (1963)
Pig	Cortex	Carboxypeptidase	YANG et al. (1968)
Rat	Lysosomal	Endopeptidase	SAITO et al. (1969)
Rat	Lysosomal	Endopeptidase and Carboxypeptidase	MATSUNAGA (1971)
Rat	Microsomal	Aminopeptidase	MATSUNAGA and MASSON (1970)

been identified by chromatography (REGOLI et al., 1963; SAITO et al., 1969; MATSUNAGA et al., 1969; MATSUNAGA, 1971).

Data collected from these studies is presented in Table 3.

Intact Organ Experiments. The probability that nonspecific intracellular enzymes with limited access to perfusing blood are released in the preparation of tissue homogenates has stimulated the development of other techniques for the measurement of angiotensinases in the kidney.

HODGE et al. (1967) used the superfusion technique of REGOLI and VANE (1966) to study angiotensin metabolism in anaesthetized dogs. Blood drawn from the renal vein superfused a series of assay organs before returning to the dog's circulation. Ang. II was infused into the renal artery or directly into blood perfusing the assay organs. Comparison of the assay responses to peptide infused by these two routes allowed the calculation of angiotensin loss during passage through the intact kidney. BIRON et al. (1968) studied renal angiotensinase activity in the anaesthetized rat and dog, using the animals own blood pressure response to assay the peptide. Angiotensin analogues were infused into the renal vein at a rate producing a stable elevation of 20 to 25 mmHg in arterial pressure. The same analogue was then infused into the renal artery at gradually increasing rates to produce the same diastolic B.P. response. Both HODGE et al. (1967) and BIRON et al. (1968) were able to show significant inactivation of angiotensin in the intact kidney, but did not prove that this was due to angiotensinases. In a similar study, OSBORN et al. (1969) found renal inactivation of [Asn^1-Val^5]-Ang. II and (^{35}S) Phenylthiocarbamyl-Ang. II in the sheep and dog. These findings were confirmed in the rat by LEARY (1970) who measured pressor responses to [Asp[1]-Ileu[5]]-Ang. II infused into the renal artery, jugular vein and inferior vena — cava in the same animal.

The technique of isolated organ perfusion has been applied to the study of renal angiotensinases in several species by BAKHLE et al. (1969) and LEARY and LEDINGHAM (1969). BAKHLE et al. (1969) studied Ang. II metabolism in isolated kidneys perfused with Krebs' solution to distinguish angiotensinase activity in the renal vascular bed from activation of plasma or erythrocyte peptidases during passage through the organ. Isolated kidneys from cats and dogs were perfused through the directly cannulated renal artery. Renal veins were cut to allow perfusate to escape from the organ. In rats both kidneys were perfused by tying a cannula into the aorta below the origin of the renal arteries. The aorta was tied above the renal arteries and kidneys and aorta then excised. The excised preparation was suspended in a perspex chamber and perfused with Krebs' solution gassed with 95% O_2 and 5% CO_2 at 37 °C. Angiotensin inactivation was measured by comparing the responses of rat colon to [Asn[1]-Val-]-Ang. II infused proximal or distal to the perfused kidney.

LEARY and LEDINGHAM (1969) perfused isolated rat kidney by the methods of NISHIITSUTSUJE-Uwo et al. (1967) with certain modifications [LEARY, 1970; LEARY and LEDINGHAM, 1970 (1)]. Rat kidney was isolated from the general circulation by ligation of appropriate vessels and perfused *in situ* for periods of not less than 6 min with an oxygenated artificial medium at pH 7.4 and 37 °C. The time course of Ang. II destruction by perfusate alone and by the isolated kidney was determined by a rat bioassay technique (PEART, 1955; LEE, 1965). BAKHLE et al. and LEARY and LEDINGHAM both reported inactivation of [Asn[1]-Val[5]]-Ang. II in the isolated perfused rat kidney and their results have been confirmed by BIRON and CAMPEAU (1971). BAKHLE et al. (1969) also described inactivation of the peptide by cat and dog kidneys and LEARY and LEDINGHAM (1969) found that angiotensin loss in their preparation was partially inhibited by edetic acid 3×10 ^{3}M. Later it was demonstrated that α-[Asp[1]-Val[5]]-Ang. II and α-[Asp[1]-Ileu[5]]-Ang. II were inactivated by isolated rat kidney whereas the β-Asp[1]-Val[5] analogue was not [LEARY and LEDINGHAM, 1970 (2)]. OSBORNE et al. (1970) have also perfused isolated rat kidneys by the method of NISHIITSUTSUJI-Uwo et al. (1967) using [Asp[1]-H_3-Tyr[4]-Val-]-Ang. II as substrate and the superfusion technique of REGOLI and VANE (1966) to assay biological activity of the peptide. Identification of radioactive compounds in the effluent perfusate was achieved by Sephadex filtration, immunoabsorption, paper chromatography and immunoassay. Disappearance of Ang. II during perfusion was found to be due to enzymatic hydrolysis rather than to specific or non-specific binding to receptor sites. The presence of 2-8 heptapeptide, 3-8 hexapeptide and 1-4 tetrapeptide in the perfusate suggests predominant aminopeptidase and endopeptidase activity in the isolated perfused kidney.

Indirect evidence for the importance of the kidney in angiotensin inactivation has been presented by several workers. BUMPUS et al. (1964) showed that in rats infused with tritiated angiotensin, the radioactivity was concentrated largely in kidney, uterus and the adrenals. BOURGOIGNIE et a. (1969) reported an increased sensitivity to infused angiotensin in nephrectomized rats. Using an immunoassay technique in the dog BAILIE et al. (1971) have found that Ang. II in the renal vein plasma is less than that in arterial plasma, indicating renal extraction of the peptide from plasma. Since no evidence was found to indicate significant plasma angiotensin entry into renal lymph, it was suggested that hydrolysis of the peptide occurred in the kidney.

Conclusions. Inactivation of Ang. II analogues by the kidney has been measured in a variety of circumstances. Methods of study include incubation of the peptide with kidney homogenates or sub-cellular fragments and perfusion of intact organs in vivo and in vitro. Inactivation has been expressed in biological terms and, in some studies, peptide fragments have been identified by chromatography. This evidence, taken in conjunction with the behaviour of kidney peptidases in the presence of enzyme inhibitors, suggests that an aminopeptidase and one or more other angiotensinases exist in mammalian kidney.

Liver Angiotensinases

Tissue Extracts. In a study comparing angiotensinase activities from various tissues in the rat ITSKOVITZ and MILLER (1967) found extracts of intestinal mucosa, kidney cortex and liver to be the most potent sources. MATSUNAGA and his colleagues, in their investigation of microsomal and lysosomal angiotensinases in rat tissues, have found liver extracts second only to kidney in content of acid and neutral angiotensinases (MATSUNAGA et al., 1969). JOHNSON and RYAN (1968) investigated the degradation of [Asn^1-Val^5]-Ang. II and its Ileu^5 analogue by aqueous extracts of rabbit liver, buffered at pH 7.4. Chromatography after incubation showed hydrolysis of all bonds in each peptide, implying the presence of several enzymes. When aminopeptidases were inhibited by dialysis of the extract against ethylene-diamine-tetraacetic acid (EDTA), angiotensinase was reduced by 60%. The residual peptidase activity was shown to be due to a carboxy peptidase, similar to pancreatic Carboxypeptidase A.

Intact Organ Experiments. Following the claim that experimental renal hypertension in dogs can be reversed by anastamoses of the renal and portal veins, METHOT et al. (1964) in the rat and CHAMBERLAIN et al. (1964), in dogs and man, performed experiments to show whether or not intact liver was capable of destroying Ang. II. Both groups compared portal with systemic venous injections of [Asn^1-Val^5]-Ang. II, and both found considerable reduction in blood-pressure response when the peptide was given via the portal vein. WERNZE and FUJII (1966), using the same technique in rats confirmed hepatic inactivation of [Asn^1-Val^5]-Ang. II when injected into the portal vein, but found no difference between the pressor effects of the β-Asp^1-Val^5-peptide given by femoral or portal vein. LEARY and LEDINGHAM (1968) also compared pressor responses to injections of angiotensin given by portal and jugular veins of rats but used small doses (5 to 15 ng) of [Asp^1-Ileu^5]-Ang. II in contrast to the much larger doses (500 to 1000 ng) of Asn^1 analogue given by both METHOT et al. and WERNZE and FUJII. No difference was found in pressor response to portal and jugular vein injections between 5 ng and 15 ng; but as the doses of angiotensin were increased from 20 ng to 200 ng there was an increasing and significant deficit in the portal vein pressor response. The failure to detect loss of angiotensin in the hepatic circulation of the rat when small amounts of peptide were injected, may reflect the insensitivity of pressor assay used. BIRON et al. (1968) report 60 to 70% inactivation of [Asn^1-Val^5]-Ang. II and of its 86% pure β-Asn^1 analogue in the hepatoportal circulation of both rats and dogs.

The *in vivo* studies so far discussed necessitate the use of very large amounts of Ang. II. More physiological doses can be assessed by the superfusion techniques of REGOLI and VANE (1966). Losses of about 70% were found during infusions containing 1 to 5 ng/ml of [Asn^1-Val^5]-Ang. II into the hepatic circulation of dogs (HODGE et al., 1967).

The isolated liver perfusion technique of LEARY and LEDINGHAM [1969; 1970 (1)] allows the effects of peptidase inhibitors to be assessed in the inactivation of angiotensin analogues by the intact rat liver. Livers perfused with an artificial Krebs' medium are very active in extracting α-[Asn^1-Val^5]-, α-[Asp^1-Val^5]-, α-[Asp^1-Ileu^5]- and β-[Asp^1-Val^5]-Ang. II (LEARY and LEDINGHAM 1970 (2)]. Inactivation of α-[Asn^1-Val^5]-Ang. II is partially inhibited by EDTA, 3×10^{-3}M, and dimercaprol 4×10^{-4}M in the medium completely prevented hepatic extraction of this analogue (LEARY and LEDINGHAM, 1969).

Conclusions. A variety of experimental techniques indicate conclusively that the liver is an important site of Ang. II catabolism. The precise nature of the angiotensinases concerned is not yet known, but the large number of analogues inactivated by the liver, and the effects of inhibitors suggest the presence of a number of different enzymes.

Lung Angiotensinases

Tissue Extracts. Ang. II is inactivated when incubated with extracts of rat and dog lung (ITSKOVITZ and MILLER, 1967; BAKHLE, 1968; MATSUNAGA et al., 1969).

Intact-Organ Experiments. Inactivation of Ang. II in the intact lung has been studied in man and animals by a variety of methods. No change in systemic-pressor response to the peptide was observed in rats by GOFFINET and MULROW (1965) in rats and dogs by BIRON et al. (1968) or in sheep and dogs by OSBORN et al. (1969) whether they infused the peptide proximal or distal to the pulmonary circulation. Subsequently BIRON et al. (1969) repeated these experiments in man and found that the pressor potency of Ang. II given into the pulmonary artery was equivalent to that obtained from aortic injection of the peptide.

HODGE et al. (1967) detected no apparent inactivation of Ang. II in the lungs of anaesthetized dogs investigated by the infusion — superfusion technique of REGOLI and VANE (1966).

BAKHLE et al. (1969), LEARY and LEDINGHAM (1969) and BIRON and CAMPEAU (1971) reported negligible losses of Ang. II biological activity during passage of the peptide through isolated lung of several species perfused with erythrocyte free solutions.

In the studies reported above, angiotensinase activity was measured in the lung by bioassay only. The fact that Ang. II loses no biological activity during passage through the lung does not rule out the possibility that some hydrolysis of the peptide occurs, coupled with the release of a second biologically active substance by the perfused organ. RYAN et al. (1970) and TÜRKER et al. (1971) have both reported the presence of substances in effluent from isolated rat lung preparations that support this possibility. These results are not conclusive. Before studying the metabolism of Ang. II in the lung TÜRKER et al. (1971) excised the organ and perfused it for 30 to 40 min. This prolonged period of perfusion might have damaged the lung with release of intracellular enzymes not normally active in vivo. RYAN et al. (1970) perfused lung by the method of LEARY and SMITH (1970) which causes negligible tissue damage as assessed by electron microscopy, but used highly unphysiological concentrations of peptide in their experiments.

Conclusions. Peptidases capable of hydrolysing Ang. II are present in lung tissue. Evidence from *in-vivo* lung perfusion studies indicates that only negligible inactivation of the peptide occurs during passage through the lung. Recent studies suggest that peptidase activity coupled with more complex changes, including the release of a hitherto unidentified vaso-active substance, may occur within the lung.

Cardiac Angiotensinases

Homogenates of cardiac tissue are capable of hydrolyzing Ang. II, but the angiotensinase content is low compared with homogenates of intestinal mucosa, kidney and liver (FASCIOLO et al., 1940; ITSKOVITZ and MILLER, 1967). Rat coronary vascular bed perfused with modified Kreb's solution is active in extracting [Asp^1-Val^5]-Ang. II, hydrolyzing some 30 to 70% of injected peptide in a single circulation (BIRON, 1969; OSBORNE et al., 1970; TÜRKER et al., 1971).

Hind Quarter Angiotensinases

The metabolism of Ang. II in isolated hindquarter preparations has been studied in dogs (HODGE et al., 1967; BIRON et al., 1968), rats (BIRON et al., 1968; BAKHLE et al., 1969; BIRON and CAMPEAU, 1971), and sheep (OSBORN et al., 1969). Hind limbs were perfused through femoral artery catheters and peptide in the effluent blood or Krebs' solution was assayed by superfusion (HODGE et al., 1967; BAKHLE et al., 1969) rat colon bioassay (BIRON and CAMPEAU, 1971) or monitoring of the pressor response in the experimental animal (BIRON et al., 1968; OSBORN et al., 1969). All groups reported that 50 to 70% of the peptide was inactivated during a single passage through the limbs.

Changes in Angiotensinase Activity in Various States

Changes in Plasma and Serum

There have been many attempts to correlate changes in plasma angiotensinase activity with disease or altered physiology, but results have been largely inconsistent (PAGE and McCUBBIN, 1968). The lack of a standardized method of angiotensinase assay and the relative unimportance of plasma enzymes in angiotensin catabolism (HODGE et al., 1967), lessen the significance of the findings reviewed below.

1. *Hypertension*. There is no consistent evidence of altered angiotensinase activity in plasma in various forms of spontaneous and experimental hypertension in man or animals (DEXTER, 1942; HAYNES and DEXTER, 1945, 1947; WOLF et al., 1961; WOOD, 1962; KLAUS, 1962; HICKLER et al., 1963; LAGRUE and MEYER, 1963; BIRON et al., 1964; NAGATSU et al., 1965; ITSKOVITZ et al., 1957; LUBASH et al., 1967).

2. *Liver Disorders*. Marked increases in plasma angiotensinase activity in patients with cirrhosis and other hepatic disorders have been reported from many laboratories (HICKLER et al., 1963; KLAUS et al., 1963; BIRON et al., 1964; KOKUBU et al., 1965; HIRASAWA, 1968; PAGE and McCUBBIN, 1968). It has been suggested that such increased activity might contribute to the improvement of arterial blood pressure in some hypertensive patients who have developed liver disease. (KOKUBU et al., 1965; HIRASAWA, 1968; PAGE and McCUBBIN, 1968). More recent studies comparing α-[Asn^1-Val^5]-Ang. II and α-L-aspartyl-β-naphthalmide (α-ANA) as substrates in serum from normal and cirrhotic patients, suggest the increased enzyme activity found in liver disease may relate only to angiotensinase A_1 and not to the peptidase more specific to naturally occurring Ang. II [NAGATSU et al., 1965 (2); LUBASH et al., 1968). A physiologically important change in plasma angiotensinase activity in cirrhosis remains unproven.

3. *Pregnancy*. KLAUS et al. (1963) and LANDESMAN et al. (1963) were unable to find differences in the rates of destruction of [Asn^1-Val^5]-Ang. II in the plasma of pregnant women compared with non-pregnant controls. NAGATSU et al. [1965 (2)]

also found inactivation of [Asn^1-Val^5]-Ang. II to be normal, while α-ANA was more rapidly destroyed in the serum of pregnant women in the third trimester, suggesting a selective increase in Angiotensinase A_2 activity. LUBASH et al. (1969) differ from NAGATSU et al., claiming not only increased hydrolysis rates of α-ANA but also of [Asn^1-Val^5]-Ang. II in the third trimester sera. It is unlikely that such changes, even if consistently detected, are of serious importance.

4. *Shock*. ITSKOVITZ et al. (1969) have reported enhanced inactivation of both [Asn^1] and [Asp^1]-Ang. II analogues by plasma from dogs shocked by haemorrhage or by E. coli endotoxin.

Effects of Changes in Sodium Balance and Other Conditions on Angiotensin-II Catabolism

Sodium balance. LEARY and LEDINGHAM [1970 (1 and 2)] have perfused isolated rat liver and kidney from animals previously fed on low- and high-sodium diets. [Asn^1-Val^5]-Ang. II or its Asp^1-Val^5- and Asp^1-Ileu^5-analogues were added to the perfusion medium, and the time course of destruction of peptide determined by bioassay of serial samples over a 6-min period. Hepatic inactivation was not altered by changes in sodium balance. In contrast the capacity of the isolated kidney for to inactivation of Ang. II analogues was markedly reduced after sodium loading and significantly increased after depletion of salt. BIRON and CAMPEAU (1971), using a different technique, have found a 20% increase in inactivation of Ang. II analogues in kidneys from adrenalectomized salt-depleted rats, and a 20% decrease when the animals had previously been salt loaded, but their results were not statistically significant.

There is other evidence that changes in sodium balance may alter angiotensin catabolism. JOHNSTON et al. (1972) have examined the metabolic clearance rate (MCR) of Ang. II in hypertensive and normotensive man in states of sodium loading and depletion. In normotensives, the MCR increased significantly from 2.23 ± 0.36 L/min in repletion, to 3.19 ± 0.34 L/min in depletion of sodium. MCR in hypertensive patients on a high salt intake was significantly higher than in normotensives and did not increase with sodium depletion. BRUNNER et al. (1972) infused rabbit Ang. II anti-body intravenously in anaesthetized rats, and determined the amount required to prevent the pressor response to exogenous Ang. II. This amount was found to be 8-fold higher in sodium-loaded animals than in those on a low-salt diet. Although BRUNNER et al. (1972) have suggested their data may indicate to changes in the affinity of vascular receptors to Ang. II, with changes in sodium balance, their results, and those of JOHNSTON et al. (1972), are also compatible with a reduction of tissue-angiotensin degradation in sodium-loaded animals. LUBASH et al. (1971) report results differing from those of JOHNSTON et al. The latter found plasma Ang. II levels to rise less in sodium depletion than in sodium repletion, during infusion of Ang. II amide: LUBASH et al. report the opposite, and found the half-life of Ang. II prolonged in the presence of salt depletion.

JELINEK et al. (1971) have recently reported that the angiotensinase content of rat kidney homogenates is lower than normal in both sodium-depleted and sodium-loaded animals. These results are difficult to interpret, since the capacity of organs to destroy angiotensin in vivo is unlikely to be reflected accurately by work using tissue homogenates [JOHNSON and RYAN, 1968; LEARY and LEDINGHAM, 1970 (1); OSBORNE et al., 1970; BIRON and CAMPEAU, 1971)].

Conclusion. There is now suggestive but not conclusive evidence that renal angiotensin catabolism may be reduced in salt loading and increased in salt depletion, perhaps selectively in the renal vascular bed. This hypothesis is compatible with the long recognized variation in pressor sensitively to angiotensin with changes in salt balance in man and animals (REID and LARAGH, 1965; OSTROVSKY and GORNALL, 1964; KUCHEL et al., 1964; LARAGH, 1962; KAPLAN and SILAH, 1964; AMES et al., 1965).

Experimental Hypertension. LEARY and LEDINGHAM [1970 (1)] examined the effects of unilateral renal artery clips with or without contralateral nephrectomy on the capacity of isolated perfused rat kidneys to inactivate [Asn^1-Val^5]-Ang. II. In rats with one renal artery constricted and the other intact, considerably less peptide was removed by the intact kidney than the ischaemic kidney: in this situation the ischaemic kidney inactivated angiotensin at the same rate as control normal organs. In rats with one kidney removed and the remaining renal artery constricted by a silver clip, the ischaemic kidney removed less peptide from perfusate than its controls. Thus the overall capacity of the renal vascular beds to inactivate angiotensin is reduced in both experimental hypertensive situations, perhaps relating to sodium retention at least in the uninephrectomized rats. BRUNNER et al. (1972) also studied renovascular hypertension with or without contralateral nephrectomy in rats, and showed a 2-fold increase in the amount of rabbit anti-angiotensin II antibody required to block the pressor effects of exogeneous angiotensin. Taken together, the data suggest the possibility that a decreased catabolism of Ang. II may contribute to GOLDBLATT hypertension in the rat.

Experiments relating kidney homogenate angiotensinase to experimental renal hypertension have not produced consistent results (BLAQUIER et al., 1961; BING, 1962; HIRASAWA, 1969; JELINEK et al., 1971).

Effects of Carbon Tetrachloride in Rat Liver. WERNZE and FUJII (1966) found the pressor sensitivity to [Asn^1]-Ang. II of rats was reduced if they had previously been given carbon tetrachloride (CCl_4), but the response to portal vein versus femoral vein injections indicated that the capacity of the liver to inactivate angiotensin was not impaired. BIRON and MEYER (1968) confirmed reduced pressor sensitivity in CCl--treated rats, but also reported a partial or total loss of the capacity of the poisoned livers to destroy either α-Asp^1 or β-[Asp$_4$]-Ang. II. HIRASAWA (1968) in contrast found evidence of increased angiotensinase activity in liver homogenates, intact infused livers, and the plasma of rats previously given CCl_4. Data so far is therefore conflicting: the different doses of carbon tetrachloride used, and the poor and variable state of health of the animals may account for these discrepancies.

Angiotensinase Assays

In ideal circumstances, enzymes are assayed after purification, in conditions of constant pH, temperature, ionic strength, specific ionic concentration and amount of substrate present. The rate of the reaction may then be taken as an index of the activity of the enzyme, and such activity may be expressed as units per mg of protein or per mg nitrogen. The kinetics of the reaction between the enzymes and its substrate should be determined by a series of estimations of substrate or reaction product concentrations, with time, in the presence of a standard amount of enzyme. In zero-order kinetics, the reaction is linear with time and rate is simply estimated. In first-order kinetics, when the reaction rate depends on the substrate concentration, the equation describing the first -order reaction may be used to express enzyme activity. When higher-order or more complex reactions occur the empirical device often used to establish an assay is the measurement of the *initial* rate of the reaction, which tends to approach zero order.

In the assay of angiotensinases in vitro or in vivo, these simple principles of enzyme assay (Mehler, 1957) either cannot be, or too often have not been, observed. Most estimates of angiotensinase activity in vitro have depended upon the incubation under standard conditions of a known concentration of Ang. II (or an analogue), with plasma, serum or tissue extract, and assay of residual pressor activity after variable time intervals. It cannot be over-emphasized that single-point assay systems are valueless in the assessment of enzyme activity, unless the reaction kinetics have been studied, and it is known whether zero-, first- or higher-order kinetics pertain. Estimates of enzyme activity based on single-point assay systems occur all too frequently in the literature on angiotensinases. This kind of error is easily avoided but there are other difficulties which are not so easily solved.

In-Vitro Assays: plasma, serum and tissues contain a variety of peptidases, so that more than one enzyme is always present, and pure preparations of angiotensinase enzymes have only very rarely been achieved (Nagatsu et al., 1970). In spite of these difficulties some useful estimate of angiotensinase activity in vitro can be achieved provided samples are assayed at frequent intervals after incubation and rates are calculated from the linear part of the curve relating angiotensin survival with time. The time taken for a 50-percent loss of substrate (T50%) may be the best index, and has been successfully used by Johnson (1967), Johnson and Ryan (1968), Yang et al. (1968) and Jelinek et al. (1971). Substrates other than Ang. II may occasionally be of value in the assay of individual angiotensinases [Nagatsu et al., 1965 (2), 1970] and reaction rates may be estimated from rate of yield of individual amino acids [Nagatsu et al., 1965 (1)].

In-Vivo Assays: The single-pass superfusion assay of angiotensinase activity (Hodge et al., 1967; Bahkle et al., 1969; Biron et al., 1968; Biron and Campeau, 1971; Osborne et al., 1970) whether applied to anaesthetized animals, or to isolated perfused organs does not allow any estimate of rate of loss of angiotensin with time. Activity of angiotensinases in organ vascular beds can therefore only be assessed in terms of percentage loss of angiotensins in a single circulation. Change of activity in altered physiological or in pathological states may therefore be difficult or impossible to quantitate.

The isolated perfused organ techniques of Leary and Ledingham [1961, 1970 (1 and 2)] allow recirculating medium to be assayed for residual angiotensin at regular intervals over relatively prolonged periods. [Asn^1-Val^5], [Asp^1-Val^5] and [Asp^1-Ileu^5]-Ang. II in concentrations of 66 or 133 ng/ml were destroyed by the perfused rat liver or kidney at a rate linear with time up to 6 min. Between 6 and 14 min there was evidence of substrate concentration becoming rate-limiting (Leary and Ledingham — unpublished observations). This technique therefore allows rates of inactivation to be compared in various physiological and pathological states, with or without the addition of enzyme inhibitors to the medium. Application of immunoassay methods to this technique, so that more physiological concentrations of angiotensin can be used, will offer obvious advantages over the bioassay methods so far employed.

Metabolic clearance rates of angiotensin. Johnston et al. (1972) have devised a method of estimating the metabolic clearance rate (MCR) of Ang. II in man. [Asn^1-Val-]-Ang. II (Hypertensin Ciba) was infused intravenously at a subpressor dose of 100 ng per min for 2 h. Plasma renin and angiotensin levels were measured before and after the infusion and the clearance rate calculated with a correction applied for the renin-suppressing effect of the infusion. The MCR was shown to be constant over infusion rates of 100 to 1000 ng/min and was not therefore altered by the infusion itself.

Difficulties particular to Ang. II metabolism arise in the accurate estimation of MCR, and these have been discussed by JOHNSTON et al. Moreover clearance data data do not distinguish receptor uptake (LIN and GOODFRIEND, 1970; GOODFRIEND and LIN, 1970) from tissue degradation of angiotensin.

Summary

The term angiotensinase is used to describe a number of enzymes capable of hydrolyzing Ang. II, but not proven to be specific to it.

Tissue extract and homogenate experiments have been helpful in the detection of separate aminopeptidases, endopeptidases and carboxypeptidases, but cannot be taken to reflect angiotensin catabolism in vivo.

The techniques devised over the last 5 years for the study of angiotensin inactivation by intact organs have been productive. There is now more than a hint that angiotensin catabolism in tissue vascular beds may be as important as its rate of formation in determining physiological activity at receptor sites.

References

AMES, R. P., BORKOWSKI, A. J., SICINSKI, A. M., LARAGH, J. H.: Prolonged infusions of angiotensin II and norepinephrine and blood pressure, electrolyte balance, aldosterone and cortisol secretion in normal man. J. clin. Invest. **44**, 1171—1186 (1965).

BAKHLE, Y. S.: Conversion of angiotensin I to angiotensin II by cell free extracts of dog lung. Nature (Lond.) **220**, 919—921 (1968).

BAKHLE, Y. S., REYNARD, A. M., VANE, J. R.: Metabolism of the angiotensins in isolated perfused tissues. Nature (Lond.) **222**, 956—959 (1969).

BAILIE, M. D., RECTOR, F. C., SELDIN, D. W.: Angiotensin II in arterial and renal venous plasma and renal lymph in the dog. J. clin. Invest. **50**, 119—126 (1971).

BING, J.: Angiotensinase content of kidneys of normal and hypertensive rats. Acta path. microbiol. Scand. **56**, 385—387 (1962).

BIRON, P., CAMPEAU, L.: Pulmonary and extra-pulmonary fate of angiotensin I. Rev. canad. Biol. **30**, 27—34 (1971).

BIRON, P., CAMPEAU, L., DAVID, P.: Fate of angiotensin I and II in the human pulmonary circulation. Amer. J. Cardiol. **24**, 544—547 (1969).

BIRON, P., LANDESMAN, R., HUNT, J. C.: Plasma angiotensinase activity in human hypertension. Nature (Lond.) **204**, 1096 (1964).

BIRON, P., MEYER, P.: Hepatic Extraction of angiotensin after carbon tetrachloride intoxication. Rev. canad. Biol. **27**, 277—279 (1968).

BIRON, P., MEYER, P., PANISSET, J. C.: Removal of angiotensins from the systemic circulation. Canad. J. Physiol. Pharmacol. **46**, 175—178 (1968).

BLAQUIER, P., BOHR, D. F., TAQUINI, A. C., HOOBLER, S. W.: Renin and angiotensinase content of the kidney of normal and hypertensive rats. Proc. Soc. exp. Biol. (N. Y.) **108**, 711—715 (1961).

BOURGOIGNIE, J., KURZ, S., PERRY, H. M.: Control of vascular reactivity to angiotensin in rats. Absh. Proc. IV. Internat. Congress Nephrol. Stockholm (1969), 196.

BRAUN-MENENDEZ, E., FASCIOLO, J. C.: Accion vasocontrictora e hipertensora de la sangre venosa del rinou en isquenianicompleta agnda. Rev. Soc. argent. Biol. **15**, 161—172 (1939).

BRUNNER, H. R., CHANG, P., WALLACH, R., SEALEY, J. E., LARAGH, J. H.: Angiotensin II vascular receptors: their avidity in relationship to sodium balance, the autonomic nervous system and hypertension. J. clin. Invest. (in press).

BUMPUS, F. M., SMEBY, P. R., PAGE, I. H., KHAIRALLAH, P. A.: Distribution and Metabolic Fate of Angiotensin II and various Derivatives .Canad. med. Ass. J. **90**, 190—193 (1964).

CHAMBERLAIN, M. S., BROWSE, N. L., GIBSON, D. G., GLEESON, J. A.: Angiotensin and renoportal Anastomosis. Brit. med. J. **1964 II**, 1507—1508.

CROXATTO, H., CROXATTO, R., ILLANES, G., SALVESTINI, H.: Action de la quimotrepsinia y de la tripsina sobre la Hypertensina y los principios presor y ocitocico de la post hypotisio. Rev. Med. Aliment. (Santiago) **5**, 300—302 (1965).

CROXATTO, R., CROXATTO, H.: Destruction of hypertensin and pepsitensin by an aminopeptidase obtained from yeast. Science **96**, 519—520 (1942).

DENGLER, H., REICHEL, G.: Untersuchungen zur intrazellulären Lokalisation der Renin- und Hypertensinase-Aktivität. Experientia (Basel) **16**, 36—38 (1960).

DEXTER, L.: The hypertensinase content of plasma of normal, hypertensive and nephrectomised dogs. Ann. intern. Med. **17**, 447—450 (1942).

DOYLE, A. E., LOUIS, W. J., OSBORN, E. C.: Plasma angiotensinase activity on angiotensin II and analogues. Aust. J. exp. Biol. med. Sci. **45**, 41—50 (1967).

FASCIOLO, J. C., LELOIR, L. F., MUNOZ, J. M., BRAUN-MENEDEZ, E.: La hipertensinasa, su dosaje y distribucion. Rev. Soc. argent. Biol. **16**, 643—649 (1940).

GADDUM, J. H.: Technique of superfusion. Brit. J. Pharmacol. 8, 321—326 (1953).

GLENNER, G. G., MCMILLAN, P. H. J., FOLK, L. F.: A mammalian peptidase specific for the hydrolysis of N-terminal L-L glutamyl and aspartyl residues. Nature (Lond.) **194**, 867 (1962).

GOFFINET, J. A., MULROW, P. J.: Estimation of angiotensin clearance by an in vivo assay. Clin. Res. **1965 II**, 408.

HAYNES, F. W., DEXTER, L.: Renal humoral pressor mechanism in man III. hypertensinase content of plasma of control subjects, and of patients with hypertension and other diseases. J. clin. Invest. **24**, 78—81 (1945).

HAYNES, F. W., DEXTER, L.: Renin, hypertensinogen, and hypertensinase concentrations of blood of dogs during the development of hypertension by constriction of the renal artery. Amer. J. Physiol. **150**, 190—197 (1947).

HICKLER, R. B., LANLER, D. P., THORN, G. W.: Plasma angiotensinase activity in patients with hypertension and oedema. J. clin. Invest. **42**, 635—648 (1963).

HIRASAWA, K.: Studies on renin — angiotensin system (I) studies on angiotensinase activity in liver disease. Jap. Circulat. J. **32**, 355—356, 407—415 (1968).

HIRASAWA, K.: Studies on renin — angiotensin system. (II) studies on renal angiotensinase activity. Jap. Circulat. J. **33**, 979—980, 985—990 (1969).

HODGE, R. L., NG, K. K. F., VANE, J. R.: Disappearance of angiotensin from the circulation of the dog. Nature (Lond.) **215**, 138—141 (1967).

ITSKOVITZ, H. D., MILLER, L. D.: Differential studies of angiotensinase: Activities from several tissue sources. Amer. J. med. Sci. **254**, 659—666 (1967).

ITSKOVITZ, H. D., MILLER, L., URAL, W., ZAPP, J., WHITE, R.: Inactivation of angiotensin in shock. Amer. J. Physiol. **216**, 5—10 (1969).

JELINEK, J., MANNEL, H., GROSS, F.: Inactivation of angiotensin II by rat kidney homogenates. Arch. Pharmak. **268**, 446—457 (1971).

JOHNSON, D. C.: Bsc Thesis. Univ. of Oxford (1967).

JOHNSON, D. C., RYAN, J. W.: Degradation of angiotensin II by a carboxypeptidase of rabbit liver. Biochim. biophys. Acta (Amst.) **160**, 196—203 (1968).

JOHNSTON, C. I., MENDELSOHN, F. A. O., DOYLE, A. E.: The metabolism of angiotensin II in sodium deplution and hypertension in humans. Circulat. Res. (in press).

KAPLAN, N. M., SILAH, J. G.: The effects of angiotensin II on the blood pressure of humans with hypertensive disease. J. clin. Invest. **43**, 659—669 (1964).

KHAIRALLAH, P. A., BUMPUS, F. M., PAGE, I. H., SMEBY, R. R.: Angiotensinase with a high degree of specificity in plasma and red cells. Science **140**, 672—674 (1963).

KHAIRALLAH, P. A., PAGE, I. H.: Plasma angiotensinases. Biochem. Med. **1**, 1—8 (1967).

KLAUS, D.: Untersuchungen über die Angiotensinase in Serum Gesunder und Kranker. Klin. Wschr. **40**, 701—702 (1962).

KLAUS, D., KAFFARNICK, H., PFEIL, H.: Untersuchungen über die Serum-Angiotensinase II. Klinische Ergebnisse beim Hochdruck und bei Lebererkrankungen. Klin. Wschr. **41**, 380—385 (1963).

KOKUBU, T., UEDA, E., FUJIMOTO, S., HIWADA, K., SANGA, M., YAMAMURA, Y.: Plasma Angiotensinase activity in liver disease. Clin. chim. Acta **12**, 484—488 (1965).

KUCHEL, O., HORNKY, K., PAZOUREK, M., GREGOROVUA, I.: Pressor hyporeactivity to angiotensin in addisons disease. Lancet **1964 II**, 1316—1317.

LAGRUE, G., MEYER, P.: Dosage biologique de l'angiotensinase plasmatique. Technique et premiers resultats. Path. et Biol. **1963 II**, 895—897.

LANDESMAN, R., BIRON, P., CASTELLANOS, R., LA RUSSA, R., WILSON, K. H.: Plasma angiotensinase activity in normal and toxaemic pregnancy. Obstet. and Gynec. **22**, 316—323 (1963).

LARAGH, J. H.: Hormones and the pathogenesis of congestive heart failure: Vasopressor aldosterione, and angiotensin II. Further evidence for renal-adrenal interaction from studies in hypertension and cirrhosis. Circulation **25**, 1015—1023 (1962).

LEARY, W. P., LEDINGHAM, J. G.: Pressor response to infusion of angiotensin in the portal vein of the Rat. Nature (Lond.) **220**, 180—181 (1968).

LEARY, W. P., LEDINGHAM, J. G.: Removal of angiotensin by isolated perfused organs of the Rat. Nature (Lond.) **222**, 959—960 (1969).
LEARY, W. P., SMITH, U.: In-situ perfusion of isolated rat lung. Life Sciences **9**, 1321—1326 (1970).
LEARY, W. P. P.: Aspects of the renin-angiotensin system D. Phil. Thesis, Univ. of Oxford (1970).
LEARY, W. P. P., LEDINGHAM, J. G. G.: (1) Renal and hepatic inactivation of angiotensin in Rats. Influence of sodium balance and renal artery compression. Clin. Sci. **38**, 573—582 (1970).
LEARY, W. P. P., LEDINGHAM, J. G.: (2) Inactivation of angiotensin II. analogues by isolated perfused rat Liver and kidney. Nature (Lond.) **227**, 178—179 (1970).
LEE, M. R.: The estimation of renin in biological fluids. D. Phil. Thesis Univ. of Oxford (1965).
LENTZ, K. E., SKEGGS, L. T., WOODS, K. R., KAHN, J. R., SHUMWAY, N. P.: The aminoacid composition of hypertensin II and its biochemical relationship to angiotensin I. J. exp. Med. **104**, 183—191 (1956).
LUBASH, G. D., BARD, R. H., KLINE, J. A.: Serum „angiotensinase activity" and female steroidal hormones. Amer J. med. Sci. **257**, 155—163 (1969).
LUBASH, G. D., HAMMEL, E. C., MEARLES, R. J.: Serum angiotensinase activity in hypertension. Clin. Chim. Acta **18**, 439—445 (1967).
LUBASH, G. D., HAMMEL, E. C., MEARLES, R. J.: Serum angiotensinase activity in cirrhosis. Amer. J. med. Sci. **255**, 105—112 (1968).
LUBASH, G. D., MUIESAN, G. E., ALICANDRI, C. L., GARFINKEL, D. J., SIEKIERSKI, E. C., MCCONNAUGHEY, C. K.: Plasma angiotensin, serum angiotensinase activity and blood pressure response during angiotensin II amide infusions in normal volunteers. Experientia (Basel) **27**, 68—69 (1971).
MATSUNAGA, M.: Nature of lysosomal angiotensinase activity. Jap. Circulat. J. **35**, 333—338 (1971).
MATSUNAGA, M., KIRA, J., SAITO, N., OGINO, K., TAKAYASU, M.: Acid angiotensinase, renin, and acid adenosine triphosphatase in rat kidney lysosomes. Jap. Circulat. J. **32**, 137—143 (1968).
MATSUNAGA, M., MASSON, G. M. C.: Hepatic and renal neutral angiotensinases. Experientia (Basel) **26**, 1297—1298 (1970).
MATSUNAGA, M., SAITO, N., KIRA, J., OGINO, K., TAKAYASU, M.: Acid angiotensinase as a lysosomal enzyme. Jap. Circulat. J. **33**, 545—551 (1969).
METHOT, A. L., MEYER, P., BIRON, P., LORAIN, M. F., LAGRUE, G., MILLIEZ, P.: Hepatic inactivation of angiotensin. Nature (Lond.) **203**, 531—532 (1964).
NAGATSU, I. T., GILLESPIE, I. L., FOLK, J. E., GLENNER, G. G.: Serum Aminopeptidase, "Angiotensinase", and hypertensin I degradation of Angiotensin II by Human Serum. Biochem. Pharmacol. **14**, 721—728 (1965).
NAGATSU, I.. T, GILLESPIE, I. L., GEORGE, J. M., FOLK, J. E., GLENNER, G. G.: Serum Aminopeptidase "Angiotensinase" and Hypertension-II. Aminoacid B-Naphthylamide Hydrolysis by Normal and Hypertensive Serum. Biochem. Pharmacol. **14**, 853—861 (1965).
NAGATSU, I. T., YAMAMOTO, T., GLENNER, G. G., MEHL, J. W.: Purification of aminopeptidase A in human serum and degradation of angiotensin II by the purified enzyme. Biochim. biophys. Acta (Amst.) **198**, 255—270 (1970).
NG, K. K. F., VANE, J. R.: Fate of angiotensin I in the circulation. Nature (Lond.) **218**, 144—150 (1968).
OSBORNE, M. J., D'AURIAC, G. A., MEYER, P., WORCEL, M.: Mechanism of extraction of angiotensin II in coronary and renal circulations. Life Sci. **9**, 859—867 (1970).
OSBORN, E. C., HUGHES, S. G., PURIE, A. T., WILLICOMBE, P. R., MAHLER, R. F.: Clearance studies of angiotensin II and (^{35}S) phenylthiocarbanyl-angiotensin II in the sheep and dog. Cardiovasc. Res. **3**, 134—146 (1969).
OSTROVSKY, D., GORNALL, A. G.: Effects of aldosterone and other adrenal hormones on the blood pressure responses to renin and angiotensin. Canad. med. Ass. J. **90**, 180—184 (1964).
PAGE, I. H., HELMER, O. M.: A crystaline pressor substance (angiotonin) resulting from the reaction between renin and reninactivator. J. exp. Med. **71**, 29—42 (1940).
PAGE, I. H., MCCUBBIN, J. W.: Renal Hypertension. Year Book Medical Publishers. Chicago 1968.
PEART, W. S.: A new method of large scale preparation of hypertensin with a role on its assay. Biochem. J. **59**, 300—302 (1955).
PICKENS, P. T., BUMPUS, F. M., LLOYD, A. M., SMEBY, R. R., PAGE, I. H.: Measurement of renin activity in human plasma. Circulat. Res. **17**, 438—448 (1965).
PLENTL, A. A., PAGE, I. H.: Enzymatic nature of angiotensin formation from renin and renin activator. J. biol. Chem. **147**, 135—141 (1943).

REGOLI, D., RINIKER, B., BRUNNER, H. R.: The enzymatic degradation of various angiotensin II derivatives by serum, plasma or kidney homogenates. Biochem. Pharmacol. **12**, 637—646 (1963).

REGOLI, D., VANE, J. R.: The continuous estimation of angiotensin formed in the circulation of the dog. J. Physiol. (Lond.) **183**, 513—531 (1966).

REID, W. D., LARAGH, J. H.: Sodium and potassium intake, blood pressure and pressor response to angiotensin. Proc. Soc. exp. Biol. (N. Y.) **120**, 26—29 (1965).

RYAN, J. W., STEWART, J. M., LEARY, W. P., LEDINGHAM, J. G.: Metabolism of angiotensin I in the pulmonary circulation. Biochem. J. **120**, 221—223 (1970).

SAITO, N., SANADA, A. K., MATSUNAGA, M., KIRA, J., MUKAINO, S., OGINO, K., TAKAYASU, M.: Amino-acid analysis after degradation of angiotensin II by rat kidney lysosomes. Jap. Circulat. J. **33**, 87—93 (1969).

TÜRKER, R. K., YAMAMOTO, M., BUMPUS, F. M., KHAIRALLAH, P. A.: Lung perfusion with angiotensin I and II. Evidence of release of myotropic and inhibition substances. Circulat. Res. **28**, 559—567 (1971).

WERNZE, H., FUJII, J.: Hepatische Inaktivierung und Pressorische Wirkung von Angiotensin. Z. ges. exp. Med. **140**, 128—235 (1966).

WOLF, R. L., MENDLOWITZ, M., GITLOW, S. E., NAFTCHI, N. E.: Metabolism of angiotensin II I^{131} in normotensive and hypertensive human subjects. Circulation **23**, 754—758 (1961).

YANG, H. Y. T., ERDÖS, E. G., CHIANG, T. S.: New Enzymatic route for the inactivation of angiotensin. Nature (Lond.) **218**, 1224—1225 (1968).

Structure-Activity Relationship in Angiotensin II Analogs

M. C. KHOSLA, R. R. SMEBY, and F. M. BUMPUS

The octapeptide, [5-isoleucine]-Angiotensin II which is specific to human, equine, rat and porcine species was synthesized by BUMPUS et al. (1957) and SCHWARZ et al. (1957), while RITTEL et al. (1957) synthesized [1-asparagine, 5-valine]-Ang. II, an analog of bovine Ang. II. These syntheses formed the basis for extensive studies of the biologic actions and structure-activity relationships of this hormone. The outcome of these efforts was the synthesis of over 90 analogs by early 1966. BUMPUS and SMEBY (1968) discussed the results in an earlier review and concluded that: a) the carboxyl terminal hexapeptide 3-8 sequence [Val-Tyr-Ile(Val)-His-Pro-Phe], composed of amino-acid residues with alternate aliphatic and aromatic side chains, carries the essential features of the hormone; b) all aromatic residues (4-tyrosine, 6-histidine, 8-phenylalanine) are essential for pressor activity while the aliphatic residues may be necessary either to stabilize a preferred conformation relative to the aromatic residues or to facilitate a favorable hydrophobic bonding on the receptor; and c) the carboxyl group at the C-terminus must be free.

Since the publication of their review, many additional Ang. II analogs have been synthesized. This rapid progress, partially due to the ease with which analogs can now be synthesized by MERRIFIELD's solid-phase procedure, has culminated in some new developments in this field.

Analogs which will probably compete for the active site and antagonize the biological response of the native hormone have been sought for many years (PAGE and BUMPUS, 1962). A number have now been synthesized [PARK et al., 1967; BUMPUS, 1971 (2); KHOSLA et al., 1971, 1972 (1), 1972 (2); GAGNON et al., 1971; RIOUX et al., 1971; PALS et al., 1971 (1), 1971 (2); REGOLI et al., 1971, 1972; REGOLI and PARK, 1972; SMEBY et al., 1972; FESSLER et al., 1972] which competitively antagonize the myotropic and pressor response of Ang. II at very low dose levels. It has been observed that pressor activity is diminished while antagonistic activity is enhanced when the side chain of phenylalanine in position 8 of Ang. II is dislocated from its relative position, when its spatial orientation is changed, or when the aromatic ring is replaced by an aliphatic or alicyclic side chain. Similarly, transposition of positions 4 and 8 in angiotensin produces an analog which when given in high doses antagonizes the action of Ang. II (MARSHALL et al., 1970).

The structure of human Ang. I has been confirmed by the synthesis of [Ile^5]-Ang. I by AOYAGI et al. (1967).

Because angiotensin had never before been obtained in crystalline form, conformational studies by X-ray have been limited and those obtained by other means have been the subject of dispute. Recently, FERMANDJIAN et al. [1971 (1)] crystallized Ang. II and observed that it has a marked tendency to adopt an antiparallel β-conformation in organic solvents as well as in aqueous solution. FERREIRA et al.

(1969) found two dializable forms of Ang. II at low ionic concentrations. WEINKAM and JORGENSEN [1971 (1), 1971 (2)] proposed that a steric effect on the peptide backbone is the primary role of the amino-acid residue in the 5 position, and it is because of this steric effect that the peptide assumes a conformation capable of interacting with the biological receptor. The present review aims to give a unified view of the recent advances and some earlier achievements in this field.

Pressor and Myotropic Response

Table 1 lists various analogs and homologs of angiotensin with their corresponding pressor and myotropic activities as compared to [Ile^5]-, [Val^5]- or [Asn^1, Val^5]-angiotensins. To facilitate comparison, the pressor activity of the naturally occurring octapeptide has been set arbitrarily at 100. Comparative competitive inhibition of myotropic response (guinea-pig ileum and rat stomach strips) of Ang. II have been expressed in terms of PA_2 and PA_{10} values (SCHILD's criteria). It was not feasible to include all the other criteria used to study reversible and irreversible inhibition on various isolated tissues or in intact animals. Unless stated otherwise, all compounds are analogous to Ang. II containing aspartic acid in position 1 and isoleucine in position 5.

Variations in the comparative biological data from different laboratories could be due to varying degree of impurities accompanying the desired peptide (KHAIRALLAH et al., 1963; BUMPUS and SMEBY, 1968; VANE, 1971). Of recent interest is the finding (WINDRIDGE and JORGENSEN, 1971) that solid-phase synthesis of angiotensin analogs yielded a much higher degree of racemization of histidine than the solution method. KHOSLA et al. (1972) isolated the octapeptide containing D-histidine from the L-histidine analogs by ion-exchange chromatography with buffers of varying pH followed by partition chromatography on Sephadex G-25. Biological evaluation indicated that the analogs containing D-histidine had very low pressor and antagonistic properties as compared to those containing L-histidine. For example, [Ile^5, D-His^6]-Ang. II possessed 4% of the pressor response of the parent hormone. Such impurities could lead to discrepancies in the correlation of structure-activity relationships. Before the compound is evaluated biologically, chemical and stereochemical homogeneity of the new compounds should be determined by amino-acid analysis, thin-layer chromatography in at least 3 solvent systems, electrophoresis at different pH values, elemental analysis and incubation of acid hydrolysates with L-or D-amino acid oxidase. Optical purity has also been indicated by showing complete hydrolysis by several enzymes.

Variations in position 1. Replacement of the β-carboxyl group of aspartic acid by a neutral amide group has no effect on pressor activity but it reduces the activity on the rabbit aorta slightly. There is no decrease in pressor activity even when the length of the side chain is increased by one carbon atom or when it is cyclized into a pyrrolidone ring. When aspartic acid is replaced by glycine, so that the acidic side chain is replaced by a hydrogen atom, the pressor activity retained is about 40% that of the natural hormone. Similarly, the N-terminal amino group does not appear to be important since 50% activity is retained when it is either blocked or totally removed. Removal of aspartic acid yields a heptapeptide with similar activity. However, when β-carboxyl group is replaced by the positively charged basic guanidine group, pressor activity drops to 33% while the oxytocic activity drops to 79% of the natural hormone level. By contrast, the duration of the pressor response is enhanced by two to three times (BRUNNER and REGOLI, 1962; REGOLI et al., 1963) when either the spatial orientation of aspartic acid is changed to α-D- or β-D-isomers or the chain of the peptide is lengthened by a methylene group

(β-carboxyl linkage). It has been reported that a single intramuscular injection of [β-Asp^1]-Ang. II (50 to 100 μg) causes a definite prolongation of action and leads to a rise in blood pressure that persists for 30 to 60 min (IMHOF et al., 1964). These differences could be due to either varying rates of enzymatic degradation or different affinities for the receptor. However, this difference between α- or β-linked aspartic acid Ang. II was less pronounced when the compounds were tested for pressor assays on intact dogs (REGOLI et al., 1963; RINIKER, 1964), or for the vasoconstrictor effects on perfused kidneys. Thus, the amino terminus of Ang. II exhibits little structural specificity for activity and can be altered without major changes in pressor or myotropic activity.

Variations in position 2. Since removal of N-terminal aspartyl residue diminishes the pressor activity of Ang. II by 2 to 4 times while removal of the N-terminal dipeptide, aspartylarginine, decreases the activity of the hormone by a factor of about three hundred, arginine in position 2 could be thought to contribute to the pressor activity through the following:

a) Positive charge of the guanidinium group.

b) Hydrogen-bonding capacity of the guanidinium group with some bidentate ionic site.

c) Hydrophobicity of the side chain and its length.

d) Spatial arrangement around the α-carbon atom.

e) Prolonged peptide chain for stabilization of some essential conformation.

The guanidinium group has a positive charge distributed over a large area of this residue and it is logical to expect a correlation between the basicity of this group and biological activity. However, nitroarginine which is not appreciably basic in character due to nitro substitution, yields a peptide which is still 50% as active as the natural hormone. Ornithine in this position lowered the activity to 20% while lysine reduced it to about 1%. In other words, a guanidinium group on carbon atom 3 (arginine) gives much more activity than an amino group on carbon atom 3 (ornithine) and this in turn gives more activity than an amino group on carbon atom 4 (lysine). Substitution of L-arginine by D-arginine reduces the pressor activity to 4%. When the basic chain is replaced by an aliphatic side chain such as in valine, or by a neutral side chain having a carbamyl group at carbon atom 3 (analogous to arginine) as in citrulline, the pressor activity is reduced to approximately 5% and 2% respectively.

These results indicate that positive charge is not important for biological activity, but it was not decided which other factors are responsible for imparting pressor avtivity. To shed further light, DE GRAAF et al. (1971) synthesized a series of over 30 analogs of [Des-Asp^1]-Ang. II. In the meantime, JORGENSEN et al. [1970 (1)] had also synthesized some analogs of [Des-Asp^1]-Ang. II. Some of the conclusions based on rat pressor assays of the analogs by both these groups were controversial. DE GRAAF et al. (1971) therefore postulated that structural alterations at the amino end of the peptide chain are likely to make the data for the *in-vivo* assays erratic because of the influence of aminopeptidase action on the peptides. To avoid this difficulty they tested all their heptapeptide analogs for myotropic activity on isolated terminal ileum. The following conclusions were reached (DE GRAAF, 1970; DE GRAAF et al., 1971):

a) Comparison of the ratios between myotropic activity and pressor activity of the heptapeptide analogs investigated revealed that aminopeptidase action played an important role in rat pressor assays.

b) The heptapeptides containing a guanidinium group in the side chain of position 2 have higher activity than those with an ammonium group in a comparable position.

c) With some exceptions, analogs with an N-terminal D-α-amino acid residue have a higher activity than all the corresponding L-analogs.

d) On the basis of a comparison of the polar groups (cationic or neutral), the hydrogen-bonding capacity seems to have a greater influence than charge, though it is difficult to exclude steric effects. Yet the nitroarginyl heptapeptides have much higher affinities than the less acidic citrullyl analogs, even though the nitroguanidyl group is about twice as large as the ureido moiety.

e) A comparison involving the distance between peptide chain and polar group suggests the length of the side chain is somehow important. If length is the crucial feature, however, it cannot be explained why, for instance, the [D-Lys^2]- and the [D-Orn^2]-heptapeptides are equally active and the L-analogs are not.

Table 1. *Analogs of angiotensin (see pages 130—145)*

Biological data

A Pressor response, nephrectomized rats
B Pressor response, non-nephrectomized rats
C Pressor response, anesthetized dogs
D Oxytocic effect, isolated rat uterus
E Oxytocic effect, guinea-pig ileum (G), rat terminal ileum (R) rabbit aorta (A), rat colon (C)
F Antagonistic effect, rabbit aortic strips: PA_2, PA_{10}
G Antagonistic effect, rat stomach strips: PA_2, PA_{10}
H Antagonistic effect to pressor response in rats (R), cats (C), and dogs (D)

Abbreviations

Abu = α-Aminobutyric acid
Ac = Acetic acid
Ach = Cyclohexane 1-amino, 1-carboxylic acid
εAcp = ε-Aminocaproic acid
Adh = 2-Amino-6-dimethylamino-4-hexynoic acid
Aev = α-Amino-β-ethylvaleric acid
Aht = Aza-α-homo tyrosine
Aib = α-Aminoisobutyric acid
*a*Ile = *allo*-Isoleucine
Amb = *p*-Aminomethyl benzoic acid
ηAoc = η-Aminooctanoic acid
Apb = 3-Amino-4-phenylbutyric acid
Apib = 3-Amino-2-benzylpropionic acid
ωApm = ωAmidopimelic acid
Atc = α-Amino-ε-trimethylammonio-caproic acid
δAvl = δ-Aminovaleric acid
Bu = Butyric acid
Bz = Benzoic acid
Car = Carbamic acid
Cha = Cyclohexylalanine
Chg = Cyclohexylglycine
Chl = p-[N,N-bis(2-chloroethyl)amino] phenylbutyric acid
Cit = Citrulline
Cpa = Cyclopentane 1-amino, 1-carboxylic acid (Cycloleucine)
Cpg = Cyclopentylglycine
Dhy = 2,6-diamino-4-hexynoic acid
δGvl = δ-Guanidinovaleric acid
δGvl (NO_2) = δNitroguanidinovaleric acid
Har = Homoarginine
Hly = Homolysine
(*hv*) = Product formed due to ultraviolet irradiation
Hyd = Hydantoic acid
Hyp = 3-Hydroxyproline
Ipc = 2-Isopropyl carbazic acid
MeAla = N-methylalanine
Nle = Norleucine
Pip = Pipecolic acid
Pr = Propionic acid
Pyr = Pyroglutamic acid
Pza = β-(Pyrazolyl-3)-alanine
Sar = Sarcosine
Suc = Succinic acid
Sun = Succinamic acid
Tal = β-2-Thienylalanine
εTcp = ε-Trimethylammonio-caproic acid
δUvl = δ-Ureidovaleric acid

No.	Ang.-II analog	1 Asp	2 Arg	3 Val	4 Tyr	5 Ile	6 His	7 Pro	8 Phe
1	[Ile[5]]- (equine, porcine and human								
2	[Val[5]]- (Bovine)					Val			
3	[Asp(OMe)[1], Val[5]]-	Asp(OMe)				Val			
4	[Asn[1]]-	Asn							
5	[Asn[1], Val[5]]-	Asn				Val			
6	[Asp(NHMe)[1], Val[5]]-	Asp(NHMe)				Val			
7	[Ac-Asn[1], Val[5]]-	Ac-Asn				Val			
8	[Bz(NO_2)-Asn[1], Val[5]]-	Bz(NO_2)-Asn				Val			
9	[Bz(NH_2)-Asn[1], Val[5]]-	Bz(NH_2)-Asn				Val			
10	[PolySer(Ac)[1]]-	PolySer(Ac)-Asp							
11	[Suc[1]]-	Suc							
12	[Suc[1], Val[5]]-	Suc				Val			
13	[Suc(OMe)[1], Val[5]]-	Suc(OMe)				Val			
14	[Sun[1], Val[5]]-	Sun				Val			
15	[Suc(NHMe)[1], Val[5]]-	Suc(NHMe)				Val			
16	[Suc(NMe_2)[1], Val[5]]-	Suc(NMe_2)				Val			
17	[D-Asp[1], Val[5]]-	D-Asp				Val			
18	[D-Asn[1]]-	D-Asn							
19	[D-Asn[1], Val[5]]-	D-Asn				Val			
20	[β-Asp[1]]-	β-Asp							
21	[β-Asp[1], Val[5]]-	β-Asp				Val			
22	[β-Asp(NH_2)[1], Val[5]]-	β-Asp(NH_2)				Val			
23	[β-D-Asp[1], Val[5]]-	β-D-Asp				Val			
24	[Glu[1], Val[5]]-	Glu				Val			
25	[Gln[1], Val[5]]-	Gln				Val			
26	[Pyr[1], Val[5]]-	Pyr				Val			
27	[γ-Glu[1], Val[5]]-	γ-Glu				Val			
28	[Arg[1]]-	Arg							

Pressor response			Myotropic response		Antagonistic activity			References
A	B	C	D	E	F	G	H	
100	100	100	100					Bumpus et al., 1957; Schwarz et al., 1957; Rittel et al., 1957; Arakawa and Bumpus, 1961; Schwyzer, 1961; Paul and Anderson, 1962; Marshall and Merrifield, 1965; Fuji and Sakakibara, 1970; Schwyzer et al., 1957 (1)
100	100		100					Schwyzer et al., 1958; Garner and Young, 1969; Grava and Cipens, 1969
								Romanovskii et al., 1971
100	50		33					Rittel et al., 1957; Paul and Anderson, 1962; Marshall and Merrifield, 1965; Visser et al., 1964
100	100		100					Schwyzer et al., 1958; Schwyzer, 1961, Kisfaludy and Korensky, 1962; Schröder, 1964; Romanovskii et al., 1971
								Romanovskii et al., 1971
35—50								Haber et al., 1965
40—50								Deodhar, 1960
40—50								Doedhar, 1960
40								Arakawa et al., 1962
	60							Arakawa et al., 1962
	50		51					Riniker and Schwyzer, 1964
								Romanovskii et al., 1971
								Romanovskii et al., 1971
								Romanovskii et al., 1971
								Romanovskii et al., 1971
100—150								Riniker and Schwyzer, 1964
91								Schattenkerk and Havinga, 1965
100								Schröder, 1966
80—100			111					Khairallah et al., 1963; Marshall and Merrifild, 1965
150								Riniker et al., 1962, Romanovskaya et al., 1971
								Romanovskii et al., 1971
150								Riniker and Schwyzer, 1964
150								Schröder, 1966; Cresswell et al., 1967
100								Schröder, 1966
150								Schröder, 1966; Cresswell et al., 1967
100								Cresswell et al., 1967, 1969
33	14.7		79					Bumpus et al., 1961; Page and Bumpus, 1961

No.	Ang.-II analog	1 Asp	2 Arg	3 Val	4 Tyr	5 Ile	6 His	7 Pro	8 Phe
29	[Gly^{1}]-	Gly							
30	[Ile^{1}]-	Ile							
31	[Gly^{1}, Val^{5}]-	Gly				Val			
32	[Des-Asp^{1}]-	□							
33	[Des-Asp^{1}, Val^{5}]-	□				Val			
34	[Asn^{1}, D-Arg^{2}]-	Asn	D-Arg						
35	[Asn^{1}, D-Arg^{2}, Val^{5}]-	Asn	D-Arg			Val			
36	[D-Asn^{1}, D-Arg^{2}]-	D-Asn	D-Arg						
37	[Gly^{1}, D-Arg^{2}]-	Gly	D-Arg						
38	[Asn^{1}, Arg(NO$_2$)^{2}, Val^{5}]-	Asn	Arg(NO$_2$)			Val			
39	[Orn^{2}, Val^{5}]-		Orn			Val			
40	[Asn^{1}, Orn^{2}, Val^{5}]-	Asn	Orn			Val			
41	[Asn^{1}, Lys^{2}, Val^{5}]-	Asn	Lys			Val			
42	[Asn^{1}, Cit^{2}]-	Asn	Cit						
43	[Asn^{1}, Val^{2}, Val^{5}]-	Asn	Val			Val			
44	[Des-Asp^{1}, Des-Arg^{2}]-	□	□						
45	[Des-Asp^{1}, Des-Arg^{2}, Val^{5}]-	□	□			Val			
46	[Gly^{2}]-		Gly						
47	[Asn^{1}, Gly^{2}]-	Asn	Gly						
48	[Asn^{1}, Gly^{2}, Val^{5}]-	Asn	Gly			Val			
49	[Gly^{1}, Gly^{2}]-	Gly	Gly						
50	[Gly^{1}, Gly^{2}, Val^{5}]-	Gly	Gly			Val			
51	[Ac-Gly^{1}, Gly^{2}]-	Ac-Gly	Gly						
52	[Suc^{1}, Gly^{2}]-	Suc	Gly						
53	[Sun^{1}, Gly^{2}]-	Sun	Gly						
54	[Hyd^{1}, Gly^{2}, Val^{5}]-	Hyd	Gly			Val			
55	[Des-Asp^{1}, Ac-Gly^{2}]-	□	Ac-Gly						
56	[Pr-Gly^{2}, Val^{5}]-		Pr-Gly			Val			

Pressor response			Myotropic response		Antagonistic activity			References
A	B	C	D	E	F	G	H	
42								Visser et al., 1964
25			50					Khosla et al., 1968
50	36		27					Gross and Turrian, 1960; Riniker and Schwyzer, 1961 (3)
15	21.6		18	47.42 (R)				Bumpus et al., 1961; Havinga et al., 1964; Visser et al., 1964; De Graaf et al., 1971
50	26		23 ± 3					Gross and Turrian, 1960; Schwyzer and Turrian, 1960; Paiva and Paiva, 1961; Riniker and Schwyzer, 1961 (4)
4	3							Visser et al., 1964
4								Riniker and Schwyzer (unpublished)
4.3								Schattenkerk and Havinga, 1965
14								Schattenkerk and Havinga, 1965
50	25		3.1					Schwyzer and Turrian, 1960; Gross and Turrian, 1960; Riniker and Schwyzer, 1961 (2)
20	8.9		1.6					Riniker and Schwyzer, 1961 (3); Schwyzer and Turrian, 1960
20	8.9		1.6					Riniker and Schwyzer, 1961 (3); Schwyzer and Turrian, 1960; Gross and Turrian, 1960
10	5							Schröder, 1964 (1)
1.7								Schattenkerk and Havinga, 1965
5	0.66							Schröder, 1964 (1)
0.3	2.3		6	0.84 (R)				Schattenkerk et al., 1964; Bumpus et al., 1961; Page and Bumpus, 1961; Smeby et al., 1962; Jorgensen and Patton, 1969 (2); De Graaf et al., 1971
0.1—0.6	<1		<0.1					Gross and Turrian, 1960; Schwyzer and Turrian, 1960; Schwyzer, 1961; Pavars and Cipens, 1970 (1); Ovchinnikov et al., 1968
10								Jorgensen et al., 1971 (1)
3								Jorgensen et al., 1971 (1)
3—5								Pavars and Cipens, 1970 (2); Pavars et al., 1971
16—20		16						Jorgensen et al., 1969
15								Pavars and Cipens, 1970 (1)
0.00		0.4						Jorgensen et al., 1969 (1)
1								Jorgensen et al., 1971 (1)
2								Jorgensen et al., 1971 (1)
1.5								Pavars et al., 1970, 1971
1								Jorgensen et al., 1970 (1)
1.3								Pavars et al., 1970, 1971

No.	Ang.-II analog	1 Asp	2 Arg	3 Val	4 Tyr	5 Ile	6 His	7 Pro	8 Phe
57	[Des-Asp^1, Gly^2]-	□	Gly						
58	[Des-Asp^1, Gly^2, Val^5]-	□	Gly			Val			
59	[Des-Asp^1, D-Arg^2]-	□	D-Arg						
60	[Des-Asp^1, Arg(NO_2)^2]-	□	Arg(NO_2)						
61	[Des-Asp^1, D-Arg(NO_2)^2]-	□	D-Arg(NO_2)						
62	[Des-Asp^1, Orn^2]-	□	Orn						
63	[Des-Asp^1, D-Orn^2]-	□	D-Orn						
64	[Des-Asp^1, Lys^2]-	□	Lys						
65	[Des-Asp^1, D-Lys^2]-	□	D-Lys						
66	[Des-Asp^1, Cit^2]-	□	Cit						
67	[Des-Asp^1, D-Cit^2]-	□	D-Cit						
68	[Des-Asp^1, Har^2]-	□	Har						
69	[Des-Asp^1, D-Har^2]-	□	D-Har						
70	[Des-Asp^1, Hly^2]-	□	Hly						
71	[Des-Asp^1, D-Hly^2]-	□	D-Hly						
72	[Des-Asp^1, δGvl^2]-	□	δGvl						
73	[Des-Asp^1-δGvl(NO_2)^2]-	□	δGvl(NO_2)						
74	[Des-Asp^1, εAcp^2]-	□	εAcp						
75	[Des-Asp^1, δAvl^2]-	□	δAvl						
76	[Des-Asp^1, Dhy^2]-	□	Dhy						
77	[Des-Asp^1, D-Dhy^2]-	□	D-Dhy						
78	[Des-Asp^1, Adh^2]-	□	Adh						
79	[Des-Asp^1, D-Adh^2]-	□	D-Adh						
80	[Des-Asp^1, Atc^2]-	□	Atc						
81	[Des-Asp^1, εTcp^2]-	□	εTcp						
82	[Des-Asp^1, δUvl^2]-	□	δUvl						

Pressor response			Myotropic response		Antagonistic activity			References
A	B	C	D	E	F	G	H	
10				18 (R)				JORGENSEN et al., 1970 (1)
5								PAVARS et al., 1970
33				45.36 (R)				HAVINGA et al., 1964 (1), 1964 (2); VISSER et al., 1964; DE GRAAF et al., 1971
1.3				6.39 (R)				SCHATTENKERK and HAVINGA, 1965; DE GRAAF et al., 1971
4.2				7.42 (R)				SCHATTENKERK and HAVINGA, 1965; DE GRAAF et al., 1971
2.7				5.98 (R)				HAVINGA et al., 1964 (1), 1964 (b); SCHATTENKERK et al., 1964; DE GRAAF et al., 1971
23				20.00 (R)				DE GRAAF et al., 1971
3—3.4				10.92 (R)				HAVINGA et al., 1964 (1), 1964 (2); SCHATTENKERK et al., 1964; DE GRAAF et al., 1971
18—23				20.62 (R)				HAVINGA et al., 1964 (1), 1964 (2); SCHATTENKERK et al., 1964; DE GRAAF et al., 1971
0.5				1.44 (R)				HAVINGA et al., 1964 (1), 1964 (2); SCHATTENKERK et al., 1964; DE GRAAF et al., 1971
11.04				6.39 (R)				DE GRAAF et al., 1971
2				25.16 (R)				HAVINGA et al., 1964 (1), 1964 (2); VISSER et al., 1964; DE GRAAF et al., 1971
11				26.80 (R)				HAVINGA et al., 1964 (1), 1964 (2); VISSER et al., 1964; DE GRAAF et al., 1971
2				6.60 (R)				HAVINGA et al., 1964 (1), 1964 (2); DE GRAAF et al., 1971
7				11.34 (R)				HAVINGA et al., 1964 (1), 1964 (2); DE GRAAF, et al. 1971
37.95				40.21 (R)				DE GRAAF et al., 1971
7.59				9.89				DE GRAAF et al., 1971
3.9—5				4.95 (R)				DE GRAAF et al., 1971; JORGENSEN et al., 1970 (1)
5—5.75				7.42 (R)				DE GRAAF et al., 1971; JORGENSEN et al., 1970 (1)
14.95				21.03 (R)				DE GRAAF et al., 1971
7.82				11.95 (R)				DE GRAAF et al., 1971
3.91				8.04 (R)				DE GRAAF et al., 1971
2.30				5.36 (R)				DE GRAAF et al., 1971
0.30				0.99 (R)				DE GRAAF et al., 1971
1.49				0.76 (R)				DE GRAAF et al., 1971
1.40				2.10				DE GRAAF et al., 1971

No.	Ang.-II analog	1 Asp	2 Arg	3 Val	4 Tyr	5 Ile	6 His	7 Pro	8 Phe
83	[Des-Asp^{1}, ωApm^{2}]-	▭	ωApm						
84	[Des-Asp^{1}, Leu^{2}]-	▭	Leu						
85	[Des-Asp^{1}, D-Leu^{2}]-	▭	D-Leu						
86	[Des-Asp^{1}, Abu^{2}]-	▭	Abu						
87	[Des-Asp^{1}, D-Abu^{2}]-	▭	D-Abu						
88	[Des-(Asp^{1}, Arg^{2}), Bu-Val^{3}]-	▭	▭	Bu-Val					
89	[Des-(Asp^{1}, Arg^{2}, Val^{3})]-	▭	▭	▭					
90	[Gly^{1}, Gly^{2}, Gly^{3}]-	Gly	Gly	Gly					
91	[Gly^{1}, Gly^{2}, Gly^{3}, Val^{5}]-	Gly	Gly	Gly		Val			
92	[Leu^{3}]-			Leu					
93	[Asn^{1}, Leu^{3}]-	Asn		Leu					
94	[Ala^{3}]-			Ala					
95	[Pro^{3}]-			Pro					
96	[Asn^{1}, Pro^{3}, Val^{5}]-	Asn		Pro		Val			
97	[Asn^{1}, Tyr^{3}, Val^{5}]-	Asn		Tyr		Val			
98	[Ipc^{3}, Val^{5}]-			Ipc		Val			
99	[Des-(Asp^{1}, Arg^{2},) ηAoc^{3}]-	▭	▭	η-Aoc					
100	[Des-(Asp^{1}, Arg^{2}), Car^{3}, Val^{5}]-	▭	▭	Car		Val			
101	[Gly^{1}, Gly^{2}, Gly^{3}, Gly^{4}, Val^{5}]-	Gly	Gly	Gly	Gly	Val			
102	[Des-(Asp^{1}, Arg^{2}, Val^{3}]-	▭	▭	▭					
103	[Des-(Asp^{1}, Arg^{2}, Val^{3}, Tyr^{4}), Val^{5}]-	▭	▭	▭	▭	Val			
104	[Tyr(Me)^{4}]-				Tyr(Me)				
105	[Tyr(Me)^{4}, Val^{5}]-				Tyr-(Me)	Val			
106	[Asn^{1}, Tyr(Me)^{4}, Val^{5}]-	Asn			Tyr-(Me)	Val			
107	[Phe^{4}, Val^{5}]-				Phe	Val			
108	[Asn^{1}, Phe^{4}, Val^{5}]-	Asn			Phe	Val			
109	[Ala^{4}]-				Ala				
110	[Asn^{1}, Glu^{4}, Val^{5}]-	Asn			Glu	Val			
111	[Asn^{1}, D-Tyr^{4}, Val^{5}]-	Asn			D-Tyr	Val			
112	[Asn^{1}, Aht^{4}, Val^{5}]-	Asn			Aht	Val			
113	[β-Asp^{1}, Aht^{4}, Val^{5}]-	β-Asp			Aht	Val			
114	[Asn^{1}, Tyr^{3}, Val^{4}, Val^{5}]-	Asn		Tyr	Val	Val			
115	[Endo-Tyr^{4a}, Val^{5}]-				(Tyr)$_{2}$	Val			

Pressor response			Myotropic response		Antagonistic activity			References
A	B	C	D	E	F	G	H	
0.69				1.56				De Graaf et al., 1971
0.39				2.16				De Graaf et al., 1971
2.99				4.33				De Graaf et al., 1971
1								Jorgensen et al., 1970 (1)
23								Jorgensen et al., 1970 (1)
1								Jorgensen et al., 1970 (1)
0								Bumpus et al., 1961; Page and Bumpus, 1961
0.1								Jorgensen et al., 1970 (2)
0.3								Pavars and Cipens, 1970 (1)
100								Schwyzer et al., 1957 (2)
100								Schwyzer and Turrian, 1960; Schwyzer et al., 1957 (2)
68								Khosla et al., 1967
53			80		6.87			Khosla et al., 1968; Khosla et al. (unpublished results)
75								Cipens et al., 1970
12	3.7		10					Schröder and Hempel, 1965
								Hess et al., 1963
0.1								Jorgensen et al., 1970 (2)
1.1								Pavars et al., 1970
0.01								Pavars and Cipens, 1970 (1)
0.00								Bumpus et al., 1961
0.01								Pavars and Cipens, 1970 (1)
1.00								Chaturvedi et al., 1970
0.9								Chaturvedi et al., 1970
0.2—0.4	0.2		0.1					Schröder and Hempel, 1965; Cresswell et al., 1967; Chaturvedi et al., 1970
10								Schwyzer and Turrian, 1960; Riniker and Schwyzer, 1961 (3)
10	4.9		2.5					Schwyzer and Turrian, 1960; Riniker and Schwyzer, 1961 (3)
0.31			0.06					Seu et al., 1962 (2)
<0.1								Cresswell et al., 1967
0.025								Riniker and Schwyzer (unpublished)
25								Riniker and Schwyzer, 1964 (2)
40								Riniker and Schwyzer, 1964 (2)
<0.1	0.02		0.037					Schröder, 1964 (2)
1								Schwyzer and Turrian, 1960; Riniker and Schwyzer, 1961 (4)

No.	Ang.-II analog	1 Asp	2 Arg	3 Val	4 Tyr	5 Ile	6 His	7 Pro	8 Phe
116	[Asn^1, Endo-Tyr^{4a}, Val^5]-	Asn			$(Tyr)_2$	Val			
117	[Asn^1, Tyr(I)^4, Val^5]-	Asn			Tyr(I)	Val			
118	[Asn^1, Tyr$(I_2)^4$, Val^5]-	Asn			Tyr(I_2)	Val			
119	[Asn^1, Phe^4, Val^5, Tyr^8]-	Asn			Phe	Val			Tyr
120	[His^4, Tyr^6]-				His		Tyr		
121	[Des-(Asp^1, Arg^2), Ala^4]-	□	□		Ala				
122	[Des-(Asp^1, Arg^2), Phe^4]-	□	□		Phe				
123	[Des-(Asp^1, Arg^2, Tal^4]-	□	□		Tal				
124	[Des-(Asp^1, Arg^2), Phe(F)^4]-	□	□		Phe(F)				
125	[Des-(Asp^1, Arg^2), Endo-Tyr^{4a}, Phe-OMe^8]-	□	□		$(Tyr)_2$				Phe-OMe
126	[Des-Arg^2), Pro^3]-		□	Pro					
127	[Des-(Asp^1, Arg^2, Val^3, Tyr^4), Val^5]-	□	□	□	□	Val			
128	[Des-(Asp^1, Arg^2, Val^3, Tyr^4), Ile^5]-	□	□	□	□	Ile			
129	[Leu^5]-					Leu			
130	[Asn^1, Leu^5]-	Asn				Leu			
131	[Ala^5]-					Ala			
132	[Asn^1, Ala^5]-	Asn				Ala			
133	[Asn^1, Abu^5]-	Asn				Abu			
134	[Asn^1, Nle^5]-	Asn				Nle			
135	[Asn, *a*Ile^5]-	Asn				*a*Ile			
136	[Asn^1, Aev^5]-	Asn				Aev			
137	[Asn^1, Cpg^5]-	Asn				Cpg			
138	[Asn^1, Chg^5]-	Asn				Chg			
139	[Asn^1, Aib^5]-	Asn				Aib			
140	[Asn^1, Sar^5]-	Asn				Sar			
141	[Asn^1, Pro^5]-	Asn				Pro			
142	[Asn^1, D-Pro^5]-	Asn				D-Pro			
143	[Asn^1, Cpa^5]-	Asn				Cpa			
144	[Asn^1, His^5]-	Asn				His			
145	[Asn^1, Arg^5]-	Asn				Arg			
146	[Asn^1, Tyr^5]-	Asn				Tyr			
147	[Asn^1, Ser^5]-	Asn				Ser			
148	[Asn^1, Amb^5]-	Asn				Amb			

Pressor response			Myotropic response		Antagonistic activity			References
A	B	C	D	E	F	G	H	
1	0.33		0.10					Schwyzer and Turrian, 1960; Riniker and Schwyzer, 1961 (4)
33				25	80(c)			Lin et al., 1970
13			2	24(c)				Lin et al., 1970
0.2	0.2		0.1					Schröder, 1964 (2)
0.0			0.0		0.0	0.0		Khosla et al., 1971, 1972 (1)
	0.0		0.0					Bumpus et al., 1961
	0.0		0.0					Bumpus et al., 1961
	0.0		0.0					Page and Bumpus, 1961
	0.0		0.0					Page and Bumpus, 1961
								Walton et al., 1961
1			4					Khosla et al., 1968
0.01								Pavars and Cipens, 1970 (1)
0.00								Bumpus et al., 1961
25								Schwyzer et al., 1957 (2)
25								Schwyzer et al., 1957 (2); Schwyzer and Turrian, 1960
5								Khosla et al., 1968
3								Jorgensen et al., 1971 (2)
16								Jorgensen et al., 1971 (2)
21								Jorgensen et al., 1971 (2)
100								Jorgensen et al., 1971 (2)
75								Jorgensen et al., 1971 (2)
89								Jorgensen et al., 1971 (2)
114								Jorgensen et al., 1971 (2)
0.9								Jorgensen et al., 1971 (3)
1								Jorgensen et al., 1971 (3)
10								Jorgensen et al., 1971 (3); Paruszewski, 1971
0.05								Jorgensen et al., 1971 (3)
24								Jorgensen et al., 1971 (3)
0								Paruszewski, 1971
0								Paruszewski, 1971
0								Paruszewski, 1971
14								Paruszewski, 1971
19								Paruszewski, 1971

No.	Ang.-II analog	1 Asp	2 Arg	3 Val	4 Tyr	5 Ile	6 His	7 Pro	8 Phe
149	[Asn^{1}, Lys^{2}, Leu^{5}]-	Asn	Lys			Leu			
150	[Asn^{1}, Val^{5}, (*hv*)^{6}]-	Asn				Val	(*hv*)		
151	[Asn^{1}, Val^{5}, Lys^{6}]-	Asn				Val	Lys		
152	[Arg^{6}]-						Arg		
153	[Asn^{1}, Val^{5}, Phe^{6}]-	Asn				Val	Phe		
154	[Asn^{1}, Val^{5}, D-His^{6}]-	Asn				Val	D-His		
155	[Val^{5}, Pza^{6}]-					Val	Pza		
156	[Tal^{6}]-						Tal		
157	[Orn^{6}]-						Orn		
158	[Met^{6}]-						Met		
159	[Ala^{6}]-						Ala		
160	[Ala^{4}, Ile^{8}]-				Ala				Ile
161	[Ala^{7}]-							Ala	
162	[Hyp^{7}]-							Hyp	
163	[Pip^{7}]-							Pip	
164	[Val^{5}, MeAla^{7}]-					Val		MeAla	
165	[Des-Asp^{1}, Endo-Tyr^{4a}, Phe(OMe)^{8}]-	□			(Tyr)$_2$				Phe-OMe
166	[Des-Asp^{1}, D-Phe^{8}]-	□							D-Phe
167	[Asn^{1}, Val^{5}, Des-Phe^{8}]-	Asn			Val				□
168	[Des-Phe^{8}]-								□
169	[Des-(Pro^{7}, Phe^{8})]-							□	□
170	[Asn^{1}, Val^{5}, Phe(OMe)^{8}]-	Asn				Val			Phe-OMe
171	[Asn^{1}, Val^{5}, Phe(NH$_2$)^{8}]-	Asn				Val			Phe-(NH$_2$)
172	[Tyr^{8}]-								Tyr
173	[Asn^{1}, Val^{5}, Tyr^{8}]-	Asn				Val			Tyr
174	[Val^{5}, Phe(Br)^{8}]-					Val			Phe-(Br)
175	[Asn^{1}, Val^{5}, Phe(Br)^{8}]-	Asn				Val			Phe-(Br)
176	[D-Asp^{1}, Val^{5}, Phe(NH$_2$)^{8}]-	D-Asp				Val			Phe-(NH$_2$)
177	[Ac-Asn^{1}, Val^{5}]-(Lys)$_n$-	Ac-Asn				Val			Phe-(Lys)$_n$

Pressor response			Myotropic response		Antagonistic activity			References
A	B	C	D	E	F	G	H	
<1								Schwyzer et al., 1957 (2); Schwyzer and Turrian, 1960
	1.0		1.0					Paiva and Paiva, 1961
0.1	0.02		0.02					Schröder and Hempel, 1965
0.0								Khosla et al., 1971, 1972 (1) Stewart, 1971
1.0								Schröder, 1964 (2)
1.0	0.04		0.04					Riniker and Schwyzer (unpublished results)
56.6	78.9	53		52.0 (G)				Hofmann et al., 1968; Andreatta et al., 1968; Hageman et al., 1969
1.0			5.00					Stewart, 1971
			0.08					Stewart, 1971
			0.13					Stewart, 1971
0.8				0.1 (G)				Khairallah et al., 1970
0.0					6.65			Khosla et al. (unpublished work)
0.83	0.00		1.4					Seu et al., 1962 (1)
9.80			10.0					Sivanandaiah et al., 1966
1.00								Chaturvedi et al., 1970
16.00	22.00			4.3(G)				Andreatta and Scheraga, 1971
								Walton et al., 1961
0.2								Schwyzer, 1961
0.05								Schwyzer and Turrian, 1960; Riniker and Schwyzer, 1961 (4)
0.00								Page and Bumpus, 1961
0.04					0.00		0.00	Khosla et al., 1972 (3)
10.00								Schwyzer et al., 1958 (1); Schwyzer and Turrian, 1960
1—3								Gross and Turrian, 1960; Schwyzer and Turrian, 1960; Riniker and Schwyzer, 1961 (2)
83			100					Sivanandaiah et al., 1966
10—20	10		3.7					Schröder and Hempel, 1965
50.00								Schwyzer and Turrian, 1960; Schwyzer, 1961
50.00								Schwyzer and Turrian, 1960; Schwyzer, 1961
0.33								Hess and Constantine, 1964
10—30								Haber et al., 1965

No.	Ang.-II analog	1 Asp	2 Arg	3 Val	4 Tyr	5 Ile	6 His	7 Pro	8 Phe
178	[Ala^{8}]-								Ala
179	[Asn^{1}, Val^{5}, Ala^{8}]-	Asn				Val			Ala
180	[Sar^{1}, Val^{5}, Ala^{8}]-	Sar				Val			Ala
181	[Phe^{4}, Val^{5}, Tyr^{8}]-				Phe	Val			Tyr
182	[D-Phe^{8}]-								D-Phe
183	[Ile^{8}]-								Ile
184	[D-*a*Ile^{8}]-								D-*a*Ile
185	[Sar^{1}, Ile^{8}]-	Sar							Ile
186	[Val^{8}]-								Val
187	[Leu^{8}]-								Leu
188	[Cha^{8}]-								Cha
189	[Suc^{1}, Phe^{4}, Tyr^{8}]-	Suc			Phe				Tyr
190	[Phe^{4}, Ala^{8}]-				Phe				Ala
191	[Ala^{4}, Ile^{8}]-				Ala				Ile
192	[Apb^{8}]-								Apb
193	[DL-Apib^{8}]-								DL-Apib
194	[Cpa^{8}]-								Cpa
195	[Ach^{8}]-								Ach
196	[Abu^{8}]-								Abu
197	[Pro^{8}]-								Pro
198	[Chl-Asp^{1}]-	Chl-Asp							
199	[Des-(Asp^{1}), Chl-Arg^{2}]-	□	Chl-Arg						

Pressor response			Myotropic response		Antagonistic activity			References
A	B	C	D	E	F	G	H	
0.10	0.00		0.00	<0.1	8.32 7.41	6.86 5.81		Bumpus et al., 1961; Park et al., 1967; Page and Bumpus, 1961; Khairallah et al., 1970; Türker et al., 1971; Gagnon et al., 1971; Rioux et al., 1971; Regoli et al., 1971; Regoli and Park, 1972
								Pals et al., 1971 (1) Fessler et al., 1972
								Pals et al., 1971 (2) Brunner et al., 1971
								Marshall et al., 1970
0.1				0.1		6.13 5.21		Gagnon et al., 1971; Rioux et al., 1971; Regoli and Park, 1972
					9.21 8.25		5 ng/g (R,C)	Bumpus, 1971 (2); Khosla et al., 1971, 1972 (1); Smeby et al., 1972; Yamamoto et al., 1972; Regoli et al., 1971
0.72					7.32			Khosla et al. (unpublished results)
1.0					9.33 8.43			Khosla et al., 1972 (2); Smeby et al., 1972; Turker et al., 1972 (1)
0.5								Khosla et al., 1972 (2); Regoli et al., 1971
								Khosla et al., 1972 (2); Regoli et al., 1971
20.0							0.9 ng/g (R, C, D)	Khosla et al., 1972 (2)
0.19					10 µg /ml		weak	Khosla et al., 1971, 1972 (2)
0.001					1 µg ml			Khosla et al., 1971, 1972 (2)
0.011					6.65			Khosla et al. (unpublished results)
10								Khosla et al., 1972 (2); Chaturvedi et al., 1970
1					5.57 4.73		weak	Chaturvedi et al., 1970; Turker et al., 1972; Khosla et al., 1972 (2)
<0.1				<0.1(C)		5.66 4.80		Rioux et al., 1971; Regoli and Park, 1972
<0.1				<0.1(C)		5.33 4.50		Rioux et al., 1971; Regoli and Park, 1972
								Rioux et al., 1971; Regoli et al., 1971
—						—		Paiva et al., 1972 (1)
								Paiva et al., 1972
								Paiva et al., 1972

No.	Ang.-II analog	1 Asp	2 Arg	3 Val	4 Tyr	5 Ile	6 His	7 Pro	8 Phe
200	[Des-(Asp^1, Arg^2), Chl-Val^3]-	□	□	Chl-Val					
201	[Des-(Asp^1, Arg^2, Val^3), Chl-Tyr^4]-	□	□	□	Chl-Tyr				
202	[Des-(Asp^1, Arg^2, Val^3, Tyr^4), Chl-Ile^5]-	□	□	□	□	Chl-Ile			
203	[Des-(Asp^1, Arg^2, Val^3, Tyr^4, Ile^5), Chl-His^6]-	□	□	□	□	□	Chl-His		
204	[Val^8]-Ang.-I								Val-His-Leu
205	[Ile^8]-Ang.-I								Ile-His-Leu
206	[Asn^1, Val^5]-Ang.-I	Asn				Val			His-Leu
207	[Val^5]-Ang.-I					Val			His-Leu
208	[Val^5, D-Phe^8]-Ang.-I					Val			D-Phe-His-Leu
209	[Asn^1, Val^5, Pro^9, Phe^{10}]-Ang.-I	Asn				Val			Phe-Pro-Phe
210	[Asn^1, Val^5, Leu(NH$_2$)^{10}]-Ang.-I	Asn				Val			Phe-His-Leu-(NH$_2$)
211	Ang.-I (human, horse)								Phe-His-Leu
212	[^{14}C-Leu^{10}]-Ang.-I								Phe-His-^{14}C-Leu
213	All D-[Asn^1, Val^5]-	D-	D-	D-	D-	D-	D-	D-	D-
214	Cyclo-[Des-(Asp^1, Arg^2)]-	□	□	Val	Tyr	Ile	His	Pro	Phe
215	[Sar^1, Leu^8]-	Sar							Leu
216	[Cpa^1]-	Cpa							
217	[Cpa^2]-		Cpa						
218	[Cpa^3]-			Cpa					
219	[Cpa^4]-				Cpa				
220	[Cpa^5]-					Cpa			
221	[Cpa^6]-						Cpa		
222	[Cpa^7]-							Cpa	
223	[Des-Asp^1, Chl-Arg^2, Val^8]-Ang.-I	□	Chl-Arg						Val-His-Leu
224	[Asn^1, Val^5, Gly^8]-	Asn				Val			Gly
225	[Asn^1, Val^5, β-Ala^8]-	Asn				Val			β-Ala
226	[Asn^1, Val^5, Abu^8]-	Asn				Val			Abu
227	[Asn^1, Val^5, Val^8]-	Asn				Val			Val
228	[Asn^1, Val^5, Leu^8]-	Asn				Val			Leu
229	[Suc^1, Ala^8]-	Suc							Ala

Pressor response			Myotropic response		Antagonistic activity			References
A	B	C	D	E	F	G	H	
								Paiva et al., 1972
								Paiva et al., 1972
								Paiva et al., 1972
								Paiva et al., 1972
					8.6		5 µg/kg	Paiva et al., 1972 (1)
					8.20		10 µg/kg	Paiva et al., 1972 (1)
50—100								Schwyzer and Turrian, 1960
100								Guttmann, 1961
1	0	0						Guttmann, 1961
0.002								Schwyzer, 1961
0.5—1								Schwyzer, 1961
100								Aoyagi et al., 1967; Thampi et al., 1968
100								Thampi et al., 1968
0					0	0	0	Vogler et al., 1965
0.03				0.1(G)				Jorgensen and Patton, 1969 (2)
0.005						+	+	Regoli et al., 1972
70				70 (C)				Regoli and Park, 1972
0.7				1.0(C)				Regoli and Park, 1972
4.0				1.0(C)				Regoli and Park, 1972
0.1				0.5(C)				Regoli and Park, 1972
100				10(C)				Regoli and Park, 1972
<0.1				0.1(C)				Regoli and Park, 1972
1.0				2.0(C)				Regoli and Park, 1972
					7.6			Paiva et al., 1972 (1)
					6.54			Fessler et al., 1972
					5.08			Fessler et al., 1972
					7.93			Fessler et al., 1972
					8.31			Fessler et al., 1972
					8.26			Fessler et al., 1972
0.20					7.07			Khosla et al. (unpublished results)

f) In analogs not containing the guanidinium group, the other interactions may become increasingly important, involving the spatial arrangement around the α-carbon atom.

From the foregoing conclusions one is tempted to believe that not one but a number of factors appear to play a role in placing the polar group in a proper position. BUMPUS et al. (1970) hold the view that the prolonged peptide chain is the important feature necessary for the stabilization of some essential conformation. This is evident from the fact that the carboxyl terminal hexapeptide of angiotensin, Val-Tyr-Ile-His-Pro-Phe, has 0.1 to 1% pressor activity of the parent octapeptide, and this low activity is significantly enhanced by extension of the peptide at the amino end by a variety of amino acids. JORGENSEN et al. [1970 (3)] have suggested that incorporation of a single basic group separated by five carbons atoms from the valine nitrogen is sufficient to enhance the activity of the hexapeptide significantly.

Variations in position 3. Contrary to the earlier belief, the aliphatic side chain in this position appears to make a considerable contribution (steric or hydrophobic) to the determination of the pressor and myotropic activity of Ang. II. Complete removal of the first three amino acids destroys the biological activity, suggesting that the chain length in Ang. II-(3-8)-hexapeptide is minimum for pressor or myotropic activity of the compound. Replacement of each of the first three amino acids with glycine yields an analog which, in spite of full-length backbone, has very little activity (0.1%) as compared to 10% obtained for [Gly^1, Gly^2]-Ang. II. This indicates the importance of side chain in this position.

When the side-chain branching of valine in this position is shifted from β- to γ-carbon atom (leucine) there is no loss of activity. Considerable activity (68%) is also retained when the isopropyl side chain is replaced with a methyl group as in alanine. High pressor activity (40%) obtained with proline in this position was somewhat surprising because of the marked effect this amino acid may have on limiting possible conformations of a peptide. However, the pressor activity is reduced to $<$ 12% when the aliphatic side chain is replaced with an aromatic moiety (hydroxyphenyl). Similarly, replacement of an α-CH of valine with a nitrogen atom, diminishes the activity to 0.5 to 1% of that of Ang. II.

Variations in position 4. Replacement of the first four amino acids with glycine almost completely destroys the pressor activity of this analog. Pressor activity is also reduced considerably either when the *p*-hydroxyl group of tyrosine is removed (Phe, 10%) or is masked by methylation ($<$ 1%), or when the aromatic side chain is dislocated through spatial orientation (D-Phe, 0.025%) or replaced with an H atom (Ala, $<$ 0.31%). Transposition of tyrosine with valine (position 3), with histidine (position 6), or with phenylalanine (position 8), or replacement of tyrosine with glutamic acid or insertion of another tyrosine residue (Endo 4 a), reduces the pressor activity in each case to less than 1%. Iodination of aromatic nucleus also leads to reduction in pressor activity; monoiodo homolog has 33% of the pressor activity of the parent hormone, while the diiodo derivative possesses only 13% activity. It appears therefore that the aromatic side chain in tyrosine (L-configuration) with a *p*-phenolic hydroxyl group is essential for vasopressor activity of the compound. Present knowledge of the conformation of angiotensin (FERMANDJIAN et al., 1971) precludes the possibility of secondary intramolecular hydrogen bonding with the phenolic hydroxyl group; it is, therefore, possible that this function may be involved in the intermolecular interaction with the receptor site.

Variations in position 5. In the two biologically identical natural variants, position 5 is occupied either by isoleucine (human, equine or porcine species) or by valine (bovine species). In both these amino acids the side chain is branched in β-position. High pressor activity was present in all the 5-substituted analogs with β-branched substituents such as L-alloisoleucine (100%), L-α-amino-β-ethylvaleric acid (75%), L-α-cyclopentylglycine (89%) and L-α-cyclohexylglycine (114%). However, the pressor activity was lowered when this branching was shifted to γ-position as in leucine (25%) or when this position was occupied by an unbranched aliphatic amino acid; L-alanine (5%), L-α-amino-butyric acid (16%), L-norleucine (21%). These results indicated that a steric effect on the peptide backbone was the primary role of the amino-acid residues in the 5-position which contributes to the pressor effect of Ang. II. α-Amino acids with little steric constraint such as sarcosine (1%) and α-amino-isobutyric acid (0.9%) in this position showed low activity, while the related rigid-ring analogs containing the proper sterochemical elements showed significant activity; L-proline (10%) and cycloleucine (24%). On the other hand, [Asn^1, D-Pro^5]-Ang. II was almost inactive (0.05%) as a pressor agent. It is interesting to not that similar steric changes in position 3 did not exert any influence on the pressor or myotropic activity of Ang. II.

Variations in position 6. PAIVA and PAIVA (1961) photolyzed [Asn^1, Val^5]-Ang. II in an oxygen atmosphere in the presence of methylene blue and observed that the decrease in pressor, oxytocic or myotropic activity of the hormone is proportional to the destruction of the imidazole ring of the histidine residue; the biological activity of the compound is reduced to less than 1% within 1 h of ultraviolet irradiation. These results suggest the importance of an imidazole ring in this position for the biological activity of the molecule. However, it is likely that one or more of the properties such as aromaticity, nucleophilicity, chelatibility with divalent cations, steriostructure or ionic interactions in the imidazole ring, may be responsible for the pressor or myotropic response of the hormone. Further work has been carried out to investigate the significance of these facets. Peptides with very low activity are obtained when the imidazole ring in the side chain of histidine is replaced by a hydrogen atom as in alanine (0.83%), by a thiophene ring as in β-2-thienylalanine (1%), by an aromatic ring such as in phenylalanine or by a basic chain as in lysine (0.1%) or arginine (completely inactive). Similarly, spatial orientation at this center by replacement of L-histidine with D-histidine residue reduced the pressor activity of the peptide to 1%. These studies suggest that neither the aromaticity alone nor the charge are responsible for the biological response of the compound. HOFMANN et al. (1968) replaced histidine in Ang. II by the isosteric β-(pyrazolyl)-L-alanine to assess the acid-base requirements for the side chain in position 6. High pressor (57%) and myotropic (79%) response obtained with this analog led these authors to believe that the stereo structure of the five-membered heterocyclic ring of histidine, and not its charge, is of crucial significance for high level angiotensin activity. In contrast to these conclusions, [Phe^4, Tyr^8]-Ang. II (MARSHALL et al., 1970) has been reported to inhibit the response of the isolated rat uterus to Ang. II when the pH of the medium was 7.4 or less. Since at this pH a significant amount of histidine imidazole is protonated (pK imidazole = 6.3; PAIVA et al., 1963), it appears that it may be the protonated form of histidine residue that interacts with the receptor. STEWART (1971) undertook a study to determine the effect of pH on rat-uterus response to Ang. II and the extent to which substituents for the histidine residue could alter the pH effects. The results indicated that the presence of a positive charge on the side chain in position 6 in the angiotensin molecule reduces the effectiveness of the peptide, both by lowering the inherent activity of the molecule and by causing it to rapidly produce tachyphylaxis. [Orn^6]-, and [Arg^6]-analogs which would bear a positive charge at all pH values studied were completely inactive and showed marked tachyphylaxis. On the basis of proton magnetic resonance studies, WEINKAM and JORGENSEN (1971) have postulated that the carboxyl of the C-terminal is associated with the imidazole ring of histidine and an intramolecular hydrogen bond between the phenylalanine amide NH and the histidine carbonyl function may stabilize the conformation of Ang. II. KHOSLA et al. [1972 (1)] have recently studied the effect of transposition of side chains in positions 4 and 6 and the compound obtained, [His^4, Tyr^6]-Ang. II is neither an agonist nor an antagonist. It appears that transposition of the side chains in positions 4 and 6 must place histidine and tyrosine in a position relative to one another which are not compatible with the receptor, or that the transposition destroys the stereo structure which is necessary for intramolecular interactions or for chelation of Ca^{++}.

Variations in position 7. Replacement of the pyrrolidine ring system in position 7 of Ang. II with an open-chain primary aliphatic amino acid such as alanine abolished the pressor activity. These results led PAGE and BUMPUS (1961) to conclude that proline in this position is essential for pressor and myotropic response of Ang. II. However, the importance of the proline residue may be due to a) the ability of the rigid pyrrolidine ring to bring the functionally essential amino acids 4-tyrosine, 6-histidine and 8-phenylalanine into proper stereo-structure (SMEBY et al., 1962) when the peptide reacts with its receptor, b) the lack of a potential H-bonding site in this residue which favors the stabilization of biologically active conformation, and c) an increase in the occurrence of cis-peptide bonds, which is perhaps a prerequisite for the required conformation. It is not possible at this stage to assess which of these factors is primarily responsible for the observed biological behavior but any deviation from these rigid requirements results in inactive peptides. Whereas the replacement of proline with alanine gives an inactive peptide, due perhaps to alteration in the chemical nature of the imide N and steric hindrance, the inactivity of [6-pipecolic acid]-Ang. II may be explained by loss of rigidity because of ring expansion. Similarly, the lowering of pressor activity in [7-hydroxyproline]-Ang. II may be explained by possible intramolecular interaction of this additional hydroxyl group with another essential group, leading to a change in the required conformation or steric hindrance. On the other hand, replacement of proline with a secondary amino acid, such as N-methyl alanine, results in a biologically active analog.

Variations in position 8. Complete removal of either phenylalanine (position 8) or the dipeptide, Pro-Phe (positions 7 and 8) completely destroys the pressor or myotropic activity of the hormone. Amide formation or esterification of the C-terminal free carboxyl group reduces the pressor activity to 3% and 10% respectively. Pressor activity is also decreased when position 8 is replaced with 3-amino-4-phenylbutyric acid (10%), DL-3-amino-2-benzyl propionic acid (1%) or cyclohexylalanine (20%). Almost inactive analogs are obtained when the aromatic ring of phenylalanine is replaced by an aliphatic chain (as in alanine, leucine, isoleucine, norleucine) or when L-phenylalanine is replaced by the corresponding D-isomer. Substitution by bromine or hydroxy group in *p*-position of the phenyl ring reduces the activity to 50% and 83% respectively. These results indicate the importance of C-terminal sequence of angiotensin for biological activity. It appears that for a good pressor and myotropic response, the amino-acid residue in this position should have the L-configuration, an aromatic ring in the side chain and a free carboxyl group. Furthermore, the length of the peptide backbone and the relative positions of the carboxyl group and the aromatic side chain should be retained. Relatively high pressor potency obtained with [8-cyclohexylalanine]-Ang. II indicates that the cyclohexyl ring may be able to mimic the aromatic ring of phenylalanine to some extent in delivering the message onto the receptor.

Synthesis of Analogs of Angiotensin II as Specific Antagonists of the Parent Hormone

The structure-activity relationships discussed in the last section were primarily concerned with the pressor and myotropic response of Ang. II. Apart from these and the vasoconstrictor effect in vessels of the skin, kidney and ventricular muscle of the heart, Ang. II is now well known for its multiplicity of direct and indirect physiological actions, e.g., antidiuretic effect, inhibition of sodium transport in renal tissue, release of aldosterone from the adrenal cortex, release of catecholamines from the adrenal medulla, reduction of mesenteric blood flow, and stimulant effects on various components of the autonomic nervous system.

Table 2. *A comparison of biologic activities of Ang. II analogs*

Ang. II analog	Concentration ng/ml	Pressor response %	Inhibition norepinephrine uptake %
Ang. II	0.2	100	80
[Ile^1]-	2.0	20	25
[Ala^3]-	2.0	65	70
[Ala^4]-	2.0	0	0
[Ala^6]-	2.0	1	0
[Ala^7]-	2.0	2	0
[Asn^1, Phe $(NH_2)^8$]-	2.0	0	0
[Tyr^8]-	2.0	85	80
[Apb^8]-	2.0	10	80
[Apib^8]-	2.0	0.1	40
[Ala^8]-	0.2	2	50
	2.0	2	80

Attempts to correlate the above diversified effects of Ang. II with the etiology of hypertension has caused the need for a specific antagonist of angiotensin to be felt more than ever before (PAGE and BUMPUS, 1962). In this connection, considerable attention has been focused recently on the release and reuptake of norepinephrine by the sympathetic nerve endings (PEACH, BUMPUS and KHAIRALLAH, 1971). In an analysis (Table 2) of structure-activity relationships of the various analogs studied by this latter group, BUMPUS (1971) concluded:

1. There was a close correlation between inhibition of uptake of norepinephrine and pressor response of all analogs with substitution in positions 1 through 7. All those analogs which had reasonable pressor response also showed corresponding inhibition of norepinephrine uptake.

2. Significant differences were evident with changes made in position 8. The aromatic ring in the side chain of phenylalanine was not necessary for inhibition of norepinephrine uptake while it was absolutely essential for pressor activity. The free C-terminal carboxyl group is required for both activities, but the location of this group is more important for pressor activity.

3. Substitution of aromatic residue in position 8 with an aliphatic group, such as in [Ala^8]-angiotensin, reduced the pressor response to 2% of the parent hormone without corresponding reduction of inhibition of norepinephrine reuptake. Similar

results were obtained when the aromatic ring was dislocated by increasing the chain length by one carbon atom.

On the basis of the foregoing results, BUMPUS [1971 (1)] suggested that position 8 was of great importance for the pressor and myotropic response to Ang. II, for the development of potent antagonists of this hormone, and for the study of the mechanism for the release and reuptake of norepinephrine by the nerve endings. This led to a reassessment of [Ala^8]-Ang. II as an antagonist of the parent hormone [BUMBUS 1971 (1); KHAIRALLAH et al., 1970], followed by synthesis of [Ile^8]-Ang. II as a potent antagonist of Ang. II in both *in-vitro* and *in-vivo* studies [BUMPUS 1971 (2); KHOSLA et al., 1971; 1972 (1)]. This was a breakthrough in structure-activity relationships in angiotensin and was the first important discovery leading to the development of numerous angiotensin antagonists.

[Ala^8]-Ang. II was found to antagonize the action of Ang. II on strips of guinea-pig ileum (KHAIRALLAH et al., 1970). In an attempt to obtain a better understanding of the mechanism, this analog was tested on isolated rabbit aorta and rat colon and it was found that its antagonistic potency was very high and that it antagonized Ang. I equally well. However, this compound did not inhibit the myotropic action of norepinephrine, serotonin or prostaglandin, nor did it antagonize the effects of Ang. II *in vivo* at levels reported by TÜRKER et al. (1971). According to GAGNON et al. (1971), [Ala^8]-Ang. II does show antagonism to angiotensin *in vivo* at high dose levels. Similarly, PALS et al. [1971 (1)] reported that [Asn^1, Val^5, Ala^8]-Ang. II, when infused at 200 μg/kg/min, inhibited the action of Ang. II on the blood pressure of rat. While reporting these results PALS et al. [1971 (1)] ignored the above developments thus claiming to be the first group to recognize the antagonistic properties in alanine-8 derivative of Ang. II. In fact, [alanine^8]-Ang. II was first reported by BUMPUS et al. in 1961. It was again synthesized by a solid-phase procedure in 1967 (PARK et al.), and its antagonistic properties on guinea-pig ileum (KHAIRALLAH et al., 1970) and rabbit aortic strips (TÜRKER et al., 1971) had already been reported in the literature before PALS et al. [1971 (2)] published their results.

[Ile^8]-Ang. II [KHOSLA et al., 1971, 1972 (1); YAMAMOTO et al., 1972; SMEBY et al., 1972] was found to have a specific competitive effect against Ang. II both *in vitro* on isolated rabbit aortic strips and rat uterus, the ganglion-stimulating action, as measured by contraction of cat nictitating membranes, and *in vivo* on blood pressure of rat, cat and dog. Infusion of this analog into rats with acute renal-clip hypertension, both with contralateral kidney intact (2 kidneys) and with the contralateral kidney removed (1 kidney), caused a fall in blood pressure (SMEBY et al., 1972). [Ile^8]-Ang. II has a pA_2 value of 9.21 as compared to 8.3 obtained for [Ala^8]-Ang. II, and satisfies the criteria established by SCHILD (1947, 1949) for competitive antagonism (TÜRKER et al., 1971).

To evaluate the potential of modification of position 8 further, phenylalanine in position 8 was replaced (KHOSLA et al., 1972 (2)] by: a) cyclohexylalanine (V) to delineate the contribution of aromaticity or ring size for myotropic response; b) valine (VII), leucine (VIII), and norleucine (IX) to investigate the nature of aliphatic side chain required for a potent antagonist; c) 3-amino-4-phenyl butyric acid (III) or DL-3-amino-2-benzyl propionic acid (IV), to study the importance of the position of the aromatic side chain in relation to the remainder of the peptide chain for myotropic activity; d) D-isoleucine (XI) to study the effect of a change of spatial orientation in position 8.

PALS et al. [1971 (2)] reported the synthesis of [Sar^1, Ala^8]-Ang. II and showed it to be more active *in vivo* than the Ala^8 analog. KHOSLA et al. [1972 (2)] synthesized [Sar^1, Ile^8]-Ang. II, an even more potent *in-vivo* antagonist, while REGOLI et al. (1972) synthesized [Sar^1, Leu^8]-Ang. II. The potentiation of the *in-vivo* potency by the substitution of sarcosine in the one position is possibly due to increased stability toward hydrolysis by amino peptidases.

MARSHALL et al. (1970) reported that [Phe^4, Tyr^8]-Ang. II, in high doses, competitively antagonizes the myotropic effect of Ang. II on isolated rat uterus and the pressor effect in anesthetized nephrectomized normotensive and hypertensive rats. The *in-vitro* inhibition, however, is pH-dependent, and is not observed

Variations in position 8 of angiotensin II

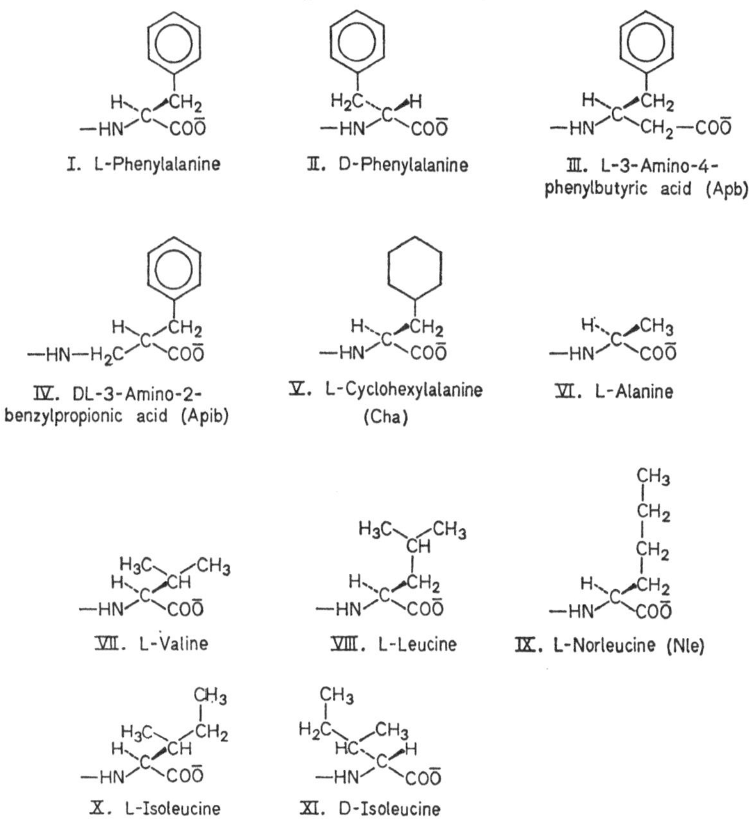

I. L-Phenylalanine; II. D-Phenylalanine; III. L-3-Amino-4-phenylbutyric acid (Apb); IV. DL-3-Amino-2-benzylpropionic acid (Apib); V. L-Cyclohexylalanine (Cha); VI. L-Alanine; VII. L-Valine; VIII. L-Leucine; IX. L-Norleucine (Nle); X. L-Isoleucine; XI. D-Isoleucine

at pH 8, where [Phe^4, Tyr^8]-Ang. II behaves only as an agonist, unless Mg^{++} is added. KHOSLA et al. [1972 (2)] therefore synthesized [Phe^4, Ala^8], and [Ala^8, Ile^4] to study the contribution of position 4 in relation to position 8 for antagonistic effect; similarly [Suc^1, Phe^4, Tyr^8]-Ang. II was synthesized in an attempt to improve the antagonistic properties of the parent analog.

The biological results obtained indicate that [Val^8] and [Leu^8]-Ang. II have 0.5 and 1.3% of the pressor activity of Ang. II respectively, and both these analogs have a specific, competitive antagonistic effect against Ang. II which is comparable to [Ile^8]-Ang. II in both *in-vitro* and *in-vivo* studies. However, [D-Ile^8]-Ang. II (XI) (KHOSLA et al., unpublished results) shows very low antagonistic activity as compared to the corresponding L-isoleucine congener and it has a pA_2 value of 7.32. PAIVA et al. [1972 (1)] have reported that [Pro⁸]-Ang. II does not show antagonistic properties.

[Cha⁸]-Ang. II (V) shows agonistic activity which is equal to 20% of that of Ang. II, both *in vitro* and *in vivo*. Continued administration, however, completely blocks the myotropic effect due to Ang. II and [Cha⁸]-Ang. II on rabbit aortic strips. In intact rats, [Cha⁸]-Ang. II antagonizes the pressor response to Ang. II at a dose level of 0.9 ng/g body weight. Similar antagonistic activity has also been observed in dogs and cats. This antagonistic activity may possibly be related to tachyphylaxis.

[Apb⁸]-Ang. II (III) shows approximately 10% pressor activity of Ang. II but no antagonistic activity, whereas [DL-Apib⁸]-Ang. II (IV) has 1% pressor activity and antagonizes the myotropic response of Ang. II on rabbit aortic strip at a dose level of approximately 5 µg/ml. The pA_2 value of this analog is 5.57 and the pA_{10} value 4.73. Its duration of action is very short and the antagonistic effect is overcome in 5 min [KHOSLA et al., 1972 (2); TÜRKER et al., 1973]. Both [Apb⁸] and [Apib⁸]-Ang. II have been found to be highly active in inhibiting uptake of catecholamines by sympathetic nerve endings and causing release of catecholamines from adrenal medulla [PEACH, 1972 (2)].

[Sar¹, Ile⁸]-Ang. II [KHOSLA et al., 1972 (2)] has been found to be the most potent and long-lasting competitive antagonist of this series. It has an almost equal antagonistic potency to that of [Ile⁸]-Ang. II when tested on isolated muscle strips but it is ten times more potent in the *in-vivo* systems. It has a pA_2 value of 9.33 as compared to 9.21 for [Ile⁸]-Ang. II and 8.32 for [Ala⁸]-Ang. II [TÜRKER et al., 1972 (1)]. Blockage of the pressor response of Ang. II in anesthetized cats and dogs was still present 100 min after discontinuation of the infusion in the case of this compound. The corresponding recovery time for [Ile⁸]-Ang. II is 30 to 65 min. When tested in dogs with acute renal artery constriction, [Sar¹, Ile⁸]-Ang. II (400 ng/kg/min × 20 min) completely reversed the hypertensive response to acute renal artery constriction and the direct vasoconstrictor response to exogenous Ang. II. It also produces a specific antagonism of the vascular actions of Ang. II in dogs without altering vasoconstrictor effects of norepinephrine. When infused into the vertebral artery, this analog significantly reduces the cardiovascular response to intravertebral infusion of Ang. II (SWEET et al., in press).

[Sar¹, Leu⁸]-Ang. II when tested on isolated rat stomach strips, (REGOLI et al., 1972) has been found to be 100 times as active than [Ala⁸]-Ang. II and 1.5 to 2 times as active than [Sar¹, Ala⁸]-Ang. II. The *in-vivo* experiments on nephrectomized rats as well as the *in-vitro* experiments on isolated rat stomach strips demonstrate the irreversible character of the inhibition by [Sar¹, Leu⁸]-Ang. II, a phenomenon which cannot be reproduced in other laboratories.

[Suc¹, Phe⁴, Tyr⁸]-Ang. II antagonizes the myotropic effect of Ang. II on rabbit aortic strips above a concentration of 10 µg/ml. It has 0.19% pressor response and negligible antagonistic effect in the *in-vivo* pressor assays on rats.

[Phe⁴, Ala⁸]-Ang. II shows 0.001% pressor activity of Ang. II and negligible myotropic activity. When tested on rabbit aortic strips this compound blocks the myotropic response to Ang. II at a dose level above 1 µg/ml. Similarly [Ala⁴, Ile⁸], and [Pro³]-Ang. II possess very low pressor response (0.0112%) and antagonistic properties. In general, the antagonists listed above inhibit a) myocardial contractile responses to Ang. II and other Ang. II analogs with inotropic activity; b) stimulation of adrenal chromaffin tissue by Ang. II; c) stimulation of aldosterone biosynthesis and d) the increase in capillary permeability in rabbit skin promoted by Ang. II. However, in isolated frog skin, where Ang. II increases the rate of sodium transport, [Ile^8]-Ang. II has been found to be twice as active an agonist as the natural peptide (WIDEMAN et al., 1972).

The above structural modifications indicate an interesting correlation for both agonistic and antagonistic properties of Ang. II and its analogs. Pressor activity is reduced while the antagonistic activity is progressively enhanced when either the spatial orientation of the side chain of L-phenylalanine in position 8 is changed, as in the substitution with D-phenylalanine (II) (GAGNON et al., 1971) or when the carboxyl group is shifted by 1C atom towards the C-terminal as in 3-amino-4-phenylbutyric acid (III) or when the aromatic residue is replaced by an aliphatic (VI, VII, VIII, IX, X) or alicyclic residue (V). Further, amide formation or esterification of the free carboxylic acid are known to reduce the pressor activity to 3% and 10% respectively. It appears, therefore, that for good pressor and myotropic response, the amino-acid residue in position 8 should have the L-configuration, an aromatic ring in the side chain, and a free carboxyl group. Moreover, length of the peptide backbone and juxtaposition of the carboxyl group in relation to the aromatic side chain should be retained. On the other hand, for antagonistic properties to myotropic response, the aromatic ring in position 8 should be either shifted by 1C atom (3-amino-2-benzylpropionic acid), dislocated through spatial orientation (D-Phe) or replaced with an H atom (L-Ala). Present information suggests that to produce potent antagonistic properties to both the myotropic and the pressor responses of Ang. II, the aromatic ring in position 8 should be replaced either with an alicyclic ring (cyclohexylalanine) or an aliphatic side chain branched at the β or γ position (Ile, Leu, Val); the aliphatic amino acid in this position, however, should have L-configuration. Since [8-cyclohexylalanine]-Ang. II initially shows agonistic properties, it appears that cyclohexyl ring may be able to deliver the message by partial imitation of the aromatic ring of phenylalanine but once the receptor has been occupied the peptide no longer acts as an agonist. Low antagonistic activity obtained with [Ala^4, Ile^8] and [Phe^4, Ala^8]-Ang. II indicate that the antagonistic properties of the antagonists obtained, due to variation in position 8, is influenced by substituents in position 4. Since replacement of the phenolic hydroxyl group by either an aliphatic or an unsubstituted aromatic residue in position 4 lowers the antagonistic properties of these antagonists, it appears that a phenolic hydroxyl group is essential to reveal the potent antagonistic properties in these compounds. On the other hand, depending upon the nature of substituents in position 1, the antagonistic property is either enhanced, as in [Sar^1, Ile^8]-Ang. II, or is decreased, as in [Suc^1, Phe^4, Tyr^8]-Ang. II.

Recently, PAIVA et al. [1972 (1)] have reported the synthesis of two analogs of Ang. I in which position 8 has been replaced by valine and isoleucine and both analogs have been found to be potent antagonists of Ang. I and II. However, [Val^8]-Ang. I has been reported to be more potent than [Ile^8]-Ang. I. Very large shifts of the dose-response curves for the pressor activity of Ang. I and II have been observed during infusion of 5 μg/kg/min of [Val^8]-Ang. I. Similar results with [Ile^8]-Ang. I are obtained with a dose of 10 μg/kg/min. [Ile^8]-Ang. I antagonized the action of angiotensin on guinea-pig ileum (pA_2, 8.03 for Ang. II and 8.31 for Ang. I) but not on the rat uterus.

The antagonistic activity obtained with the various 8-substituted analogs may prove useful in understanding the mode of action of angiotensin itself. A competitive inhibitor of angiotensin is an important tool in the study of "biologically active" conformation of Ang. II, its mechanism of action and the identification of its various receptors. However, such compounds may afford little knowledge about the nature of the cellular receptor for angiotensin. Conversely, an irreversible specific inhibitor may bind covalently with nucleophilic sites on the receptor and may be useful in the identification and characterization of receptor substances. The first attempt in this direction was made by LIN and GOODFRIEND (1970), who found that radioactive monoiodoangiotensin binds to several so-called "specific angiotensin receptors". Recently PAIVA et al. (1972) incorporated the nitrogen mustard chlorambucil, *p*-[N, N-bis (2-chloroethyl) amino] phenylbutyric acid (XII), into Ang. II and various C-terminal fragments of Ang. II.

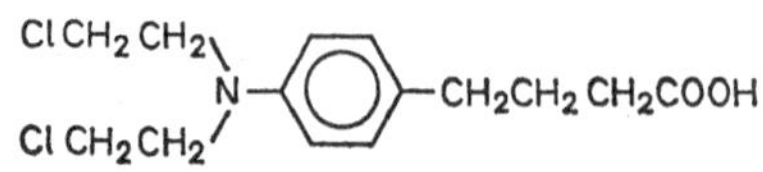

XII Chlorambucil

Chlorambucil Ang. II and chlorambucil-[Des-Asp^1, Ile^5]-Ang. II caused non-competitive inhibition of the action of angiotensin on guinea-pig ileum which was not reversed after 8 h. These compounds also showed pressor activity in the rat, but it was not possible to demonstrate an antiangiotensin action of the chlorambucil peptides on rat blood pressure. According to the authors, this failure may be due to low solubility of these peptides in water which made it impractical to infuse large doses; with the low concentration and slow infusion rate, most of the alkylating moiety of the compounds reacted with water and the plasma proteins before reaching the angiotensin receptors responsible for pressor activity. Contrary to expectation, [Des-Asp^1, Chl-Arg^2, Val^8]-Ang. I was found to be a competitive and reversible inhibitor of Ang. II.

Conformation of Angiotensin II

The initial studies on Ang. II conformation using optical rotary dispersion (o.r.d.) suggested that in aqueous solution the octapeptide had a center of assymetry not found in the C-terminal hexapeptide or C-terminal tetrapeptide (SMEBY et al., 1962). The o.r.d. data obtainable at that time were limited due to restrictions on the instrumentation available, but the data were consistent with an α-helical conformation. It was also shown by titration that the phenolic group of tyrosine was free in the native peptide. On the basis of these limited data the hypothesis was advanced that Ang. II existed in aqueous solution as an α-helix. While this was a risky suggestion and has subsequently been shown to be incorrect, it proved valuable for it stimulated further interest in this problem.

In a more detailed study, PAIVA, PAIVA and SCHERAGA (1963) demonstrated that the C-terminal carboxyl, the imidazole group of histidine, the N-terminal amino group, the β-carboxyl of aspartic acid and the phenolic group of tyrosine were free and not associated with other groups. Recently WEINKAM and JORGENSEN (1971) concluded from n.m.r. spectra and e.s.r. spectra of nitronylnitroxylalanylprolylphenylalanine derivatives that the C-terminal carboxyl group interacts with the imidazole ring of histidine. However, this observation cannot be confirmed by natural abundance ^{13}C n.m.r. spectra (ZIMMER et al., 1972) or other n.m.r. spectral studies (GLICKSON et al., 1972). It was also demonstrated (PAIVA et al., 1963) that all exchangeable hydrogen atoms of Ang. II exchanged rapidly with deuterium and their o.r.d. data were not consistent with a helical structure or a stable conformation in aqueous solution. They therefore concluded that Ang. II existed in a random conformation.

Using thin-film dialysis CRAIG et al. (1964) found that Ang. II passed through cellophane membranes significantly faster than could be predicted by molecular weight. They therefore concluded that this peptide had some type of folded conformation and could not be random. In a more detailed study of the dialysis behavior of the peptide, FERREIRA et al. (1969) found evidence for two forms of Ang. II in solutions of low ionic strength (less than 0.1) in the pH range of 2 to 9.

Recently PRINTZ et al. (1972) restudied the rate of exchange of the exchangeable hydrogen atoms of Ang. II with tritium at 0°. In contrast to the previous results, they found that some N-H hydrogen atoms did exchange slowly with solvent and concluded that this peptide was capable of forming stable, intramolecular hydrogen bonds. They further concluded that the side chain of asparagine is freely accessible to solvent, two of six backbone peptide N-H bonds are involved in secondary structure; and that the peptide N-H bond of Asp-Arg is not involved in secondary structure.

Investigations of Ang. II using circular dichroism (CD) (FERMANDJIAN et al., 1971) have demonstrated that there is an increase in structural order when proline is added onto the N-terminal hexapeptide. However, there is a further marked increase in order when the eighth amino acid is added and the shape of the CD spectrum is dependent on the structure of the eighth amino acid. When phenylalanine, in the natural peptide, occupies the 8 position, the CD curve obtained is significantly different from that obtained when alanine, which produces an analog with Ang. II antagonistic properties [FERMANDJIAN et al., 1971 (1)] occupies the 8 position. This observation suggests the C-terminal amino acid of Ang. II has a strong influence on peptide conformation. Heating aqueous solutions of Ang. II increases structural order of the peptide, as measured by CD, indicating that hydrophobic forces play a very important role in the peptide conformation. The CD curves are consistent with an antiparallel β-pleated sheet structure for Ang. II and this seems to be favored by heating and in solvents such as trifluoroethanol.

Having observed the decrease in unordered structure of Ang. II in trifluoroethanol, FERMANDJIAN et al. [1971 (1)] were able to crystallize the peptide from this solvent. The X-ray crystallographic data obtained from these crystals were consistent with the antiparallel β-pleated sheet structure (FROMAGEOT, private communication). Energy calculations have suggested two models in which the peptide chain is folded back onto itself to form the antiparallel β-structure are favorable [PRINTZ et al., 1972 (1)]. Both models yield a very hydrophobic side-group region with the ionic side groups arranged to give minimum interaction and freely accessible to solvent.

These experimental results have led to the following conclusions about the conformation of Ang. II in aqueous solution [PRINTZ et al., 1972 (1)].

1. The most probable structure represents an atiparallel β-pleated sheet. Such a structure may be formed either by the peptide chain turning back onto itself or by combination of 2 peptide chains. The latter possibility seems unlikely because molecular weight determinations in solutions gave no evidence of dimer formation (PAIVA et al., 1963).

2. Two peptide N-H hydrogens are probably involved in secondary structure and one of these is involved in an intramolecular hydrogen bond.

3. The peptide N-H bond in Asp-Arg is probably not H bonded.

4. Asparagine side chain is accessible to solvent although the situation with the natural aspartic-acid side chain is not known.

5. The ionic side groups, with the possible exception of arginine are probably not involved in secondary structure. Data are not available for the arginine side chain.

6. Hydrophobic bonding plays an important role in the conformational stability of Ang. II.

These studies give some concept of the structure of the peptide in solution but do not give us the conformation on the receptor. While the receptor may greatly modify the structure of a peptide, it is generally assumed that such distortion will be minimal. Thus, there has been speculation [PRINTZ et al., 1972 (1)] that the receptor structure is a complimentary structure to the peptide. However, there are several questions to be settled. First the conformation proposed for Ang. II cannot be considered a fixed structure. The peptide chain remains flexible and the proposed conformation probably represents only one of several conformers present in solution but it is the one present in greatest concentration. For example, under certain conditions there is some evidence for both the β-pleated sheet structure and traces of a helical structure (FERMANDJIAN, 1971). For such speculations it must be assumed that only the major conformer will react with the receptor and not a minor one. Second, we do not know which side groups react with the receptor. Thus, when speculating about the receptor structure, we do not know which portion of the peptide to use for the design of the complimentary structure. Third, the chemical nature of the receptor is not known. It is generally assumed that the receptor is a protein but since all β-pleated sheet models have a very hydrophobic region in their structures it is conceivable that the receptor is a polar lipid such as a phospholipid of a combination of protein and lipids. However, once the major conformation of Ang. II in aqueous solution is known, the more difficult question of the structure of the receptor and the chemical nature of the peptide-receptor interaction can be approached.

References

ANDREATTA, R., HOFMANN, K.: Studies on polypeptides XLI. The synthesis of [5-Valine, 6-β-(pyrazolyl-3)-alanine]-angiotensin II, a potent hypertensive peptide. J. Amer. chem. Soc. **90**, 7334 (1968).

ANDREATTA, R. H., SCHERAGA, H. A.: Synthesis of [5-Valine, 7-N-methylalanine]-angiotensin II, a hypertensive peptide. J. Med. Chem. **14**, 489 (1971).

AOYAGI, H., ARAKAWA, K., IZUMIYA, N.: Synthesis of human Angiotensin I. J. Amer. chem. Soc. **89**, 4239 (1967).

ARAKAWA, K., BUMPUS, F. M.: An improved synthesis of isoleucine[5] angiotensin octapeptide. J. Amer. chem. Soc. **83**, 728 (1961).

ARAKAWA, K., SMEBY, R. R., BUMPUS, F. M.: Synthesis of succinyl[1]-isoleucyl[5]-Angiotensin II and N-(Poly-O-acetylseryl)-isoleucyl[5]-angiotensin II. J. Amer. chem. Soc. **84**, 1424 (1962).

BRUNNER, H., REGOLI, D.: Unterschiedliche Empfindlichkeit verschiedener Angiotensin-Derivative gegen Abbau durch Plasma oder Nierenhomogenat. Experientia (Basel) 18, 504 (1962).

BRUNNER, H. R., KIRSHMAN, J. D., SEALEY, J. E., LARAGH, J. H.: Hypertension of Renal Origin: Evidence for two different mechanisms. Science **174**, 1344 (1971).

BUMPUS, F. M.: (1) Angiotensin, structure-activity relationships. In: Structure-activity relationships of protein and polypeptide hormones, p. 18. (MARGOULIES, M., GREENWOOD, F. C., Eds.). Amsterdam: Excerpta Medica 1971.

BUMPUS, F. M.: (2) [8-isoleucine]-angiotensin II, a potent competitive antagonist of angiotensin II. Annual Fall Conference of the Council for High Blood Pressure Research. Cleveland: Oct. 1971.

BUMPUS, F. M., SMEBY, R. R.: Angiotensin. In: Renal Hypertension, p. 62 (PAGE, I. H., MCCUBBIN, J. W., Eds.). Chicago: Year Book Publishers 1968.

BUMPUS, F. M., SCHWARZ, H., PAGE, I. H.: Synthesis and pharmacology of the octapeptide angiotensin. Science **125**, 3253 (1957).

BUMPUS, F. M., KHAIRALLAH, P. A., ARAKAWA, K., PAGE, I. H., SMEBY, R. R.: The relationship of structure to pressor and oxytocic actions of isoleucine[5] angiotensin octapeptide and various analogues. Biochim. biophys. Acta (Amst.) **46**, 38 (1961).

BUMPUS, F. M., SMEBY, R. R., KHAIRALLAH, P. A.: Synthesis and biological properties of angiotensin II analogs. In: Peptides, Chemistry and Biochemistry, Proceedings 1st American Peptide Symposium, p. 127 (WEINSTEIN, B., LANDE, S., Eds.). New York: Marcel Dekker 1970.

CHATURVEDI, N. C., PARK, W. K., SMEBY, R. R., BUMPUS, F. M.: Analogs of Angiotensin II. Solid Phase Synthesis. J. Med. Chem. **13**, 177 (1970).

CIPENS, G. E., VEGNERS, R., LICLAIS, J., PAPSUEVICH, O. S., ROMANOVSKIS, P.: Identity of the signatures of the end fragments of angiotensin and some neurohypophysoric hormones. Latv. PSR Zinat. Akad. Vestis, Kim. Ser. 1969, 629, Chem. Abstr. **72**, 39425 d.

CRAIG, L. C., HARFENIST, E. J., PALADINI, A. C.: Dialysis Studies VII. The behavior of angiotensin, oxytocin, vasopressin, and some of their analogs. Biochemistry **3**, 764 (1964).

CRESSWELL, M. A., HANSON, R. W., LAW, H. D.: The synthesis and properties of analogues of angiotensin modified in the 1- or the 4-position. J. chem. Soc., C, 2669 (1967).

DE GRAAF, J. S.: Angiotensin II, myotropic activities of some des-Asp[1]-analogues. Thesis, Leiden Univ., 1970.

DE GRAAF, J. S., JANSEN, A. C. A., KERLING, K. E. T., SCHATTENKERK, C., HAVINGA, E.: Studies on Polypeptides. Part XII: Myotropic activities of some des-Asp[1]-[Ile[5]]-Angiotensin analogues. Data and a working hypothesis on the contributions of the arginine residue to activity. Rec. Trav. chim. Pays-Bas **90**, 301 (1971).

DEODHAR, S. D.: Immunologic production of antiangiotensin I. Preparation of angiotensin-protein complex antigen. J. exp. Med. **111**, 419 (1960).

FERMANDJIAN, S., MORGAT, J. L., FROMAGEOT, P.: Studies of angiotensin II conformations by Circular Dichroism. Europ. J. Biochem. **24**, 252 (1971).

FERMANDJIAN, S., MORGAT, J. L., FROMAGEOT, P., LEGRESSUS, C., MAIRE, P.: (1) Crystallization of angiotensinamide II. FEBS Letters **16**, 192 (1971).

FERREIRA, A. T., HAMPE, O. G., PAIVA, A. C. M.: The conformation of angiotensin II in aqueous solution. II. Dialysis and Gel filtration behavior of [Asn[1], Val[5]] angiotensin II. Biochemistry **8**, 3483 (1969).

FESSLER, D. C., SIPOS, F., DENNING, G. S., Jr., PALS, D. T., MASUCCI, F. D.: Angiotensin II antagonism. Structure-activity relationships of 8-substituted angiotensin II analogs. J. Med. Chem. **15**, 1015 (1972).

FUJI, T., SAKAKIBARA, S.: The solid-phase synthesis of Ile[5]-Angiotensin II to demonstrate the use of N[im]-Tosyl-histidine. Bull. chem. Soc. Jap. **43**, 3954 (1970).

GAGNON, D., PARK, W. K., REGOLI, D.: Specific antagonists for the myotropic action of angiotensin II and angiotensin I on the isolated rat colon. Brit. J. Pharmacol. **43**, 409 (1971).

GARNER, R., YOUNG, G. T.: Facilitation of peptide synthesis by the use of 4-picolyl esters; synthesis of 5-valine angiotensin II. Nature (Lond.) **222**, 177 (1969).

GLICKSON, J. D., CUNNINGHAM, W. D., MARSHALL, G. R.: Proton magnetic resonance study of angiotensinamide in aqueous solution. In: Chemistry and Biology of Peptides. Proc. 3rd Amer. Peptide Symposium, June 18—23, 1972, p. 563 (MEIENHOFER, J., Ed.). Ann. Arbor: Ann Arbor Publishers 1972.

GRAVA, I., CIPENS, G.: Synthesis of [Val[5]]-angiotensin II. Latv. PSR Zinat. Akad. Vestis, Kim. Ser., 230 (1969). Chem. Abstr. **71**, 91848 n.

GROSS, F., TURRIAN, H.: Pharmacology of hypertensin and synthetic analogues. In: Polypeptides which Affect Smooth Muscles and Blood Vessels (SCHACHTER, M., Ed.). Oxford: Pergamon Press 1960.

GUTTMANN, S.: Synthese de la Val[5]-D-Phe[8]-angiotensin I et nouvelle synthese de la Val[5]-angiotensin I. Helv. chim. Acta **44**, 721 (1961).

HABER, E., PAGE, L. B., JACOBY, G. A.: Synthesis of antigenic branch-chain copolymers of angiotensin and poly-l-lysine. Biochemistry **4**, 693 (1965).

HAGEMAN, W. E., HOFMANN, K., ERTEL, R. J., BUCKLEY, J. P.: Pharmacology of valyl[5]-(3-pyrazolyl)-L-alanyl[6]-angiotensin II. J. Pharmacol. exp. Ther. **168**, 295 (1969).

HAVINGA, E., SCHATTENKERK, C., VISSER, G. H., KERLING, K. E. T.: (1) Polypeptides I. Synthesis and activity of angiotensin analogs (mostly heptapeptides) in which the arginine moiety is replaced by similar residues of varied structure and configuration. Rec. Trav. chim. Pays-Bas **83**, 672 (1964).

HAVINGA, E., SCHATTENKERK, C., VISSER, G. H., KERLING, K. E. T.: (2) Polypeptides II. Synthesis of the heptapeptides (de-Asp[1]) Lys[2]-Ileu[5]-angiotensin II, (de-Asp[1]) D-Lys[2]-Ileu[5]-angiotensin II, (de-Asp[1])-Orn[2]-Ileu[5]-angiotensin II, (de-Asp[1])-Cit[2]-Ileu[5]-angiotensin II, and the hexapeptide Val-Tyr-Ileu-His-Pro-Phe. Rec. Trav. chim. Pays-Bas **83**, 677 (1964).

HESS, H. J., MORELAND, W. T., LAUBACH, G. D.: N-[2-Isopropyl-3-(L-aspartyl-L-arginyl)-carbazoyl]-L-tyrosyl-L-valyl-L-histidyl-L-prolyl-L-phenylalanine, an isostere of bovine angiotensin II. J. Amer. chem. Soc. **85**, 4040 (1963).

HESS, H. J., CONSTANTINE, J. W.: D-aspartyl[1]-valyl[5]-phenylalanine[8] amide angiotensin II. J. Med. Chem. **7**, 602 (1964).

HOFMANN, K., ANDREATTA, R., BUCKLEY, J. P., HAGEMAN, W. E., SHAPIRO, A. P.: Studies on polypeptides. XXXIX.: Elimination of the imidazole portion of histidine as an essential site for biological function of angiotensin. J. Amer. chem. Soc. **90**, 1654 (1968).

IMHOF, P., BRUNNER, H., QUITT, J., STEINMANN, B., JACONO, A.: Experimentelle und klinische Untersuchungen mit β-Angiotensin II (Präparat Ciba 33902-Ba), einem neuen Angiotensin II-Analogen mit verstärkter und verlängerter pressorischer Wirkung. Schweiz. med. Wschr. **94**, 1199 (1964).

JORGENSEN, E. C., WINDRIDGE, G. C., PATTON, W., LEE, T. C.: (1) Angiotensin II Analogs. I. Synthesis and biological evaluation of [Gly^1, Gly^2, Ile^5]-angiotensin II, [Ac-Gly^1, Gly^2, Ile^5]-angiotensin II, and [Gly^1, Gly^2, Ile^5, His $(Bzl)^6$]-angiotensin II. J. Med. Chem. **12**, 733 (1969).

JORGENSEN, E. C., PATTON, W.: (2) Angiotensin II Analogs. II. Cyclo (-Val-Tyr-Ile-His-Pro-Phe-). J. Med. Chem. **12**, 935 (1969).

JORGENSEN, E. C., WINDRIDGE, G. C., LEE, T. C.: (1) Angiotensin II Analogs. III. Synthesis and biological evaluation of some Des-aspartyl-angiotensins. J. Med. Chem. **13**, 352 (1970).

JORGENSEN, E. C., WINDRIDGE, G. C., LEE, T. C.: (2) Angiotensin II Analogs. IV. Synthesis and biological evaluation of simplified angiotensins. J. Med. Chem. **13**, **744** (1970).

JORGENSEN, E. C., WINDRIDGE, G. C., PATTON, W., LEE, T. C.: (3) Structure-Action Relationships in Angiotensin II: Some new data on the contribution of aspartic acid and arginine to the Biological Activity. In: Chemistry and Biochemistry of Peptides. Proceedings 1st Amer. Peptide Symposium p. 113 (WEINSTEIN B., LANDE, S., Eds.). New York: Marcel Dekker 1970.

JORGENSEN, E. C., WINDRIDGE, G. C., LEE, T. C.: (1) Angiotensin II Analogs. 5. [2-Glycine]-angiotensin II and related analogs. J. Med. Chem. **14**, 631 (1971).

JORGENSEN, E. C., RAPAKA, S. R., WINDRIDGE, G. C., LEE, T. C.: (2) Angiotensin Analogs. 6. Stereochemical factors in the 5 position influencing pressor activity 1. J. Med. Chem. **14**, 899 (1971).

JORGENSEN, E. C., RAPAKA, S. R., WINDRIDGE, G. C., LEE, T. C.: (3) Angiotensin II analogs. 7. Stereochemical factors in the 5 position influencing pressor activity 2. J. Med. Chem. **14**, 904 (1971).

KHAIRALLAH, P. A., BUMPUS, F. M., PAGE, I. H., SMEBY, R. R.: Unitage and suggested designation of angiotensin activity. Nature (Lond.) **196**, 1059 (1962).

KHAIRALLAH, P. A., BUMPUS, F. M., PAGE, I. H., SMEBY, R. R.: Angiotensinase with a high degree of specificity in plasma and red cells. Science **140**, 672 (1963).

KHAIRALLAH, P. A., TOTH, A., BUMPUS, F. M.: Analogs of angiotensin II. II. Mechanism of receptor interactions. J. Med. Chem. **13**, 181 (1970).

KHOSLA, M. C., SMEBY, R. R., BUMPUS, F. M.: Solid phase peptide synthesis of [L-$alanine^3$-L-$isoleucine^5$]-angiotensin II. Biochemistry **6**, 754 (1967).

KHOSLA, M. C., CHATURVEDI, N. C., SMEBY, R. R., BUMPUS, F. M.: Synthesis of [1-Isoleucine-, 3 Proline-, and 5-Alanine]-angiotensins II. Biochemistry **7**, 3417 (1968).

KHOSLA, M. C., SMEBY, R. R., BUMPUS, F. M.: Synthesis of some angiotensin analogs. Proc. 162nd National Meeting of the American Chemical Society, Washington, D. C., (Sept. 12—17, 1971), Abstract No. MEDI-64.

KHOSLA, M. C., SMEBY, R. R., BUMPUS, F. M.: Difficulties in solid phase peptide synthesis of some analogs of angiotensin II. In: Chemistry and Biology of Peptides. Proc. 3rd Amer. Peptide Symposium, June 18—23, 1972, p. 227 (MEIENHOFER, J., Ed.). Ann. Arbor: Ann Arbor Publishers 1972.

KHOSLA, M. C., KUMAR, S., SMEBY, R. R., BUMPUS, F. M.: (1) Solid Phase Synthesis of [Arg^6]-, [His^4, Tyr^6]-, and [Ile^8]-angiotensins II. J. Med. Chem. **15**, 627 (1972).

KHOSLA, M. C., LEESE, R. A., MALOY, W. L., FERREIRA, A. T., SMEBY, R. R., BUMPUS, F. M.: (2) Synthesis of some analogs of angiotensin II as specific antagonists of the parent hormone. J. Med. Chem. **15**, 792 (1972).

KHOSLA, M. C., SMEBY, R. R., BUMPUS, F. M.: (3) Failure sequence in solid phase peptide synthesis due to the presence of an N-alkylamino acid. J. Amer. chem. Soc. **94**, 4721 (1972).

KISFALUDY, L., KORENCZKY, F.: Hypertensin II. Hung. 150, 735, Appl. Aug. 17, 1971. Chem. Abstr. **60**, P 5638 h (1964).

LIN, S. Y., GOODFRIEND, T. L.: Angiotensin receptors. Amer. J. Physiol. **218**, 1319 (1970).

LIN, S. Y., ELLIS, H., WEISBLUM, B., GOODFRIEND, T. L.: Preparation and properties of iodinatedangiotensins. Biochem. Pharmacol. **19**, 651 (1970).

MARSHALL, G. R., MERRIFIELD, R. B.: Synthesis of angiotensins by the solid-phase method. Biochemistry **4**, 2394 (1965).

MARSHALL, G. R., VINE, W., NEEDLEMAN, P.: A specific competitive inhibitor of angiotensin II. Proc. nat. Acad. Sci. (Wash.) **67**, 1624 (1970).

OPARIL, S., TREGEAR, G., HABER, E.: Role of the C-terminal sequence of angiotensic I on immunologic reactivity and on conversion to angiotensin II *in vivo* and *in vitro*. Abstracts: 2nd Amer. Peptide Symposium, Cleveland (Aug. 17—19, 1970).

OVCHINNIKOV, YU. A., KIRYUSHKIN, A. A., KOZHEVNIKOVA, I. V.: Synthesis of peptides on a polymer carrier in solution II. Synthesis of L-valyl-L-tyrosyl-L-valyl-L-histidyl-L-prolyl-L-phenylalanine and Gly^5-Gly^5-Gly^{10}-gramicidin S. Zh. obshch. Khim. **38**, 2636 (1968). Chem. Abstr. **70**, 78358 n.

PAGE, I. H., BUMPUS, F. M.: Angiotensin. Physiol. Rev. **41**, 331 (1961).

PAGE, I. H., BUMPUS, F. M.: A new hormone, angiotensin. Clin. Pharmacol. Ther. **3**, 758 (1962).

PAIVA, A. C. M., PAIVA, T. B.: The photo-oxidative inactivation of angiotensinamide. Biochem. biophys. Acta (Amst.) **48**, 412 (1961).

PAIVA, T. B., PAIVA, A. C. M., SCHERAGA, H. A.: The conformation of angiotensin II in aqueous solution. Biochemistry **2**, 1327 (1963).

PAIVA, T. B., PAIVA, A. C. M., FREER, R. J., STEWART, J. M.: Alkylating analogs of peptide hormones 2. Synthesis and properties of p-[N-, N-Bis (2-Chloroethyl) amino]-phenylbutyryl derivatives of angiotensin II. J. Med. Chem. **15**, 6 (1972).

PAIVA, A. C. M., NOUAILHETAS, V. L. A., MIYAMOTO, M. E., BERGSTEN, G., PAIVA, T. B.: (1) New specific angiotensin antagonists: [8-Val]- and [8-Ile] angiotensin I. Abstracts: Satellite symposium on the molecular pharmacology of angiotensin. San Francisco, July 29—30, 1972.

PALS, D. T., MASUCCI, F. D., SIPOS, F., DENNING, G. S., Jr.: (1) A specific competitive antagonist of the vascular action of angiotensin II. Circulat. Res. **29**, 664 (1971).

PALS, D. T., MASUCCI, F. D., DENNING, G. S., Jr., SIPOS, F., FESSLER, D. C.: (2) Role of the pressor action of angiotensin II in experimental hypertension. Circulat. Res. **29**, 673 (1971).

PARK, W. K., SMEBY, R. R., BUMPUS, F. M.: Synthesis of [5-isoleucine, 8-alanine]-angiotensin II by the solution method synthesis and the solid-phase method synthesis. Biochemistry **6**, 3458 (1967).

PARUSZEWSKI, R.: Obtaining analogs of Aspβ-Amide-angiotensin II. Roczniki Chemii, Ann. Soc. Chim. Polonorum, **45**, 289 (1971). Chem. Abstr. **75**, 64244 p (1971).

PAUL, R., ANDERSON, G. W.: N, N^1-carbonyl-diimidazole in peptide synthesis III. A synthesis of isoleucine-5 angiotensin II amide-1. J. org. Chem. **27**, 2094 (1962).

PAVARS, A. P., CIPENS, G. E.: (1) Synthesis of fragments of angiotensin II and its glycine containing analogs. Latv. PSR Zinat. Akad. Vestis, Kim. Ser. 121 (1970).

PAVARS, A. P., CIPENS, G. E.: (2) Synthesis of [Asn^1, Gly^2, Val^5]-angiotensin II. Latv. PSR Zinat. Akad. Vestis, Kim. Ser. 250 (1970), Chem. Abstr. **73**, 56406 m (1970).

PAVARS, A. P., CIPENS, G. E., AUNA, Z. P.: Some derivatives of [Gly^2, Val^5]-angiotensin II. Latv. PSR Zinat. Akad. Vestis, Kim. Ser. 737 (1970).

PAVARS, A. P., AUNA, Z., CIPENS, G.: Synthesis of [2-glycyl-5-valyl]-angiotensin II and some of its derivatives. Zh. Obshch. Khim. **41**, 1859 (1971). Chem. Abstr. **76**, 4152 t (1972).

PEACH, M. J.: Physiological roles of angiotensin. In: Chemistry and Biology of Peptides. Proc. 3rd Amer. Peptide Symposium, June 18—23, 1972, p. 471 (MEIENHOFER, J., Ed.). Ann Arbor: Ann Arbor Publishers 1972.

PEACH, M. J.: (2) Structure-activity relationships of angiotensin analogs in the adrenal, uterus and papillary muscle. Abstracts: Satellite symposium on the molecular pharmacology of angiotensin. San Francisco, July 29—30, 1972.

PEACH, M. J., BUMPUS, F. M., KHAIRALLAH, P. A.: Release of catecholamines by angiotensin I. J. Pharmacol. exp. Ther. **176**, 366 (1971).

PRINTZ, M. P., HAZEL, P. W., CRAIG, L. C.: Evidence for the presence of hydrogen bonded secondary structure in angiotensin II in aqueous solution. Proc. nat. Acad. Sci. (Wash.) **69**, 378 (1972).

PRINTZ, M. P., NEMETHY, G., BLEICH, H.: (1) Proposed models for angiotensin II in aqueous solution and conclusions about receptor topography. Nature (Lond.) New Biology **237**, 135 (1972).

REGOLI, D., RINIKER, B., BRUNNER, H.: The enzymatic degradation of various angiotensin II derivatives by serum, plasma or kidney homogenate. Biochem. Pharmacol. **12**, 637 (1963).

REGOLI, D., PARK, W. K., RIOUX, F., CHAN, C. S.: Antagonists of angiotensin, substitution of an aliphatic chain to phenyl ring in position 8. Rev. canad. Biol. **30**, 319 (1971).

REGOLI, D., PARK, W. K.: The pressor and myotropic effects and the antagonistic properties of several analogs of angiotensin II. Canad. J. Physiol. Pharmacol. **50**, 99 (1972).

REGOLI, D., RIOUX, F., PARK, W. K.: Dissociation constant of angiotensin II as determined by the use of an irreversible specific inhibitor. Rev. canad. Biol. **31**, 73 (1972).

RINIKER, B.: Recent work on the chemistry and biochemistry of angiotensin II. Metabolism **13**, 1248 (1964).

RINIKER, B., SCHWYZER, R.: (1) Die sterische Einheitlichkeit des synthetischen Val^5-hypertensin II-Asp^1-β-amids. Helv. chim. Acta **44**, 658 (1961).

RINIKER, B., SCHWYZER, R.: (2) Synthetische Analoge des Hypertensins. II. Arg (NO_2)-Val^5-hypertensin II-Asp^1-β-amid und Val^5-hypertensin II-Asp^1-β-Phe^8-diamid. Helv. chim. Acta **44**, 674 (1961).

RINIKER, B., SCHWYZER, R.: (3) Synthetische Analoge des Hypertensins. III. Gly^1-Val^5-hypertensin II, Orn^2-Val^5-hypertensin II, Phe^4-Val^5-hypertensin II, und Derivat. Helv. chim. Acta **44**, 677 (1961).

RINIKER, B., SCHWYZER, R.: (4) Synthetische Analoge des Hypertensins. IV. Synthese kettenhomologer Peptide. Helv. chim. Acta **44**, 685 (1961).

RINIKER, B., SCHWYZER, R.: (1) Synthetische Analoge des Hypertensin. V. α-L-, β-L^5-, α-D-, und β-D-Asp^1-Val^5-hypertensin II; desamino-Val^5-hypertensin II. Helv. chim. Acta **47**, 2357 (1964).

RINIKER, B., SCHWYZER, R.: (2) Synthetische Analoge des Hypertensins. VI. α-L-Asp $(NH_2)^1$-Aza-α-homo-Tyr^4-Val^5-hypertensin II, und β-L-Asp^1-Aza-α^1-homo-Tyr^4-Val^5-hypertensin II. Helv. chim. Acta **47**, 2375 (1964).

RINIKER, B., BRUNNER, H., SCHWYZER, R.: β-Asp^1-Val^5-hypertensin II, ein Hypertensin-Analoges mit besonders hoher biologischer Aktivität. Angew. Chem. **74**, 469 (1962).

RIOUX, F., REGOLI, D., PARK, W. K.: Competitive antagonists of angiotensin II on the isolated rat stomach strip. Rev. canad. Biol. **30**, 333 (1971).

RITTEL, W., ISELIN, B., KAPPELER, H., RINIKER, B., SCHWYZER, R.: Synthese eines hochwirksamen Hypertensin II-Amids. Helv. chim. Acta **40**, 614 (1957).

ROMANOVSKAII, I. K., CIPENS, G. E.: Solid-phase synthesis of [1-(β-aspartyl)-5-valyl]-angiotensin II. Zh. Obshch. Khim. **41**, 1856 (1971). Chem. Abstr. **76**, 4151 S (1972).

ROMANOVSKAII, Z. P. YA., CIPENS, G., AUNA, Z. P.: Analogs of 5-valylangiotensin II containing a modified asparaginic acid residue. Latv. PSR Zinat. Akad. Vestis, Kim. Ser. 503 (1971). Chem. Abstr. **75**, 118597 b.

SCHATTENKERK, C., HAVINGA, E.: Studies on polypeptides. IV. Syntheses and activities of some angiotensin-like peptides. Rev. Trav, chim. Pays-Bas **84**, 653 (1965).

SCHATTENKERK, C., VISSER, G. H., KERLING, K. E. T., HAVINGA, E.: Studies on Polypeptides II. Synthesis of the hexapeptide (des-Asp^1)-Lys^2-Ile^5-angiotensin II, (des-Asp^1)-D-Lys^2-Ile^5-angiotensin II, (des-Asp^1)-Orn^2-Ile^5-angiotensin II, (des-Asp^1)-Cit^2-Ile^5-angiotensin II and the hexapeptide Val-Tyr-Ile-His-Pro-Phe. Rec. Trav. chim. Pays-Bas, **83**, 677 (1964).

SCHILD, H. O.: pA, a new scale of the measurement of drug antagonism. Brit. J. Pharmacol. Chemother. **2**, 189 (1947).

SCHILD, H. O.: pAx and competitive drug antagonism. Brit. J. Pharmacol. **4**, 277 (1949).

SCHRÖDER, E.: (1) Synthese von Val^5-angiotensin II-Asp^1-β-amid, von Lys^2-Val^5-, und von Val^2-Val^5-angiotensin II-Asp^1-β-amide. Justus Liebigs Ann. Chem. **680**, 132 (1964).

SCHRÖDER, E.: (2) Synthese von Tyr^3-Val^4-Val^5-, von Phe^6-Val^5-, und von Phe^4-Tyr^8-Val^5-angiotensin II-Asp β-Amid. Justus Liebigs Ann. Chem. **680**, 142 (1964).

SCHRÖDER, E.: Synthese von *d*-Asp^1-, Glu^1, Glu $(NH_2)^1$-, und Pyroglu^1-Val^5-angiotensin II. Justus Liebigs Ann. Chem. **691**, 232 (1966).

SCHRÖDER, E., HEMPEL, R.: Synthese von Lys^6-Val^5-, von Tyr^3-Val^5-, von Tyr (Me)^4-Val^5-und von Tyr^8-Val^5-angiotensin II-Asp^1-β-amid. Justus Liebigs Ann. Chem. **684**, 243 (1965).

SCHWARZ, H., BUMPUS, F. M., PAGE, I. H.: Synthesis of a biologically active octapeptide similar to natural isoleucine angiotensin octapeptide. J. Amer. chem. Soc. **79**, 5697 (1957).

SCHWYZER, R.: Synthetische Analogs des Hypertensins. I. Einleitung. Helv. chim. Acta **44**, 667 (1961).

SCHWYZER, R., TURRIAN, H.: Chemistry and pharmacology of angiotensin. In: Vitamins and Hormones, Vol. 18, p. 237 (HARRIS, R. S., THIMANN, K. V., Eds.). New York: Academic Press 1960.

SCHWYZER, R., ISELIN, B., KAPPELER, H., RINIKER, B., RITTEL, W., ZUBER, H.: (1) Synthese von Hypertensin-Peptiden. Chimia (Switz.) **11**, 335 (1957).

SCHWYZER, R., ISELIN, B., KAPPELER, H., RITTEL, W., RINIKER, B.: (2) Ciba Ag. Basel, D.A.S., 1, 125, 942 (Sept. 2, 1957).

SCHWYZER, R., ISELIN, B., KAPPELER, H., RINIKER, B., RITTEL, W., ZUBER, H.: (1) Synthese hochwirksamer Dekapeptide mit der Aminosäuresequenz des Val^5-hypertensins I. Helv. chim. Acta **41**, 1273 (1958).

SCHWYZER, R., ISELIN, B., KAPPELER, H., RINIKER, B., RITTEL, W., ZUBER, H.: (2) Synthese hochwirksamer Octapeptide mit der Aminosäuresequenz des Hypertensins II aus Rinderserum. Helv. chim. Acta **41**, 1287 (1958).

SEU, J. H., SMEBY, R. R., BUMPUS, F. M.: (1) Synthesis of isoleucyl^5-alanyl^7-angiotensin II. J. Amer. chem. Soc. **84**, 3883 (1962).

SEU, J. H., SMEBY, R. R., BUMPUS, F. M.: (2) Synthesis of alanyl^4-isoleucyl^5-angiotensin II. J. Amer. chem. Soc. **84**, 4948 (1962).

SIVANANDAIAH, K. M., SMEBY, R. R., BUMPUS, F. M.: Synthesis of isoleucine^5-tyrosine^8-angiotensin II and isoleucine^5-hydroxyproline^7-angiotensin II. Biochemistry **5**, 1224 (1966).

SMEBY, R. R., ARAKAWA, K., BUMPUS, F. M., MARSH, M. M.: A proposed conformation of Ileu^5-angiotensin II. Biochim. biophys. Acta (Amst.) **58**, 550 (1962).

SMEBY, R. R., KHOSLA, M. C., BUMPUS, F. M.: Highlights of recent structure-activity studies with angiotensin II. In: Chemistry and Biology of Peptides. Proc. 3rd Amer. Peptide Symposium, June 18—23, 1972, 509 (MEIENHOFER, J., Ed.). Ann. Arbor: Ann. Arbor Publishers 1972.

STEWART, J. M.: Structure-activity relationships of proteins and polypeptide hormones. The 2nd International Symposium, Liege (Belgium), sept. 28—Oct. 1, 1971.

SWEET, C. S., FERRARIO, C. M., KHOSLA, M. C., BUMPUS, F. M.: Effect of [1-sarcosine, 8-isoleucine] angiotensin II in normotensive, acute renal hypertensive and chronic perinephritic hypertensive dogs. Proc. Amer. Physiology Society, Pennsylvania, August 28—31, 1972.

SWEET, C. S., FERRARIO, C. M., KHOSLA, M. C., BUMPUS, F. M.: Antagonism of peripheral and central effects of angiotensin II by [1-sarcosine-8-isoleucine]-angiotensin II. J. Pharmacol. exptl. Ther. (in press).

THAMPI, N. S., SCHOLLMAN, G., HURST, M. W., HUGGINS, C. G.: The solid-phase synthesis of 5-isoleucine angiotensin I and 5-isoleucine [10-^{14}C (U)-leucine]-angiotensin I. Life Sci. (Oxford) **7**, 641 (1968).

TÜRKER, R. K., YAMAMOTO, M., KHAIRALLAH, P. A., BUMPUS, F. M.: Competitive antagonism of 8-Ala angiotensin II to angiotensins I and II on isolated rabbit aorta and rat ascending colon. Europ. J. Pharmacol. **15**, 285 (1971).

TÜRKER, R. K., YAMAMOTO, M., BUMPUS, F. M.: A new short-acting antagonist of angiotensin II. Arch. int. Pharmacodyn. **201**, 162 (1973).

TÜRKER, R. K., HALL, M. M., YAMAMOTO, M., SWEET, C. S., BUMPUS, F. M.: A new long lasting competitive inhibitor of angiotensin II. Science **177**, 1203 (1972).

VANE, J. R.: Purity and stability of synthetic peptides such as angiotensin and kinins. Nature (Lond.) **230**, 382 (1971).

VISSER, G. H., SCHATTENKERK, C., KERLING, K. E. T., HAVINGA, E.: Studies on polypeptides. Rec. Trav. chim. Pays-Bas **83**, 684 (1964).

VOGLER, K., STUDER, R. O., LERGIER, W., LANZ, P.: Synthese von all D-Val^5-angiotensin II-Asp^1-β-amid. Helv. chim. Acta 48, 1047 (1965).

WALTON, E., RODIN, J. O., STAMMER, C. H., HOLLY, F. W.: Synthesis of L-valyl-L-tyrosyl-L-tyrosyl-L-isoleucyl-L-histidyl-L-prolyl-L-phenylalanine methyl ester dihydrochloride. J. org. Chem. **26**, 1657 (1961).

WEINKAM, R. J., JORGENSEN, E. C.: (1) Angiotensin II analogs. VIII. The use of free radical containing peptides to indicate the conformation of the carboxyl terminal region of angiotensin II. J. Amer. chem. Soc. **93**, 7033 (1971).

WEINKAM, R. J., JORGENSEN, E. C.: (2) Angiotensin II analogs. IX. Conformational studies of angiotensin II by proton magnetic resonance. J. Amer. chem. Soc. **93**, 7038 (1971).

WIDEMAN, C. H., KHOSLA, M. C., SMEBY, R. R.: Effect of analogs of angiotensin II on isolated frog skin, 56th Annual meeting FASEB, Atlantic City, New Jersey, (April 9—14, 1972). Federation Proceedings 31 (No. 2), 228 (1972). Abstract. N. 101.

WINDRIDGE, G. C., JORGENSEN, E. C.: Racemization in the solid phase synthesis of histidine-containing peptides. Intra. Sci. Chem. Rep. **5**, 375 (1971).

YAMAMOTO, M., TÜRKER, R. K., KHAIRALLAH, P. A., BUMPUS, F. M.: A potent competitive antagonist of angiotensin II. Europ. J. Pharmacol. **18**, 316 (1972).

ZIMMER, S., HAAR, W., MAURER, W., RUTERJANS, H., FERMANDJIAN, S., FROMAGEOT, P.: ^{13}C-NMR investigation of the structure of angiotensin II. Europ. J. Biochem. **29**, 80 (1972).

Antagonists of Angiotensin II

R. K. TÜRKER, I. H. PAGE, and F. M. BUMPUS

Recently, interest in specific pharmacological antagonists to angiotensin has grown (GODFRAIND, 1968). Since angiotensin has a wide spectrum of actions and stimulates smooth muscle both directly and indirectly it is convenient to describe the antagonists in two categories:

1. Drugs which antagonize the indirect effects of angiotensin,
2. Drugs which antagonize the direct effects of angiotensin.

1. Antagonists Blocking the Indirect Actions

KHAIRALLAH and PAGE (1961) and ROBERTSON and RUBIN (1962) showed that atropine and other antimuscarinic agents were able to partially block the contractile effect of angiotensin on the isolated guinea-pig ileum: They suggested that part of the action of angiotensin on smooth muscle is mediated by a cholinergic pathway. Cholinergic pathways have also been described in nictitating membrane of cats (TÜRKER et al., 1969). Atropine and hemicholinium can block angiotensin in chronically denervated nictitating membranes.

Hexamethonium partially blocks the effect of angiotensin in the isolated perfused cat terminal ileum, suggesting that angiotensin has a preganglionic cholinergic effect (TÜRKER, 1969). Such an effect has also been observed in sympathetic ganglia (HAEFELY et al., 1965; PANISSET et al., 1966). REGOLI and VANE (1964) and ELLIS and REIT (1969) found the ascending colon of rat a sensitive preparation for assay of angiotensin. Apparently no cholinergic pathways were present since antimuscarinic agents did not block the response to angiotensin.

Angiotensin also affects the sympathetic nervous system at different levels and it has been shown that adrenergic blocking agents can partially abolish some of the pharmacological effects of angiotensin at different levels. For example, the ability of angiotensin to release catecholamines from the adrenal medulla (BRAUN-MENENDEZ et al., 1940; KANEKO et al., 1961; FELDBERG and LEWIS, 1964, 1965) is reduced by adrenergic blocking agents. Angiotensin also stimulates sympathetic ganglia (LEWIS and REIT, 1965, 1966; TRENDELENBURG, 1966) and releases catecholamines from postganglionic adrenergic neurons (DISTLER et al., 1965; SCHÜMANN and GUTHER, 1967).

α-Adrenergic blocking agents have been reported to reduce the vascular response to angiotensin (BICKERTON and BUCKLEY, 1961; JOHNSON et al., 1965), although this has not been confirmed by others (MCGIFF and FASY, 1965; RENSON et al., 1959). SCROOP and WHELAN (1966) showed that phenoxybenzamine abolishes the vascular response of angiotensin on the blood vessels of the hand.

Bretylium and β-adrenergic blockers (pronethalol and propranolol) prevent the cardioacceleration induced by angiotensin in anesthetized dogs (KRASNEY et al., 1965). PANISSET et al. (1966) observed that small doses of angiotensin II injected into the superior cervival ganglion decreased the response of nictitating membrane to preganglionic stimulation. In addition, dihydroergotamine pretreatment abolished this effect of angiotensin and it was proposed that angiotensin released catecholamines locally which then inhibited presynaptic transmission.

The intestinal inhibitory action of angiotensin is mainly due to the effect of angiotensin on sympathetic ganglia and not to catecholamines released from the adrenals; acute bilateral adrenalectomy does not alter the response as does pretreatment with morphine [TÜRKER and KAYAALP, 1967 (1)], which blocks the ganglion-stimulating effect of angiotensin.

2. Drugs Which Antagonize Direct Effects of Angiotensin

These drugs can be divided into two subgroups:

a) Physiologic antagonists of angiotensin,

b) Direct pharmacologic antagonists of angiotensin.

A. Physiologic (Indirect) Antagonists

The response to angiotensin can be diminished, or abolished, by a group of drugs which have the opposite effect to that of angiotensin in a particular preparation. Many vasodilator drugs reduce the pressor effect of angiotensin (BIANCHI et al., 1960; BARER, 1963). Contractile responses of isolated guinea-pig ileum are inhibited by adrenergic drugs (KHAIRALLAH and PAGE, 1962). Aldosterone pretreatment has been reported to reduce the sensitivity of angiotensin in rabbits (KATZ et al., 1963). Pressor responsiveness to angiotensin is reduced by pretreatment with thiazide diuretics in dogs (BOCK and GROSS, 1960), but acute administration of chlorothiazide does not affect this response in man (SILAH et al., 1965). Antagonism has been reported by TÜRKER et al. [1967 (1)] between ouabain and angiotensin, who concluded that angiotensin stimulates Na^+-K^+ activated ATPase since it increased Na^+ efflux in isolated rat uterus and dog carotid artery. This effect was blocked by ouabain. Ouabain also blocks the contractile action of angiotensin on isolated rat uterus. Further, ouabain-induced cardiac arrhythmia can be blocked by angiotensin in guinea-pigs (TÜRKER, 1965).

Biologically active peptides and lipids which have the opposite action can also reduce the effect of angiotensin. Bradykinin has been shown to decrease the renal vasoconstrictor effect of angiotensin in cats (BARER, 1963). Also, prostaglandin E_1, when given intravenously to anesthetized rats, decreases the pressor response to angiotensin without changing that to norepinephrine [TÜRKER et al., 1968 (2)].

B. Direct Pharmacological Antagonists of Angiotensin

1. Non-Competive Antagonists

LEWIS and REIT (1965) and TRENDELENBURG (1966) reported that mepyramine, morphine and cocaine reduced the ganglion-stimulating action of angiotensin in the superior cervical ganglion of the cat. The effects of angiotensin in increasing capillary permeability in guinea-pig skin can be blocked by mepyramine (BISSET and LEWIS, 1962), Since mepyramine is an antihistamine, it was assumed that angiotensin increased the capillary permeability by causing release of histamine. However, this effect of the octapeptide was not observed in other species (BISSET and LEWIS, 1962). Recent observations (ROBERTSON and KHAIRALLAH, unpublished) have shown that angiotensin also has the effect of increasing the capillary permeability in rabbit skin. This effect is blocked by [Ala^8] and [Ile^8]-Ang. II and is not affected by Benedryl (2[diphenylmethoxy]-N,N-dimethylethylamine HCl). The actions of morphine and cocaine are apparently not specific, for they can also abolish other "non-nicotinic-like" ganglion-stimulating agents such as bradykinin, histamine and serotonin on the superior cervical ganglion of the cat.

Hydralazine does not affect the vasoconstrictor response of angiotensin in perfused innervated dog kidneys (PAGE and McCUBBIN, 1953) but appears to reduce responsiveness of angiotensin in rats, in the isolated rabbit hind limb (MEIER et al., 1957, 1958) and the dog kidney *in vivo* (McGIFF and FASY, 1965).

Another compound which non-competitively blocks the pressor effect of angiotensin is guancidine (CUMMINGS et al., 1968; WORCEL et al., 1971). A specific antagonist described by GASCON and WALASZEK (1966) is an isoflavone derivative, osajin, which was isolated from hedge apples or osage oranges and which blocks the myotropic effect of angiotensin on guinea-pig ileum.

Cinnarizine, a piperazine derivative, antagonizes angiotensin, blocking the effect of both angiotensin and histamine on isolated guinea-pig ileum and cat papillary muscle (SCHAPER et al., 1963; VAN NUETEN et al., 1964), indicating that it is not specific for angiotensin. Large numbers of piperazine derivatives were studied as inhibitors of angiotensin (GODFRAIND, 1968). One of these compounds, lidoflazine, has been shown to be effective, especially in its direct myotropic effect on guinea-pig ileum (GODFRAIND et al., 1966). It did not, however, antagonize angiotensin action on rabbit isolated aorta [TÜRKER and KAYAALP, 1967 (2)], cat ileum *in vivo* [TÜRKER et al., 1968 (1)] and isolated ascending colon of rats (ELLIS and REIT, 1969).

2. Competitive Antagonists of Angiotensin

Within the last year a number of investigators have studied the pharmacological properties of some synthetic angiotensin analogs. KHAIRALLAH et al. (1970) observed that [Ala^8]-Ang. II, given in concentrations $>$ 500 ng/ml, specifically blocked the contractile response of angiotensin on the isolated guinea-pig ileum without affecting the response to vasopressin or serotonin. Comparison of the action of several angiotensin analogs on release of catecholamines from the adrenals and their ability to contract smooth muscle suggests the existence of different receptor mechanisms. For example, the aromatic side group in position 8 and the location of the C-terminal carboxyl group seem to be less significant for norepinephrine release (PEACH et al., 1970) than for myotropic activity. They reported that Ang. II inhibited uptake of norepinephrine into sympathetic nerve endings at peptide concentrations of less than 0.05 ng/ml. This receptor site resembled that of adrenal medulla, differing in specificity from that of smooth muscle. These observations suggest the importance of the 8 position of Ang. II, not only as necessary for binding but also as a part of the molecule with transcribed information [KHOSLA et al., 1972 (1, 2)].

MARSHALL et al. (1970) prepared [4-phenylalanine, 8-tyrosine]-Ang. II ([Phe^4, Tyr^8]-Ang. II) and showed that it inhibited the effects of Ang. II on isolated uterus and blood pressure of rat. [Phe^4, Tyr^8]-Ang. II itself had myotropic, as well as pressor properties. This analog produced antagonism in a competitive manner since the dose-response curve of angiotensin was shifted to the right parallel to the control curve. Other criteria for the establishment of competitive antagonism were not studied. This analog is an effective competitive inhibitor of angiotensin, as well as a specific one, since it does not inhibit other spasmogenic peptides, or amines. TÜRKER et al. (1971) observed that [Ala^8]-Ang. II has a specific competitive inhibitory effect against both Ang. I and Ang. II on rabbit aortic strips and rat ascending colon, but it has no inhibitory effect against the pressor response to

Ang. II on blood pressure or intestinal motility of cat. These results were confirmed by GAGNON et al. (1971) and by REGOLI and PARK (1971). The latter workers presented evidence that the 8-alanine derivative does not only antagonize the effects of Ang. II in the isolated smooth muscle preparations but also blocks the pressor response to angiotensin in rats.

Other synthetic analogs of angiotensin (8-substituted) [8-α-amino-n-butyl]-[8-valine]-[8-isoleucine]- and [8-leucine]-Ang. II were shown to be competitive antagonists to the myotropic effect of the parent peptide. Recently, YAMAMOTO et al. (1972) found that [8-isoleucine]-Ang. II was the most potent competitive inhibitor of any 8-substituted analog of Ang. II reported thus far. It also blocked the pressor effect of angiotensin in rats, cats and dogs.

Another analog of angiotensin [8-aminophenylisobutyric acid]-Ang. II ([APIB^8] Ang. II) was shown to inhibit specifically the myotropic as well as the pressor activity of angiotensin. The agonistic activity of this analog was 1000 times less than that of the parent peptide (TÜRKER et al., 1971).

PALS et al. [1971 (1)] reported that another modification of the [8-alanine]-Ang. II analog, [1-sarcosine, 8-alanine]-Ang. II competitively blocks the myotropic and pressor effect of angiotensin. All the peptide analogs mentioned above have been shown to be specific antagonists for angiotensin since they have no inhibitory effect against the myotropic and the pressor actions of other agonists.

These analogs have primary structures similar to the parent peptide and may be degraded by the same enzyme system(s) which metabolize angiotensin. The antagonistic potencies on different smooth muscle preparations and the duration of the antagonistic effect have been tested in various species. The potency of [Ala^8]-Ang. II, [Ile^8]-Ang. II and [Sar^1-Ala^8]-Ang. II can be compared if pA_2 values (SCHILD, 1947) of each compound in the aortic strip are calculated.

Table 1 shows pA_2 and pA_{10} values of these analogs against Ang. II on the rabbit aortic strips.

This table shows that [Ile^8]-Ang. II and [Sar^1, Ile^8]-Ang. II have the highest pA_2 values of the analogs reported and indicates that [Ile^8]-Ang. II and [Sar^1, Ile^8]-Ang. II are the most potent competitive antagonists of angiotensin. The other analogs are also competitive inhibitors of angiotensin since pA_2-pA_{10} was found to be near the hypothetical value of 0.95 in each case (SCHILD, 1947, 1957). Of the compounds in Table 1, [APIB^8]-Ang. II has the lowest pA_2 value, which indicates that it has a lower antagonistic potency than the others. However, it is a competitive antagonist of the parent peptide since the value of pA_2-pA_{10} was found to be 0.843 which is not significantly different from 0.95.

[Sar^1, Ile^8]-Ang. II has been shown to be a more potent competitive inhibitor than [Ile^8]-Ang. II in *in-vivo* preparations even though their pA_2 values determined on the aortic strip are very similar. The difference between the results of *in-vivo* and *in-vitro* experiments could be explained if sarcosine attached to the N-terminus position stabilized the compound so that it was degraded more slowly *in vivo*. Comparison of agonist properties of [Sar^1]-Ang. II with the parent peptide will yield more information on this matter.

The duration of the antagonistic effect of these 8-substituted analogs has been estimated in different pharmacological preparations. TÜRKER et al. (1971) demonstrated that complete recovery of the response to Ang. II in aortic strips occurred within 30 to 45 min after a single exposure of the muscle to [Ala^8]-Ang. II. During this period the muscle was washed several times with buffer. The same recovery time was found in rat ascending colon. Complete recovery of response of aortic strip and rat uterus to Ang. II occurred at least 2 h after treatment of the muscles with [Ile^8]-Ang. II (YAMAMOTO et al., 1972).

Table 1

Compound	pA_2 (Mean + S.E.M.)	pA_{10} (Mean + S.E.M.)	pA_2-pA_{10}	References
Ala^8-Ang. II	8.32 ± 0.08 (10)	7.41 ± 0.07	0.91	Türker et al. (1971)
Ile^8-Ang. II	9.21 ± 1.02 (14)	8.25 ± 0.8 (14)	0.96	Yamamoto et al. (1972)
APIB^8-Ang. II	5.576 ± 0.004 (9)	4.733 ± 0.23 (9)	0.843	Türker et al. [1972 (1)]
Sar^1, Ala^8-Ang. II	8.61 ± 0.03 (12)	—	—	Pals et al. (1971)
Sar^1, Ile^1-Ang. II	9.48 ± 0.08 (7)	—	—	Türker et al. [1972 (2)]

Table 2. *The pharmacological properties of various 8-substituted analogs of Ang. II against parent peptide in different pharmacologigal preparations*

Compound	Preparations	Antagonistic Activity (pA_2 value)	Agonistic Activity	Duration of Action
Phe^4,Tyr^8-Ang.II	isolated uterus	competitive inhibition pA_2 is not measured	+ +	short
	rat blood pressure	competitive inhibition	+ +	short
Ala^8-Ang.II	isolated rat uterus	competitive inhibition	– –	30 to 45 min
	isolated rat colon	competitive inhibition	– –	30 to 45 min
	isolated rabbit aorta	competitive inhibition 8.32	– –	30 to 45 min
	cat blood pressure	no inhibition	– –	
Ile^8-Ang.II	rat uterus	competitive inhibition	– –	1.5 to 2 h
	rat colon	competitive inhibition	– –	1.5 to 2 h
	rabbit aorta	competitive inhibition 9.21	– –	1.5 to 2 h
	rat blood pressure	competitive inhibition	+ +	1.5 to 2 h
	cat blood pressure	competitive inhibition	+ +	30 to 45 min
	cat intestinal motility	competitive inhibition	– –	30 to 45 min
	cat nictitating membrane	competitive inhibition	– –	30 to 45 min
APIB^8-Ang.II	rat uterus	competitive inhibition	+ +	5 to 10 min
	rat colon	competitive inhibition	+ +	5 to 10 min
	rabbit aorta	competitive inhibition 5.576	+ +	5 to 10 min
	rat blood pressure	no inhibition	+ +	
	cat blood pressure	competitive inhibition	+ +	5 to 10 min
	cat intestinal motility	competitive inhibition	no effect	5 to 10 min
	cat nictitating membrane	competitive inhibition	no effect	5 to 10 min
Sar^1,Ile^8-Ang.II	rat colon	competitive inhibition	no effect	long-lasting
	rabbit aorta	competitive inhibition 9.48	no effect	more than 2 h
	rat blood pressure	competitive inhibition	no effect	more than 2 h
	cat blood pressure	competitive inhibition	no effect	more than 2 h
	cat nictitating membrane	competitive inhibition	no effect	more than 2 h

Following single i.v. injection of [Ile^8]-Ang. II the pressor response to angiotensin was blocked for at least 2 h in anesthetized rats and 30 min in cats. These results indicate that [Ile^8]-Ang. II was a longer-lasting antagonist than [Ala]-

Ang. II. [APIB[8]]-Ang. II produced a short-lived blockade (5 to 10 min) in isolated smooth muscle preparations and in cat blood pressure. [Phe[4], Tyr[8]]-Ang. II (MARSHALL et al., 1970) has similar effects. Table 2 summarizes the pharmacological properties of 8-substituted analogs of Ang. II.

Recently, YAMAMOTO et al. (1972) and TÜRKER et al. (1972) found that [Ile[8]]-Ang. II and [APIB[8]]-Ang. II competitively blocked the pressor action of angiotensin in cats as well as the ganglion-stimulating effect tested on the motility of terminal ileum in cat. The latter responds to the systemic injection of Ang. II by relaxation in bilaterally adrenalectomized cats. The competitive blockers of angiotensin inhibit this ganglion-stimulating effect, indicating the receptors in smooth muscles and ganglia might be the same or that the 8-substituted analogs may also specifically occupy the receptors for angiotensin in autonomic ganglia.

Summary

The action of angiotensin has been antagonized by numerous drugs which inhibit the indirect actions of the peptide. This type of blockade is non-specific for the peptide but has been useful in determining its mode of action. The response to Ang. II has also been reduced by drugs which possess opposing action but are not inhibitory in a pharmacologic sense. Non-competitive antagonists have also been found but are all very non-specific. Competitive antagonists of Ang. II reported so far, however, are all very specific. They are all analogs of angiotensin with modifications in the 8 position with or without other position modifications.

References

BARER, G. R.: The action of vasopressin, a vasopressin analog (PLV_2), oxytocin, angiotensin, bradykinin and theophylline ethylene diamine on renal blood flow in the anesthetized cat. J. Physiol. **169**, 67 (1963).

BIANCHI, A., DE SCHAEPDRYVER, A. F., DE VLEESCHHOUVER, G. R., PREZIOSI, P.: On the pharmacology of synthetic hypertensine. Arch. int. Pharmacodyn. **124**, 21 (1960).

BICKERTON, R. K., BUCKLEY, J. P.: Evidence for a central mechanism in angiotensin-induced hypertensin. Proc. Soc. exp. Biol. (N. Y.) **106**, 834 (1961).

BISSET, G. W., LEWIS, G. P.: A spectrum of pharmacological activity in some biologically active peptides. Brit. J. Pharmacol. **19**, 168 (1962).

BOCK, K. D., GROSS, F.: Venous pressor changes after administration of renin, angiotensin and noradrenaline. Naunyn-Schmiedebergs Arch. Pharmakol. exp. Path. **242**, 188 (1961).

BRAUN-MENEDEZ, E., FASCIOLI, J. C., LELOIR, L. F., MUNOZ, J. M., TAQUINI, A. C.: Renal hypertension, p. 157. Springfield/Illinois: Charles C. Thomas 1946.

CUMMINGS, J. R., WELTER, A. N., GRACE, J. L., Jr., GRAY, W. D.: Angiotensin blocking actions of guaneydine. J. Pharmacol. exp. Therap. **170**, 334 (1969).

DISTLER, A., LIEBAU, H., WOLFF, H. P.: Action of angiotensin on sympathetic nerve endings in isolated blood vessels. Nature (Lond.) **207**, 764 (1965).

ELLIS, D. E., REIT, E.: Inhibition of lidoflazine of the contractile response of the rat isolated colon to angiotensin. Brit. Pharmacol. **35**, 132 (1969).

FELDBERG, W., LEWIS, G. P.: The action of peptides on the adrenal medulla. Release of adrenaline by bradykinin and angiotensin. J. Physiol. **171**, 98 (1964).

FELDBERG, W., LEWIS, G. P.: Further studies on the effects of peptides on the suprarenal medulla of the cats. J. Physiol. **178**, 239 (1965).

GAGNON, D., PARK, W. K., REGOLI, D.: Specific antagonists for the myotropic action of angiotensin II and angiotensin I on the isolated rat colon. Brit. J. Pharmacol. **43**, 409 (1971).

GASCON, A. L., WALASZEK, E. J.: Inhibition of valyl[5]-angiotensinamide II by osajin. J. Pharm. Pharmacol. **18**, 497 (1966).

GODFRAIND, T.: Pharmacology of angiotensin antagonists: Pharmacology of hormonal polypeptides and proteins. New York: Plenum Press 1968.

GODFRAIND, T., KABA, A., POLSTER, P.: Specific antagonism to the direct and indirect action of angiotensin on isolated guinea-pig ileum. Brit. J. Pharmacol. **28**, 93 (1966).

HAEFELY, W. A., HURLIMANN, A., THOENEN, H.: The effect of bradykinin and angiotensin on ganglionic transmission. Biochem. Pharmacol. **14**, 1393 (1965).

Johnson, G., Henning, M., Ablad, B.: Studies on the mechanism of the vasoconstrictor effects of angiotensin II in man. Life Sci. 4, 1549 (1965).
Kaneko, Y., McCubbin, J. W., Page, I. H.: Ability of vasoconstrictor drugs to cause adrenal medullary discharge after "sensitization" by ganglion stimulating agents. Circulat. Res. 9, 1247 (1961).
Katz, Y. J., Moore, R. S., Velasquez, A. M., Tamosaitis, I. T.: Angiotensin pressor inhibition by aldosterone in the rabbit. Science 141, 725 (1963).
Khairallah, P. A., Page, I. H.: Mechanisms of action of angiotensin and bradykinin on smooth muscle in situ. Amer. J. Physiol. 200, 51 (1961).
Khairallah, P. A., Page, I. H.: Effect of adrenergic agents on responses of smooth muscle to angiotensin. Amer. J. Physiol. 202, 841 (1962).
Khairallah, P. A., Toth, A., Bumpus, F. M.: Analogs of angiotensin II. Mechanism of receptor interaction. J. med. Chem. 13, 181 (1970).
Khosla, M. C., Kumar, S., Smeby, R. R., Bumpus, F. M.: (1) Solid phase synthesis of [6-arginine]-, [4-histidine, 6-tyrosine]- and [8-isoleucine]-angiotensin II. J. med. Chem. 15, 627 (1972).
Khosla, M. C., Leese, R. A., Maloy, W. L., Ferreira, A. T., Smeby, R. R., Bumpus, F. M.: (2) Synthesis of some analogs of angiotensin II as specific antagonists of the parent hormone. J. med. Chem. 15, 792 (1972).
Krasney, J. A., Paudler, F. J., Smith, D. C., Davis, L. D., Youmans, W. B.: Mechanisms of cardioaccelerator action of angiotensin. Amer. J. Physiol. 209, 539 (1965).
Lewis, G. P., Reit, E.: The action of angiotensin and bradykinin on the superior cervival ganglion of the cat. J. Physiol. 179, 538 (1965).
Lewis, G. P., Reit, E.: Further studies on the actions of peptides on the superior cervival ganglion and suprarenal medulla. Brit. J. Pharmacol. 26, 444 (1966).
Marshall, G. R., Vine, W., Needleman, P.: A specific competitive inhibitor of angiotensin II. Proc. nat. Acad. Sci. (Wash.) 67, 1624 (1970).
McGiff, J. C., Fasy, T. M.: The relationship of the renalvascular activity of angiotensin II to the autonomic nervous system. J. clin. Invest. 44, 1911 (1965).
Meier, R., Gross, F., Tripod, J., Turrian, H.: Pharmakologische Charakterisierung von synthetischer Hypertension. Experientia (Basel) 13, 361 (1957).
Meier, R., Tripod, J., Studer, A.: Comparison des proprietes vasculaires peripheriques de l'hypertensive synthetique et de divers vasoconstricteurs. Arch. int. Pharmacodyn. 117, 185 (1958).
Page, I. H., McCubbin, J. W.: Renal vascular and systemic arterial pressure responses to nervous and chemical stimulation of the kidney. Amer. J. Physiol. 173, 411 (1953).
Pals, D. T., Masucci, F. D., Denning, G. S., Jr., Sipos, F., Fessler, D. C.: Role of the pressor action of angiotensin II in experimental hypertension. Circulat. Res. 29, 673 (1971).
Pals, D. T., Masucci, F. D., Sipos, F., Denning, G. S., Jr.: (1) specific competitive antagonist of the vascular action of angiotensin II. Circulat. Res. 29, 664 (1971).
Panisset, J. C., Biron, P., Beaulnes, A.: Effect of angiotensin on the superior cervical ganglion of the cat. Experientia (Basel) 22, 394 (1966).
Peach, M. J., Bumpus, F. M., Khairallah, P. A.: Release of catecholamines by angiotensin I. J. Pharmacol. exp. Ther. 176, 366 (1970).
Regoli, D., Park, W. K.: The pressor and myotropic effects and the antagonistic properties of several analogues of angiotensin II. Canad. J. Physiol. Pharmacol. 50, 99 (1972).
Regoli, D., Park, W. K., Rioux, F., Chan, C. S.: Antagonists of angiotensin, substitution of an aliphatic chain to phenyl ring in position 8. Rev. canad. Biol. 30, 319 (1971).
Regoli, D., Vane, J. R.: A sensitive method for the assay of angiotensin. Brit. J. Pharmacol. 23, 351 (1964).
Renson, J., Barae, G., Bacq, Z. U.: Effect of two synthetic angiotensins on the arterial pressure and nictitating membrane of the cat. C. R. Soc. Biol. (Paris) 153, 1621 (1959).
Robertson, A. L., Khairallah, P. A.: Effects of angiotensin II and some analogs on vascular permeability in the rabbit. Circulat. Res. XXXI, 923 (1972).
Robertson, P. A., Rubin, D.: Stimulation of intestinal nervous elements by angiotensin. Brit. J. Pharmacol. 19, 5 (1962).
Schaper, W. K. A., Jageneau, A. H. M., Xhonneux, R., Van Nueten, J., Jansseu, P. A. J.: Cinnarizine (R516) a specific angiotensin-blocking coronary vasodilator. Life Sci. 2, 963 (1963).
Schild, H. O.: pA. A new scale of the measurement of drug antagonism. Brit. J. Pharmacol. 2, 189 (1947).
Schild, H. O.: Drug antagonism and pA_x. Pharmacol. Rev. 9, 242 (1957).
Schümann, H. J., Guther, W.: Untersuchungen zum Wirkungsmechanismus von Angiotensin am solierten Aortenpräparat und am Blutdruck von Ratten und Meerschweinchen. Nauinyn-Schmiedebergs Arch. Pharmak. exp. Path. 256, 169 (1968).

SCROOP, G. C., WHELAN, R. F.: A central vasomotor action of angiotensin in man. Clin. Sci. **30**, 79 (1966).

SILAH, J. G., JONES, R. E., BASHOUR, F. A., KAPLAN, N. M.: The effect of acute administration of chlorothiazide upon the pressor responsiveness to angiotensin and norepinephrine. Amer. Heart J. **69**, 301 (1965).

TRENDELENBURG, U.: Observation on the ganglion stimulating action of angiotensin and bradykinin. J. Pharmacol. exp. Therap. **154**, 418 (1966).

TÜRKER, R. K.: Action of angiotensin on the cardiac arrhytmias induced by G-Strophanthine. Experientia (Basel) **20**, 707 (1965).

TÜRKER, R. K.: Possible postganglionic effect of angiotensin in the isolated perfused cat intestinal segment. Arch. int. Physiol. **77**, 587 (1969).

TÜRKER, R. K., HALL, M. M., YAMAMOTO, M., SWEET, C. S., BUMPUS, F. M.: A new long-lasting competitive inhibitor of angiotensin. Science **177**, 1203 (1972).

TÜRKER, R. K., KAYAALP, S. O.: (1) Inhibitory effect of angiotensin on intestinal motility of the cat and its relation to sympathetic nervous system. Arch. int. Physiol. Biochim. **75**, 735 (1967).

TÜRKER, R. K., KAYAALP, S. O.: (2) Effects of lidoflazine on norepinephrine, angiotensin and serotonin responses in isolated smooth muscle preparations. Experientia (Basel) **23**, 647 (1967).

TÜRKER, R. K., KAYAALP, S. O., ÖZER, A.: (1) Further studies on lidoflazine (RA7904). Arzneimittel-Forsch. **18**, 1209 (1968).

TÜRKER, R. K., KAYMAKCALAN, S., AYHAN, I. H.: (2) Effect of prostaglandin E_1 (PGE_1) on the vascular responsiveness to norepinephrine and angiotensin in the anesthetized rat. Arzneimittel-Forsch. **18**, 1310 (1968).

TÜRKER, R. K., KHAIRALLAH, P. A., KAYAALP, S. O., KAYMAKCALAN, S.: Responses of the nictitating membrane to prostaglandin E_1 and angiotensin. Europ. J. Pharmacol. **5**, 173 (1969).

TÜRKER, R. K., YAMAMOTO, M., BUMPUS, F. M.: (1) A new short-acting antagonist of angiotensin II. Arch. int. Pharmacodyn. **201**, 162 (1963).

TÜRKER, R. K., YAMAMOTO, M., KHAIRALLAH, P. A., BUMPUS, F. M.: Competitive antagonism of 8-Ala-angiotensin II to angiotensin I and II on the isolated rabbit aorta and rat ascending colon. Europ. J. Pharmacol. **15**, 285 (1971).

VAN NUETEN, J., DRESSE, A., DONY, J.: Action antagoniste de la cinnarizine vis-à-vis de l'angiotensin in vitro. C. R. Soc. Biol. (Paris) **158**, 1750 (1964).

WORCEL, M., PAPADIMITRIOU, A., MEYER, P.: Blockade of the effects of angiotensin, oxytocin, norepinephrine, 5-hydroxytryptamine and acetylcholine by guancydine. J. Pharmacol. exp. Ther. **179**, 42 (1971).

YAMAMOTO, M., TÜRKER, R. K., KHAIRALLAH, P. A., BUMPUS, F. M.: A potent competitive antagonist of angiotensin II. Europ. J. Pharmacol. **18**, 316 (1972).

Tachyphylaxis to Angiotensin

JOHN M. STEWART

With 8 Figures

If dose-response curves are determined for Angiotensin II and norepinephrine (NE) on isolated strips of guinea-pig aorta, it will be observed that the maximum response obtained to Ang. II is significantly lower than that to NE. Furthermore, if repeated maximal doses of Ang. II are given at fairly short intervals, the response diminishes rapidly, and the tissue becomes unresponsive. If at this time a further challenge of NE is given, the response of the tissue will be normal, or even enhanced. On the other hand, if the tissue is challenged with Ang. I, the tissue will not respond. Washing the tissue several times and allowing time to pass, and again challenging it with Ang. II results in a normal response. This is an example of tachyphylaxis, and shows several of the characteristics of the phenomenon.

Tachyphylaxis, or "acute tolerance", is a special case of the general phenomenon of tolerance to drugs (GOLDSTEIN et al., 1968). Tolerance to drugs developed over a long period of time may involve enzyme induction or other metabolic changes. This is probably not the case with tachyphylaxis, which can occur fully within a very short time.

A. Characteristics of Tachyphylaxis

1. Dose and Time Dependence

The degree of tachyphylaxis to drugs depends upon the size of the dose, the time schedule under which the drug is administered, the drug, the species and the organ. Its onset is faster and its degree is more extensive when large doses are given at short time intervals, or when large doses of drugs are administered continuously. The entire range of sensitivity to tachyphylaxis induction has been observed with angiotensin. In certain tissues a single dose capable to producing only a moderate effect will make the tissue completely refractory to further doses of peptide, whereas in other tissues it is not possible to demonstrate tachyphylaxis even with rapidly-repeated doses of large amounts.

Tachyphylaxis in different tissues can perhaps best be understood by study of the onset and recovery characteristics. In a given tissue, both the rate of onset and the degree produced depend upon the size of the dose. Recovery is time- and specific tissue-dependent. These characteristics are illustrated in Fig. 1. Curve A represents a situation where the dose administered produces only a moderate degree of tachyphylaxis, and the recovery is rapid. In this case subsequent doses (administered at the arrows) will produce the full response. In curve B the situation with a more tachyphylactogenic tissue is represented. Here, due to the greater degree of insensitivity produced and the large amount of time required for recovery, successive doses administered will produce less than full responses, and the response will diminish with each successive dose. The extreme case is represented by curve C where a single application of a drug produces complete refractoriness and recovery is so slow that no further useful responses can be obtained from the tissue. These considerations are extremely important in the performance of bioassays of angiotensin or other substances which produce tachyphylaxis.

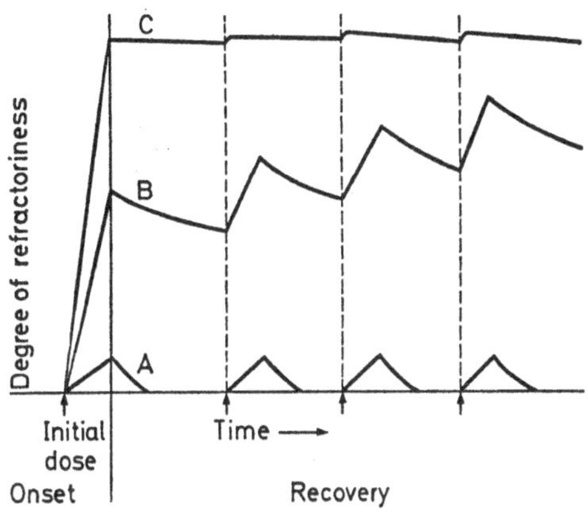

Fig. 1. Characteristics of tachyphylaxis. Effect of repeated equal doses of agonist, administrated at the arrows. Curve *A*: Slight tachyphylaxis, *B*: moderate tachyphylaxis, *C*: severe tachyphylaxis

2. Drug Specificity

Tachyphylaxis is specific for a given drug or a class of drugs. For example, when a tissue has been made tachyphylactic to Ang. II it will also be tachyphylactic to Ang. II analogs and to Ang. I, but not to bradykinin or to non-peptide agonists. We understand these observations by assuming that Ang. II and its analogs all act upon the same receptor, while other unrelated agonists act upon separate receptors. Cross-tachyphylaxis, then, is a useful tool for analyzing the mechanism of action of drugs. A special type of cross-tachyphylaxis is encountered when two separate drugs, each acting upon its own receptor, produce the same ultimate effect by liberation of a common mediator. If tachyphylaxis to one such drug is due to exhaustion of stores of the mediator, the tissue will then be tachyphylactic to the other drug. In this type of tachyphylaxis, no inference can be made concerning a common receptor for the two drugs. This latter type of tachyphylaxis appears to be important in the action of Ang. II on some tissues, and is further discussed below.

3. Species and Tissue Specificity

Development of tachyphylaxis to drugs varies greatly from species to species. In addition, differences are observed between the response of the entire animal and isolated tissues from the same species. Among various isolated tissues from one animal (e.g. response of various smooth muscles to Ang. II), wide variability may be encountered in the development of tachyphylaxis. Another important consideration in the production of tachyphylaxis, particularly in isolated tissues, is the

Table 1. *Examples of Tachyphylaxis to Angiotensin*

Species	Tissue	Response measured	Comments	Reference
Dog	Whole animal	Blood pressure	Renin, Angiotensin	TIGERSTEDT and BERGMANN (1898), PAGE et al. (1957), BOCK and GROSS (1961)
	Kidney	Blood flow	Renin and Ang. II cross-tachyphylaxis	PAGE and McCUBBIN (1953)
	Paw	Perfusion pressure	See Footnote[a]	LIAO and ZIMMERMAN (1972)
	Hindquarters	Perfusion pressure		
	Arteries	Contraction	Coronary, renal, carotid	WALTER and BASSENGE (1969)
Cat	Whole animal	Blood pressure	Cross-tachyphylaxis to renin	GROSS and TURRIAN (1960)
	Carotid artery	Contraction		KHAIRALLAH et al. (1966)
	Aorta	Contraction		KHAIRALLAH et al. (1966)
	Vena cava	Contraction		KHAIRALLAH et al. (1966)
	Isolated atrium	Inotropic effect	Reversed by NE	BEAULNES (1963)
	Perfused adrenal	Catecholamine release	Cross-tachyphylaxis to all Ang. II analogs and Ang. I	PEACH et al. (1971)
	Spleen	Contraction		BENELLI et al. (1964)
Guinea pig	Aorta	Contraction		WALTER and BASSENGE (1969), PALAIC and LE MORVAN (1971)
	Ileum	Contraction	Very variable	HOLLENBERG et al. (1971)
	Seminal vesicle	Contraction	Contracts only after pretreatment with NE	GASCON and WALASZEK (1968)
	Vas deferens	Potentiation of nerve stimulation		BENELLI et al. (1964)
Rat	Whole animal	Blood pressure	Renin and Ang. II showed cross tachyphylaxis, but not NE	GROSS et al. (1961)
	Aorta	Contraction		KHAIRALLAH et al. (1966), WALTER and BASSENGE (1969), HOLLENBERG et al. (1971)
	Caudal artery	Perfusion pressure	See footnote-	NICHOLAS (1970)
	Hindlimb	Perfusion pressure	Reversed by NE	SATO and MASUYAMA (1971)
	Uterus	Contraction		PAIVA and PAIVA (1960)

Table 1 (continued)

Species	Tissue	Response measured	Comments	Reference
Rabbit	Whole animal	Blood pressure		Bianchi et al. (1960)
	Heart	Coronary blood flow		Bianchi et al. (1960)
	Isolated atrium	Inotropic effect	Reversed by NE	Beaulnes (1963)
	Vena cava	Contraction		Kairallah et al. (1966)
	Ear	Flow rate	Complete tachyphylaxis by single dose	Page and Helmer (1940)
	Ear vein	Perfusion pressure	Complete tachyphylaxis by single dose	Horowitz and Mashford (1969)
Human	Intact	Blood pressure		Lubash et al. (1971)
	Artery strip	Contraction	Reversed by NE	Liebau et al. (1965)
	Forearm	Perfusion pressure	Very little	Lumbers and Whelan (1970)
	Colon	Contraction	*In vitro*	Fishlock and Gunn (1970)
Cow	Artery strip	Contraction	Reversed by NE	Liebau et al. (1965)
Pig	Artery strip	Contraction	Reversed by NE	Liebau et al. (1965)
Hamster	Isolated smooth muscles	Contraction	Severe in all tissues	Daum and Lembeck (1969)
Sheep	Whole animal	Blood pressure		Osborn et al. (1969)
	Artery strip	Contraction		Khairallah et al. (1966)

[a] Tachyphylaxis developed to constrictor effect of Ang. II, but not to its potentiation of response to sympathetic stimulation and NE.

concentration of various ions, including hydrogen ion, in the medium. Alteration in ionic composition and balance have also been implicated in the response of whole animals to Ang. II. This may be particularly important with Ang. II, since its action on whole animals involves changes in ionic flux. Sodium, potassium, and calcium have been the principal ions implicated.

B. Occurrence of Tachyphylaxis to Angiotensin

In theory, tachyphylaxis to the pressor effect of angiotensin was first reported by TIGERSTEDT and BERGMAN (1898), who observed that administration of a moderate dose of renin caused a diminished response to subsequent doses administered soon afterward. The discovery that renin was an enzyme producing the agonist angiotensin made it clear that the tachyphylaxis being produced was to Ang. II, and that Ang. I and renin exerted their effect by production of Ang. II. Subsequent studies in a wide variety of species and tissues have shown that Ang. II produces tachyphylaxis very readily in most systems. In general, production of tachyphylaxis to Ang. II is more severe than to other peptide or small molecule agonists. Some of these observations are summarized in Table 1.

Certain tissues have been reported to respond to Ang. II without production of tachyphylaxis. Among these are rabbit arteries (KHAIRALLAH et al., 1966; HOLLENBERG et al., 1971), rat stomach strip (HOLLENBERG et al., 1971), and cat papillary muscle (BEAULNES, 1963). Failure to produce tachyphylaxis may be misleading, since it is possible that the doses used were not high enough. Guinea-pig aorta was originally reported (KHAIRALLAH et al., 1966) not to become tachyphylactic to Ang. II, but later PALAIC and LEMORVAN (1971) showed that Ang. II reliably produces tachyphylaxis at high doses.

Not all peptides structurally related to Ang. II are equally able to induce tachyphylaxis. Using rat blood pressure as an assay, [Asp^1]-Ang. II was found to produce tachyphylaxis at lower doses than [Asn^1]-Ang. II (SAMBHI and BARRETT, 1967). This correlates with the known greater resistance of [Asp^1]-Ang. II to plasma and tissue angiotensinases (REGOLI et al., 1963). Similarly, [β-Asp^1]-Ang. II produced tachyphylaxis in the perfused dog hindquarter (LOUIS and JERUMS, 1968) at lower concentrations than did [Asp^1]-Ang. II. The involvement of angiotensinases in the development of tachyphylaxis is discussed further in Section C below. The importance of a positive charge on the imidazole of the histidine residue in Ang. II for production of tachyphylaxis in rat uterus has recently been discovered, and is described in detail in Section C.

C. Mechanism of Tachyphylaxis

1. Possible Mechanisms for Production of Tachyphylaxis

Involvement of several different mechanisms has been suggested or demonstrated in the production of tachyphylaxis to angiotensin and other drugs. Among these are:

1. Receptor saturation.
2. Increased destruction of agonist.
3. Change in the receptor; "receptor fatigue".
4. Exhaustion of a transmitter.
5. Increased sequestration of the agonist or activation of storage mechanisms.

6. Abnormal strong binding of the agonist to the receptor in such a way that entry of new agonist is blocked.

Of these mechanisms, only (5) has not been suggested as an explanation for tachyphylaxis to Ang. II. Work done previously on the first four mechanisms will be summarized, and a new explanation (6), will be described in detail.

2. Receptor Saturation and Agonist Destruction

In all systems the degree of tachyphylaxis produced to Ang. II is proportional to the dose of Ang. II given or the concentration of Ang. II in the medium. This has led to the suggestion that production of tachyphylaxis is due to saturation of the receptors with agonist, which prevents entry of additional agonist into effective combination with the receptors. If one adheres to the classical concept of pharmacology, which states that combination of the agonist with the receptor produces the response, this mechanism of tachyphylaxis production is difficult to understand. Receptor saturation should lead to a maximal response, rather than maximum inhibition of the response. On the other hand, if PATON's theory of receptor function is correct, receptor saturation is a possible mechanism for production of tachyphylaxis. PATON (1961) has proposed that the pharmacological response of a receptor is proportional to the rate at which agonist combines with the receptor, rather than to the fraction of receptors occupied by agonist. If PATON's theory is true and the rate of dissociation of Ang. II receptor complexes is slow relative to the rate of combination, then with repeated doses or in sustained high concentrations of the agonist, receptors would be expected to become saturated and no longer respond. In this case obviously any force which decreases the concentration of Ang. II or removes it from the biophase would help prevent the formation of tachyphylaxis and should accelerate its reversal, once established.

KHAIRALLAH et al. (1966) found that isolated artery strips from several species made tachyphylactic to Ang. II recovered more rapidly when treated with Dowex 50 or with angiotensinase from plasma. Dowex 50, an anion exchange resin, binds Ang. II very strongly, and evidently functions by removing all Ang. II from the medium. Thus any Ang. II which dissociated from tissue could not reassociate to help maintain tachyphylaxis. Angiotensinase could act similarly to destroy any Ang. II dissociated, or might additionally destroy Ang. II while it was still bound to the receptor. The greater efficacy of these agents over simple washing for reversal of tachyphylaxis probably means that dissociation of Ang. II from the tissue is absolutely irreversible in their presence. It is difficult to visualize a large resin bead coming into such intimate contact with peptide-receptor complexes that it might actually remove the hormone from the receptors. Dowex and angiotensinase may also accelerate removal of Ang. II from "silent" receptors and other non-receptor tissue binding sites; such sites may serve as hormone pools to help maintain tachyphylaxis. One other possible complication of the Dowex experiment may be alteration of calcium-ion concentration in the medium. KHAIRALLAH et al. (1966) used the Ca^{++} salt of Dowex 50 to avoid removing Ca^{++} from the medium. However, some ion exchange may have occurred under the conditions of the experiment, and the Ca^{++} concentration may have increased; this would be expected to accelerate recovery from tachyphylaxis (see section V below).

HOLLENBERG et al. (1971) examined total tissue angiotensinase in homogenates of several smooth muscles with very different propensities for tachyphylaxis induction, and found no correlation between the tendency of the tissue to develop tachyphylaxis and its content of angiotensinase. It is important to realize, as these authors pointed out, that total angiotensinase may not be a meaningful measure of the significant destruction of the peptide which takes place in the intact tissue. Active angiotensinase at, or near, the receptor may be different from concentrations observed in homogenates of whole tissue. Differences have also been observed between physiological destruction of bradykinin in a tissue and destruction of the peptide by homogenates of the same tissue (RYAN et al., 1968). The demonstration that removal of angiotensin from the medium — whether by adsorption to an ion exchange resin or by enzymatic destruction — accelerates recovery from tachyphylaxis really sheds little light on the question of the actual mechanism of tachyphylaxis production. At any rate, it seems unlikely that sufficient angiotensinase could be formed or liberated during the few seconds onset of tachyphylaxis to play a significant role in development of tachyphylaxis in isolated tissues.

Angiotensinases may be much more important in the prevention of tachyphylaxis *in vivo*, for in that case very active angiotensinases could prevent formation of a high concentration of the agonist. LUBASH et al. (1971), studying the action of Ang. II in human beings, found a correlation between angiotensinase levels and response to Ang. II, and agreed with the mechanism proposed by KHAIRALLAH et al. (1966) for inhibition of tachyphylaxis. In contrast, SAMBHI and BARRETT (1968) found no correlation in rats between plasma angiotensinase and the level of tachyphylaxis produced in the animal by administration of Ang. II. Studying Ang. II tachyphylaxis *in vivo* in sheep and dogs, OSBORN et al. (1969), concluded that plasma angiotensinase was not an essential factor in recovery from tachyphylaxis in these species. They considered that the rapid recovery from tachyphylaxis after infusion of Ang. II into sheep, as well as derivatives not susceptible to angiotensinase, made involvement of angiotensinase unlikely. They also observed that the principal loss of Ang. II was by removal in tissue rather than destruction by plasma angiotensinase. In attempting to evaluate these conflicting observations, one must always keep in mind that species and tissue differences, as well as the difference between acute and chronic experiments, and *in-vivo* versus isolated tissue experiments, may mean that different mechanisms are involved and that no general rule can be applied.

3. Receptor Modification as a Mechanism for Tachyphylaxis Production

Guinea-pig aorta has been extensively studied by PALAIC and LEMORVAN (1971) as a model for tachyphylaxis production. Their recent observation that tachyphylactic aortic strips bind more [^{14}C]-Ang. II than do non-tachyphylactic controls would appear to be in conflict with the proposal that tachyphylaxis is due to receptor saturation. They suggest that in tachyphylaxis new binding sites are exposed. This experiment is difficult to assess since it is difficult to distinguish between binding of radioactive Ang. II to receptors and nonspecific binding to tissue. In addition, EDTA was included in the medium in order to inhibit angiotensinase; this may have drastically altered the calcium concentration available to the tissue, and changed the state of tachyphylaxis. The effect of calcium concentration has recently been found to be important in Ang. II tachyphylaxis [FREER and STEWART, 1972 (2, 3)], and influences the rate of recovery of rabbit aorta from nicotine tachyphylaxis (SHIBATA et al., 1971).

Due to the difficulty of correlating tachyphylaxis production with angiotensinase, several authors have proposed changes in receptor conformation as a mechanism for tachyphylaxis production. For example, SAMBHI and BARRETT

(1968) suggested the difference in tachyphylaxis production by [Asp[1]]-Ang. II and [Asn[1]]-Ang. II was due to the presence of the anionic charge at the N-terminus of the peptide which induced a change in the receptor conformation. This work was done *in vivo* in rats. OSBORN et al. (1969), working with sheep and dogs, felt that similar response patterns and rates of removal of Ang. II and derivatives resistant to angiotensinase action ruled out an angiotensinase mechanism for tachyphylaxis, and tended to support the proposal of SAMBHI and BARRETT.

Changes in ion flux induced by Ang. II action may induce changes in receptor conformation, and thus facilitate tachyphylaxis. Profound ion fluxes are produced by Ang. II in many tissues, and were suggested by PEART (1965) as a possible mechanism for tachyphylaxis. GODFRAIND (1970) has shown that Ang. II produces significant calcium fluxes in smooth muscle. This calcium translocation may reflect a change due to a primary alteration of the sodium pump. It has recently been shown that Ang. II accelerates the Na-K ATPase of cell membranes (GUTMAN et al., 1972). It has also been suggested (CIER et al., 1969) that ion balance may be a significant factor in Ang. II tachyphylaxis in human beings. The mechanism proposed for Ang. II tachyphylaxis in rat uterus and guinea-pig ileum by FREER and STEWART [1972 (2, 3)] (see below) suggests that tachyphylaxis occurs when Ang. II binds abnormally to an anionic site near the receptor normally occupied by calcium. An alternative explanation of these observations is that low Ca^{++} concentration may alter the receptor conformation to make the anionic site more readily accessible to the peptide molecule.

4. Transmitter Exhaustion and Tachyphylaxis

Angiotensin not only has a direct action on smooth muscles, but also acts indirectly through mediation of cholinergic or adrenergic mechanisms. For example, part of the effect of Ang. II on guinea-pig ileum can be blocked by atropine and is therefore presumably mediated via a cholinergic process. However, exhaustion of acetylcholine has not been implicated in the tachyphylaxis to Ang. II which develops in this tissue. *In vivo*, a significant part of the pressor action of Ang. II might be mediated by catecholamine released from the adrenals, and PEACH et al. (1971) have shown that in retrogradely perfused cat adrenals tachyphylaxis to this action of Ang. II occurs readily. CLINE (1971) showed that in dogs, tachyphylaxis to catecholamine (CA) release paralleled that of tachyphylaxis to the pressor effect of Ang. II. CLINE concluded that CA release was not significant in the pressor effect of Ang. II in the dog, although the baseline pressure of his experimental animals was not controlled and his results may be invalid for this reason. There is clear evidence that in rats [FREER and STEWART, 1972 (4)] CA release contributes significantly (40 to 60%) to the pressor action of Ang. II. CLINE's conclusion was that since CA release was not significant in the pressor action of Ang. II, tachyphylaxis to CA release could not be the explanation for tachyphylaxis to the pressor effect of Ang. II.

The question of the involvement of NE in the action of Ang. II on isolated vascular smooth muscles is by no means settled at present. There is some degree of involvement in some tissues, but the mechanism and the extent are not clear. Guinea-pig seminal vesicle, which does not normally contract to angiotensin, after treatment with NE exhibits one or two contractions when treated with Ang. II, after which it no longer responds. But the tissue will still respond to tyramine, again with one or two contractions. Evidently, Ang. II is exerting its action by liberation of NE from some stores distinct from those depleted by tyramine.

The situation with respect to isolated tissues which normally respond to Ang. II and develop tachyphylaxis is less clear. The literature is replete with conflicting claims from which no overall picture emerges concerning the role of NE as a mediator of Ang. II. The question of Ang. II tachyphylaxis in various smooth muscles needs systematic re-investigation.

The response to NE of arterial tissue made tachyphylactic to Ang. II is either normal or enhanced. This has been demonstrated in perfused dog hindquarters (Louis and Jerums, 1968) and isolated guinea-pig aorta (Palaic and Lemorvan, 1971). However, tachyphylaxis to Ang. II also inhibits the response to tyramine in guinea-pig aorta and in arteries from cow, pig, rat and human beings (Liebau et al., 1965). Reversal of tachyphylaxis by NE was inhibited by cocaine. Tachyphylaxis to tyramine in guinea-pig aorta did not inhibit the response of the tissue to Ang. II (Palaic and Lemorvan, 1971). In dog hindquarters Ang. II tachyphylaxis did not decrease the response of the tissue to tyramine. Reversal of Ang. II tachyphylaxis by incubation with NE has been reported for cow, pig, rat and human arteries (Liebau et al., 1965), perfused rat hind limb (Sato and Masuyama, 1971), and for isolated atria and heart of cat and rabbit (Beaulnes, 1963). The response of the perfused central artery of rabbit ear to sympathetic stimulation was inhibited by Ang. II (Day and Owen, 1968), while that of perfused rat caudal artery (Nicholas, 1970) and rabbit portal vein and celiac artery (Hughes and Roth, 1971) were enhanced. The response of the perfused rabbit ear central artery to NE was potentiated by Ang. II (Khairallah et al., 1971).

These mixed data would seem to indicate that in some tissues and in some species NE is clearly involved in the action of Ang. II, and may participate in the mechanism of tachyphylaxis production. Its participation in other tissues and other species is questionable. It may be that the mechanism of action in Ang. II in the different tissues and species differs as widely as indicated, or that other experimental variables such as ion concentrations are responsible for at least some of the differences.

5. A Suggested Mechanism for Angiotensin Tachyphylaxis in Smooth Muscle

Recent work [Freer and Stewart, 1972 (2, 3)] has indicated that tachyphylaxis to angiotensin in smooth muscle (rat uterus, guinea-pig ileum) may be due to combination of Ang. II with the receptor in an abnormal way which is stronger than the normal hormone-receptor interaction, and blocks the receptor to the advent of additional Ang. II. Data from experiments on the effects of changes in pH and Ca^{++} concentration on the response of smooth muscles to Ang. II, from a study of the effect of amino-acid substitutions at position 6 in Ang. II, and results of experiments with alkylating (affinity-labeled) peptide derivatives have been combined to provide the basis for a hypothetical model of the topography of the Ang. II receptor of smooth muscle, and to suggest a mechanism for the production of tachyphylaxis at low pH and Ca^{++} concentration.

The response of rat uterus to Ang. II in low Ca^{++} (0.18 mM) de Jalon's solution is maximal at pH 8.0, and decreased at higher and lower pH. The decreased activity is most marked below pH 7, due to the production of a rapid and severe tachyphylaxis. This observation suggested that the tachyphylaxis might be due to protonation of the imidazole of the histidine residue (pK 6.3). Several 6-substituted analogs of Ang. II were synthesized and assayed to test this hypothesis. The results (Table 2) showed that for maximum Ang. II activity the side chain at position 6 must have both aromatic and nucleophilic character, and that when a strongly basic residue was present in this position, production of tachyphylaxis was severe [Freer and Stewart, 1972 (2)]. In contrast to the earlier work of Rocha e Silva [1969 (1)] on histamine, these data suggest that the response is determined by protonation of the imidazole in the hormone, rather than in the receptor.

Development of tachyphylaxis to Ang. II in rat uterus was dependent not only on pH of the medium but also on Ca^{++} concentration. When the concentration of Ca^{++} was 1.0 m*M* or greater, tachyphylaxis was never seen at any pH when rat uterus was used. Recovery from tachyphylaxis in a medium with low pH and low Ca^{++} was slow, requiring about 1 h. However, recovery could be greatly accelerated by raising either the pH or the Ca^{++} concentration of the medium. Guinea-pig ileum responds to changes in pH and [Ca^{++}] in a similar but less clear-cut manner. This prolongation of tachyphylaxis by low Ca^{++} concentration is reminiscent of

Table 2. *Biological properties of Ang. II analogs*

Compound	Relative potency[a]	Tachyphylaxis at pH 6.8
[Ile^5]-Ang. II	100	+
[Asn^1-Val^5]-Ang. II	100	+
[Val^5-Pza^6]-Ang. II	5.0	–
[Ile^5-Thi^6]-Ang. II	5.0	–
[Ile^5-Orn^6]-Ang. II	0.08	+
[Ile^5-Arg^6]-Ang. II	0.004	+
[Ile^5-Phe^6]-Ang. II	0.25	+ –
[Ile^5-Met^6]-Ang. II	0.13	+ –

[a] Calculated by comparison of the dose necessary to give a 50% maximal contraction of isolated rat uterus at pH 8.9. Abbreviations: *Pza* pyrazolylalanine, *Thi* thienylalanine.

the results of Shibata et al. (1971), who observed a similar effect in the recovery of rabbit aorta to nicotine tachyphylaxis.

Figure 2 depicts schematically the structure of Ang. II, showing those functional groups which are known to be important for biological activity. In the adjacent rectangle are suggested functional groups on the receptor which could most logically interact with the important groups on the peptide. The anionic site near the receptor adjacent to the locus of combination with the histidine of Ang. II is probably normally occupied by Ca^{++}. Fig. 3 depicts a suggested peptide-receptor interaction in tachyphylaxis. In low Ca^{++} medium, the anionic site would no longer be saturated with Ca^{++}, and would be available to combine strongly with the protonated form of the imidazole to anchor the peptide firmly and probably abnormally to the receptor. This would prevent normal agonist action of the adsorbed peptide, and would also inhibit entry of additional agonist to the receptor.

Two peptides containing the nitrogen mustard chlorambucil (*p*-[N, N-bis-(2-chloroethyl)amino]phenylbutyric acid) (Chl) were used to provide additional information about the Ang. II receptor. [Chl^1]-Ang. II specifically and irreversibly inhibited the action of Ang. II on isolated guinea-pig ileum, without affecting the response of the tissue to bradykinin, histamine, or ions (Paiva et al., 1972). This result suggests that the nitrogen-mustard moiety of the hormone derivative is

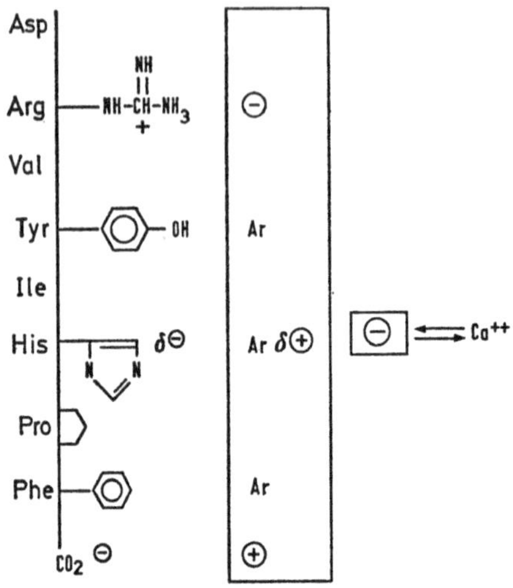

Fig. 2

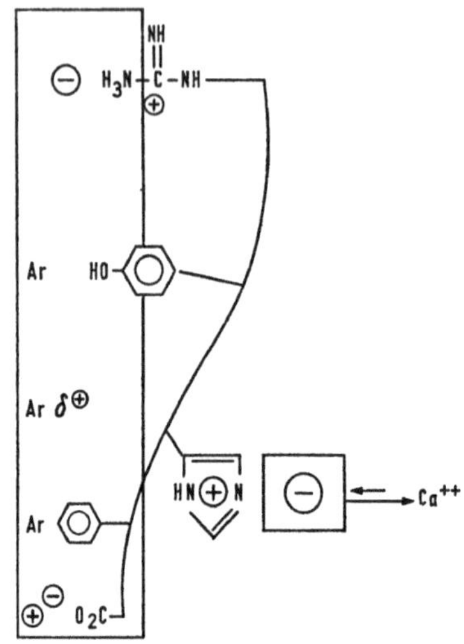

Fig. 3

Fig. 2. Suggested normal angiotensin-receptor interaction. The receptor area is indicated by the large vertical rectangle. The anionic site to the right of the receptor is normally occupied by Ca^{++}

Fig. 3. Suggested peptide-receptor interaction in tachyphylaxis

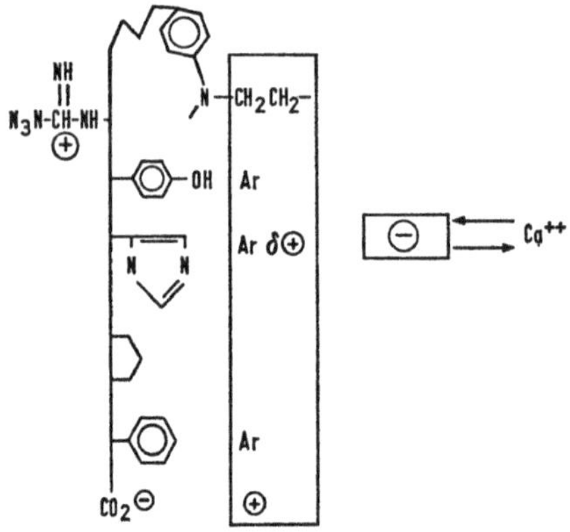

Fig. 4

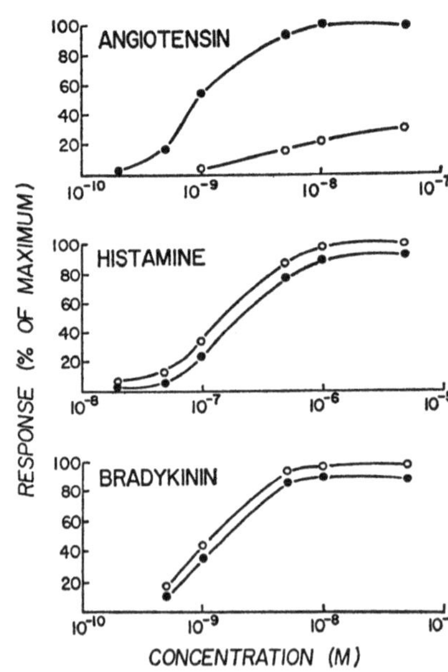

Fig. 5

Fig. 4. Alkylation of angiotensin receptor by [Chl[1]]-Ang. II

Fig. 5. Dose-response curves for three agonists on isolated guinea pig ileum before (●—●) and after (○—○) treatment with [Chl[1]]-angiotensin. (From PAIVA et al., 1972)

alkylating an anionic site on the receptor which normally combines with the guanidinium side chain of the Arg[2]-residue. Fig. 4 shows how [Chl[1]]-Ang. II might alkylate the receptor in this way to block it noncompetitively and irreversibly to the action of Ang. II. Fig. 5 shows dose-response curves which depict this inhibition. Repetition of the alkylation further decreased the Ang. II response without affecting those of bradykinin and histamine. The inhibition of the Ang. II response persisted as long as the experiment was continued (more than 8 h). Chl-Pro-Phe-Arg also produces a permanent inhibition of the response of ileum to Ang. II [FREER and STEWART, 1972 (1)], but this inhibition is quite different from that produced by [Chl[1]]-Ang. II. After treatment of the tissue with the larger derivative, no amount of Ang. II could produce a maximal response, (noncompe-

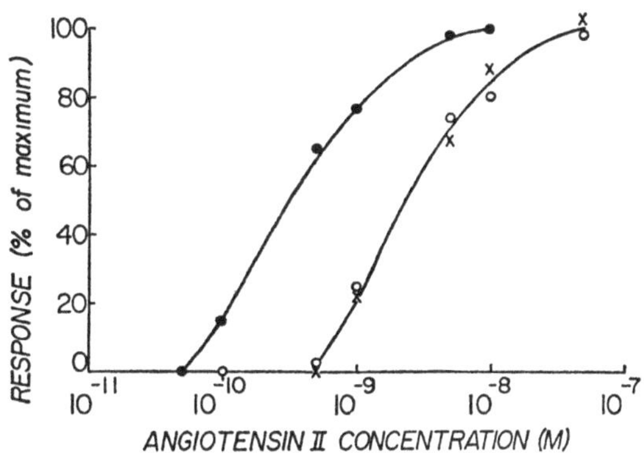

Fig. 6

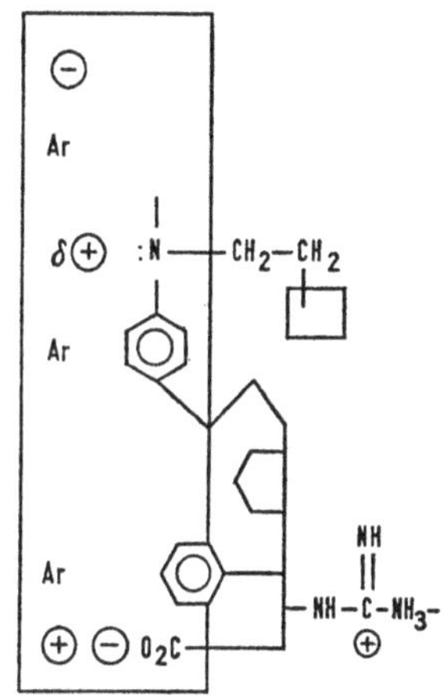

Fig. 7

Fig. 6. Dose-response curves for Ang. II on guinea pig ileum before (●—●), immediately after (○—○), and 3 h after (×—×) treatment with Chl-Pro-Phe-Arg [From FREER and STEWART, 1972 (1)]

Fig. 7. Suggested mode of alkylation of angiotensin receptor by Chl-Pro-Phe-Arg

titive inhibition) but after treatment with the small derivative, the dose response curves obtained had the characteristics of competitive inhibition; that is, the dose-response curve was parallel to and displaced to the right of the control curve. A maximal response could always be evoked by large doses of Ang. II. However, the inhibition persisted after washing. Fig. 6 shows the dose-response curve for this tissue. The responses to bradykinin and histamine were not affected. Repeated treatment with the inhibitor did not reduce the maximum response of the tissue, ruling out the possibility that unalkylated spare receptors might be adequate to produce the full response. A suggestion describing this type of inhibition [ROCHA E SILVA, 1969 (2)] is that the inhibitor is bound to the tissue by attachment to a site not directly on the receptor, but adjacent to it, so that the receptor is partially occluded. Fig. 7 suggests that alkylation of the Ang. II receptor by Chl-Pro-Phe-Arg may involve the proposed anionic Ca^{++} binding site adjacent to the receptor near the imidazole binding site. High concentrations of Ang. II could displace that part of the derivative which lay directly over the receptor, and allow complete receptor occupation and a full response of the tissue. Since the derivative is covalently attached to the tissue, once the high concentration of Ang. II was washed out the peptide part of the inhibitor would return to occlude the receptor.

The model for tachyphylaxis proposed above on the basis of the analog studies suggests that tachyphylaxis is due to an abnormal combination of Ang. II with this same anionic site alkylated by Chl-Pro-Phe-Arg. If this is true, it follows that alkylation of guinea-pig ileum with Chl-Pro-Phe-Arg should prevent tachyphylaxis at low pH and Ca^{++} concentration. An experiment which validates this hypothesis is shown in Fig. 8. A guinea-pig ileum which did not develop tachyphylaxis under the conditions of the experiment at physiological [Ca^{++}] became tachyphylactic at low pH and [Ca^{++}]. After treatment with Chl-Pro-Phe-Arg, tachyphylaxis was no longer developed at low [Ca^{++}]. This experiment confirms the prediction.

While the experiments were done in tissues where tachyphylaxis developed strongly only at low pH and Ca^{++} concentration, the same mechanism of tachy-

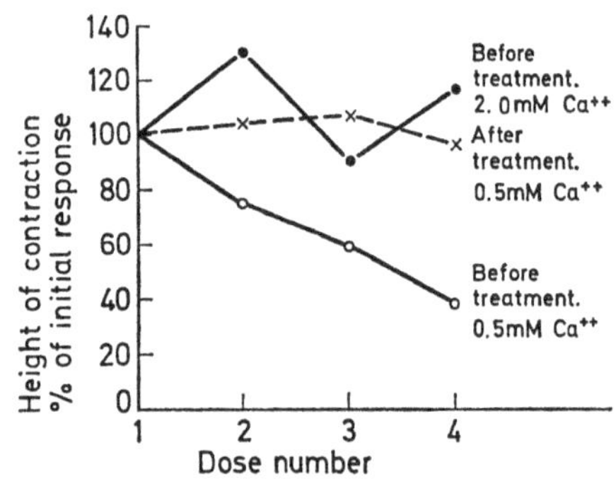

Fig. 8. Inhibition of tachyphylaxis in guinea pig ileum by alkylation with Chl-Pro-Phe-Arg

phylaxis production may also apply to other tissues where tachyphylaxis occurs at physiological pH and Ca^{++} concentration. In those tissues the conformation of the receptor site may be such that the tachyphylactogenic anionic site is much closer to the normal receptor combining site, or Ca^{++} may not be as tightly bound to the anionic site, making it more accessible to the peptide. If the pK of the histidine imidazole is 6.3 (PAIVA et al., 1963), approximately 10% of the Ang. II molecules will be protonated at physiological pH and able to bind strongly to the anionic site. Since this tachyphylactogenic binding presumably has a much longer dissociation time than the normal Ang. II-receptor binding, a progressively larger fraction of the receptor would become inactivated as the tissue is exposed to the peptide. In addition, very close proximity of the anionic site to the receptor-bound Ang. II could alter the pK of the imidazole or induce a dipole in the peptide, thus increasing the tendency to tachyphylactogenic binding.

In those tissues which develop tachyphylaxis only at low Ca^{++} concentration, removal of Ca^{++} from the medium may alter the conformation to move the tachyphylactogenic anionic site closer to the receptor, while in those tissues which develop tachyphylaxis at physiological Ca^{++} concentration the anionic site may normally be quite close to the receptor so that Ang. II is readily trapped.

In considering mechanisms of tachyphylaxis production one must remember that different mechanisms may be acting in different tissues. The situation in the whole animal may be very different from that in isolated tissues. Variables which have not heretofore been adequately controlled or examined (pH, concentrations of ions, ion fluxes) may influence the results or even change the mechanism of action of Ang. II in various tissues or species.

Acknowledgement. Original research reported in this chapter was supported by grants from USPHS (HE-12325) and the Population Council (M71.81C), and by NHLI Contract 71-2497.

References

BEAULNES, A.: Effets de l'angiotensine sur le coeur. Biochem. Pharmacol. **12** (suppl.), 181 (1963).
BENELLI, G., DELLABELLA, D., GANDINI, A.: Angiotensin and peripheral sympathetic nerve activity. Brit. J. Pharmacol. **22**, 211 (1964).
BIANCHI, A., DE SCHAEPDRYVER, A. F., DE VLEESCHOUWER, G. R., PREZIOSI, P.: On the pharmacology of synthetic hypertensine. Arch. int. Pharmacodyn. **124**, 21 (1960).
BOCK, K. D., GROSS, F.: Renin and angiotensin tachyphylaxis. Circulat. Res. **9**, 1044 (1961).
CIER, J. F., SASSARD, J., ZECH, P., VINCENT, M., GHARIB, C.: Influence des facteurs ioniques sur l'action pressive de l'angiotensine exogene chez l'homme. Arch. int. Pharmacodyn. **178**, 357 (1969).
CLINE, W. H., Jr.: Release of catecholamines during the induction of and recovery from tachyphylaxis to angiotensin II. J. Pharmacol. exp. Ther. **179**, 532 (1971).
DAUM, A., LEMBECK, F.: Pharmakologische Untersuchungen an isolierten glattmuskulären Organen des Goldhamsters. Arzneimittel-Forsch. **19**, 1603 (1969).
DAY, M. D., OWEN, D. A. A.: The interaction between angiotensin and sympathetic vasoconstriction in the isolated artery of the rabbit ear. Brit. J. Pharmacol. **34**, 499 (1968).
FISHLOCK, D. J., GUNN, A.: The action of angiotensin on the human colon in vitro. Brit. J. Pharmacol. **39**, 34 (1970).
FREER, R. J., STEWART, J. M.: (1) Alkylating analogs of peptide hormones. I. Synthesis and properties of *p*-[N,N-Bis(2-chloroethyl)-amino] phenylbutryryl derivatives of bradykinin and bradykinin potentiating factor. J. Med. Chem. **15**, 1 (1972).
FREER, R. J., STEWART, J. M.: (2) Synthesis and pharmacology of position 6 analogs of angiotensin II. J. Med. Chem. (1972), (in press).
FREER, R. J., STEWART, J. M.: (3) Some characteristics of uterine angiotensin receptors. Proceedings of the Second International Symposium on Protein and Polypeptide Hormones (MARGOULIES, M., GREENWOOD, F. C., Eds.). Excerpta med. (Amst.), part 2, 480 (1972).
FREER, R. J., STEWART, J. M.: (4) Unpublished data (1972).
GASCON, A. L., WALASZEK, E. J.: Mechanism of the Musculotropic activity of angiotensin on the isolated guinea pig seminal vesicle. Arch. int. Pharmacodyn. **175**, 265 (1968).
GODFRAIND, T.: Angiotensin autopotentiation. Brit. J. Pharmacol. **40**, 542P (1970).
GOLDSTEIN, A., ARONOW, L., KALMAN, S. M.: Principles of Drug Action, p. 558. New York: Harper and Row 1968.
GROSS, F., BOCK, K. D., TURRIAN, H.: Untersuchungen über die Blutdruckwirkung von Angiotensin. Helv. physiol. pharmacol. acta **19**, 42 (1961).
GROSS, F., TURRIAN, H.: Pharmacology of hypertensin and synthetic analogs. In: Polypeptides which Affect Smooth Muscles and BloodVessels (SCHACHTER, M., Ed.), p. 137. Oxford: Pergamon Press 1960.
GUTMAN, Y., SHAMIR, Y., GLUSHEVITZKY, D., HOCHMAN, S.: Angiotensin increases microsomal (Na^+-K^+)-ATPase activity in several tissues. Biochim. biophys. Acta (Amst.) **273**, 401 (1972).
HOLLENBERG, N. K., BARBERO, L. R., HINRICHS, K. P.: Angiotensin tachyphylaxis and vascular angiotensinase activity. Experientia (Basel) **27**, 1032 (1971).
HOROWITZ, J. D., MASHFORD, M. L.: A perfused vein preparation sensitive to plasma kinins. Naunyn-Schmiedeberg Arch. Pharmak. exp. Path. **263**, 332 (1969).
HUGHES, J., ROTH, R. H.: Evidence that angiotensin enhances transmitter release during sympathetic nerve stimulation. Brit. J. Pharmacol. **41**, 239 (1971).
KHAIRALLAH, P. A., DAVILA, D., PAPANICOLAOU, N., GLENDE, N. M., MEYER, P.: Effects of angiotensin infusion on catecholamine uptake and reactivity in blood vessels. Circulat. Res. **28**, Suppl. II, 96 (1971).
KHAIRALLAH, P. A., PAGE, I. H., BUMPUS, F. M., TÜRKER, R. K.: Angiotensin tachyphylaxis and its reversal. Circulat. Res. **19**, 247 (1966).

LIAO, J. C., ZIMMERMAN, B. G.: Response to sympathetic stimulation during angiotensin tachyphylaxis in dog's paw. Arch. int. Pharmacodyn. **197**, 362 (1972).
LIEBAU, H., DISTLER, A., WOLFF, H. P.: The noradrenoline releasing effect of angiotensin II in isolated blood vessels. Acta Endocr. (Kbh.) Suppl. **100**, 138 (1965).
LOUIS, W. S., JERUMS, G.: Tachyphylaxis to alpha- and beta-angiotensin in dogs perfused with Ringer's solution or blood. Circulat. Res. **22**, 75 (1968).
LUBASH, G. D., MUIESAN, G. E., ALICANDRI, C. L., GARFINKEL, D. J., SIEKIERSKI, E. C., LUMBERS, E. R., WHELAN, R. F.: Tachyphylaxis to angiotensin in man. Cardiovasc. Res. **4**, 312 (1970).
MCCONNAUGHEY, C. K.: Plasma angiotensin, serum angiotensinase activity and blood pressure response during angiotensin II amide infusions in normal volunteers. Experientia (Basel) **27**, 68 (1971).
NICHOLAS, T. E.: Potentiation of the effects of noradrenaline and of sympathetic nerve stimulation of the perfused rat caudal artery by angiotensin. J. Pharm. Pharmacol. **22**, 37 (1970).
OSBORN, E. C., HUGHES, S. G., PIRIE, A. T., WILLICOMBE, P. R., MAHLER, R. F.: Clearance studies of angiotensin II and ^{35}S-phenylthiocarbamyl-angiotin II in the sheep and dog. Cardiovasc. Res. **3**, 134 (1969).
PAGE, I. H., HELMER, O. M.: Angiotonin activator, renin and angiotonin-inhibitor and the mechanism of angiotonin tachyphylaxis in normal, hypertensive and nephrectomized animals. J. exp. Med. **71**, 495 (1940).
PAGE, I. H., MCCUBBIN, J. W.: Renal vascular and systemic arterial pressure responses to nervous and chemical stimulation of the kidney. Amer. J. Physiol. **173**, 411 (1953).
PAGE, I. H., MCCUBBIN, J. W., SCHWARTZ, H., BUMPUS, F. M.: Pharmacologic aspects of synthetic angiotonin. Circulat. Res. **5**, 552 (1957).
PAIVA, T. B., PAIVA, A. C. M.: The oxytocic activity of synthetic angiotensinamide. J. Pharmacol. exp. Ther. **130**, 177 (1960).
PAIVA, T. B., PAIVA, A. C. M., FREER, R. J., STEWART, J. M.: Alkylating analogs of peptide hormones. 2. Synthesis and properties of *p*-*p*-[N, N-Bis(2-chloroethyl)amino) phenylbutyryl derivatives of angiotensin II. J. Med. Chem. **15**, 6 (1972).
PAIVA, T. B., PAIVA, A. C. M., SCHERAGA, H.: The conformation of Angiotensin II in aqueous solution. Biochemistry **2**, 1327 (1963).
PALAIC, D., LE MORVAN, P.: Angiotensin tachyphylaxis in guinea pig aortic strips. J. Pharmacol. exp. Ther. **179**, 522 (1971).
PATON, W. D. M.: A theory of drug action based on the rate of drug receptor combination. Proc. roy. Soc. B **154**, 21 (1961).
PEACH, M. J., BUMPUS, F. M., KHAIRALLAH, P. A.: Release of adrenal catecholamines by angiotensin II. J. Pharmacol. exp. Ther. **176**, 366 (1971).
PEART, W. S.: The renin-angiotensin system. Pharmacol. Rev. **17**, 143 (1965).
REGOLI, D., RINIKER, B., BRUNNER, H.: The enzymatic degradation of various angiotensin II derivatives by serum, plasma or kidney homogenate. Biochem. Pharmacol. **12**, 637 (1963).
ROCHA E SILVA, M.: (1) Concerning the histamine receptor. J. Pharm. Pharmacol. **21**, 778 (1969).
ROCHA E SILVA, M.: (2) A thermodynamic approach to problems of drug antagonism. I. The "Charniere theory". Europ. J. Pharmacol. **6**, 294 (1969).
RYAN, J. W., ROBLERO, J., STEWART, J. M.: Inactivation of bradykinin in the pulmonary circulation. Biochem. J. **110**, 795 (1968).
SAMBHI, M. P., BARRETT, J. D.: Plasma "angiotensinase" activity as a determinant of angiotensin pressor action and tachyphylaxis in the rat. Biochem. Pharmacol. **17**, 787 (1968).
SATO, R., MASUYAMA, Y.: Interaction of angiotension and noradrenaline in rat's hindlimb preparation. A possible mechanism of experimental renal hypertension. Jap. Circulat. J. **35**, 505 (1971).
SHIBATA, S., HATTORI, K., SANDERS, B.: Relationship between external calcium concentration and recovery rate of aortic strips from nicotine tachyphylaxis. Europ. J. Pharmacol. **16**, 109 (1971).
TIGERSTEDT, R., BERGMANN, P. G.: Niere und Kreislauf. Skand. Arch. Physiol. **8**, 223 (1898).
WALTER, P., BASSENGE, E.: Effect of angiotensin on vascular smooth muscles. Pflügers Arch. ges. Physiol. **307**, 70 (1969).

Immunogenicity and Antigenicity of Angiotensin I and II*

M. B. Vallotton**

Introduction

Numerous studies on synthetic homopolymers have indicated a sequence of 6 to 7 residues as the minimal requirement for immunogenicity[1], somewhat less being required for antigenicity[1], although exceptions such as the series of "arsenyl"-N-acetyltyrosine (MW = 450) have been described (Borek et al., 1965). The small polypeptide hormones comprising the octapeptide Angiotensin II (MW = 1030), the decapeptide Ang. I (MW = 1280), the nonapeptide bradykinin (MW = 1060) and the neurohypophyseal hormones oxytocin, lysine and arginine-vasopressine (MW = 1007 to 1084) are among the smallest natural polypeptides to have immunogenic and/or antigenic properties. These small polypeptide hormones have been used as model haptens for immunochemical studies because they offer the following advantages: a) their primary structure is well established, b) they can be synthesized and are consequently available free of other protein contaminants, c) a large number of analogues are available in which single or multiple amino acids have been exchanged or modified, d) they are easily manipulated chemically, which allows their attachment to carriers or the obtention of well-defined fragments. Each of these polypeptides appears to behave as an integral whole dotted with a defined secondary structure or conformation if not in solution at least in contact with the complementary steric pattern of the antibody's combining site and of the target cell's receptor (binding, recognition) site.

Immunogenicity of Angiotensin I and II

Attempts at immunization against Ang. II have been made in cats, mongrel dogs (Hedwall and Dietrich, 1967), guinea pigs (Dietrich and Hedwall, 1967; Gocke et al., 1969), chickens and rabbits [Dietrich and Frischknecht, 1968 (1)] and rats [Hedwall and Dietrich, 1967; Dietrich and Frischknecht, 1968 (1), Oken and Biber, 1968; Johnston et al., 1970], while in all other studies reviewed below rabbits were selected as the most suitable and convenient animal for immunization. In cats and dogs no *in-vitro* antibody activity was found by Hedwall and Dietrich (1967) and the antibody level after immunization of dogs was reported by Deodhar et al. (1964) as very low.

Although Dietrich (1966), using guinea pig, and more recently Pierach et al. (1969), using rabbits, have succeeded in immunizing animals with free Ang. II

* Supported by a grant (No. 3.427.70) from the Fonds National Suisse de la Recherche Scientifique.

** Assistant Professor of Medicine, Chief of the Endocrine Division, Department of Medicine, Hôpital Cantonal, Geneva, Switzerland.

[1] The term *immunogenicity* is defined as the capacity of a compound to provoke an immune response and the term *antigenicity* as its specific ability to combine with antibody (Sela, 1969).

suspended in complete Freund's adjuvant, angiotensin, like other small polypeptide hormones [VALLOTTON, 1969 (2)], has a very low immunogenicity [DEODHAR, 1960 (2)], which has thus to be enhanced artificially by attachment of the molecule to a carrier. The procedure of binding an antigen covalently to a carrier has become a classic one since LANDSTEINER's generalized use of synthetic organic haptens covalently attached to serum proteins. In the case of angiotensin a variety of carriers have been chosen. Originally Ang. II was coupled to bovine gamma-globulin [DEODHAR, 1960 (1), 1960 (2); DIETRICH, 1966], rabbit gamma-globulin (GOODFRIEND et al., 1964), poly-L-lysine [HABER et al., 1965 (1), 1965 (2), 1968; PAGE et al., 1965 (1), 1965 (2), 1967; GOODFRIEND et al., 1966; HABER, 1967; STASON et al., 1967; VALLOTTON et al., 1967 (1), 1967 (2); HOLLEMANS et al., 1968 (1), 1968 (2); VALLOTTON, 1970, 1971 (1)], human gamma-globulin (DIETRICH, 1967), rat serum albumin (OKEN and BIBER, 1968), rabbit serum albumin (DIETRICH, 1966; GOODFRIEND et al., 1966, 1968; DIETRICH and HEDWALL, 1967; HEDWALL and DIETRICH, 1967), porcine gamma-globulin [CATT and COGHLAN, 1967 (1); CATT et al., 1967 (2), 1967 (3), 1968] to edestin, gliadin, zein, maleic anhydride and ethylene polymer (GOODFRIEND et al., 1968), and to erythrocytes [DIETRICH and FRISCHKNECHT, 1968 (1)]. BOYD et al. (1967) showed that Ang. II could also be rendered immunogenic by adsorbing it onto charcoal particles [BOYD and PEART, 1968; VALLOTTON, 1970, 1971 (2)]. Immunization was also possible with Ang. II adsorbed onto bentonite [DIETRICH and FRISCHKNECHT, 1968 (1)].

In the light of the experience gained with Ang. II, antibodies against Ang. I were first raised after adsorption onto charcoal (BOYD et al., 1968, 1969; HOLLEMANS et al., 1969), and coupling to poly-L-lysine [HABER et al., 1969; VALLOTTON, 1969 (1), 1969 (2), 1969 (3), 1970, 1971 (1), 1971 (2)] and to porcine gamma-globulin (GIESE et al., 1970).

Since then a fast-increasing number of authors have succeeded in raising antibodies against Ang. II, either coupled to rabbit serum albumin (GOCKE et al., 1969; COHEN et al., 1971; DÜSTERDIECK and MCELWEE, 1971), rabbit gamma-globulin (STOCKIGT et al., 1971), bovine serum albumin (EIDE and AARS, 1970; JOHNSTON et al., 1970; AARS et al., 1971) porcine gamma-globulin (POULSEN, 1969; WORCEL et al., 1970; FUKUCHI and KATSUSHIMA, 1971), or poly-L-lysine (SUNDSFJORD, 1970; ROSSKAMP and KAUFMANN, 1971), or adsorbed onto charcoal (WILMSHURST et al., 1971), or against Ang. I coupled to rabbit serum albumin (LEHFELDT and HUTCHENS, 1971), bovine serum albumin (JOHNSTON et al., 1970) or poly-L-lysine (ROSSLER et al., 1971).

In all these studies the immunogen was emulsified with complete Freund's adjuvant for at least the first course of immunization. Injections were given according to classical immunological methods in the toe-pads, subcutaneously and/or intra-muscularly. BOYD et al. (1968) introduced the immunogen directly into inguineal lymph nodes and into the spleen.

Comparative reports on various modes of immunization are scarce. DIETRICH (1966) observed both immediate and delayed reaction by skin-testing after sensitization of guinea pigs with one of the following preparations: Ang. II alone, angiotensin coupled to rabbit serum albumin or to bovine gamma-globulin by carbodiimide, alum-precipitated angiotensin and p-azobenzenearsenate-Ang. II. The last two preparations did not enhance the immunogenicity. Complete Freund's adjuvant was found to cause a marked increase in the immunogenicity. DIETRICH and FRISCHKNECHT [1968 (1), 1968 (2)] also compared the responses of rabbits immunized to Ang. II-protein conjugates, Ang. II-erythrocytes conjugates and Ang. II adsorbed on to bentonite. The titers of the antiserum, as judged by the hemagglutination technique, were similar but the inhibition of hemagglutination by Ang. II revealed marked differences in their affinity. Again the use of complete Freund's adjuvant was found to promote immunogenicity. GOODFRIEND et al. (1968) followed the antibody titers in the sera of four rabbits injected successively with Ang. II coupled to rabbit or bovine albumin, edestin, zein, gliadin and to maleic anhydride and ethylene copolymer. HABER et al. (1967) showed that antibodies raised with Ang. II coupled in a uniform and strictly defined orientation by its N-terminus to succinylated poly-L-lysine, gave an index of heterogeneity equal to unity according to the Sips equation, indicating that the antibodies population was monodisperse as far as its association constant was concerned. This observation has since been found to hold true for all antisera raised with angiotensin coupled to succinylated poly-L-lysine which we have tested (VALLOTTON, unpublished results). Studies performed with bradykinin coupled to a great variety of carrier-proteins indicated that the method of coupling had a pronounced effect on the association constant and the specificity of the antibody obtained (TALAMO et al., 1968; HABER, 1971); the lowest affinity was observed when the polypeptide was randomly coupled by either end through carbodiimide reaction to albumin. The specificity of their antibody was also less restricted, as was to be expected since a large number of amino acids from the carrier protein around the point of attachment of the polypeptide may participate in forming heterogeneous antigenic determinants. With a non-immunogenic homopolymer such as poly-L-lysine or inert charcoal particle, immunogens of restricted heterogeneity can be prepared and have been compared (HABER et al., 1967; VALLOTTON, 1970).

Various coupling procedures have been used. DEODHAR [1960 (1)] coupled p-Aminobenzoyl-Ang. II to bovine gamma-globulin by diazotation. GOODFRIEND et al. (1966) synthesized a copolymer of angiotensin and poly-L-lysine by the use of N-ethyl-benzisoxazole in the form of a fluoroborate salt. Gluteraldehyde was used by JOHNSTON et al. (1970) to attach Ang. I and II to bovine serum albumin. In all the syntheses mentioned carbodiimide in the form of 1-ethyl-3-(3-dimethyl aminopropyl)carbodiimide hydrochloride or exceptionally in the form of 1-cyclohexyl-3-(2-morpholinyl(4)ethyl)-carbodiimide metho-p-toluene sulfonate (GOODFRIEND et al., 1964, 1966; DIETRICH, 1966) was used. Two bifunctional reagents have been used to couple the N-terminus of angiotensin selectively to poly-L-lysine, m-xylylene diisocyanate [HABER et al., 1965 (2)] and succinic anhydride (STASON et al., 1967).

Numerous authors have reported that antibodies raised against angiotensin neutralized the hypertensive effect of Ang. II whether injected or generated *in vivo* after injection of renin in immunized animals or mixed with the antiserum before injection in non-immunized test-animals [BOYD and PEART, 1968; BOYD et al., 1968 (1); OKEN and BIBER, 1968; PIERACH et al., 1969; EIDE and AARS, 1970; GOODFRIEND et al., 1970; JOHNSTON et al., 1970; MACDONALD et al., 1970; AARS et al., 1971; ROSSKAMP and KAUFMANN, 1971; RÖSSLER et al., 1971).

It could thus be concluded that Ang. I and II, although endowed with a low intrinsic immunogenicity, can elicit antibodies in many animals, and particularly the rabbit, with relative ease when they are attached to a carrier — serum proteins, homopolymer or inert particles — and injected emulsified in complete Freund's adjuvant. These antibodies proved to be biologically effective in neutralizing the pressure effect of angiotensin. This encouraged their use as tools to study the structural requirements for binding to the receptors or combining sites.

Antigenicity of Angiotensin I and II and their Analogues

Of some 100 synthesized analogues of angiotensin, 44 have been tested for their ability to bind to antibody directed against Ang. II (Table 1) or to antibody directed against Ang. I (Table 2). In most cases the method used was one of the variants of the radioimmunological assay in which the ability of the analogue to compete with ^{125}I-Ang. II or I for the antibody binding-site is being measured. But microcomplement fixation (GOODFRIEND et al., 1966) and passive hemagglutination [DIETRICH and FRISCHKNECHT, 1968 (1), 1968 (2)] have also been used. With rare exceptions, which will be mentioned, a rather similar pattern for the role of each individual amino acid toward the overall antigenicity of the molecule emerged from these studies[2].

Position 1: aspartic acid does not appear to play a dominant role in either the biological or the immunological activity of the molecule. The 2 to 8 heptapeptide retains 30 to 50% pressor activity of the natural hormone, has a very similar stimulatory effect on aldosterone secretion (BLAIR-WEST et al., 1971), and maintains 24 to 65% binding activity. Other modifications of this N-terminal amino acid, as found in analogues 1 through 5 (Table 1), barely affect the antigenicity.

Position 2: modifications or deletion of the arginine residue cause the greatest dissociation between biological and immunological activity. Thus the hexapeptide 3 to 8 has no stimulatory effect on aldosterone and retains minimal pressure effect, while retaining full or only partially decreased antigenicity (Tables 1 and 4). Another remarkable feature of this residue is that removal of the positively charged guanidino side chain (replacement of arginine by alanine), *increases* binding activity, as seen with the majority of the antisera tested (Table 3). This is all the more interesting in that the same phenomenon was observed following replacement of Arg^9 by Ala^9 in bradykinin (SPRAGG et al., 1968).

Position 3: the hexapeptide 3 to 8 seems to be the smallest fragment of angiotensin retaining any significant antigenicity. The pentapeptide 4 to 8 was generally found to be unreactive except in one recent study (STOCKIGT et al., 1972). On the other hand, position 3 can be occupied either by an amino acid with a shorter aliphatic side chain or by a bulky aromatic side chain without much change in the antigenicity (analogue 8 and 9, Table 1).

Position 4: the exact positioning of tyrosine at this point appeared of crucial importance to us since the mere permutation of Val^3 and Tyr^4 brought about an important decrease in antigenicity despite identical overall amino-acid composition (VALLOTTON, 1970). It was considered one the main immunological arguments in favor of the three-dimensional model of the angiotensin molecule proposed by SMEBY et al. (1962) [VALLOTTON, 1970, 1971 (1)], although these data would also fit a molecular model in which the two aromatic residues tyrosine and phenylalanine were on the same side of the molecule but not after permutation of Val^3 and Tyr^4. Not only the aromatic side chain but also the hydroxyl group of tyrosine appears to play a role since substitution by phenylalanine does diminish both the biological and the immunological properties in about the same proportion. Substitution by D-tyrosine or by alanine abolishes both activities. The introduction of a single atom of iodine appears to affect the antigenicity only minimally, while the data for the biological activity indicate a wide range from 25 to 80%. Yet the introduction of a second atom of iodine has a much more profound effect (analogue 17 and 18, Table 1) (LIN et al., 1970).

---

[2] In this section references to studies of individual analogues, when not specifically mentionned in the text, are to be found in Table 1 and 2.

Table 1. *Biological activity and immunological binding activity (to anti-Ang. II antiserum) of various Angiotensin analogues compared to Val^5-Ang. II-Asp^1-β-amide*

No.	Analogue	1	2	3	4	5	6	7	8	9	10	Biological activity[a]	Immunological activity[b]
1	Val^5-Ang. II-Asp^1-β-amide	β-L-Asp(NH_2)	Arg	Val	Tyr	Val	His	Pro	Phe			100	100
2	β-L-Asp^1-Ang. II	β-L-Asp										100—150	66—122
3	β-D-Asp^1-Ang. II	β-D-Asp										150	12.2—108
4	α-L-Asp-Ang. II	α-L-Asp										100	72—100
5	Succinyl^1-Val^5-Ang. II	Succinyl										50— >100	92.5
6	Ala^2-Val^5-Ang. II-Asp^1-β-amide		Ala									—	100—166
7	Orn^2-Val^5-Ang. II-Asp^1-β-amide		Orn									20	24—40
8	Ala^3-Ileu^5-Ang. II	Asp		Ala		Ileu						30—68	21.7—100
9	Tyr^{3}Val^5-Ang. II-Asp^1-β-amide			Tyr								12	15.6—61.8
10	Tyr^3-Val^4-Val^5-Ang. II-Asp^1-β-amide			Tyr	Val							<0.1	0.26—1.05
11	Ala^4-Ileu^5-Ang. II	Asp			Ala	Ileu						0.3—3	0.5
12	Phe^4-Val^5-Ang. II-Asp^1-β-amide				Phe							10	8—25.5
13	Phe^4-Val^5-Ang. II	Asp			Phe							10	0.133—10
14	Homo-(Tyr$^{4'}$), Val^5-Ang. II	Asp			Tyr (Tyr')							1	0.6—5.5
15	D-Tyr^4-Val^5-Ang. II-Asp^1-β-amide				D-Tyr							0—0.025	0.072—3
16	D-Tyr^4-Val^5-Ang. II	Asp			D-Tyr							2.5	1.6 —3
17	Monoiodo-Tyr^4-Val^5-Ang. II-Asp^1-β-amide				Tyr(I)							25—80	75—116
18	Diiodo-Tyr^4-Val^5-Ang. II-Asp^1-β-amide				Tyr(I_2)							1—13	2.9—56.6
19	Ileu^5-Ang. II-Asp^1-β-amide					Ileu						100	26.5—100
20	Ileu^5-Ang. II	Asp				Ileu						100	66.6—100
21	Ileu^5-Ang. II-Asp^1-α-amide	α-L-Asp(NH_2)				Ileu						100	67—70
22	α-L-Asp^1-Ileu^5-Ang. II	α-L-Asp				Ileu						100	60—73
23	Tyr^5-Ang. II-Asp^1-β-amide					Tyr						—	5—10
24	Tyr^5-Ang. II	Asp				Tyr						—	5—14
25	Ala^6-Val^5-Ang. II	Asp					Ala					0.3—0.83	0.3
26	Val^5-Pyr(3)Ala^6-Ang. II	Asp					Pyr(3) Ala					56.6	0.5—62.5
27	Ala^7-Ileu^5-Ang. II	Asp				Ileu		Ala				0—0.83	0.06—0.6
28	OH Pro^7-Ileu^5-Ang. II	Asp				Ileu		OH Pro				7—9.8	100

Table 1 (continued)

No.	Analogue	1	2	3	4	5	6	7	8	9	10	Biological activity[a]	Immunological activity[b]
29	Ala^8-$Ileu^5$-Ang. II	Asp				Ileu			Ala			0—0.3	<0—0.024
30	Tyr^8-Ang. II								Tyr			10—30	8
31	All-D-Val^5-Ang. II-Asp^1-β-amide	D-Asp (NH_2)	D-Arg	D-Val	D-Tyr	D-Val	D-His	D-Pro	D-Phe			0	0.0025—0.005
32	Des-(Asp^1)-D-Phe^8-$Ileu^5$-Ang. II-$Ileu^5$-D-Phe^8-heptapeptide 2-8	—				Ileu			D-Phe			0.2	0.63
33	Heptapeptide 2-8	—										30—50	23.8—81
34	Hexapeptide 3-8	—	—									<0.1—2	1.69—2
													32.9—123
35	Pentapeptide 4-8	—	—	—								0	0.635
36	Tetrapeptide 5-8	—	—	—	—							0	<0.005—0.366
37	Tetrapeptide 1-4					—	—	—	—			<0.1	0.021—0.3
38	Heptapeptide 1-7								—			<0.1	<0.059—0.12
39	Val^5-Ang. I-Asp^1-β-amide					Val				His	Leu	25	0.054—2.4
40	$Ileu^5$-Ang. I					Ileu				His	Leu	0—125	0.013—0.5
41	Pro^9-$Phe^{10}$$Val^5$-Ang. I-$Asp^1$-$\beta$-amide									Pro	Phe	0—0.2	20
42	Tetradecapeptide 1-14											0—83.5	0.86—2.38
43	Asp^1-$Ileu^5$-D-Leu^{10}-Ang. I	Asp				Ileu				His	D-Leu	0	1.5
44	Asp^1-$Ileu^5$-des-Leu^{10}-Ang. I	Asp				Ileu				His	—	0	10

All data have been calculated on the base of 100% activity for Val^5-Ang. II-Asp^1-β-amide.

[a] Data for biological activity (pressor activity in nephrectomized rat) taken from SCHRÖDER and LÜBKE (1966), from PAGE and MCCUBBIN (1968) or from works on immunological activity as refered below. Data for coumpound 8 comes from KHOSLA, SMEBY and BUMPUS (1967), for compound 26 from ANDREATTA and HOFMANN (1968).

[b] Data taken from following references given with the number of the analogue tested: BOYD et al. (1968): 1, 2, 4, 8, 11, 25, 28, 29, 30, 36, 37, 38, 40. CATT et al. (1967): 1, 34, 39, 42. CATT et al. (1968): 1, 19, 20. DIETRICH (1967): 1, 2, 3, 5, 12, 17, 18, 19, 32, 33, 34, 35, 36, 37, 38. DÜSTERDIECK et al. (1971): 1, 2, 20, 33, 34, 40. GOODFRIEND (1966, 1968): 1, 2, 3, 13, 14, 15. HOLLEMANS et al. (1968): 1, 19, 33. HOLLEMANS et al. (1969): 1, 39. LIN et al. (1970): 17, 18. OPARIL et al. (1972): 43, 44. STOCKIGT et al. (1972): 1, 20, 33, 34, 35, 36, 37, 38, 39, 40. SUNDSFJORD (1970): 1, 20, 40. VALLOTTON et al. (1967): 1, 2, 20, 34, 36, 37, 38, 39. VALLOTTON (1970): 1, 2, 6, 8, 9, 10, 19, 20, 26, 27, 29, 31, 34, 39, 40, 42. WORCEL et al. (1970): 1, 2, 4, 7, 12, 13, 15, 16, 21, 22, 23, 24, 34, 40, 41.

Position 5: the only known natural variation of angiotensin with valine in beef and dog angiotensins and isoleucine in horse, hog and human angiotensins is in this position. Although an antiserum may exceptionally distinguish between these two forms of angiotensins [DIETRICH, 1967; CATT et al., 1968; HOLLEMANS et al., 1968 (2)], antisera raised against angiotensin generally have the same affinity for these two variants of angiotensins. Substitution in this position by tyrosine does induce a greater decrease in antigenicity than a similar exchange in position 3. Thus positions 3 and 5, which in some species are both occupied by valine on either side of tyrosine ,may not be of equivalent importance antigenically, the residue closer to the C-terminus being more significant.

Position 6: histidine in this position is one of the features of angiotensin deemed essential for biological activity. Actually, substitution by alanine almost abolishes both biological and immunological activity (analogue 25). This group bears one of the positive charges of the molecule of angiotensin and at neutral pH shows approximately 5% ionization (FERNANDEZ et al., 1968). However this charge does not seem to be the contributing factor but rather the conformation of the side-chain, since its isosteric replacement by β-(Pyrazolyl-3) alanine yields an analogue with considerable biological activity (ANDREATTA and HOFMANN, 1968); the greatest variation of affinity among antisera was observed with this analogue (Table 3). With some antisera this analogue had almost the same affinity as the natural hormone while with the others its affinity was considerably reduced.

Position 7: proline is unique among the amino acids in that the inclusion of nitrogen in the pyrroline group impedes the freedom of rotation around the α-carbon and thus rigidly fixes the direction of the backbone of the polypeptide. Replacement of this residue by alanine is followed by a considerable loss of both biological and immunological activity. Histidine has thus been recognized as an essential feature of the angiotensin molecule. However, ANDREATTA and SCHERAGA (1971) recently demonstrated that [Val^5-Mal^7]-Ang. II (in which proline is replaced by N-methylalanine) retained 22% pressor activity. The authors concluded that what was required in this position was an imide nitrogen. No data are available on the antigenicity of this analogue.

Position 8: phenylalanine at the C-terminus of Ang. II is the last feature estimated as essential for the characteristic action of this hormone. The heptapeptide has no biological activity and is also devoid of binding activity (with one exception during a transitory phase of immunization observed by STOCKIGT et al., 1972). Substitution by alanine or by D-phenylalanine has almost the same effect as its deletion. Substitution by tyrosine is already sufficient to decrease both activities to approximately one tenth.

Position 9 and 10: these two residues, which account for the difference between Ang. I and II, will be dealt with together. Few analogues differing in these positions have been prepared. While up to residue in position 8 the antigenicity of the compounds was estimated with antiserum raised against the octapeptide, with the addition of these two residues the affinity toward antibodies raised against the decapeptide has to be considered. This elongation at the C-terminus by two amino acids completely changes the immunogenicity and antigenicity so that practically no cross-reaction between Ang. II and I and their respective antisera is observed (Table 1 and 2) and parallel assay of these two compounds is possible [BOYD et al., 1967, 1969; HABER et al., 1969; HOLLEMANS et al., 1969; PAGE et al., 1969; VALLOTTON, 1969 (2), 1969 (3), 1971]. Actually, further elongation, as with the tetradecapeptide 1 to 14, transforms the antigenic site again so that only a weak cross-reaction with antiserum raised against Ang. I is observed [VALLOTTON, 1971 (2)].

Table 2. *Immunological binding activity to anti-Ang. I antiserum of analogues of Ang. I, Ang. II and fragments of renin substrate compared to Ileu⁵-Ang. I*

No.	Compound	1	2	3	4	5	6	7	8	9	10	11	12	13	14	Immunological activity
1	$Ileu^5$-Ang. I	Asp	Arg	Val	Tyr	Ileu	His	Pro	Phe	His	Leu					100
2	Val^5-Ang. I-Asp^1-β-amide	$Asp(NH_2)$				Val										25—100
3	Val^5-Ang. II-Asp^1-β-amide	$Asp(NH_2)$				Val				—	—					0.12—0.25
4	$Ileu^5$-Ang. II									—	—					0.12—0.25
5	Ala^2-Ang. II		Ala							—	—					<0.5
6	Ala^3-$Ileu^5$-Ang. II			Ala						—	—					<0.5
7	Tyr^3-Ang. II			Tyr						—	—					<0.5
8	Tyr^3-Val^4-Ang. II			Tyr	Val					—	—					<0.5
9	Pyr(3) Ala^6-Ang. II						Pyr(3) Ala			—	—					<0.5
10	Ala^7-$Ileu^5$ Ang. II							Ala		—	—					<0.5
11	Ala^8-$Ileu^5$-Ang. II								Ala	—	—					0.5
12	All-D-Val^5-Ang. II									—	—					0.5
13	Tetrapeptide 7-10	—	—	—	—	—	—									0.01
14	Tetradecapeptide 1-14											Leu	Val	Tyr	Ser	0.5—10
15	Nonapeptide 6-14	—	—	—	—	—						Leu	Val	Tyr	Ser	0
16	Octapeptide 7-14	—	—	—	—	—	—					Leu	Val	Tyr	Ser	0
17	Asp^1-$Ileu^5$-D-Leu^{10}-Ang. I										D-Leu					44
18	Asp^1-$Ileu^5$-des-Leu^{10}-Ang. I										—					10

In this table the relative biological activity is not reported since either it is already given in Table 1 or the compounds are precursors of the final active octapeptide. Data for individual compounds are taken from following references: BOYD et al. (1969): 1, 2, 3, 15, 16. HABER et al. (1969): 3, 4. HOLLEMANS et al. (1969): 3, 4. OPARIL et al. (1972): 17, 18. VALLOTTON (1970): 1—14.

Table 3. *Immunological binding activity of various angiotensin analogues to antisera raised in different rabbits by various procedures*

No.[a]	Analogue[b]	Rabbit identification number[c]									
		302	410	411	412	413	501	502	503	504	505
1	Val^5-Ang. II-Asp^1-β-amide	100	100	100	100	100	100	100	100	100	100
20	$Ileu^5$-Ang. II	96	81.2	92.2	93.3	84	101.9	109.4	95.7	97.9	99.1
6	Ala^2-Val^5-Ang. II-Asp^1-β-amide	113.1	77.6	107.7	91.8	95	110.8	117.9	107	107.4	103.6
8	Ala^3-$Ileu^5$-Ang. II	98.6	16.8	98.2	94.1	62	95.5	105.9	94.3	96.5	100
9	Tyr^3-Val^5-Ang. II-Asp^1-β-amide	85.5	36.2	66.3	70.7	33	82.8	73.5	71.8	79.6	84.7
26	Val^5-Pyr(3)-Ala^6-Ang. II	96.8	4.5	3.4	1.5	71.2	<1	82.0	2.8	13.6	21.5
39	Val^5-Ang. I-Asp^1-β-amide	48.7	98.9	46.5	4.5	7.0	15.9	63.2	4.2	8.2	10.1
40	$Ileu^5$-Ang. I	35.5	74.2	27.5	1.5	7.0	22.9	71.8	<1	13.6	11.4
29	Ala^8-$Ileu^5$-Ang. II	21.0	9.6	9.4	1.5	2.4	1.2	17.1	<1	<1	<1
10	Tyr^3-Val^4-Val^5-Ang. II-Asp^1-β-amide	67.1	23.8	91.3	<1	68.4	3.2	105.9	<1	<1	<1
27	Ala^7-$Ileu^5$-Ang. II	46.0	55.6	70.6	4.5	68.4	68.1	87.2	5.6	15.6	11.4
31	All-D-Val^5-Ang. II-Asp^1-β-amide	<1	0.98	<1	1.5	<1	<1	<1	<1	<1	3.8

[a] This number refers to analogues listed in Table 1.

[b] Analogues above the horizontal line used at a concentration of 1 ng/ml and under the line at a concentration of 100 ng/ml, except for analogue 31 used at a concentration of 1000 ng/ml.

[c] Rabbits No. 302, 410, 411, 501, 502, 503 immunized with Ang. II coupled to succinyl-poly-L-lysine. Rabbits No. 412, 413 immunized first with angiotensin I coupled to succinyl-poly-L-lysine then boosted with Ang. II adsorbed on to charcoal particle. Rabbits No. 504, 505 immunized with Ang. II adsorbed on to charcoal particle. All these sera were used at the lowest dilution (varying from 1:100 to 1:6400) enabling to achieve displacement of the tracer by the analogues used.

All displacement data calculated on the base of 100% binding activity for Val^5-Ang. II-Asp^1-β-amide.

Table 4. *Relative binding activity of the hexapeptide 3-8 to various antisera anti-Ang. II compared to Val^5-Ang. II (= 100%)*

Antisera	PLA5	XCPLA	301	302	411	412	413
Hexapeptide 3-8	108	87	50	112	100	105	35

Antisera	502	501	504	505	512	513	514	515
Hexapeptide 3-8	123	117	112	122	114	123	118	114

The role of the residue in position 10 has been studied by OPARIL et al. (1972), both from the point of view of antigenicity and from that of reactivity as substrate for converting enzyme. The intermediate nonapeptide 1 to 9 or des-[Leu]-Ang. I showed only 10% reactivity with either antiserum against Ang. I or II. The substitution of D-leucine for L-leucine induced a loss of 56% in binding with anti-angiotensin I antiserum. Neither of these analogues could function as substrate for pulmonary converting enzyme.

Discussion and Conclusion

The cellular mechanism of protein synthesis provides only information for the chemical sequence of amino acids in proteins (their primary structure) through colinear transfer of sequential information. The conformation stabilized by non-covalent interaction between groups along the same sequence of amino acids (secondary and tertiary structures) or between two or more sequences (quaternary structure) depends uniquely on the amino-acid sequence and the environment surrounding the molecule. No other source of information seems to be necessary. Yet so far, very few rules for this folding of the peptides upon themselves have been discovered and it is still not possible to predict the thermodynamically most stable conformation in a given medium from a given amino-acid sequence. X-ray diffraction studies of protein crystals, when available, are the most precise methods of elucidating conformation. When this is not feasible the means to approach this goal include optical rotary dispersion (ORD), nuclear magnetic resonance (NMR) and circular dichroism (CD) spectra, dialysis escape-time measurement, denaturation studies and immunochemical studies. All these approaches have their limitations and they do not all give the same sort of information, but are complementary in helping to decipher the relationship between structure and activity of the peptides.

The advantages of the immunochemical methods lay in their extreme sensitivity, facilitating the study of the molecule at or near its physiological concentration, avoiding intermolecular interaction, and also of analogues available in minute quantities. Another great advantage is that they rely upon the conformation of the peptide at the combining site of the antibody, while physicochemical methods study the behavior of the isolated molecule in solution and often in an unphysiological solvent. This is very important indeed since the conformation may not be the same in the two situations (SCHWYZER, 1963, 1971; VALLOTTON, 1970). From work done during recent years it appears more and more likely that the interaction of the peptide hormone with its receptor induces a conformational change in one or both (RASMUSSEN, 1971; RODBELL et al., 1971). Studies with heterologous substituted benzenearsenates in which different substituents were exchanged in position ortho-, meta- or para- showed that the combining sites of antibodies were able to accommodate different haptens by some deformation (PAULING and PRESSMAN, 1945). Thus, a certain flexibility of both the antibody's combining sites and the target cell's receptor or binding site appears possible. This conformational flexibility or the transconformation induced by the receptor may in some case be calcium-dependent as found by LIBERTI et al. (1971) and MAURER et al. (1970) with antibodies to poly-α-amino acids and by BOYD et al. [1967, 1968 (1)] and FAVRE and VALLOTTON (1972) with antibodies to Ang. II. The calcium requirement for binding or expression of hormone at the receptor site of the target cell may play a similar role (RODBELL et al., 1971; HECHTER and BRAUN, 1971). Sodium chloride may exert an analogous effect (BERGMANN et al., 1971).

Immunochemical methods also have their limitations and disadvantages, however, the main ones being variation of specificity of antiserum from animal to animal and the heterogeneity of the antibody population within an antiserum. This variation may not be random but has been found to be genetically controlled (MOZES et al., 1969; ARQUILLA and FINN, 1965).

Furthermore, this heterogeneity may be turned to advantage in the future since recent studies tend to demonstrate that heterogeneity of the biological receptor for hormones may also exist. There is still some uncertainty about whether or not different receptors for the same hormone exist at the surface of the same target cell (HECHTER and BRAUN, 1971), but in the case of Ang. II the receptor sites on smooth muscle and on parasympathetic nerves have been found to have different specificity and thus probably to represent different conformations (KHAIRALLAH et al., 1970). The combination of results obtained by radioimmunoassay and results obtained by radioreceptor assay should make this aspect of the problem much clearer.

This variation restricts the number of conclusions which could be drawn and should render one cautious of any generalization. However, taking this in to account, and assuming that a sufficient number of antisera have been tested, a similar overall pattern of inhibition (Table 1 to 4) is obtained which allows some conclusions (VALLOTTON, 1970, 1971 (2); DIETRICH and FRISCHKNECHT, 1968; HABER et al., 1967).

The antigenic determinant of Ang. II encompasses the hexapeptide 3 to 8, comprising the C-terminus. Four of the residues included in this sequence are immunodominant: tyrosine^4, histidine^6, proline^7 and phenylalanine^8. It is not surprising to find these amino acids include two aromatic ones, since the importance of the aromatic ring for immunogenicity and antigenicity has been recognized since the appearance of LANDSTEINER's work (1936). SELA et al. (1956), SELA and ARNON (1960) showed that tyrosine or phenylalanine were unique among amino acids in that they were able to render gelatin immunogenic even when as little as 2% tyrosine was attached to it. The fact that neither tyrosine nor phenylalanine can be interchanged without a significant loss of antigenicity proves that their exact spatial location is important and indicates a conformational orientation of the determinant. The charge of histidine does not appear to be as important as the presence of the five-membered ring of the side chain. Proline was thought to play a definitive role in fixing the orientation of the backbone of the molecule, yet the recent demonstration that the opening of the ring while the imide nitrogen is maintained does not affect the biological effect too dramatically (ANDREATTA and SCHERAGA, 1971) forces one to reconsider this point; no immunochemical data are yet available.

These requirements for antigenicity so far are in complete agreement with the requirement for biological activity except for the fact that the latter requires an extension up to the heptapeptide 2 to 8. It is not surprising that the biological site overlaps the antigenic site almost completely in such a small polypeptide (VALLOTTON, 1971 (2)]. In future it will be interesting to study the role of the arginine residue which is essential for binding to target-cell receptor but not to antibody's combining site. This amino acid is certainly not "immunologically indifferent" since removal of its guanidino group *increased* the binding activity, as if this rather bulky side chain or the positive charge impeded a perfect fit into the combining site in some way. Two amino acids — Val^3 and Val^5(Ileu^5) — seem unessential both for biological and for immunological activities.

It is probably still debatable for such a small polypeptide to conclude that the antigenic determinant is a conformational one and not a sequential one in the definition of SELA (1969) or, speaking in term of biological activity, to conclude that one is dealing with a "discontinuate" word and not with a "continuate" one in the terminology used by SCHWYZER et al. (1971). An overall definite conformation appears to be necessary for a proper interaction of angiotensin with its receptor site and it seems that conformational models will have to fit such data. The one proposed by SMEBY et al. (1962), with one and a half turns of α helix and the juxtaposition of the two aromatic residues fitted in well with both biological and immunological data (VALLOTTON, 1970). A more recent model suggested by FERMANDJIAN et al. (1972), a β-structure with the two aromatic amino acids apart from each other but with their side chains on the same side of the molecule, has now also to be considered. From circular-dichroism spectra these authors conclude that in dilute aqueous solution angiotensin exhibits polymorphism with both unordered and ordered conformations; these ordered conformations include both antiparallel-β and helical structures. As changing environments modified the relative proportion of these various forms, it is quite conceivable that a specific conformation is induced in the microenvironment of the receptor sites, favoring the best molding and thus probably the highest binding of the peptide to the receptor site.

Using another technique, automated tritium-hydrogen exchange, PRINTZ et al. [1972 (1), 1972 (2)] proposed two models, a γ-turn and a β-turn model, for Ang. II in aqueous solution, the peptide chain being folded upon itself with two of the six backbone peptide hydrogens involved in secondary structure and at least one of these two hydrogens participating in an intramolecular hydrogen bond.

These recent studies thus support the idea that angiotensin, despite its small size, may indeed adopt a limited number of ordered conformations dependent on the environment.

Acknowledgements

The author wishes to thank Mrs. D. SCHOLER-MARKOVIC for her invaluable technical help and Miss V. NICOLET for her skilful secretarial assistance in preparing this manuscript.

This work is dedicated to Professor F. LEUTHARDT at the occasion of his 70th birthday.

References

AARS, H., EIDE, I., AKRE, S.: Abolished sympathetic stimulating effect of angiotensin in rabbits immunized with angiotensin II. Scand. J. clin. Lab. Invest. **27**, 47 (1971).

ANDREATTA, R., HOFMANN, K.: Studies on polypeptide. XLI. The synthesis of [5-Valine, 6-β-)-(pyrazolyl-3)-alanine]-angiotensin II, a potent hypertensive peptide. J. Amer. chem. Soc. **90**, 7334 (1968).

ANDREATTA, R. H., SCHERAGA, H. A.: Synthesis of [5-Valine, 7-N-methylalanine]-angiotensin II, a hypertensive peptide. J. Med. Chem. **14**, 489 (1971).

ARQUILLA, E. R., FINN, J.: Genetic control of combining sites of insulin antibodies produced by guinea pigs. J. exp. Med. **122**, 771 (1965).

BERGMANN, J., OEHME, P., JELINEK, J., CORT, J. H.: Potentiation of angiotensin and eledoisin activities by sodium chloride. Life Sci. **10**, 969 (1971).

BLAIR-WEST, J. R., COGHLAN, J. P., DENTON, D. A., FUNDER, J. W., SCOGGINS, B. A., WRIGHT, R. D.: The effect of the heptapeptide (2-8) and hexapeptide (3-8) fragments of angiotensin II on aldosterone secretion. J. clin. Endocrin. **32**, 575 (1971).

BOREK, F., STUPP, Y., SELA, M.: Immunogenicity and role of size: Response of Guinea Pigs to oligotyrosine and tyrosine derivatives. Science **150**, 1177 (1965).

BOYD, G. W.: In: Protein and Polypeptide Hormones, Proceedings of the International Symposium Liège 1968 (MARGOULIES, M., Ed.). ICS 161. Excerpta med. (Amst.) **3**, 558 (1969).

BOYD, G. W., ADAMSON, A. R., FITZ, A. E., PEART, W. S.: Radioimmunoassay determination of plasma-renin activity. Lancet **1969 I**, 213.

BOYD, G. W., FITZ, A. E., PEART, W. S.: (1) The measurement of plasma renin by radioimmunoassay of generated angiotensin I. In: Protein and Polypeptide Hormones, Proceedings of the International Symposium, Liège 1968 (MARGOULIES, M., Ed.). ICS 1961. Excerpta med. (Amst.) **3**, 896 (1969).

BOYD, G. W., LANDON, J., PEART, W. S.: Radioimmunoassay for determining plasma-levels of angiotensin in man. Lancet **1967 II**, 1002.

BOYD, G. W., LANDON, J., PEART, W. S.: (2) Some problems encountered in the radioimmunoassay of circulating angiotensin II. In: Protein and Polypeptide Hormones, Proceedings of the International Symposium, Liège 1968 (MARGOULIES, M., Ed.). ICS 161. Excerpta med. (Amst.) **2**, 365 (1968).

BOYD, G. W., PEART, W. S.: The production of high-titre antibody against free angiotensinII. Lancet **1968 II**, 129.

CATT, K. J., CAIN, M. C., COGHLAN, J. P.: (2) Measurement of angiotensin II in blood. Lancet **1967 II**, 1005.

CATT, K. J., CAIN, M. D., COGHLAN, J. P.: Radioimmunoassay of angiotensin II in blood. In: Protein and Polypeptide Hormones, Proceedings of the International Symposium, Liège 1968 (MARGOULIES, M., Ed.). ICS 161, Excerpta med. (Amst.) **1**, 77 (1968).

CATT, K., COGHLAN, J. P.: (1) Generation and use of antibodies to angiotensin II. Aust. J. exp. Biol. med. Sci. **45**, 269 (1967).

CATT, K. J., COGHLAN, J. P., ROMBERG, B.: (3) Immunological reactivity of peptides related to angiotensin. Nature (Lond.) **215**, 395 (1967).

COHEN, E. L., GRIM, C. E., CONN, J. W., BLOUGH, W. M., GUYER, R. B., KEM, D. C., LUCAS, C. P.: Accurate and rapid measurement of plasma renin activity by radioimmunoassay. Results in normal and hypertensive people. J. Lab. clin. Med. **78**, 1025 (1971).

DEODHAR, S. D.: (1) Immunologic production of antiangiotensin. I. Preparation of angiotensin protein complex. J. exp. Med. **111**, 419 (1960).

DEODHAR, S. D.: (2) Immunologic production of angiotensin. II. Production and detection of antiangiotensin. J. exp. Med. **111**, 429 (1960).

DEODHAR, S. D., HAAS, E., GOLDBLATT, H.: Production of antirenin to homologous renin and its effect on experimental renal hypertension. J. exp. Med. **119**, 425 (1964).

DIETRICH, F. M.: Immunogenicity of synthetic angiotensin II. Int. Arch. Allergy **30**, 497 (1966).

DIETRICH, F. M.: Immunological analysis of rabbit antibodies against angiotensin II. Immunochemistry **4**, 65 (1967).

DIETRICH, F. M., FRISCHKNECHT, H.: (1) Immunogenicity of synthetic angiotensin II octapeptide and analysis of antibodies by passive haemagglutination. Intern. Arch. Allergy **34**, 597 (1968).

DIETRICH, F. M., FRISCHKNECHT, H.: (2) Analysis of antibodies against synthetic angiotensin II by the passive haemagglutination technique. Nature (Lond.) **217**, 264 (1968).

DIETRICH, F. M., HEDWALL, P. R.: Antikörper-Produktion gegen synthetisches Angiotensin bei verschiedenen Tierarten. Naunyn-Schmiedeberg's Arch. Pharmak. exp. Path. **257**, 273 (1967).

DÜSTERDIECK, G., MCELWEE, G.: Estimation of angiotensin II concentration in human plasma by radioimmunoassay. Some applications to physiological and clinical states. Europ. J. clin. Invest. **2**, 32 (1971).

EIDE, I., AARS, H.: Renal hypertension in rabbits immunized with angiotensin II. Scand. J. clin. Lab. Invest. **25**, 119 (1970).

FAVRE, L., VALLOTTON, M. B.: Influence of calcium on angiotensin II — antibody reaction. Immunochemistry **10**, 43 (1973).

FERMANDJIAN, S., MORGAT, J. L., FROMAGEOT, P.: Studies of angiotensin-II conformations by circular dichroism. Europ. J. Biochem. **24**, 252 (1971).

FRANZE DE FERNANDEZ, M. T., DELIUS, A. E., PALADINI, A. C.: Influence of pH on the conformation of angiotensin II and analog peptides. Biochim. biophys. Acta (Amst.) **154**, 223 (1968).

FUKUCHI, S., KATSUSHIMA, I.: Measurement of plasma angiotensin II by radioimmunoassay. Tohoku J. exp. Med. **103**, 185 (1971).

GIESE, J., JORGENSEN, M., NIELSEN, M. D., LUND, J. O., MUNCK, O.: Plasma renin concentration measured by use of radioimmunoassay for angiotensin I. Scand. J. clin. Lab. Invest. **26**, 355 (1970).

GOCKE, D. J., GERTEN, J., SHERWOOD, L. M., LARAGH, J. H.: Physiological and pathological variations of plasma angiotensin II in man. Correlation with renin activity and sodium balance. Circulat. Res. Suppl. **1**, **24**, **25**, I—131 (1969).

GOODFRIEND, T. L., FASMAN, G., KEMP, D., LEVINE, L.: Immunochemical studies of angiotensin. Immunochemistry **3**, 223 (1966).

GOODFRIEND, T. L., BALL, D. L., FARLEY, D. B.: Radioimmunoassay of angiotensin. J. Lab. clin. Med. **72**, 648 (1968).

GOODFRIEND, T. L., LEVINE, L., FASMAN, G. D.: Antibodies to bradykinin and angiotensin: A use of carbodiimides in immunology. Science **144**, 1344 (1964).

GOODFRIEND, T. L., WEBSTER, M. E., MCGUIRE, J. S.: Complex effects of antibodies to polypeptide hormones. J. clin. Endocr. **30**, 565 (1970).

HABER, E.: Enhancement of immunogenicity of small polypeptides (angiotensin) and use of antibodies in their measurement. Pharmacologist **9**, 177 (1967).

HABER, E.: Bradykinin: Structural requirements of binding to antibody in relation to biological activity. In: Protein and Polypeptide Hormones, Proceedings of the International Symposium, Liège 1971 (MARGOULIES, M., GREENWOOD, F. C., Eds.). ICS 241. Excerpta med. (Amst.) **1**, 66 (1971).

HABER, E., KOERNER, T., PAGE, L. B., KLIMAN, B., PURNODE, A.: Application of a radioimmunoassay for angiotensin I to the physiologic measurements of plasma renin activity in normal human subjects. J. clin. Endocr. 29, 1349 (1969).
HABER, E., PAGE, L. B., JACOBY, G. A.: (2) Synthesis of antigenic branch-chain copolymers of angiotensin and poly-L-lysine. Biochemistry 4, 693 (1965).
HABER, E., PAGE, L. B., RICHARDS, F. F.: (1) Radioimmunoassay employing gel filtration. Analyt. Biochem. 12, 163 (1965).
HABER, E., RICHARDS, F. F., SPRAGG, J., AUSTEN, K. F., VALLOTTON, M. B., PAGE, L. B.: Modifications in the heterogeneity of the antibody response. Cold Spr. Harb. Symp. quant. Biol. Antibodies 32, 299 (1967).
HABER, E., VALLOTTON, M. B., KIMURA, A., PAGE, L. B.: Immunoassay for angiotensin II. In: Protein and Polypeptide Hormones, Proceedings of the International Symposium, Liège 1968 (MARGOULIES, M., Ed.). ICS 161. Excerpta med. (Amst.) 3, 359 (1969).
HECHTER, O., BRAUN, TH.: Peptide hormone-receptor interactions: an informational transaction. In: Protein and Polypeptide Hormones, Proceedings of the International Symposium, Liège 1971 (MARGOULIES, M., GREENWOOD, F. C., Eds.). ICS 241. Excerpta med. (Amst.) 1, 212 (1971).
HEDWALL, P. R., DIETRICH, F. M.: Production of antibodies against synthetic angiotensin II in various animal species. Experientia (Basel) 23, 952 (1967).
HOLLEMANS, H. J. G., VAN DER MEER, J., KLOOSTERZIEL, W.: Identification of the incubation product of Boucher's renin activity assay, by means of radioimmunoassays for angiotensin I and angiotensin II, and a converting enzyme preparation from lung tissue. Clin. chim. Acta 23, 7 (1969).
HOLLEMANS, H. J. G., VAN DER MEER, J., TOUBER, J. L.: (1) A radioimmunoassay of angiotensin, its use in the measurement of renin activity in plasma. In: Protein and Polypeptide Hormones, Proceedings of the International Symposium, Liège 1968 (MARGOULIES, M., Ed.). ICS 161. Excerpta med. (Amst.) 2, 370 (1968).
HOLLEMANS, H. J. G., VAN DER MEER, J., TOUBER, J. L.: (2) Radioimmunoassay of angiotensin. Nature (Lond.) 217, 277 (1968).
JOHNSTON, C. I., HUTCHINSON, J. S., MENDELSOHN, F. A.: Biological significance of renin angiotensin immunization. Circulat. Res. Suppl. II, 26, 27, II—215 (1970).
KHAIRALLAH, P. A., TOTH, A., BUMPUS, F. M.: Analogs of angiotensin II. II. Mechanism of receptor interaction. J. Med. Chem. 13, 181 (1970).
KHOSLA, M. C., SMEBY, R. R., BUMPUS, F. M.: Solid phase peptide synthesis of [L-Alanine^3-L-isoleucine^5]-angiotensin II. Biochemistry 6, 754 (1967).
LANDSTEINER, K.: The specificity of serological reactions. New York: Dover publ. 1962.
LEHFELDT, D. C., HUTCHENS, T. T.: A kinetic method for determination of plasma renin activity using radioassay of angiotensin I. Amer. J. clin. Path. 55, 513 (1971).
LIBERTI, P. A., MAURER, P. H., CLARK, L. G.: Antigenicity of polypeptides (poly-α-amino acids). Physicochemical studies of a calcium-dependent antigen-antibody reaction. Biochem. 10, 1632 (1971).
LIN, S. Y., ELLIS, H., WEISBLUM, B., GOODFRIEND, T. L.: Preparation and properties of iodinated angiotensins. Biochem. Pharmacol. 19, 651 (1970).
MACDONALD, G. J., LOUIS, W. J., RENZINI, V., BOYD, G. W., PEART, W. S.: Renal-clip hypertension in rabbits immunized against angiotensin II. Circulat. Res. 27, 197 (1970).
MAURER, P. H., CLARK, L. G., LIBERTI, P. A.: Antigenicity of polypeptides (poly-α-amino acids): Calcium-dependent and independent antibodies. J. Immunol. 105, 567 (1970).
MOZES, E., MCDEVITT, H. O., JATON, J.-C., SELA, M.: The genetic control of antibody specificity. J. exp. Med. 130, 1263 (1969).
OKEN, D. E., BIBER, T. U. L.: Biologically effective immunization against angiotensin. Amer. J. Physiol. 214, 791 (1968).
OPARIL, S., TREGEAR, G., HABER, E.: Role of the C-terminal sequence of angiotensin I on immunologic reactivity and on conversion to angiotensin II in vivo and in vitro. In: Protein and Polypeptide Hormones, Proceedings of the second International Symposium, Liège 1971 (MARGOULIES, M., GREENWOOD, F. C., Eds.). ICS 241. Excerpta med. (Amst.) 2, 262 (1972).
PAGE, L. B., HABER, E., KIMURA, A. Y., PURNODE, A.: Studies with the radioimmunoassay for angiotensin II, and its application to measurement of renin activity. J. clin. Endocr. 29, 200 (1969).
PAGE, L. B., HABER, E., LAGG, S.: (1) Specific immunochemical method for quantitative determination of angiotensin. Circulation 32, Suppl. II, 167 (1965).
PAGE, L., HABER, E., LAGG, S.: (2) Quantitative immunochemical determination of angiotensin. J. clin. Invest. 44, 1083 (1965).
PAGE, L. B., VALLOTTON, M. B., HABER, E.: Radioimmunoassay determination of angiotensin and renin activity in normal and disease states. Circulation 35/36, Suppl. II, 203 (1967).

PAGE, I. H., McCUBBIN, J. W. (Edit.): Renal hypertension. Chicago: Year Book 1968.

PAULING, L., PRESSMAN, D.: The serological properties of simple substances. IX. Hapten inhibition of precipitation of antisera homologous to the o-, m-, and p-Azophenylarsonic acid groups. J. Amer. chem. Soc. **67**, 1003 (1945).

PIERACH, C. A., JACOBSON, M. E., CARLSON, K. L.: Radioimmunologische Angiotensinbestimmung. Verh. dtsch. Ges. inn. Med. **75**, 191 (1969).

POULSEN, K.: Estimation of plasma renin concentration using radioimmunoassay of angiotensin II. Scand. J. clin. Lab. Invest. **24**, 291 (1969).

PRINTZ, M. P., NEMETHY, G., BLEICH, H.: (1) Proposed models for angiotensin II in aqueous solution and conclusions about receptor topography. Nature (Lond.) New Biol. **237**, 135 (1972).

PRINTZ, M. P., WILLIAMS, H. P., CRAIG, L. C.: (2) Evidence for the presence of hydrogen-bonded secondary structure in angiotensin II in aqueous solution. Proc. nat. Acad. Sci. (Wash.) **69**, 378 (1972).

RASSMUSSEN, H.: Cell receptor sites for peptide hormones. In: Protein and Polypeptide Hormones, Proceedings of the International Symposium, Liège 1971 (MARGOULIES, M., GREENWOOD, F. C., Eds.). ICS 241. Excerpta med. (Amst.) **1**, 194 (1971).

RODBELL, M., BIRNBAUMER, L., POHL, S. L., KRANS, H. M. J.: Regulation of glucagon action at its receptor. In: Protein and Polypeptide Hormones, Proceedings of the International Symposium, Liège 1971 (MARGOULIES, M., GREENWOOD, F. C., Eds.). ICS 241. Excerpta med. (Amst.) **1**, 199 (1971).

ROSSKAMP, E., KAUFMANN, W.: Radioimmunologische Bestimmung von Angiotensin II. Klin. Wschr. **49**, 876 (1971).

RÖSSLER, R., HORNEF, W., KLAUS, D., SIMSCH, A.: Bestimmung der Plasmareninaktivität durch radioimmunologischen Nachweis von Angiotensin I. Klin. Wschr. **49**, 870 (1971).

SCHRÖDER, E., LÜBKE, K.: The Peptides, Bd. 2, pp. 52—61. New York: Academic Press 1966.

SCHWYZER, R.: Chemical structure and biological activity in the field of polypeptide hormones. Pure Appl. Chem. **6**, 265 (1963).

SCHWYZER, R., SCHILLER, P., FAUCHERE, J.-L., KARLAGANIS, G., PELICAN, G.-M.: Adrenocorticotropic hormone (ACTH): Conformations and potential receptor molecules. In: Protein and Polypeptide Hormones, Proceedings of the second international Symposium, Liège 1971 (MARGOULIES, M., GREENWOOD, F. C., Eds.). ICS 241. Excerpta med. (Amst.) **1**, 167 (1971).

SELA, M.: Antigenicity: Some molecular aspects. Science **166**, 1365 (1969).

SELA, M., ARNON, R.: Studies on the chemical basis of the antigenicity of proteins. I. Antigenicity of polypeptidyl gelatins. Biochem. J. **75**, 91 (1960).

SELA, M., KATCHALSKY, E., OLITZKI, A. L.: Anaphylactic shock in guinea pigs sensitized to polytyrosylgelatin. Science **123**, 1129 (1956).

SMEBY, R. R., ARAKAWA, K., BUMPUS, F. M., MARSH, M. M.: A proposed conformation of isoleucyl^{5}-angiotensin II. Biochim. biophys. Acta (Amst.) **58**, 550 (1962).

SPRAGG, J., TALAMO, R. C., SUZUKI, K., APPELBAUM, D. M., AUSTEN, K. F., HABER, E.: Structural requirements for binding of bradykinin to antibody. II. Studies with bradykinin fragments. Biochemistry **7**, 4086 (1968).

STASON, W. B., VALLOTTON, M., HABER, E.: Synthesis of an antigenic copolymer of angiotensin and succinylated poly-L-lysine. Biochim. biophys. Acta (Amst.) **133**, 582 (1967).

STOCKIGT, J. R., COLLINS, R. D., BIGLIERI, E. G.: Determination of plasma renin concentration by angiotensin I immunoassay. Circulat. Res. **28**, **29**, Suppl. II, II—175 (1971).

STOCKIGT, J. R., SHIZGAL, H. M., GANONG, W. F.: The immunologic activity and metabolic fate of angiotensin II and related peptides. In: Protein and Polypeptide Hormones, Proceedings of the second International Symposium, Liège 1971 (MARGOULIES, M., GREENWOOD, F. C., Eds.). ICS 241. Excerpta med. (Amst.) **2**, 290 (1972).

SUNDSFJORD, J. A.: Radioimmunoassay of angiotensin II in plasma. Acta endocr. (Kbh.) **64**, 181 (1970).

TALAMO, R. C., HABER, E., AUSTEN, K. F.: Antibody to bradykinin: effect of carrier and method of coupling on specificity and affinity. J. Immunol. **101**, 333 (1968).

VALLOTTON, M. B.: (1) Radioimmunoassay of angiotensin I and determination of endogenous renin in human plasma. Acta endocr. (Kbh.) **61**, 118 (1969).

VALLOTTON, M. B.: (2) Radioimmunoassays of angiotensin I and II and other small polypeptide hormones. 7th int. Congr. clin. Chem., Geneva/Evian 1969, Vol. 3: Hormones, Lipids and Miscellaneous, pp. 246—253. Basel/München/Paris/New York: Karger 1970.

VALLOTTON, M. B.: (3) Radioimmunoassay of angiotensin I and II for clinical evaluation of the renin-angiotensin system. 7th int. Congr. clin. Chem., Geneva/Evian 1969, Vol. 3: Hormones, Lipids and Miscellaneous, pp. 254—257. Basel/München/Paris/New York: Karger 1970.

VALLOTTON, M. B.: Relationship between chemical structure and antigenicity of angiotensin analogues. Immunochemistry 7, 529 (1970).
VALLOTTON, M. B.: (1) Parallel radioimmunoassays of angiotensin I and of angiotensin II for measurement of renin activity and of circulating active hormone in human plasma. In: Immunological Methods in Endocrinology. Proceedings of Symposium, Ulm 1970, p. 94. Stuttgart: Thieme; New York: Academic Press 1971.
VALLOTTON, M. B.: (2) Comparison of the structural requirements for antigenicity and for biological activity of angiotensin. In: Protein and Polypeptide Hormones, Proceedings of the International Symposium, Liège 1971 (MARGOULIES, M., GREENWOOD, F. C., Eds.). ICS 241. Excerpta med. (Amst.) 1, 57 (1971).
VALLOTTON, M. B., PAGE, L. B., HABER, E.: (1) Radioimmunoassay of angiotensin in human plasma. Nature (Lond.) 215, 714 (1967).
VALLOTTON, M. B., PAGE, B. L., HABER, E., LAGG, S.: (2) Determination of angiotensin II and renin activity in human plasma by radioimmunoassay. J. clin. Invest. 46, 1126 (1967).
WILMSHURST, E. G., ZEUNERT, H. A., GORDON, R. D.: Radioimmunoassay of Angiotensin II in peripheral venous plasma: Effects of diet and posture and application to measurement of renal venous renin ratio. Aust. N. Z. J. Med. 3, 228 (1971).
WORCEL, M., MEYER, M. D., ANGLES D'AURIAC, G.: The role of angiotensin. Indirect studies with antiangiotensin plasma. Circulat. Res. 27, Suppl. II, 223 (1970).

Measurement of Renin and of Angiotensin (Extraction and Bioassay)

R. BOUCHER and J. GENEST

Introduction

Anyone entering the field of the renin-angiotensin system will be faced with a choice of many techniques for the determination of the different components of the system. These are so numerous that it is impossible for one group of investigators to have had direct experience of all the methods. To sort the useful from the less useful or poor ones, could be difficult indeed. However, it is the intention of the authors first to discuss the procedures for measurement of angiotensin and to describe here in some detail some useful techniques for measurement of renin activity or renin concentration. Angiotensin I-converting enzyme, angiotensinases radioimmunoassays are discussed in another chapter.

I. Angiotensin

Ang. II, the effector hormone has been and still is considered the representative parameter of the renin-angiotensin system by many investigators.

SKEGGS et al. (1956) were the first to report a specific method for the assay of angiotensin in blood. In subsequent years, PALADINI et al. (1959); SCORNIK et al. (1960); and BOUCHER et al. (1961, 1964) reported methods for the measurement of angiotensin in blood or plasma. The main objection to these methods is the large amount of blood required for the measurement of circulating angiotensin. Furthermore, no adequate separation of Ang. II from Ang. I was achieved. A continuous assay of Ang. II on the ascending colon of the rat has been described by REGOLI and VANE (1966). When angiotensin is injected into the donor dog, only about 10 to 20% of the angiotensin is estimated in the assay preparation. The lack of sensitivity and specificity of this technique does not permit accurate measurement of circulating blood angiotensin.

Unfortunately, none of the methods currently available permits reliable measurement of low levels of this peptide in plasma or biological fluids. Though the biological assay methods are highly sensitive, they are still not efficient enough to detect the minute amounts of angiotensin which may play a physiopathological role in a reasonably small volume of blood. Recently, highly sensitive radioimmunoassay techniques have been developed. However, antibodies to Ang. I or Ang. II are not as specific as originally claimed and it must be remembered that the degree of specificity of these procedures for measurement of circulating Ang. I or Ang. II depends somewhat on the efficiency of the steps taken to purify the angiotensins and to eliminate interfering materials.

It must be emphasized that quantitative work with small amounts of angiotensin is difficult. Ang. I and Ang. II are strongly adsorbed on glass and plastic, and loss due to adsorption increases with increasing purity and dilution of the peptides. This has been overcome in various ways. SKEGGS et al. (1954) used sodium carbonate-bicarbonate buffer. Soluble casein 0.25% or 0.1% sodium lauryl sulfate (PAGE and BUMPUS, 1961) and lysozyme (VALLOTTON et al., 1967) have been reported as effective agents to eliminate this adsorption onto the walls of glass or polyethylene vessels. Siliconized containers have been used and more recently 1% bovine serum albumin in a borate buffer, final pH 7.5 (designated 1% BSA) has been extensively used, mainly in radioimmunoassay techniques, to prevent adsorption losses of angiotensins. There is great variation in recovery between the pure peptides and crude angiotensins; probably because of the detergent action of peptide or protein impurities no loss by adsorption is generally observed.

The successful separation of angiotensins from protein and peptide mixtures resulting from either enzymatic formation or chemical synthesis of these octapeptides requires the application of more than one technique. Ion-exchange resin such as Dowex 50, gel filtration, chromatography on derivative cellulose or dextran gels, or paper electrophoresis and chromatography have been used. These different methods have been well summarized in different reviews (SCHWYZER, 1960; PAGE and BUMPUS, 1961; PAGE and MCCUBBIN, 1968). More recently the behaviour of angiotensin octapeptides has been studied during chromatography on polyacrylamide (bio-gel, P-2) and dextran (Sephadex G-15) by GREGERMAN et al. (1970), and [ASP]-Ang. II was readily separatable from [ASN]-Ang. II.

The first separation of Ang. II from Ang. I was achieved by SKEGGS et al. (1954). These workers used countercurrent distribution of angiotensin produced from horse angiotensinogen with hog renin in a solvent system composed of n-butanol and 0.05 N sodium phosphate (pH 7.0).

After 50 transfers, the faster-moving material was Ang. I and the slower-moving material was Ang. II. BUMPUS et al. (1956) also used the countercurrent distribution to separate the two angiotensins. The separation of Ang. I and Ang. II by paper chromatography has been reported by SCHWYZER (1958) and WISENBAUGH et al. (1964). Though good separation of the peptides was possible, quantitative separation is extremely difficult to carry out, especially with small amounts of angiotensins. More recently the difference in isoelectric point between Ang. I (pH 7.5) and Ang. II (pH 7.0) has been utilized for their quantitative separation on ionic exchange resin by BOUCHER et al. (1970). Passage on Dowex 50W-X8 of a mixture of Ang. I and Ang. II in 0.25 M up to 0.4 M pyridine solution retained quantitatively Ang. I while Ang. II was not adsorbed under these experimental conditions. All technical steps must be executed with care to obtain high and reproducible recoveries. Because of the very short in-vivo half-life of angiotensin more sensitive analytical methods are needed. Radioimmunological assays show great promise in this direction, although it is unfortunate that up to now no serious effort has been made to eliminate interfering fragment of angiotensin or other substances distorting the radioimmunoassay.

II. Methods for Measurements of "Renin"

During recent years, the measurement of plasma-renin activity (PRA) or plasma-renin concentration (PRC) in peripheral or/and renal venous blood has become an important tool for investigators and clinicians in evaluation of hypertensive patients, mostly for the correct diagnosis of primary aldosteronism, especially of the normokalemic form, and in establishing the functional significance of renal artery stenosis.

There has been a considerable amount of discussion on methods for the measurement of "renin".

The first methods reported for the estimation of "renin" consisted of direct intravenous injection of alcohol-dried kidney powder (PICKERING and PRINZMETAL, 1938) or crude extracts obtained from incubation medium, where the angiotensin formed was not adequately protected against angiotensinases [LELOIR et al., 1940 (1, 2)], and KOHLSTAEDT and PAGE, 1940]. Needless to say, they are grossly inaccurate and could reflect variation in renin activity mostly in samples where this enzyme was markedly elevated.

Many different methods of measuring the plasma-renin values have been reported in recent years. Basically, they all depend on the incubation of plasma in vitro under predetermined conditions of time, pH and temperature, with or without added substrate to generate angiotensin. Chelating agents such as salt of ethylenediaminetetraacetate (EDTA), 2,3-dimercapto-1-propanol (BAL), 8-hydroxyquinoline or diisopropylfluorophosphate (DFP) are added to inhibit angiotensinases. Dowex 50W-X2 (NH_4^+), (BOUCHER et al. 1964) and more recently, antibodies to angiotensin (POULSEN, 1971) have been added to the incubation mixture to capture the angiotensin formed and thereby protect it against enzymatic degradation. Contamination with microorganisms may destroy the angiotensin if incubation is prolonged. This can be avoided by using appropriate antiseptics (neomycin, chlorhexidine, toluene, bacitracin, and sodium azide have been used).

It is evident that when excess substrate is not assured, the incubation time will become particularly critical in the measurement of angiotensin-production rate. Two, three and four hours are employed frequently. The angiotensin formed is then measured in a bioassay system. The most commonly employed bioassay is the blood-pressure response of nephrectomized rats which seems to be particularly indicated for an angiotensin determination, although non-nephrectomized rats with pharmacological ganglionic blockade have been widely used (PEART, 1955; BOUCHER et al., 1961; BLAQUIER et al., 1962; BING, 1964; PICKENS et al., 1965; SOKABE, 1965). Some investigators have combined nephrectomy and ganglion blockade (CONN et al., 1964; GUNNELS et al., 1967). Various methods using isolated organs and superfusion technique (REGOLI and VANE, 1964; COHN and NORTARGIACOMO, 1969; LEMIEUX and REGOLI, 1971) have been described for the quantitative evaluation of angiotensin. The lack of specificity of these methods and the variations in sensitivity encountered in the course of an assay largely counterbalance the slight advantage they may possess in simplicity and rapidity of preparation as compared with the intact animal.

When endogenous substrate in the plasma is used to generate the angiotensin, the value obtained is called "plasma-renin activity" (PRA). When exogeneous substrate is added to the incubation mixture, the value obtained is referred to as the "plasma-renin concentration" (PRC). Other attempts to control the substrate variable have been proposed, including concomitant estimation of angiotensinogen and the demonstration of the linear generation of angiotensin in the original plasma. Under extreme conditions where the renin is high and the endogenous substrate low, PRC differs from PRA. It must be emphasized that while PRC is an important parameter, PRA is easier to measure and in most cases its value is adequate for diagnostic purposes. Furthermore it does reflect the in-vivo capacity to form angiotensin to an extent.

a) Methods Proposed for Measurement of Plasma-Renin Activity

The simplicity of methods using whole plasma has brought them into more general use. Three techniques are commonly used.

1. The first is described by HELMER and JUDSON (1963). The plasma is obtained from heparinized, cooled blood. The pH of the plasma is adjusted to 5.5 and the plasma is dialyzed against cold running tap water at 13 °C for 18 to 20 h. After dialysis, plasma pH is readjusted to 5.5 and after centrifuging, the supernatant is made isotonic by addition of 0.26 ml of saturated sodium-chloride solution per 10 ml of plasma. Samples are then incubated at pH 5.5 for 1 h at 37 °C and the amount of angiotensin liberated is measured into assay preparations: 1) The spirally cut strip of rabbit aorta and 2) a pitted cat, nephrectomized two days previously. GUNNELS et al. (1967) later used essentially this method, but replaced the biological assay procedures of HELMER by a pressor assay in bilaterally nephrectomized, pentolinium-treated rats.

Although this was the first method to demonstrate clearly the feasibility of the assay of renin in human plasma, many objections can be raised. Dialysis to remove vasoactive agents might activate other enzymatic systems (kinin-releasing enzymes and others), thus adding new interfering substances. Another important point is the possibility that renin itself may be partially destroyed or inactivated during dialysis or incubation. Degradation of renin by human plasma has been clearly demonstrated in the absence of EDTA (SCHAECHTELIN et al., 1968; REGOLI, 1970) and it lowers the detection limit of the method. Finally, another criticism, which unfortunately applies to practically all the methods reported is the so-called quantitative measurement of angiotensin formed in a crude extract without purification before assay. This basic error may contribute to inaccurate results and misunderstanding of the renin-angiotensin system.

Finally, the value of this and similar techniques (FASCIOLO et al., 1964) depends largely on the pH during incubation at which angiotensinases are less active, no inhibitors of proteolytic enzymes being added. It is evident that this method is less useful or less accurate for other species where the optimum pH for renin is similar to angiotensinases.

2. The second technique was proposed by BOUCHER et al. (1964). Its essential features are the adsorption of angiotensin during incubation onto Dowex 50W-X2 (NH_4^+). The ammonium salt of EDTA is also employed as an inhibitor of many proteolytic enzymes. This procedure has the advantage over that proposed by HELMER, not only of protecting the angiotensin formed during incubation but at the same time offering a convenient way of purifying it, eliminating many known (norepinephrine, arginine vasopressine, serotonin, bradykinin, tyramine) and possibly unknown substances that could interfere in the assay. This procedure was first described some eight years ago and is still used extensively, in its original form or in one or another of its modifications (BLAUFOX et al., 1966; IWAI et al., 1970; IMAY and SOKABE, 1967; MEURER et al., 1970; MIURA, 1969).

Though the method is extremely simple, some obvious precautions often neglected by investigators should be emphasized. Dowex 50W-X2 may be obtained from Bio-Rad Laboratories (Richmond, California). The most commonly used particle-size range has the dry mesh designation of 100 to 200. The total exchange capacity (mEq/ml) of each new batch must be controlled. The resin is ready for use after it has been cycled through the 4 N NaOH distilled H_2O, 2 N HCl, and distilled H_2O and the fine particles have been removed to ensure good column flow. Finally the resin is converted to the ammonium form by washing with several volumes of 0.2 M NH_4OH followed by a final equilibration with 0.2 M $NH_4CH_3CO_2$ at pH 6. A second important point is the evaporation of the angiotensin-containing eluate under reduced pressure; this must be performed under high vacuum, to ensure complete removal of volatile salt. Obviously metallic salts formed in the metallic rotary evaporators generally used for such purposes must not reach the sample. All-glass evaporators or glass traps between the evaporating flask and the vacuum system are essential to eliminate possible contamination by metallic salt that interferes in the rat blood pressure assay. Although this method is accurate, shows good reproducibility and is suitable for routine clinical investigation, from a biochemical point of view, further purification of the final product before assay would be useful.

The third technique was reported by PICKENS et al. (1965). In this procedure, plasma is dialyzed at 0 to 4 °C for 24 h against a solution of the salt of EDTA and for another 24 h against distilled water. After addition of di-isopropylfluorophosphate (DFP) the dialyzed plasma is incubated at pH 5.5 and 37 °C for 4 h. The enzymatic reaction is stopped by heating in a boiling water bath for 10 min and the crude supernatant is injected without further processing.

Sodium (BIS) — ethylenediaminetetraacetate and DFP are used as angiotensinases inhibitors and their use yields adequate results, although protection of the end product is not complete. Direct measurement of the hormone in a crude extract is far from satisfactory and, as mentioned earlier, at least one purification step should be added before the assay. KLAUS and HEIZMANN (1968) found that BOUCHER's method was superior, as that of PICKENS often lacked precision because of interfering depressor substances. The lack of purification of the angiotensin fraction before assay could explain this finding.

A combination of the methods of BOUCHER et al. (1964) and PICKENS et al. (1965) has been proposed by MIURA (1969). The use of DFP alone is not sufficient to inhibit the activity of angiotensinases and a modification such as that proposed by GOCKE et al. (1958) cannot therefore be recommended. The methods of HELMER and JUDSON (1963); BOUCHER et al. (1964); and PICKENS et al. (1965) have been described recently by SMEBY and BUMPUS (1970).

b) Plasma Renin Concentration (PRC)

The most elaborate techniques reported for the measurement of PRC are those of BROWN et al. [1964 (1, 2)] and LEVER et al. (1964). This procedure represents an important attempt to measure "true renin concentration". This is achieved at great and variable loss (mean recovery of renin: 37% by chromatography on diethylaminoethyl cellulose (DEAE) column). The renin eluate is dialyzed at pH 3 for 24 h in order to destroy remaining traces of substrate and angiotensinases. It is well known that renin is far more stable than angiotensinogen and angiotensinases, but such treatment involves some degree of denaturation of the renin itself. Several modifications and improvements of this technique have been reported (COOK and LEE, 1965; LEE et al., 1966). Considering the relative instability of renin, and the numerous difficulties in consecutive purification of plasma renin, such approaches to the evaluation of PRC are not popular and are being used less and less. A number of workers have reported improved or simplified versions for measurement of PRC. In most cases, these include the addition of homologous or heterologous substrate to untreated plasma (GOULD et al., 1966; HAAS et al., 1968; SKINNER, 1967; DAHLHEIM et al., 1970; ARAKAWA et al., 1968; KLAULHAUSEN et al., 1970; RYAN et al., 1968).

A micromethod for repeatedly measuring PRC in small amounts of rat plasma (0.1 ml) was reported by BOUCHER et al. (1967) and later adapted to dog (GRANGER et al., 1970; HAYDUK et al., 1970).

c) Other Methods

Measurement of renin by inhibition of the enzymatically active renin as a function of the concentration of antirenin has been proposed (POULSEN, 1966;

KEUTEL et al., 1967). Problems of specificity, species differences and presence of different forms of renins introduce many pitfalls and the accuracy of such procedures is questionable.

POULSEN (1967) reported a micromethod for the measurement of renin in plasma, based on determination of the substrate concentration instead of measurement of the angiotensin produced. This method is an improvement of the procedure described by LELOIR et al. [1940 (2)] and MUÑOZ et al. (1943). The many problems in connection with this technique (two incubation periods, possible breakdowns of substrate by proteolytic enzymes different from renin, lack of purification of the final product before assay) make it cumbersome and complex.

A different approach is that of ROTH and REINHARZ [1966 (1, 2)]. The synthetic substrate N-CBO-Pro-Phe-His-Leu-Leu-Val-Tyr-Ser-β-naphthylamine has been used. Renin attacks this substituted peptide by cleaving the Leu-Leu bond. The resulting tetrapeptide is then degraded by an excess of aminopeptidase M and gives rise to β-naphthylamine which can be measured spectrophotometrically, the rate of release of β-naphthylamine being proportional to the concentration of renin. However, this method was established with purified renin; the presence of other plasma proteolytic enzymes seemed to interfere considerably and this method is not useful for PRC measurement in the form described.

An alternative approach, perhaps more promising, to the measurement of plasma renin value has been pursued by SKEGGS et al. (1969) and MENDELSOHN and JOHNSTON (1971). The rate of formation of [^{14}C Val_3]-Ang. I from the substrate ^{14}C Val_3 tetradecapeptide is proportional to the quantity of renin added. However, longer periods of incubation are needed to liberate enough ^{14}C-labelled Ang. I to give reliable measurements. This adds difficulties of assaying plasma renin because of the associated problems of non-specific breakdown of ^{14}C-labelled tetradecapeptide by non-specific plasma peptidases (MONTAGUE et al., 1966). The rapid hydrolysis of the synthetic substrate might explain, at least in part, the finding of SKEGGS et al. (1963) that, when the tetradecapeptide is added to serum its rate of hydrolysis is severely reduced. It must also be stressed that with this substrate the rate of formation of Ang. I, as compared to the natural substrate, is far greater with tissue renin than with kidney renin (SKEGGS et al., 1969; GANTEN et al., 1971). For these reasons, it seems that the use of the tetradecapeptide might have limited use in the measurement of plasma-renin activity. Further work is needed to improve the sensitivity and specificity of these methods to measure the low levels of renin in plasma.

Dog-renin substrate labelled with ^{125}I has also been tried for PRC (NASH et al., 1968).

LEVINE et al. (1970) reported an automated chemical method for measurement of renin in hog kidney extract. The method is accurate and much quicker than biological assay. Although not sufficiently sensitive to detect renin at normal plasma concentrations it is a convenient way to determine renin activity in kidney tissues.

Discussion and Conclusion

It must be borne in mind that "true renin concentration" cannot be measured. This would entail the extraction of renin followed by purification and incubation in the presence of purified substrate, which is currently unattainable especially with small amounts of renin. Furthermore, different renins with different affinities for a particular substrate are known to exist. The nature of the enzyme may also be modified by extraction procedures and acidification (SKEGGS et al., 1967). Purification attempted by some investigators in order to evaluate PRC does not rule out the possible presence of activator(s) or inhibitor(s) in the semipurified renin extract or substrate preparation. Furthermore, the occurrence of more than one renin substrate with different rates of reaction with renin and competing with each other can influence the formation of angiotensin.

It is interesting, that the optimum pH of renin varies with species and for the same enzyme depending on the substrate used. For human renin an optimum pH of 5.5 is obtained with human substrate and tetradecapeptide (HELMER and JUDSON, 1963; BOUCHER et al., 1964; and WALDHAUSL et al., 1970). The optimum pH is 7.5 to 8.5 in the presence of hog substrate (WALDHAUSL et al., 1970). Up to now, no physiological implication of the low optimum pH of human renin with the natural substrate as compared to other species has been found.

Recently it has been re-emphasized that inhibitors of angiotensinases are also effective inhibitors of the converting enzyme and that the end product of incubation is Ang. I in most cases.

However, Ang. II or a mixture of Ang. I and Ang. II may be present in certain circumstances. BOUCHER et al. (1972) reported a new Ang. I-converting enzyme (β-converting enzyme). This enzyme is not inhibited by the chelating agents currently used for renin-activity techniques, although it is inhibited by a plasma protein. It is possible that in certain physiopathological conditions this Ang. I β-converting enzyme might be activated and Ang. II formed even in presence of EDTA, or other chelating agents.

This is important, since in an individual rat used for bioassay the relative responsiveness to Ang. I as compared to Ang. II may vary by as much as 50% or more. Considering that Ang. I seems to be the end product of the enzymatic reaction with most procedures, it is important to use Ang. I for bioassay standards rather than Ang. II. On the other hand, variations in α- and β-Ang. I-converting enzymes in the plasma aliquots to be assayed may influence the ratio of the two peptides. It appears that the best way would be to complete the enzyme reaction of the final product Ang. II, and that β-Ang. I-converting enzyme would be an enzyme of choice to achieve this goal.

Up to now, [ASP (NH_2) 1-Val 5]-Ang. II, which is largely supplied by the Ciba Laboratories, is used as an unofficial standard and most measurements are expressed in terms of this synthetic preparation. The many arbitrary units used currently for expressing PRA or PRC have been a source of some confusion among clinical investigators. The establishment of international renin and angiotensin standards and assay is an important and desirable goal. The problem is obviously complicated by crude reactants and variation in methodology. In this respect, it is important to emphasize that each laboratory must have its own set of control values its own range of renin response by normal subjects to different stimuli, such as upright posture, sodium restriction or furosemide administration. Yet no angiotensin preparation has been accepted as international standard. This standard should behave identically to the generated compound, in bioassay as well as in immunoassay. Different structures of angiotensin obtained in the presence of exogenous substrate and different renin from various species complicate the problem of standardization.

The difficulties inherent in the adequat determination of renin activity, renin concentration, substrate, different forms of substrates or other parameters, which under certain physiopathological conditions might alter the rate of generation of angiotensin, are likely to remain with us for quite some time. It is therefore important that new developments in technique should permit not only accurate but also more rapid analysis of these parameters. It must be stressed that more effort should be made to purify substances to be analyzed to avoid the reliability of the method being based on the relative specificity of bioassay or immunoassay techniques. Methods reported up to now have made progress possible in this field. However, there is still a great deal of work be done in the further refinement of the methodology. It is becoming more and more evident that the control and knowledge of many formerly, unsuspected variables, enzymatic and non-enzymatic, are essential to the understanding of the renin-angiotensin system and its involvement in sodium regulation and in hypertensive diseases. Only further enzymatic and chemical advances will improve our knowledge on this complex enzymatic system.

References

ARAKAWA, K., MINOHARA, A., YAMADA, J., UEMURA, N., NAKAMURA, M.: Micro-determination of human plasma renin activity with the addition of homologous substrate. Clin. chim. Acta **22**, 309 (1968).

BING, J.: Mechanisms of the increased sensitivity to renin in nephrectomized animals. Acta path. microbiol. scand. **60**, 311 (1964).

BLAQUIER, P., HOOBLER, S. W., SCHROEDER, J., GOMEZ, A., KREULEN, T.: Effect of bilateral nephrectomy on pressor response to renin. Amer. J. Physiol. **203**, 339 (1962).

BLAUFOX, M., BIRBARI, A., HICKLER, R. B., MERRILL, J. P.: Peripheral plasma renin activity in renal homotransplant recipients. New Engl. J. Med. **275**, 1165 (1965).

BOUCHER, R., BIRON, P., GENEST, J.: Procedure for isolation and determination of human blood angiotensin. Canad. J. Biochem. **39**, 581 (1961).

BOUCHER, R., KURIHARA, H., GRISE, C., GENEST, J.: Measurement of plasma angiotensin I converting enzyme activity. Circulat. Res. **XXVI** and **XXVII**, I—83 (1970).

BOUCHER, R., MENARD, J., GENEST, J.: A micromethod for measurement of renin in the plasma and kidney of rats. Can. J. Physiol. Pharmacol. **45**, 881 (1967).

BOUCHER, R., SAIDI, M., GENEST, J.: A new "angiotensin I converting enzyme" system. In: Hypertension 1972 (GENEST, J., KOIW, E., Eds.). Berlin-Heidelberg-New York: Springer 1972.

BOUCHER, R., VEYRAT, R., DE CHAMPLAIN, J., GENEST, J.: New procedures for measurement of human plasma angiotensin and renin activity levels. Canad. med. Ass. J. **90**, 194 (1964).

BROWN, J. J., DAVIES, D. L., LEVER, A. F., ROBERTSON, J. I. S.: (1) Variations in plasma renin concentration in several physiological and pathological states. Canad. med. Ass. J. **90**, 201 (1964).

BROWN, J. J., DAVIES, D. L., LEVER, A. F., ROBERTSON, J. I. S., TREE, M.: (2) The estimation of renin in human plasma. Biochem. J. **93**, 594 (1964).

BUMPUS, F. M., SCHWARZ, H., PAGE, I. H.: Partial separation of an oxytocic principle from preparations of angiotonin. Circulat. Res. **4**, 488 (1956).

COHN, J. N., NOTARGIACOMO, A. V.: Clinical application of a simple specific bioassay technique for measuring renin activity. Amer. J. med. Sci. **257**, 344 (1969).

CONN, J. W., COHEN, E. L., ROVNER, D. R.: Suppression of plasma renin activity in primary aldosteronism. J. Amer. med. Ass. **190**, 213 (1964).

COOK, W. F., LEE, M. R.: The preparation of rabbit renin-substrate for the assay of minute amounts of renin. Biochem. J. **96**, 413 (1965).

DAHLHEIM, H., GRANGER, P., THURAU, K.: A sensitive method for determination of renin activity in the single juxtaglomerular apparatus of the rat kidney. Pflügers Arch. ges. Physiol. **34**, 303 (1970).

FASCIOLO, J. C., DE VITO, E., ROMERO, J. C., CUCCHI, J. N.: The renin content of the blood of humans and dogs under several conditions. Canad. med. Ass. J. **90**, 206 (1964).

GANTEN, D., MARQUEZ-JULIO, A., GRANGER, P., HAYDUK, K., KARSUNKY, K. P., BOUCHER, R., GENEST, J.: Renin in Dog Brain. Amer. J. Physiol. **221** (6), 1733 (1971).

GOCKE, D. J., SHERWOOD, L. M., OPENHOFF, I., GERTEN, J., LARAGH, J. H.: Measurement of plasma angiotensin II and correlation with renin activity. J. clin. Endocr. **28**, 1675 (1968).

GOULD, A. B., SKEGGS, L. T., KAHN, J. R.: Measurement of renin and substrate concentrations in human serum. Lab. Invest. **15**, 1802 (1966).

GRANGER, P., BOUCHER, R., GENEST, J.: Method for determination of renin activity in dog's plasma and renal tissue. Can. J. Physiol. Pharmacol. **48** (7), 457 (1970).

GREGERMAN, R. I., WEAVER, T., KOWATCH, M. A.: Behavior of angiotensin octapeptides and dinitrophenyl-angiotensin during chromatography on polyacrylamide and dextran gels. J. Chromatog. **47**, 369 (1970).

GUNNELS, J. C., GRIM, C. E., ROBINSON, R. R., WILDERMANN, N. M.: Plasma renin activity in healthy subjects and patients with hypertension. Arch. intern. Med. **119**, 232 (1967).

HAAS, E., GOULD, A. B., GOLDBLATT, H.: Estimation of endogenous renin in human blood. Lancet **1968 I**, 657.
HAYDUK, K., BOUCHER, R., GENEST, J.: Renin activity content in various tissues of dogs under different physiopathological states. Proc. Soc. exp. Biol. (N. Y.) **134**, 252 (1970).
HELMER, O. M., JUDSON, W. E.: The quantitative determination of renin in the plasma of patients with arterial hypertension. Circulation **27**, 1050 (1963).
IMAI, M., SOKABE, H.: A method for the determination of plasma renin activity in small samples. Jap. Heart J. **8**, 607 (1967).
IWAI, J., KNUDSEN, K. D., DAHL, L. K.: Genetic influence on the renin-angiotensin system. J. exp. Med. **131**, 543 (1970).
KAULHAUSEN, H., FILLMANN, B., BREVER, H.: Determination of renin activity in human plasma. Biochem. J. 8 (3), 254 (1970).
KEUTEL, H. J., OUTZEN, H. C., WEAVER, R. G.: Application of the renin-antirenin assay in experimental hypertension: A preliminary report. Invest. Urol. **5**, 107 (1967).
KLAUS, D., HEIZMANN, A.: Methoden für die Bestimmung der Reninaktivität im Plasma. Z. klin. Chem. **6**, 1 (1968).
KOHLSTAEDT, K. G., PAGE, I. H.: The liberation of renin by perfusion of kidneys following reduction of pulse pressure. J. exp. Med. **72**, 201 (1940).
LEE, M. R., COOK, W. F., MCKENZIE, J. K.: A sensitive method for assay of plasma renin activity. Circulat. Res. **XIX**, 260 (1966).
LELOIR, L. F., MUÑOZ, J. M., BRAUN-MENENDEZ, E., FASCIOLO, J. C.: (1) La secrecion de renina y la formacion de hypertensina. Rev. Soc. argent. Biol. **16**, 75 (1940).
LELOIR, L. F., MUÑOZ, J. M., BRAUN-MENENDEZ, E., FASCIOLO, J. C.: (2) Dosaje de la renina. Rev. Soc. argent. Biol. **16**, 635 (1940).
LEMIEUX, R., REGOLI, D.: Une méthode simple et specifique pour la mesure de l'activité réninique du plasma chez l'homme. Un. méd. Can. **100**, 727 (1971).
LEVER, A. F., ROBERTSON, J. I. S., TREE, M.: The estimation of renin in plasma by an enzyme kinetic technique. Biochem. J. **91**, 346 (1964).
LEVINE, M., DORER, F. E., KAHN, J. R., LENTZ, K. E., SKEGGS, L. T.: Chemical determination of hog kidney renin by an automated method. Ann. Biochem. **34** (2), 366 (1970).
MENDELSOHN, F. A., JOHNSTON, C. I.: A radiochemical renin assay. Biochem. J. **121**, 241 (1971).
MEURER, K. A., GANTEN, D., KAUFFMANN, W.: A test for assessing the responsiveness of plasma renin activity. Germ. Med. Mth. **V**, 606 (1970).
MIURA, Y.: Measurement of renin activity in human plasma. Tohoku J. exp. Med. **98** (2), 125 (1969).
MONTAGUE, D., RINIKER, B., BRUNNER, H., GROSS, F.: Synthesis and biological activities of a tetradecapeptide renin substrate. Amer. J. Physiol. **210** (3), 591 (1966).
MUÑOZ, J. M., TAQUINI, A. C., BRAUN-MENENDEZ, E., FASCIOLO, J. C., LELOIR, L. F.: Metodo para la medicione de la renina humana. Rev. Soc. argent. Biol. **19**, 321 (1943).
NASH, F. D., BAILIE, M. D., WATHEN, R. L., ROSTORFER, H. H.: An approach automated determination of renin activity in plasma. Automat. Anal. Chem. Technicon Symp. **1**, 599 (1968).
PAGE, I. H., BUMPUS, F. M.: Angiotensin. Physiol. Rev. **41**, 331 (1961).
PAGE, I. H., MCCUBBIN, J. W.: Angiotensin. In: Renal Hypertension, pp. 64—98. Chicago: Year Book Medical Publishers 1968.
PALADINI, A. C., BRAUN-MENENDEZ, E., DEL FRADE, I. S., MASSANI, Z. M.: The estimation of angiotensin in blood. J. Lab. clin. Med. **53**, 264 (1959).
PEART, W. S.: A new method of large scale preparation of hypertensin, with a note on its assay. Biochem. J. **59**, 300 (1955).
PICKENS, P. T., BUMPUS, F. M., LLOYD, A. M., SMEBY, R. R., PAGE, I. H.: Measurement of renin activity in human plasma. Circulat. Res. **17**, 438 (1965).
PICKERING, G. W., PRINZMETAL, M.: Some observations on renin, a pressor substance contained in normal kidney, together with a method for its biological assay. Clin. Sci. **3**, 211 (1938).
POULSEN, K.: Kinetic and measurement of the renin-antirenin system. Acta path. microbiol. scand. **68**, 197 (1966).
POULSEN, K.: Microtechnique for quantitative measurement of renin in plasma. Acta path. microbiol. scand. **69**, 19 (1967).
POULSEN, K.: Simplified method for radioimmunoassay of enzymo systems. Application on the human renin-angiotensin system. J. Lab. clin. Med. **78**, 309 (1971).
REGOLI, D.: Renin inactivation by human plasma. Can. J. Physiol. Pharmacol. **48** (6), 350 (1970).
REGOLI, D., VANE, J. R.: A sensitive method for the assay of angiotensin. Brit. J. Pharmacol. **23**, 351 (1964).

REGOLI, D., VANE, J. R.: The continuous estimation of angiotensin formed in the circulation of the dog. J. Physiol. **183**, 513 (1966).

ROTH, M., REINHARZ, A.: (1) Un dosage chimique de la rénine. Helv. physiol. pharmacol. Acta **24**, 115 (1966).

ROTH, M., REINHARZ, A.: (2) Un substrat pour le dosage chimique de la rénine. Helv. chim Acta **49**, 1903 (1966).

RYAN, J. W., MCKENZIE, J. K., LEE, M. R.: A rapid simple method for the assay of renin in rabbit plasma. Biochem. J. **108**, 679 (1968).

SCHAECHTELIN, G., BAECHTOLD, N., HAEFELI, L., REGOLI, D., GAUDRY-PAREDES, A., PETERS, G.: A renin-inactivating system in rat plasma. Amer. J. Physiol. **215**, 632 (1968).

SCHWYZER, R., TURRIAN, H.: The chemistry and pharmacology of angiotensin. Vitam. and Horm. **18**, 237 (1960).

SCORNIK, O. A., PALADINI, A. C., BRAUN-MENENDEZ, E.: Further improvements on a method for the estimation of angiotensin in blood. Acta physiol. lat.-amer. **10**, 64 (1960).

SKEGGS, L. T., KAHN, J. R., SHUMWAY, N. P.: The preparation and function of the hypertensin converting enzyme. J. exp. Med. **103**, 295 (1956).

SKEGGS, L. T., LENTZ, K. E., KAHN, J. R., HOCHSTRASSER, H.: Studies on the preparation and properties of renin. Circulat. Res. Supp. **21**, II—91 (1967).

SKEGGS, L. T., LENTZ, K. E., KAHN, J. R., DORER, F. E., LEVINE, M.: Pseudorenin. A new angiotensin-forming enzyme. Circulat. Res. **25**, 451 (1969).

SKEGGS, L. T., MARSCH, W. H., KAHN, J. R., SHUMWAY, N. P.: The existence of two forms of hypertension. J. exp. Med. **99**, 275 (1954).

SKINNER, S. L.: Improved assay methods for renin "concentration" and "activity" in human plasma. Methods using selective denaturation of renin substrate. Circulat. **1967,** Res. 391.

SMEBY, R. R., BUMPUS, F. M.: Renin. In: Proteolytic Enzymes, Vol. XIX, p. 699 (PERLMANN, G. E., LORAND, L., Eds.). New York 1970.

SOKABE, H.: Renin and euryhalinity in the Japanese eel. Internat. Cong. Physiol. Sc. **23**, 392 (1965).

VALLOTTON, M. B., PAGE, L. B., HABER, E.: Radioimmunoassay of angiotensin in human plasma. Nature (Lond.) **215**, 714 (1967).

WALDHAUSL, W. K., LUCAS, C. P., CONN, J. W., LUTZ, J. H., COHEN, E. L.: Studies on the partial isolation of human renin. Biochim. biophys. Acta (Amst.) **221**, 536 (1970).

WISENBAUGH, P. E., WILLS, N. E., HILL, R. W.: Paper chromatographic identification of angiotensins. Amer. J. Physiol. **207**, 759 (1964).

Angiotensin Immunoassay

G. W. BOYD and W. S. PEART

With 2 Figures

Introduction

In the investigation of the *aetiological role* of the renin-angiotensin system in various clinical and experimental states, direct measurement of the biologically active component of the system, viz. *angiotensin II*, would seem more relevant

Renin + Renin Substrate α_2 globulin*

↓

Angiotensin I (decapeptide)

↓ Converting enzyme (lung)

Angiotensin II (octapeptide)

↓ Tissue clearance

Metabolic degradation

Fig. 1. The renin-angiotensin system. A simplified view of its *in-vivo* mode of operation. * Recent work suggests that in some species, notably man and rat, a large part of renin substrate migrates with an electrophoretic mobility of albumin (NASJLETTI et al., 1971)

than any assessment of plasma renin itself, particularly since the relationship between these two factors is potentially so complex (see Fig. 1). However, until recently, the only practicable method of angiotensin measurement was the rat blood-pressure bioassay system (PEART, 1955), and although this method was applied to the estimation of circulating plasma Ang. II (KAHN et al., 1952; PALADINI et al., 1959; BOUCHER et al., 1964; MORRIS and ROBINSON, 1964; MULROW et al., 1966; MASSANI et al., 1966), it soon emerged that the levels of circulating angiotensin were frequently too low for precise quantitation by this method. Because of this, we and other investigators examined the possibility of radioimmunoassay of Ang. II, and in 1967 reported techniques which were sufficiently sensitive to measure Ang. II levels circulating in normal human subjects (VALLOTTON et al., 1967; BOYD et al., 1967; CATT et al., 1967). This assay has since been developed in various centres, and accumulated experience with the method will be reviewed below.

Quite apart from considerations of aetiology or pathogenesis, the renin-angiotensin system may be *secondarily* altered in various states, and here some index of the overall activity of the system may be extremely useful, particularly from the diagnostic viewpoint in clinical hypertension with suppressed activity of the system, such as occurs in cases of primary hyperaldosteronism. In such cases plasma-renin activity or concentration assays may be more convenient than the more exacting measurement of the circulating level of Ang. II itself, and with the introduction of Ang. II radioimmunoassay, it was natural to look at the application of this method to plasma renin-activity estimation, as a sensitive, specific and rather more convenient alternative to bioassay. Using Ang. II immunoassay of the generation product of plasma incubation in this sort of approach, VALLOTTON et al. (1967) found very much lower values for plasma renin activity than those previously reported by bioassay. However, in keeping with the earlier observations of SKEGGS et al. (1956), it was subsequently shown (BOYD et al., 1967) that materials such as EDTA, which are frequently added to blood for anticoagulation and for "angiotensinase" inhibition during plasma incubation (HABER et al., 1968), may give rise to serious limitation of plasma angiotensin-converting enzyme activity, so that the product of the reaction is not Ang. II but Ang. I, and this reacts only feebly with Ang. II antibodies. Subsequently, the possibility of restoring the activity of plasma-converting enzyme without interfering with the angiotensin inhibition produced by these materials was investigated in our own laboratories, but this approach also proved difficult (FITZ et al., 1971).

An alternative procedure was therefore adopted whereby the renin reaction was stopped deliberately at the Ang. I step, and the Ang. I generated measured by its own specific immunoassay. Initial studies demonstrating the feasibility of this approach were first reported in 1968 at the International Symposium on Protein and Polypeptide Hormones in Liège, Belgium [BOYD et al., 1969 (1)], followed by a more detailed report in 1969 [BOYD et al., 1969 (2)]. In contrast with the previous Ang.-II immunoassay for plasma-renin activity, this method showed good correlation with bioassay [BOYD et al., 1969 (1)]. Similar assays for this measurement of plasma renin activity, or *in-vitro* Ang.-I generation rate, have since been developed in a number of centres (HOLLEMANS et al., 1969; HABER et al., 1969; GIESE et al., 1970; STOCKIGT et al., 1971; VALLOTTON, 1971; COHEN et al., 1971). Other approaches using the application of the Ang. II immunoassay to the estimation of plasma-renin activity have been pursued by some workers (PAGE et al., 1969; POULSEN, 1969, 1971), and some of these will also be considered below.

Since the immunoassay of Ang. I and II present many features and problems in common, they will be considered together first, and later specific aspects of each assay will be reviewed in turn.

Development of Antibodies to Angiotensin

Ang. II is a small molecule (MW = 1046), and at the time of investigation into the possibility of raising antibodies, was considered unlikely to be antigenic in its own right. Therefore various groups of workers linked Ang. II chemically to larger protein or synthetic poly-amino acid molecules and used this as the immunogen. DEODHAR (1960), the first to investigate this approach, was able to show that antibodies raised against such a compound cross-reacted with Ang. II itself. Following this, GOODFRIEND et al. (1964) introduced the carbodiimide method of coupling angiotensin to protein, and this has been the method of choice for workers using this general type of approach since that time (HABER et al., 1965; CATT et al., 1967; GOCKE et al., 1969). These antibodies had a specificity directed largely towards the C-terminal 3 to 8 hexapeptide of Ang. II (see VALLOTTON, 1970, for review) with little involvement of the extreme N-terminus, and it was in an attempt to improve this specificity that we investigated the possibility of raising antibodies against free Ang. II. To this end, angiotensin was merely adsorbed onto fine micro-particles of carbon and the suspension injected with Freund's adjuvant into rabbits, either by the conventional parenteral routes, or better, directly into lymph nodes and spleen (BOYD and PEART, 1968). This resulted in the production of high-titre antibodies to angiotensin, but as it turns out, any increase in specificity over antibodies raised against chemically-linked angiotensin appears to be marginal (VALLOTTON, 1970). Even without adsorption into carbon, Ang. II has recently been shown to be immunogenic when given with Freund's adjuvant alone (DIETRICH, 1966; HEFFERMAN et al., 1967; PIERACH, 1969), with the occasional production of even quite high titres when injected into toepads (PIERACH et al., 1969).

In general, there seems to be little to choose between the method of covalent linkage of angiotensin and that of carbon adsorption in terms of the specificity, avidity or titre of the resultant antibody. In a small study, VALLOTTON et al. (1970) found that antibodies were rather slower to develop with the carbon technique, and although the differences seem marginal, our general findings are in agreement with this. Regardless of the technique, however, our initial experience that titres are higher if the primary injections are given directly into lymph nodes and spleen (BOYD and PEART, 1968) still seems to hold true.

The specificity of angiotensin antibodies is discussed elsewhere in this handbook (VALLOTTON, 1972). Suffice it to say here that most Ang.-II antibodies have a specificity directed largely towards the C-terminal hexapeptide, so that the 2-8 heptapeptide and 3-8 hexapeptide fragments may be detected by the immunoassay as well as Ang. II itself. This bears on the question of the specificity of measurements *in vivo* and this will be discussed in detail below. Most Ang. II antibodies show only slight cross-reaction with Ang. I. They are variable (25 to 100%) in their degree of cross-reaction with native human Ang. II, which is the $Ileu^5$ form (ARAKAWA et al., 1967), so that it is important to test this before using any particular antibody in human studies. Incidentally this variability of cross-reaction with $Ileu^5$ angiotensin can be used to great effect in the characterization of the form of angiotensin native to any given species (CAIN et al., 1970; MACDONALD et al., 1970). The Ang. I antibodies show very little cross-reaction with Ang. II, and again the specificity is directed more towards the C-terminal end of the molecule [BOYD et al., 1969 (2); VALLOTTON, 1970].

A finding of interest and of some practical consequence emerged during studies of our antibodies, i.e. that antibody plasmas from about half our rabbits showed a greatly reduced capacity to react with Ang. II in the presence of a low concentration of EDTA, and this was reversible by the addition of a slight molar excess of calcium or even some other divalent metal ions [BOYD et al., 1967; BOYD, 1969 (1)]. The mechanism of this effect does not appear to involve complement [BOYD, 1969 (1)], but it may be related to a similar effect observed by MAURER et al. (1970) with antibodies to poly-amino acids. These workers (LIBERTI et al., 1971) have recently suggested that their antigen may possess a different conformational structure in the presence of calcium ions, due to bridging of two glutamyl-carboxyl residues, and although such an explanation cannot be extended directly to antibodies against Ang. II *amide*, the mechanism may be related. This work makes it unlikely that our findings are related to the technique of adsorption of angiotensin onto carbon for the purposes of immunization so it will always have to be borne in mind when there is any question of non-specific interference in angiotensin immunoassays. Even the small amounts of EDTA which are carried through our plasma-Ang. II-extraction method may be sufficient to interfere with the assay, so we routinely guard against the problem by the addition of 0.02 M calcium chloride to all immunoassay buffers.

It has not usually been found necessary to purify the specific antibody globulin from plasma for use in the assay, even though quite elegant techniques are available for this purpose (HURWITZ et al., 1970). However, when low dilutions of antibody plasma are used (less than 1:200), we think it advisable to heat the plasma at 56 °C for thirty minutes to inhibit converting-enzyme and "angiotensinase" activity which could otherwise interfere with the assay.

Labelled Angiotensin

Both Ang. I and Ang. II contain a tyrosine molecule in the 4-position, and so may readily be labelled with ^{125}I or ^{131}I. Most workers have used the technique of GREENWOOD et al. (1963), and although this method has been applied widely in radioimmunoassay, there are a few features of its application to angiotensin labelling which warrant special mention. In the first place, to obtain a good quality label repeatedly with minimum "damage" (see below), we have found it important to obtain *instantaneous* mixing of the reagents chloramine T, angiotensin and ^{125}I during the iodination procedure. To achieve this, chloramine-T solution (40 μg) and angiotensin are drawn up separately into a disposable radioiodination pipette of the type described by CATT and CULROSS (1968) using a 1 ml syringe, and the reagents held separate in the pipette by an air space. For iodination of angiotensin, the reagents are expelled rapidly into the ^{125}I-solution (1 mCi, Amersham IMS 3) contained at the bottom of a small conical glass tube and mixed instantaneously by bubbling a further quantity of air through the pipette from the syringe. The incorporation of iodine into angiotensin is approximately 90% after 10 sec, when the reaction is stopped by the addition of 80 μg of sodium metabisulphite. Each of the reagents used during iodination is contained in 25 μl of 0.05 M sodium phosphate buffer pH 7.5.

Despite all precautions, most workers find some damage to the label when using the technique of GREENWOOD et al. (1963), due probably to the formation of di-iodinated angiotensin. This compound certainly may be formed during iodination (KURCBART et al., 1971; GANDOLFI et al., 1971) and has a greatly reduced immunological activity (LIN et al., 1970). However, our own experience is that iodination damage (as assessed by the percentage binding of the labelled angiotensin to an excess of a standard antibody over thirty minutes at room temperature) is reduced to a minimum by aiming only for low specific activities of the label (approximately 40 μCi ^{125}I per μg angiotensin), and this is in keeping with the observation of KURCBART et al. (1971) that the yield of di-iodinated angiotensin is also low under these circumstances. Of course the high tracer mass associated with such low specific activities does not favour optimal assay sensitivity, but it is a relatively simple matter to remove the unlabelled angiotensin (and at the same time any remaining "damage") from the product by further purification procedures. We find the technique of DÜSTERDIECK and MCELWEE [1971 (1)], using column chromatography on DEAE Sephadex at pH 7.5, both convenient and satisfactory for this purpose in purification of both Ang. I and Ang. II, and NIELSEN et al. (1971) have recently reported similar experience. Other techniques also appear satisfactory and include paper electrophoresis (VALLOTTON, 1971) and G 25 Sephadex column chromatography (GOCKE et al., 1969; GANDOLFI et al., 1971). CM-Sephadex is useful for separating out damaged angiotensin [BOYD et al., 1969 (2)], but does not give as clear a separation of labelled from unlabelled angiotensin as DEAE-Sephadex.

A possible alternative for the production of undamaged angiotensin label is suggested by the work of ROSA and his colleagues (KURCBART et al., 1971; GANDOLFI et al., 1971) who found that the yield of di-iodinated Ang. II could also be reduced by performing the iodination reaction at a higher pH than usual (pH 9.0).

Damage to labelled angiotensin can be assessed in a variety of ways, but in practical terms the most meaningful is a determination of its capacity to bind to antibody. This property may also be utilized in the purification of immunologically undamaged from damaged label (HABER et al., 1965). General experience suggests that this method does not give a complete one-stage purification (e.g. see GOCKE et al., 1969), but the reason for this may lie partly in the use of *excess* antibody, and it may perhaps be more successful under conditions of relative *antigen* excess when there would be competition for antibody molecules between undamaged and damaged labels.

Some investigators have found that iodinated angiotensin, particularly Ang. I, deteriorates on *storage* (e.g. STOCKIGT et al., 1971). However, our experience is that providing the label is prepared with the precautions outlined above, and provided also that it is diluted to assay strength before storage to avoid self-irradiation damage (YALOW and BERSON, 1957), there is no detectable deterioration over three months (see also GANDOLFI et al., 1971). After this of course, the usefulness of the label is limited by the extent of *radioactive* decay of the ^{125}I itself.

Angiotensin Standards

Since synthetic angiotensins are now available, there should be no difficulty about uniformity of standardization of radioimmunoassays of Ang. I and Ang. II. However, this is not the case, since several workers have found that commercial preparations of peptides may vary widely (VANE, 1971; NIELSEN, 1971; FREEDLENDER, 1971). In an attempt to overcome this problem, the Division of Biological Standards at the National Institute of Medical Research, London N.W. 7, has made available a standardized preparation of [Asp^1, Ileu^5]-Ang. II. In due course it is anticipated that standardized [Ileu^5]-Ang. I will also be available (BANGHAM et al., 1971). In any event it is best to check any new standard by bioassay, and to store it in aliquots of assay strength at temperature well below 0 °C.

Adsorption of angiotensin onto glass and other materials is an important source of apparent loss of activity of standards, particularly with Ang. I, and may seriously compromise the assay system (e.g. see PAGE et al., 1969). However, the problem is readily overcome by the addition of protein to all buffers used in the immunoassay system (BOYD et al., 1967).

The Standard Angiotensin Immunoassay Curve

The assay of angiotensin is based on the principles of "saturation analysis" and radioimmunoassay, which were introduced in 1960 (EKINS, 1960; YALOW and BERSON, 1960) and have since been applied to the measurement of a wide variety of hormones. These assays depend on competition between labelled and unlabelled hormone for the binding sites on a specific binding-protein (see below).

Based on an antibody-dilution curve (e.g. see BOYD et al., 1967), a dilution of antibody is first selected for use in the standard curve which binds the selected amount of labelled angiotensin. We find that approximately 70% of label bound to antibody in the absence of unlabelled angiotensin gives a good working immunoassay curve, although a lowering of the limit of detectability, together with increased sensitivity for assay of small amounts of angiotensin may be achieved by using rather less antibody. Even greater improvements in detection limit and sensitivity have been obtained in some immunoassay systems by "late addition" of labelled hormone (HALES and RANDLE, 1963; SAMOLS and BILKUS, 1964), a technique

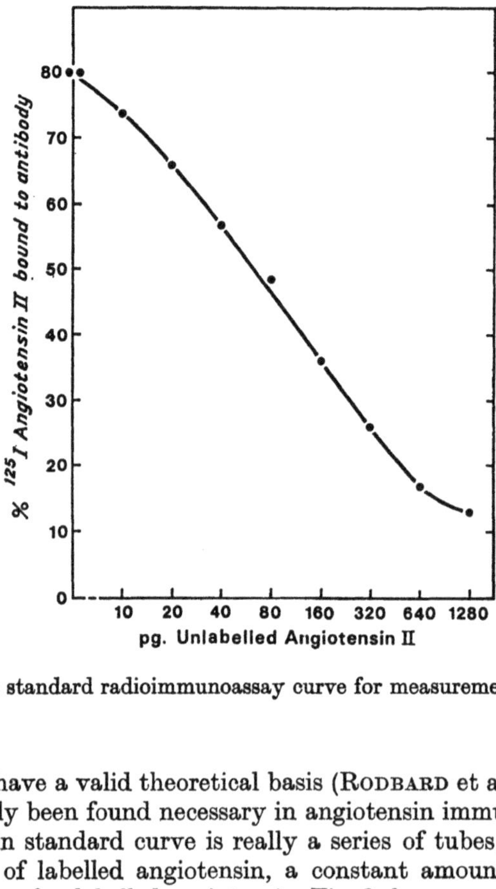

Fig. 2. The standard radioimmunoassay curve for measurement of Ang. II

which appears to have a valid theoretical basis (RODBARD et al., 1971). However, this has not usually been found necessary in angiotensin immunoassay.

The angiotensin standard curve is really a series of tubes, each containing a constant amount of labelled angiotensin, a constant amount of antibody, but increasing amounts of unlabelled angiotensin. Fig. 2 shows an example where 80% of an Ang. II-label is bound to antibody in the absence of unlabelled Ang. II. Looked at simply, the standard curve may be viewed as a series of points at which increasing amounts of *unlabelled* Ang. II cause increasing displacement of the *labelled* hormone from antibody, so that at the point where an excess of unlabelled angiotensin has been added (approximately 1.0 ng in this case) almost all the label is displaced.

In the practice of the immunoassay, we set up various tubes containing doubling dilutions of either standard or unknown angiotensins (in 0.2 ml), together with 0.05 ml labelled angiotensin (5 pg or 100 c.p.s. for Ang. II, and 200 c.p.s. for Ang. I) and 0.05 ml of a suitable dilution of antibody (see above). The pH of the incubation is not critical between 7.0 and 8.6, but we use the latter and employ barbitone HCl (0.05 M) rather than phosphate as a buffer to avoid problems with calcium-dependent antibodies (Boyd et al., 1967). In fact, to ensure an excess of calcium during incubation, 0.02 M calcium chloride is added to all immunoassay buffers. Neomycin 0.02% is also added to avoid problems from any bacterial contamination, and 2.5 mg/ml human serum albumin to prevent non-specific adsorption of angiotensin onto glassware, etc. Total counts present in each tube are conveniently counted overnight and on the following day the tubes are cooled to 4 °C, and the angiotensin bound to antibody is separated from that which is not by the addition of dextran-coated charcoal (Herbert et al., 1965).

Of all the methods of separation of bound and free angiotensin after incubation, this last method is the most widely used. It is simple, quick, very effective, and particularly convenient when large numbers of samples are being processed. We have found the final concentration of charcoal (about 1%) in the immunoassay tubes, as recommended by Herbert et al. (1965), perfectly adequate when separating bound and free angiotensin in buffer solution of standard angiotensin. However, separation in plasma extracts (see below) requires a rather higher charcoal concentration, due possibly to the presence of a large number of various peptides competing for a limited number of adsorption sites. Now although this higher concentration of charcoal overcomes this particular problem entirely, it accentuates the tendency for dissociation of the antigen-antibody complex during the time of its contact with charcoal. This problem may be reduced to an extent by performing the separation at 4 °C, but if large numbers of tubes are assayed in each run, there may still be considerable differences in contact-time (up to 5 min) within, say, 100 tubes which have their charcoal added in turn. To overcome the problem completely, we add the charcoal solution to the polyethylene caps of the immunoassay tubes, as described previously [Boyd, 1969 (2)]. When the caps are then placed on the immunoassay tubes (at 4 °C), surprising strong surface-tension effects prevent the charcoal suspension from falling into the immunoassay incubation mixture until this is determined deliberately by a brief centrifugation. The tubes are then mixed for a total time of 2 min, the charcoal spun down by centrifugation at 3,500 rpm at 4 °C, and the charcoal button counted after aspiration of the supernatant. The whole procedure is quick, simple and very effective in preventing antigen-antibody dissociation during separation.

The "Norit A" charcoal (Hopkins and Williams) used by Herbert et al. (1965) is no longer available, but we have found Norit SX1, made by the same company, a satisfactory substitute. The only point is that its affinity for angiotensin adsorption is about twice as great as that of Norit A and so rather less is needed for separation of bound and free hormone. In our procedure the addition of 0.2 ml of 2% Norit SX1 charcoal suspension in assay buffer (containing 1.25 mg/ml T40 Dextran, Pharmacia) to each immunoassay incubation mixture (of 0.3 ml volume) gives a very satisfactory separation.

Some workers have employed other techniques in the separation of bound and free angiotensin, including G25 Sephadex (Haber et al., 1965; Giese et al., 1970) and Morgan and Lazarow's (1963) double-antibody technique (Cohen et al., 1971). However, although perfectly adequate, these technique do not appear in general to be quite as convenient as the charcoal method of separation.

Angiotensin II: Immunoassay of Levels in Circulating Blood

If assay of the *circulating* level of Ang. II is to be accurate, the first essential is that Ang. II should be neither formed nor destroyed during the process of blood sampling. Complete avoidance of venous stasis and haemolysis must therefore be ensured during venous sampling, and immediately blood has been taken it is essential to stop the action of plasma angiotensin-converting enzyme and "angiotensinase" *in vitro* completely. The anticoagulant EDTA appears to be effective in preventing the conversion of any Ang. I to Ang. II in plasma *in vitro* (SKEGGS et al., 1956; GOCKE et al., 1969) but our early studies showed that it would not completely inhibit the various plasma "angiotensinases". However, RYAN et al. (1968) have shown that 2,3-dimercapto-propanol (B.A.L.) is an excellent inhibitor of "angiotensinase" activity in rabbit plasma and we have extended their observations to show equally good inhibition in human plasma (BOYD et al., 1967). Our procedure is to draw blood into syringes containing both B.A.L. and EDTA and to cool it immediately to 4 °C. This effectively eliminates "angiotensinase" and converting-enzyme activity. CATT and his colleagues (1967) have chosen the alternative technique due to KAHN et al. (1952), whereby the activities of these enzymes are prevented by taking blood immediately into ethanol. The combination of EDTA and O-phenanthroline may also prove useful [DÜSTERDIECK and McELWEE, 1971 (2)].

The results obtained for circulating-plasma levels of Ang. II in normal human subjects vary in different laboratories from 10 pg/ml to approximately 100 pg/ml. In general those workers extracting angiotensin from plasma [BOYD et al., 1967, 1972 (1); CATT et al., 1967, 1971; PAGE et al., 1969; SUNDSFJORD, 1970; DÜSTERDIECK and MCELWEE, 1971 (2)] find rather lower values than those obtained from unextracted plasma (GOODFRIEND et al., 1968; GOCKE et al., 1969). Possible reasons for this include non-specific interference by plasma protein itself in the assay (KIRKENDALL, 1969; LARAGH, 1969), the possibility of cross-reaction of plasma renin-substrate with the Ang. II antibody [DÜSTERDIECK and MCELWEE, 1971 (2)] and the other non-specific factors including, with some antibodies, the anticoagulant EDTA (BOYD et al., 1967). Not that plasma extraction necessarily ensures freedom from non-specific interference. This seems to have been particularly troublesome with Dowex resin-column extraction (PAGE et al., 1969; HOLLEMANS et al., 1969; SUNDSFJORD, 1970), necessitating repeated washing of the resin after extraction (HOLLEMANS et al., 1969), preparation of standards in angiotensin-free plasma (PAGE et al., 1969), or even the processing of these prepared standards through the extraction method (PAGE et al., 1969). If Dowex resin is used, batchwise extraction may be preferable [DÜSTERDIECK and MCELWEE, 1971 (2)]. The techniques involving Fuller's-earth extraction [BOYD et al., 1967, 1972 (1)] or ethanol-precipitation of blood followed by extraction on SE-Sephadex (CATT et al., 1967, 1971) do not appear to be associated with any appreciable degree of non-specific interference. In our own system of a simple batch extraction on Fuller's earth followed by elution with ammonia in methanol [BOYD et al., 1967, 1969 (2)], extracts of saline or of plasma from nephrectomized patients gave a reading which was below detection limit (1 to 2 pg/ml) of the assay [BOYD et al., 1972 (1)]. CATT et al. (1971) also found values at the limit of detection following nephrectomy and in patients with Conn's syndrome.

We use two other assessments for continuing *quality control* of the method. The first is a check on whether the percentage uptake of angiotensin on dextran-charcoal (97 to 100%) is the same in both plasma extracts and buffer, and consists of a tube containing the extract (or buffer), labelled angiotensin, but no antibody. There is rarely any difference between these two. The second is a "blank" and consists of a second Fuller's-earth extract of the test plasma. The level found on assay is usually substantially less than the value in the original sample, but occasionally it is not, and when this occurs the value is rejected. The *accuracy* of the plasma angiotensin assay is also maximized by setting up *duplicate* standard curves with each run, and by assaying serial dilutions of all unknowns.

In general, since the circulating plasma level of angiotensin is frequently low, it would seem preferable to extract plasma prior to assay. Although some of the methods are time-consuming, they may be quick and relatively simple, particularly when batch-wise procedures are used [Boyd et al., 1967; Düsterdieck and McElwee, 1971 (2)]. Recoveries of most methods are good (70 to 100%) and may be corrected for, if necessary by the addition of an internal indicator to each sample (Catt et al., 1967). Not only does extraction increase the amount and concentration of angiotensin in the assay, and thereby allow a more accurate estimation *at several dilutions*, but it may also avoid many of the problems of non-specific interference which are liable to occur in the assay of unextracted plasma samples.

Of course the results obtained with Ang. II immunoassays should more properly be expressed as "Ang. II-like activity" since the antibodies present are not entirely specific to the whole Ang. II molecule and may measure some non-biologically active Ang. II fragments as well. Indeed the data of Cain et al. (1969) suggest that at least one such fragment (the 3 to 8 angiotensin hexapeptide) may constitute a significant proportion of the Ang. II-like activity in venous, although not in arterial, blood[1] so that the true venous level of Ang. II is probably over-estimated by the immunoassay. As it happens however, the estimation of venous Ang. II-like activity is usually only performed as a convenient first approximation to the arterial level, which is probably more meaningful in physiological terms, and since this latter is much more nearly approximated by total venous immunoreactivity (76% of arterial level in normal man) than by the true venous Ang. II-concentration (28% of arterial level), cross-reaction af Ang. II antibodies with the hexapeptide fragment in this circumstance is to some extent fortunate (Cain et al., 1969). Nonetheless, this approximation makes the assumption that the ratio of arterial to venous angiotensin immunoreactivity is constant, and since this may not hold true under all circumstances, it is obviously preferable to measure the arterial level direct in situations where accurate physiological data are required (e.g. see MacDonald et al., 1970).

Estimation of Ang. II-Levels in Other Body Fluids

The same general principles apply when measurement of angiotensin is extended to other body fluids, but it is important to stress that where relatively slow flow occurs *in vivo* (e.g. in lymphatics), there may be destruction or even formation of angiotensin during passage to the point of sampling *in vivo*, so that caution must be observed in the extrapolation of any result to the state of affairs at a more proximal site. For example, Bailie et al. (1971) suggested that their finding of a relatively high level of Ang. II-like activity in renal lymph supported the notion that angiotensin may be formed locally within the kidney substance and act as a local renal hormone (Lever and Peart, 1962). However, renin, renin-substrate and converting enzyme have all been found in renal lymph (Lever and Peart, 1962; Horky et al., 1971), making their data difficult to assess since it is possible that the increase in measured angiotensin concentration could have resulted partly, or even wholly, from the formation of Ang. II during passage along the lymphatics themselves.

[1] Incidentally, this finding suggests strongly that the angiotensin 3-8 hexapeptide is cleared very efficiently in the lung.

Application of Angiotensin Immunoassay to the Measurement of Plasma Renin Activity

1. Angiotensin I Immunoassay

As indicated above (see "Introduction") the immunoassay of Ang. I generated during plasma incubation *in vitro* in the presence of "angiotensinase" and converting-enzyme inhibitors is probably the optimal immunoassay method for this measurement at present. We use the combination of BAL and EDTA to prevent conversion and destruction of the Ang. I formed during incubation [Boyd et al., 1969 (2)] and some workers add 8 hydroxyquinoline as well (Haber et al., 1969). We also carry out the plasma incubation (4 h, 37 °C) without altering plasma pH, in order to approximate conditions *in vivo* as nearly as possible, but where samples are assayed without extraction, the pH of incubation may have to be reduced to 5.5 in order to generate sufficient angiotensin for accurate assay (Cohen et al., 1971).

Many workers extract Ang. I from plasma after incubation, and using Fuller's earth we have not encountered any problems of non-specific interference in our method [Boyd et al., 1969 (2), 1972 (2)]; plasma from nephrectomized patients gives rates of Ang. I generation which are at or below the detection limit of the assay; a second Fuller's-earth extract of incubated plasma (plasma "blank") almost invariably gives levels of less than 10% of the original sample, and the plasma extracts themselves have not been found to interfere with the uptake of labelled angiotensin on charcoal in the immunoassay. An extract of *un*incubated plasma almost always gives levels of less than 5% of the incubated sample. However, as with Ang.-II extraction, the use of Dowex resin again appears to be associated with problems of non-specificity, as described by Hollemans et al. (1969), and although this can be minimized the resultant procedure appears rather tedious. SE-Sephadex may be a suitable alternative (Giese et al., 1970).

More recently, with improving Ang. I antibodies, investigators have looked towards the use of *un*extracted plasma in the assay of Ang. I generated during incubation (Haber et al., 1969; Stockigt et al., 1971; Cohen et al., 1971). This approach appears quite feasible where antibodies are sufficiently sensitive, but it should be stressed that with this method it is essential to assay a control *un*incubated plasma blank in order to correct for any cross-reaction of Ang. I antibodies with renin-substrate, and also to allow for any other factors causing non-specific interference. Furthermore, particularly in those important clinical cases where low amounts of angiotensin are being measured (e.g. Conn's syndrome), it is important that this level of non-specific interference (i.e. the blank) should be low, since a high level may seriously compromise the *precision* of the assay. The other word of caution is that Stockigt et al. (1971) have found this particular approach rather sensitive to any deterioration of labelled Ang. I tracer (as evidenced first by non-parallelism between standards and unknowns) and they suggest that unknowns should routinely be run in serial dilution as a continuing check on this point.

It would seem important to compare the biological and immunological assessment of the generation product of plasma incubation as a means of validating any particular immunoassay method [Boyd et al., 1967, 1969 (2)]. Further, this comparison should be made on the same samples. This point has recently been emphasized by Kritzinger et al. (1971) who compared the same samples by bioassay and the commercially-available Ang. I immunoassay kit based on the method of Haber et al. (1969), and found approximately three-fold greater levels by immunoassay. This was in apparent contrast to the previous report by HABER et al. (1969), which showed good agreement between their immunoassay results and the earlier bioassay data of GUNNELS et al. (1967). However, it seems that this agreement may have been fortuitous, since KRITZINGER et al. (1971) have pointed out that the pH of plasma incubation for the immunoassay of HABER et al. was different from that for the bioassay of GUNNELLS and his colleagues, and that correction for this factor would give values in keeping with their own observations. This suggests that there may be some degree of non-specificity with this particular method.

2. Angiotensin II Immunoassay in the Estimation of Renin Activity

Most methods which have attempted to measure plasma renin activity by immunoassay of the amount of Ang. II generated have run into the problem of inhibition of plasma converting enzyme *in vitro* by "angiotensinase" inhibitors (e.g. VALLOTTON et al., 1967), so that the generation product is Ang. I rather than Ang. II (see above). However, where workers have only Ang. II antibodies available, the technique recently described by POULSEN (1971) may prove useful. He performs plasma incubation in the presence of excess Ang. II antibody which takes up Ang. II as it is generated and so limits its degradation by "angiotensinase". Immunoassay is then carried out by addition of labelled Ang. II and dilution of the sample to produce dissociation of the antigen-antibody complex to conditions of relative antigen excess. The performance of such an assay obviously takes rather fine judgement, particularly of the amount of antibody added, and it is yet to be shown *directly* that the Ang. II antibody gives effective protection of the liberated *native* Ang. II during plasma incubation. Certainly the protection of synthetic Ang. II-amide appears far from complete. Along similar lines, it may also be possible to utilize Ang. II antibodies for the measurement of Ang. I generated during plasma incubation using the approach described recently by GIESE et al. (1971). They found that when Ang. I was used as the assay label with certain Ang. II antibodies, the standard curve became relatively more specific for Ang. I, suggesting that this label had selected antibodies from a heterogeneous population which happened to be more specific for this molecule. Another approach has been to use the "angiotensinase" inhibitor diisopropyl fluorophosphate, D.F.P. (GOCKE et al., 1969) which does not appear to inhibit converting enzyme, but it must be said that this material is highly toxic. Finally PAGE et al. (1969) have described a method which accepts much of the "angiotensinase" activity in plasma and standardizes the result by comparison with the effect of added human renin, according to the principle described by HAAS et al. (1968). However, the method is rather tedious and particularly subject to difficulties in cases where "angiotensinase" activity is sufficient to interfere with the linearity of the Ang. II-generation curve during plasma incubation.

Other Renin Assays

Recently MENDELSOHN and JOHNSTON (1971) described an assay for renin based on the rate of cleavage of ^{14}C-labelled synthetic tetradecapeptide renin-substrate. However, apart from some general problems encountered by these workers with this method, it should be remembered that this was precisely the substrate which led to the discovery of pseudorenin (SKEGGS et al., 1969), and so it would appear that this approach lacks the necessary specificity for this determination.

Angiotensin II Levels and Plasma Renin Activity in Various States

A detailed account of Ang. II levels and plasma renin activity in various conditions is beyond the scope of this chapter, but brief mention of the range of values in clinical states may be of value as a guide in determining the level of sensitivity necessary in any intended studies.

Plasma Angiotensin II

Normal values vary among different laboratories. The range in venous plasma is from 10 to 100 pg/ml, but most workers find values towards the lower end of this range. The level may be elevated in malignant human hypertension and in hypertension associated with renal artery stenosis, where values of up to 250 pg/ml have been reported [GOCKE et al., 1969; CATT et al., 1971; DÜSTERDIECK and MCELWEE, 1971 (2); BOYD et al., 1972 (2)]. Similar elevations may occur in hypertension associated with renal disease [CATT et al., 1971; BOYD et al., 1972 (2)]. Patients with Conn's syndrome have values which appear to overlap the lower limit of the normal range [CATT et al., 1971; BOYD et al., 1972 (2); DÜSTERDIECK and MCELWEE, 1971 (2)].

Plasma Angiotensin-I Generation Rate in vitro (Plasma Renin Activity)

Even more variability between laboratories has been observed with plasma-renin immunoassay methods. This is partly due to different methods of angiotensin generation, especially the incubation pH and the presence or absence of added renin substrate. However, if approximate corrections are made for these factors the values from most laboratories for the *in-vitro* generation rate of Ang. I (plasma renin *activity*) at pH 7.4 in plasma from normal recumbent human subjects would appear to be in the range of 0.1 to 1.0 ng/ml/h [BOYD et al., 1969 (2); HABER et al., 1969; STOCKIGT et al., 1971; COHEN et al., 1971]. As with Ang. II, elevated levels of plasma renin activity are frequently seen in malignant hypertension and in hypertension associated with renal artery stenosis or renal parenchymal disease [up to 40 ng/ml/h — BOYD et al., 1972 (2)]. In keeping with previous observations using bioassay, some patients with essential hypertension have reduced values and almost all patients with Conn's syndrome (aldosterone-producing adenoma) have levels well below the normal range [BOYD et al., 1969 (2), 1972 (2); STOCKIGT et al., 1971; COHEN et al., 1971].

Renin-Angiotensin II Correlations

There is a significant correlation between plasma venous Ang. II and immunoassay measurements of plasma renin activity [GOCKE et al., 1969; BOYD et al., 1972 (2)], but it is worth remembering that the correlation coefficient is only of the order of 0.4 [BOYD et al., 1972 (2)] and such a degree of scatter suggests that despite the overall trend, dissociations probably occur quite frequently in individual cases. This is hardly surprising when account is taken of the complexities of the renin-angiotensin system, and is probably due to variability in some of the factors shown in Fig. 1.

Angiotensin I Levels in Human Plasma

PAGE (1970) has reported finding unexpectedly high circulating levels of Ang. I in human plasma. Most of the activity appeared to be due to a rather obscure

"Ang. I-like protein" but even allowing for this the "free" level of Ang. I was found to be about ten times higher than the Ang. II level. We also have found higher levels of Ang. I (50 to 100 pg/ml) than Ang. II (5 to 20 pg/ml) in freshly drawn human plasma (as a control in renin activity determination), but as pointed out elsewhere (BOYD, 1970) these findings cannot be taken as a direct reflection of the *circulating* Ang. I level *in vivo* since the reaction of renin on its substrate may continue to some extent after the blood sample is taken, so that at least some of the measured Ang. I may have been generated *in vitro*. When *circulating* levels of Ang. I are to be examined it is important to stop the renin reaction immediately, and a technique such as that described by KAHN et al. (1952) whereby blood is taken into ethanol would seem more appropriate. Alternatively, the recently-described renin inhibitor "pepstatin" (GROSS et al., 1971) may be of value.

Conclusion

The advent of immunoassay of Ang. I and Ang. II has provided a tool of greater sensitivity and potentially greater specificity than bioassay for investigation of the renin-angiotensin system. However, like all methods, these immunoassays must be applied carefully and with due respect for the complexities of the renin-angiotensin system, as well as for the possible problems which may arise in immunoassay in general. With these provisos, it is our belief that angiotensin immunoassays can contribute substantially to our understanding of the role of the renin-angiotensin system in various clinical and experimental states.

References

ARAKAWA, K., NAKATANI, M., MINOHARA, A., NAKAMURA, A.: Isolation and amino acid composition of human angiotensin I. Biochem. J. **104**, 900 (1967).

BAILIE, M. D., RECTOR, F. C., SELDIN, D. W.: Angiotensin II in arterial and renal venous plasma and renal lymph in the dog. J. clin. Invest. **50**, 119 (1971).

BANGHAM, D. R., CALAM, D. H., PARSONS, J. A., ROBINSON, C. J.: Purity of synthetic peptide preparations. Nature (Lond.) **232**, 631 (1971).

BOUCHER, R., VEYRAT, R., DE CHAMPLAIN, J., GENEST, J.: New procedures for measurement of human plasma angiotensin and renin activity levels. Canad. med. Assoc. J. **90**, 194 (1961).

BOYD, G. W.: (1) In: Protein and Polypeptide Hormones, Part 3, p. 558. Amsterdam, New York, London, Paris, Milan, Tokyo, Buenos Aires: Excerpta Medica Foundation 1969.

BOYD, G. W.: (2): In: Protein and Polypeptide Hormones, Part 3, p. 636. Amsterdam, New York, London, Paris, Milan, Tokyo, Buenos Aires: Excerpta Medica Foundation 1969.

BOYD, G. W.: In discussion. Circulat. Res. Suppl. I, Vols. **26** and **27**, 105 (1970).

BOYD, G. W., ADAMSON, A. R., ARNOLD, M., JAMES, V. H. T., PEART, W. S.: (1) The role of angiotensin II in the control of aldosterone in man. Clin. Sci. **42**, 91 (1972).

BOYD, G. W., ADAMSON, A. R., FITZ, A. E., PEART, W. S.: (2) Radioimmunoaassay determination of plasma-renin activity. Lancet **1969 I**, 213.

BOYD, G. W., FITZ, A. E., PEART, W. S.: (1) The measurement of plasma renin by radioimmunoassay of generated angiotensin I. In: Proceedings of an Internat. Symposium on Protein and Polypeptide hormones, held in Liège, Belgium, May 19—25th, 1968, Part 3, p. 896. Amsterdam, New York, London, Paris, Milan, Tokyo, Buenos Aires: Excerpta Medica Foundation 1969.

BOYD, G. W., JONES, M. B. S., PEART, W. S.: (2) The radioimmunoassay of angiotensin II and plasma renin activity in human hypertension. In: Hypertension 72, p. 583. Berlin-Heidelberg-New York: Springer 1972.

BOYD, G. W., LANDON, J., PEART, W. S.: Radioimmunoassay for determining plasma levels of angiotensin II in man. Lancet **1967 II**, 1002.

BOYD, G. W., PEART, W. S.: The production of high-titre antibody against free angiotensin II. Lancet **1968 II**, 129.

CAIN, M. D., CATT, K. J., COGHLAN, J. P.: Effect of circulating fragments of angiotensin II on radioimmunoassay in arterial and venous blood. J. clin. Endocr. **29**, 1639 (1969).

CAIN, M. D., CATT, K. J., COGHLAN, J. P., BLAIR-WEST, J. R.: Evaluation of angiotensin II metabolism in sheep by radioimmunoassay. Endocrinology **86**, 955 (1970).

CATT, K. J., CAIN, M. D., COGHLAN, J. P.: Measurement of angiotensin II in blood. Lancet **1967 II**, 1005.
CATT, K. J., CRAN, E., ZIMMET, P. Z., BEST, J. B., CAIN, M. D., COGHLAN, J. P.: Angiotensin II blood-levels in human hypertension. Lancet **1971 I**, 459.
CATT, K. J., CULROSS, J.: A disposable radioiodination pipet. Analyt. Biochem. **26**, 207 (1968).
COHEN, E. L., GRIM, C. E., CONN, J. W., BLOUGH, W. M., GUYER, R. B., KEM, D. C., LUCAS, C. P.: Accurate and rapid measurement of plasma renin activity by radioimmunoassay. J. Lab. clin. Med. **77**, 1025 (1971).
DEODHAR, S. D.: Immunologic production of angiotensin. J. exp. Med. **111**, 419, 429 (1960).
DIETRICH, F. M.: Immunogenicity of synthetic angiotensin II. Int. Arch. Allergy **30**, 497 (1966).
DÜSTERDIECK, G., MCELWEE, G.: (1) Iodination of angiotensin II and purification of the labelled hormone. In: Radioimmunoassay Methods, p. 24. Edinburgh-London: Livingstone 1971.
DÜSTERDIECK, G., MCELWEE, G.: (2) Estimation of angiotensin II concentration in human plasma by radioimmunoassay. Some applications to physiological and clinical states. Europ. J. clin. Invest. **2**, 32 (1971).
EKINS, R. P.: The estimation of thyroxine in human plasma by an electrophoretic technique. Clin. chim. Acta **5**, 453 (1960).
FITZ, A., BOYD, G. W., PEART, W. S.: Converting enzyme activity in human plasma. Circulat. Res. **28**, 246 (1971).
FREEDLENDER, A.: In: Radioimmunoassay Methods, p. 387. Edinburgh-London: Livingstone 1971.
GANDOLFI, C., MALVANO, R., ROSA, U.: Preparation and Immunoreactive properties of monoiodinated angiotensin labelled at high specific activity. Biochem. biophys. Acta (Amst.) **251**, 254 (1971).
GIESE, J., JORGENSEN, M., NIELSEN, M. D., LUND, J. O., MUNCK, O.: Plasma renin concentration measured by use of radioimmunoassay for angiotensin I. Scand. J. clin. Lab. Invest. **26**, 355 (1970).
GIESE, J., NIELSEN, M. D., JORGENSEN, M.: New view of cross-reactions in anti-angiotensin sera. Nature (Lond.) New Biology **229**, 189 (1971).
GOCKE, D. J., GERTEN, J., SHERWOOD, L. M., LARAGH, J. H.: Physiological variations of plasma angiotensin II in man. Circulat. Res. Vols. **24** and **25**, Suppl. I, 131 (1969).
GOODFRIEND, T. L., BALL, D. L., FARLEY, D. B.: Radioimmunoassay of angiotensin. L. Lab. clin. Med. **72**, 648 (1968).
GOODFRIEND, T. L., LEVINE, L., FASMAN, G. D.: Antibodies to bradykinin and angiotensin. A use of carbodiimides in immunology. Science **144**, 1344 (1964).
GREENWOOD, F. C., HUNTER, W. M., GLOVER, J. S.: The preparation of ^{131}I-labelled human growth hormone of high specific radioactivity. Biochem. J. **89**, 114 (1963).
GROSS, F., LAZAR, J., ORTH, H.: Inhibition of the renin-angiotensinogen reaction by pepstatin. Science **175**, 656 (1972).
GUNNELS, J. C., GRIM, C. E., ROBINSON, R. R., WILDERMANN, N. M.: Plasma renin activity in healthy subjects and patients with hypertension. Arch. intern. Med. **119**, 232 (1967).
HAAS, E., GOULD, A. B., GOLDBLATT, H.: Estimation of endogenous renin in human blood. Lancet **1968 I**, 657.
HABER, E., KOERNER, T., PAGE, L. B., KLIMAN, B., PURNODE, A.: Application of a radioimmunoassay for angiotensin I to the physiologic measurements of plasma renin activity in normal human subjects. J. clin. Endocr. **29**, 1349 (1969).
HABER, E., PAGE, L. B., JACOBY, G. A.: Synthesis of antigenic branch-chain copolymers of angiotensin and poly-l-lysine. Biochemistry **4**, 693 (1965).
HABER, E., VALLOTTON, M. B., KIMURA, A., PAGE, L. B.: Immunoassay for angiotensin II. In: Protein and Polypeptide Hormones, Part 2, p. 359. Amsterdam, New York, London, Paris, Milan, Tokyo, Buenos Aires: Excerpta Medica Foundation 1968.
HALES, C. N., RANDLE, P. J.: Immunoassay of insulin with insulin-antibody precipitate. Biochem. J. 88, 137 (1963).
HEFFERMAN, A. G. A., GILLILAND, P. F., PROUT, T. E.: Studies on the development of a radioimmunoassay for angiotensin II. Irish J. med. Sci., Sixth Series, No. 500, 343 (1967).
HERBERT, V., LAU, K.-S., GOTTLIEB, C. W., BLEICHER, S. J.: Coated charcoal immunoassay of insulin. J. clin. Endocr. **25**, 1375 (1965).
HOLLEMANS, H. J. G., VAN DER MEER, J., KLOOSTERZIEL, W.: Measurement of renin activity in plasma by a radioimmunoassay for angiotensin I. Clin. chim. Acta **24**, 353 (1969).
HORKY, K., ROJO-ORTEGA, J. M., RODRIGUEZ, J., BOUCHER, R., GENEST, J.: Renin, renin-substrate and angiotensin I — converting enzyme in the lymph of rats. Amer. J. Physiol. **220**, 307 (1971).

HURWITZ, E., DIETRICH, F. M., SELA, M.: A sensitive technique for detecting and estimating the peptide hormone angiotensin-II-amide and its antibodies by using chemically modified bacteriophage and activated sepharose. Europ. J. Biochem. **17**, 273 (1970).
KAHN, J. R., SKEGGS, L. T., SHUMWAY, N. P., WISENBAUGH, P. E.: The assay of hypertensin from the arterial blood of normotensive and hypertensive human beings. J. exp. Med. **95**, 523 (1952).
KIRKENDALL, W. M.: In discussion. Circulat. Res. Vols. **24** and **25**, Suppl. 1, 147 (1969).
KRITZINGER, E. E., KANENGONI, E., JONES, J. J.: Plasma-renin assay. Letter to the editor. Lancet **1971 II**, 665.
KURCBART, H., COLI, A., VANCHERI, L., ROSA, U.: Chemical and Biological effects associated with the iodination of angiotensin II. Biochem. biophys. Acta (Amst.) **230**, 160 (1971).
LARAGH, J.: In discussion. Circulat. Res. Vols. **24** and **25**, Suppl. 1, 147 (1969).
LEVER, A. F., PEART, W. S.: Renin and angiotensin-like activity in renal lymph. J. Physiol. (Lond.) **160**, 548 (1962).
LIBERTI, P. A., MAURER, P. H., CLARK, L. G.: Antigenicity of polypeptides (Poly-α-amino acids). Physicochemical studies of a calcium-dependent antigen-antibody reaction. Biochemistry **10**, 1632 (1971).
LIN, S.-Y., ELLIS, H., WEISBLUM, B., GOODFRIEND, T. L.: Preparation and properties of iodinated angiotensins. Biochem. Pharmacol. **19**, 651 (1970).
MACDONALD, G. J., LOUIS, W. J., RENZINI, V., BOYD, G. W., PEART, W. S.: Renal-clip hypertension in rabbits immunized against angiotensin II. Circulat. Res. **27**, 197 (1970).
MASSANI, Z. M., FINKIELMAN, S., WORCEL, M., AGREST, A., PALADINI, A. C.: Angiotensin blood levels in hypertensive and non-hypertensive diseases. Clin. Sci. **30**, 473 (1966).
MAURER, P. H., CLARK, L. G., LIBERTI, P. A.: Antigenicity of polypeptides (poly-α-amino acids): calcium-dependent and independent antibodies. J. Immunol. **105**, 567 (1970).
MENDELSOHN, F. A., JOHNSTON, C. I.: A radiochemical renin assay. Biochem. J. **121**, 241 (1971).
MORGAN, C. R., LAZAROW, A.: Immunoassay of insulin: Two antibody system. Plasma insulin levels of normal, subdiabetic and diabetic rats. Diabetes **12**, 115 (1963).
MORRIS, R. E., ROBINSON, P. R.: A method for determination of angiotensin II in human blood. Bull. Johns Hopk. Hosp. **114**, 127 (1964).
MULROW, P. J., LYTTON, B., STANSEL, H. C.: The role of the renin-angiotensin system in the hypertension associated with renal vascular disease. In: L'Hypertension Arterielle, p. 296. Paris: L'Expansion Scientifique Français 1966.
NASJLETTI, A., LEWIS, L. A., MASSON, G. M. C.: Electrophoretic studies on renin substrate from various species. Amer. J. Physiol. **220**, 804 (1971).
NIELSEN, M. D.: In: Radioimmunoassay Methods, p. 388. Edinburgh-London: Livingstone 1971.
NIELSEN, M. D., JORGENSEN, M., GIESE, J.: ^{125}I-labelling of angiotensin I and II. Acta endocr. (Kbh.) **67**, 104 (1971).
PAGE, L. B.: In discussion. Circulat. Res., Suppl. 1, Vols. **26** and **27**, 103 (1970).
PAGE, L. B., HABER, E., KIMURA, A. Y., PURNODE, A.: Studies with the radioimmunoassay for angiotensin II, and its application to measurement of renin activity. J. clin. Endocr. **29**, 200 (1969).
PALADINI, A. C., BRAUN-MENENDEZ, E., DEL FRADE, I. S., MASSANI, Z. M.: The estimation of angiotensin in blood. J. Lab. clin. Med. **53**, 264 (1959).
PEART, W. S.: A new method of large-scale preparation of hypertensin with a note on its assay. Biochem. J. **59**, 300 (1955).
PIERACH, C. A., JACOBSON, M. E., CARLSON, K. L.: Radioimmunologische Angiotensinbestimmung. Verh. dtsch. Ges. inn. Med. **75**, 191 (1969).
POULSEN, K.: Estimation of plasma renin concentration using radioimmunoassay of angiotensin II. Scand. J. clin. Lab. Invest. **24**, 291 (1969).
POULSEN, K.: Simplified method for radioimmunoassay of enzyme systems. J. Lab. clin. Med. **78**, 309 (1971).
RODBARD, D., RUDER, H. J., VAITUKAITIS, J., JACOBS, H. S.: Mathematical analysis of kinetics of radioligand assays. Improved sensitivity obtained by delayed addition of labelled ligand. J. clin. Endocr. **33**, 343 (1971).
RYAN, J. W., MCKENZIE, J. K., LEE, M. R.: A rapid simple method for the assay of renin in rabbit plasma. Biochem. J. **108**, 679 (1968).
SAMOLS, E., BILKUS, D.: A comparison of insulin immunoassays. Proc. Soc. exp. Biol. (N. Y.) **115**, 79 (1964).
SKEGGS, L. T., KAHN, J. R., SHUMWAY, N. P.: The preparation and function of the hypertensin-converting enzyme. J. exp. Med. **103**, 295 (1956).
SKEGGS, L. T., LENTZ, K. E., KAHN, J. R., DORER, F. E., LEVINE, M.: Pseudorenin .A new angiotensin-forming enzyme. Circulat. Res. **25**, 451 (1969).

Stockigt, J. R., Collins, R. D., Biglieri, E. G.: Determination of plasma renin concentration by angiotensin I immunoassay. Circulat. Res. Vols. **28** and **29**, Suppl. II, 175 (1971).

Sundsfjord, J. A.: Radioimmunoassay of angiotensin II in plasma. Acta endocrinologica (Kbh.) **64**, 181 (1970).

Vallotton, M. B.: Relationship between chemical structure and antigenicity of angiotensin analogues. Immunochemistry **7**, 529 (1970).

Vallotton, M. B.: Parallel radioimmunoassays of angiotensin I and of angiotensin II for measurement of renin activity and of circulating active hormone in human plasma. In: Hormone and Metabolic Research, Suppl. series No. 3. New York, London: Academic Press 1971.

Vallotton, M. B.: In: Angiotensin. Handbook of Experimental Pharmacology. Berlin-Heidelberg-New York: Springer 1972 (in press).

Vallotton, M. B., Page, L. B., Haber, E.: Radioimmunoassay of angiotensin in human plasma. Nature (Lond.) **215**, 714 (1967).

Vane, J. R.: Purity and stability of synthetic peptides such as angiotensins and kinins. (Nature (Lond.) **230**, 382 (1971).

Yalow, R. S., Berson, S. A.: Chemical and biological alterations induced by irradiation of ^{131}I labelled human serum albumin. J. clin. Invest. **36**, 44 (1957).

Yalow, R. S., Berson, S. A.: Plasma insulin concentrations in non-diabetic and early diabetic subjects. Determinations by a new sensitive immunoassay technic. Diabetes **9**, 254 (1960).

Bioassay of Angiotensin

PHILIP A. KHAIRALLAH and ROBERT R. SMEBY

This chapter is not intended to be an exhaustive survey of all the bioassay techniques published relating to angiotensin. Instead it is limited to measurement of blood pressure responses, mainly on the rat, and to measurement of isolated smooth muscle contractions. Finally, brief mention is made of another technique, which has not yet been utilized as an assay system, although its sensitivity and specificity are adequate for this purpose. This method involves the measurement of catecholamines released from a perfused adrenal gland. Quantitative extraction of angiotensin from body fluids is discussed in chapter "Measurement of Renin and of Angiotensin (Extraction and Bioassay)" by R. BOUCHER and J. GENEST.

Methods of Measuring Rat Blood Pressure

One of the first actions described for angiotensin was vasoconstriction in a wide variety of vascular beds. These included, among others, the use of pithed cats [PAGE and HELMER, 1940 (1); DEXTER et al., 1945], pithed dogs (BRAUN-MENENDEZ et al., 1940), vasoconstriction in perfused rabbit ears [PAGE and HELMER, 1940 (2); PAGE, 1942], and toad hind limbs (HOUSSAY and TAQUINI, 1938). DEKANSKI (1952, 1954) described a specific and sensitive blood-pressure method for assay of the peptide. Dibenamine-pretreated rats were used because this drug effectively antagonizes pressor responses to amines while not changing responses to angiotensin or vasopressin. A stable basal blood pressure was maintained, injections of angiotensin were given every 3 to 5 min, and up to 50 injections administered to each rat. A straight log dose-response line was obtained, relating the response in mmHg to varying doses of the peptide. A four-point pressor assay was recommended for the measurement of the angiotensin content of plasma or plasma extracts. PEART (1955) slightly modified this method. He used rats weighing between 250 and 350 g, anesthetized with 100 mg/kg urethane administered intraperitoneally. Instead of dibenamine, pentapyrollidium (pentolinium) tartrate in polyvidone solution (2.5 mg/100 g subcutaneously) was used. The method was further changed by MASSON et al. (1957), who gave 3 mg pentolinium tartrate dissolved in a 20% solution of polyvinylpyrolidone (PVP) per rat subcutaneously. Urethane was replaced with sodium amytal (100 mg/kg intraperitoneally) as the anesthetic agent. The method was still further modified by KHAIRALLAH and PAGE (1960) who administered 0.6 mg atropine sulfate per rat, and performed a bilateral vagotomy. All these changes were summarized by PICKENS et al. (1965). In this method rats weighing between 150 and 200 g were used, anesthetized with sodium amytal, and were given 0.65 mg atropine and 5 mg pentolinium tartrate in 20% PVP (Type NP-K30, General Aniline and Film Corporation, Dyestuff and Chemical Division, 140 West 51 Street, New York, N. Y. 10020). In general, other ganglioplegic agents like hexamethonium, chlorisondamine and mecamylamine can be used instead of pentolinium, since all of them augment pressor responses by a mechanism which is not wholly dependent upon ganglionic blockade (PAGE and McCUBBIN,

1959, 1963). The trachea was intubated, both vagus nervus cut, and the carotid artery cannulated and connected to a mercury manometer. Angiotensin solutions were administered via a fine catheter placed in a femoral vein. A direct relationship was obtained between the logarithm of the dose administered and the response measured as elevation of blood pressure in mmHg. This relationship held when the amount of angiotensin administered was between 0.2 and 10 ng. Sensitivity of individual rats varied both initially and during the course of the day, but a linear relationship between log dose and response was maintained. A three-point assay is recommended, and at least as many injections of standard as of the unknown are administered.

Nephrectomy has been shown to specifically augment pressor responses to angiotensin (MCCUBBIN and PAGE, 1954). This has been used by BOUCHER et al. (1961, 1964) to develop a modified pressor-assay system. Rats weighing between 120 and 150 g and nephrectomized 24 h previously are used. A stable base-line blood pressure is obtained and amounts of angiotensin as low as 0.2 ng can be detected in sensitive rats. Only rats responding by a 10 mmHg rise or more to 5 ng angiotensin are used. Two dose levels of standard and two of unknown are injected. The volume of each sample administered must be kept small, since these animals cannot get rid of excess water. Most sample sizes are around 0.1 ml in the pentolinium-treated rats, and have to be kept to 0.01 to 0.02 ml in the nephrectomized ones. Otherwise, both assay methods are very similar, and results obtained with them are comparable.

A number of investigators have used combinations of these methods, giving ganglioplegics to nephrectomized animals (see e.g., ING et al., 1968). There is no evidence that such a combination of experimental techniques is better than either nephrectomy or ganglioplegia.

Isolated Organ Techniques

One of the earliest descriptions of the use of rat uterus for bioassay of smooth muscle-stimulating substances was by HOLTON (1948). She recommended that standard physiological salt solutions containing $^1/_4$ to $^1/_2$ the normal content of calcium be used, in order to reduce spontaneous contractions. These can be further minimized by lowering the temperature to 32°. Contractions are recorded isotonically by the use of a frontal writing lever exerting a tension of 1.2 g and giving a four-fold magnification. The agonist is added every 3 to 4 min, and 60 to 90 sec are allowed for contractions to develop. The muscle is then rinsed twice and allowed to recover for 1 to 2 min, before a second dose is applied. Two doses of known standard are given, one giving a supraminimal response (10 to 20% of maximal) and one giving a large response which must, however, be less than 80% of maximal. These two points are used to draw a straight line, plotting responses on a linear scale, and doses administered on a logarithmic scale. Two doses of unknown are given, producing approximately comparable effects to the standard doses, and responses are compared to the log dose-response curves plotted for the standard.

DEKANSKI (1954) first applied this method to the assay of angiotensin. He used uteri from estrus rats in a salt solution of low calcium content at 30°. Angiotensin was injected into the bath every 4 min and level of response was related to dose.

A different approach to assay was used by SCHWARZ et al. (1955). This was based on the observation of LUDUEÑA (1940) that responses of uterus to angiotensin were somewhat delayed and slow in onset compared to responses to acetylcholine. The assay method is based on the time interval between the addition of the agonist and maximal contraction. The time includes the latent period and the time of contraction. A simple linear relationship exists between this "response" time, and the dose of angiotensin administered. Estrus rat uteri were mounted in an 8 ml bath at 30°, containing physiological salt solution with decreased calcium content. Contractions were recorded by isotonic lever at a magnification of 3 to 4 times. After a 20 to 30 min equilibration time, angiotensin was injected, and the time from injection to maximal contraction (called response time) was measured with a stop watch. The time of maximal contraction was easily and accurately determined, since the uterus began to relax immediately after attainment of maximal response. Once relaxation started, the strip was washed three times and 2 to 3 min allowed for recovery before the next dose was administered. Either three doses of standard and three of unknown were given (three-point assay) or two of each (two-point assay). With this method, the response time was inversely proportional to the dose administered. With a very large dose, response time approached 40 sec, while the minimal feasible dose that could be measured gave response times of around 200 sec. Thus, when the reciprocal of any dose level, minus minimal feasible dose, was plotted against response time, a linear relationship was obtained. For quantitation, dose response-time curves were drawn for the known standard and to the unknown. Both were extended until the two lines intersected. The ratio of the slope of these two curves was directly proportional to the ratio of the dose administered.

In both cases of log dose-response curves, and dose response-time curves, a uterus in estrus responds to angiotensin at a minimal dose of 0.1 ng/ml muscle bath, while the upper limit of normal is close to 10 ng/ml bath. The methods are fairly easy to carry out and do not require extensive laboratory facilities or prolonged technical training. The greatest difficulty is to obtain repeatedly sensitive rat uteri. This has been accomplished by administration of synthetic estrogens such as diethyl stilbestrol 18 to 24 h prior to obtaining the uterine strips. However, this relatively crude procedure has an uncertain latency time, and an uncertain relationship to endogenous estrogens and progesterones. Administration of synthetic estrogens often leads to a high degree of hypersensitivity manifested by excessive spontaneous contractions in spite of reduced calcium content and temperature. The survey of a colony of virgin rats by vaginal smears in order to determine natural estrus is also tedious.

A modification of the rat uterus technique has been used for oxytocin assay (RUDINGER and KREJČÍ, 1962). The main difference is that a cumulative dose-response curve is measured. The peptide is added at dose ratios of 1, 2, 4, 8, 16, 32, etc., until maximal responses are obtained. The doses are added at 1 to 2 min intervals, just as soon as maximal response to the previous dose has been reached. The bath fluid is not washed out between injections. This technique has mainly been used to study agonist-antagonist interactions on smooth muscle [ARIENS and DE GROOT, 1954; TÜRKER et al., 1971 (2)]. As a method of assay, it allows many more responses to be obtained in a shorter period of time, but the statistical analysis of the data obtained is more complicated.

Many other smooth-muscle tissues can be used for assay, but in general they are all less sensitive to angiotensin. Almost all smooth muscle assay techniques are fairly non-specific, since many peptides and non-peptides contract smooth muscle. Thus, in many cases, preliminary extraction and purification of the peptide has to be carried out. For the assay of angiotensin not contaminated by other agonists, the smooth-muscle methods are simple, repeatable, and sensitive. However, for the assay of angiotensin in blood or plasma, other methods are probably preferable.

Continuously Superfused, Blood-Bathed Organ Techniques

As seen in the previous section, the amount of an active substance required for assay on isolated smooth muscle preparations depends to a great extent on the volume of the bath. In most cases, standard bath volumes of 5 or 10 ml are used, and it becomes very inconvenient if a bath of 2 ml or less is used, especially when the smooth muscle is a guinea-pig ileum.

FINKELMAN (1930) was the first to describe a preparation of an intestinal strip suspended in air, and kept in good condition by a stream of salt solution running over its surface. By analogy with perfusion, where the fluid runs through the tissue, this technique has been called superfusion by GADDUM (1953) since the fluid runs over the tissue. KWIATKOWSKI (1941) used this method to assay histamine, and GADDUM (1953) improved the sensitivity and reproducibility of the technique. He was able to assay 0.02 milli-units of oxytocin in 0.2 ml physiological salt solution superfused over a rat uterus in 3 to 4 sec.

Although GADDUM's superfusion technique facilitated assay of smaller amounts of active substances, one of its main limitations was that bioactive substances present in blood or tissues had first to be extracted, separated from other active or inhibitory substances and dissolved in a salt solution (which in the case of biologically active lipids and prostaglandins entailed overcoming solubility problems) before assay. To overcome extraction problems VANE (1964) developed the blood-bathed superfused organ technique.

Methods

Heparinized blood from an anesthetized animal is constantly superfused over a series of isolated smooth-muscle preparations, and then returned intravenously. The smooth muscle preparations are arranged in cascade; usually up to three tissues can conveniently be handled in one series (VANE, 1969). If more assay organs are needed two banks of tissue can be set up. Blood from the first bank can then be pumped up over the second bank. On the other hand, each bank can be superfused separately, so that hormone concentrations in arterial and venous blood from the same animal can be compared.

As described by VANE (1969), different smooth muscle preparations are used to facilitate assay of many circulating hormones. The choice of isolated organs depends upon the hormone to be assayed. Most organs respond to more than one stimulus, and thus, since there are no steps of extraction or purification of blood, more than one organ is needed for every assay of a specific hormone. The rat colon is very sensitive to angiotensin (REGOLI and VANE, 1964) while being relatively insensitive to most other hormones with the exception of prostaglandins. Thus, if rat colon were used as the only assay organ, a contraction would not be specific for angiotensin. The rat stomach strip responds to prostaglandins and other hormones (VANE, 1957), but is relatively insensitive to angiotensin. A chick rectum also responds to prostaglandins and is totally insensitive to angiotensin (ARMITAGE and VANE, 1964). Thus, a cascade with a rat colon as one organ, and a rat stomach strip or chick rectum as the second organ would allow specific measurement of the amount of Ang. II in circulating blood. Specificity can be further enhanced by using specific antagonists for certain of the circulating hormones. Since rat colon is relaxed by both epinephrine and norepinephrine, the presence of catecholamines would interfere with measurement of the peptide. This can be prevented by antagonizing this effect with a β-receptor antagonist (pronethalol or propranolol) (HODGE et al., 1966). When perfused through the lumen of the colon, the β-blocker will not circulate through the whole animal, which might interfere with the experimental procedure.

In a typical experiment (HODGE et al., 1966) dogs were anesthetized and cannulae inserted into the jugular vein, carotid artery and trachea. Each animal was ventilated mechanically, and received 1000 μ/kg heparin. Blood from the carotid artery was pumped at 15 ml/min through plastic tubing over three assay organs, the rat colon and stomach strip, and chick rectum by a roller pump. The blood returned into the jugular vein by gravity. Movements of the isolated smooth-muscle strips were recorded on a kymograph by auxotonic levers, with a resting load of 1 to 3 g and a magnification of 1:16. Rat colon is highly sensitive and responds to angiotensin at concentrations as low as 0.1 ng/ml. Rat stomach strip requires a minimum concentration of 1 ng/ml, while chick rectum is insensitive. The rat colon can be perfused intraluminally with 1 mg/ml propranolol, which abolished responses to catecholamines without changing sensitivity to angiotensin. This cascade superfusion technique detects changes in angiotensin concentrations occurring over periods of time, while absolute concentrations can only be derived from the fall in base-line tension occurring after nephrectomy, assuming that the concentration of circulating angiotensin has fallen to zero. The response of the assay organs to endogenous angiotensin can be calibrated in terms of blood angiotensin concentrations, by infusing angiotensin at a known rate into the blood passing over the assay organs.

Limitations of the Methods

Once the assay organs are prepared, they are mounted and superfused with a physiological salt solution, until the experimental animal is prepared, and blood superfusion is started. When blood first hits the tissue, the strips contract and remain in a state of higher resting tone for some time. This effect may be due to the presence of unknown myotropic substances in blood, to a change in ionic composition of the superfusion medium, or to changes in oxygen tension. A new stable base line cannot usually be obtained until 30 to 60 min after the start of blood superfusion. Since the resting tone is changed as compared to physiological salt solution superfusion, the assay organs cannot be precalibrated. The assay is valid only when *changes* in blood concentrations are measured.

Another problem is the relatively short half-life of Ang. II in incubating blood. This figure ranges from less than 100 sec to a little over 200 sec (HODGE et al., 1967). Thus, if the tubing connecting the animal to the assay organs is long or two banks of tissues are used, it may take 10 to 20 sec for the angiotensin to get to the assay organ, and 10 to 15% of the peptide would be metabolized. Any delay introduced into the circulation such as that recommended for the assay of circulating renin (VANE, 1969) simply magnifies the error.

A more serious objection is the possibility that the first tissue in the cascade may either metabolize, trap and inactivate angiotensin, or on the other hand, release substances that affect the following assay organ. VANE (1969) has reported that in his experience, these factors do not play a role. However, YAMAMOTO et al. (1972) [see also TÜRKER et al., 1971 (1)] reported that when Ang. I and II dissolved in a physiological salt solution were superfused over a rabbit aortic strip, only 50% of the activity could be measured when assayed on a second strip. Normal physiological salt-solution effluent did not metabolize angiotensin. Either the first strip inactivated the peptide, or else the peptide released a substance from the first tissue that partially inhibited responses of the second strip. No such loss was measured if the first strip was a rat colon instead of a rabbit aorta. In view of the

Table 1. *Program for evaluation of pressor assays*

```
100:   ###      * #####.#     * #####.##      * #####.##     * #####.##
110:****************************************
120 DIM X(30),Y(30),T(30),J(30)
130 FOR 1=1 TO 30
140 READ T(I)
150 NEXT I
160 DATA 25.452,6.205,4.176,3.495,3.163,2.969,2.841,2.752,2.685
170 DATA 2.634,2.593,2.560,2.533,2.510,2.490,2.473,2.458,2.445
180 DATA 2.433,2.423,2.414,2.406,2.398,2.391,2.385,2.379,2.373
190 DATA 2.368,2.364,2.360
200 PRINT
210 PRINT "MODIFIED 11/8/71"
220 PRINT
225 W1=0
230 PRINT
240 PRINT "THE DATA FOR STANDARDS"
250 PRINT "DOSE","RESPONSE (MM)"
260  A=B=C=D=E=F=G=H=K=L=0
270  N=Q=0
280 FOR I=1 TO 30
290  X(I)=Y(I)=0
300 NEXT I
310 READ Z,W
320 REM Z=DOSE,W=RESPONSE OF STD.
330 IF Z=0 THEN 450
340  N=N+1
350 PRINT Z,W
360 IF W<W1 THEN 380
370 W1=W
380  Y(N) =LOG(Z)/LOG(10)
390  X(N)=W
400  A=A+X(N)
410  B=B+Y(N)
420  C=C+Y(N)*X(N)
430 D=D+X(N)↑2
440 GO TO 310
450 E=((N*C)-(A*B))/((N*D)-A↑2)
460  F=(B/N)-(E*(A/N))
470 FOR I=1 TO N
480  G=G+(Y(I)-(B/N))↑2
490  H=H+(Y(I)-(F+(E*X(I))))↑2
500  Q=Q+(X(I)-(A/N))↑2
510 NEXT I
520  K=1-H/G
530  L=SGN(E)*SQR(K)
540 PRINT
550 PRINT "CORR. COEF. FOR STD. LINE=";L
560 IF L>0.97 THEN 630
570 PRINT
580 PRINT USING 110
```

loss in activity, care should be taken in interpreting results from superfusion techniques.

Calculation of Assay Results

Pressor Assay

To determine the assay result of an Ang. II unknown sample, the standard curve may be plotted graphically and the unknown result read from such a curve. This method has several disadvantages. First, it is time-consuming; second, it is sometimes difficult to estimate the best straight line from the plotted points; third, the results from manual plotting can vary from one person to another; fourth, the amount of variation permitted in the rat blood pressure response to a single injected standard sample can vary from one person to another.

The availability of inexpensive time-sharing computer services with very rapid response time is a valuable laboratory aid to the solution of the above problems.

Table I (continued)

Assay 1 (continued)

```
590 PRINT "CAUTION: ASSAY MAY NOT BE VALID"
600 PRINT "CORRELATION COEFF. TOO LOW"
610 PRINT USING 110
620 PRINT
630 IF E<0.055 THEN 740
640 PRINT
650 PRINT USING 110
660 PRINT "CAUTION: ASSAY MAY NOT BE VALID"
670 PRINT "RAT TOO INSENSITIVE-- IF THE RAT HAS JUST BEEN SET UP"
680 PRINT "WAIT ABOUT 45 MINUTES AND TRY AGAIN.  IF IT IS NECESSARY"
690 PRINT "TO GIVE NEM. DO THIS AT LEAST 15 MINUTES BEFORE"
700 PRINT "RE-RUNNING THE STANDARD"
710 PRINT USING 110
720 PRINT
730 PRINT
740  P=1
750 PRINT "SLOPE=";E
760 PRINT "INTERCEPT =";F,"INTERCEPT (DOSE) =";10↑F;"NG."
770 PRINT
780 PRINT "UNKNOWN NO.","RESPONSE(MM.)","NG ANGIOTENSIN",
790 PRINT "  95 PERCENT PRED. LIMITS"
800 PRINT TAB(32);"PER 0.1 ML.";TAB(51);"LOWER";TAB(65);"UPPER"
810 PRINT
820 READ J(P)
830 IF J(P)=0 THEN 960
840 REM J-RESP OF UNKNOWN
850  O1=(H/(N-2))*(1+(1/N)+(((J(P)-(A/N))↑2)/Q))
860 V=T(N)*SQR(O1)
870  O=E*J(P)+F
880  M=10↑O
890  R1=O-V
900  R2=O+V
910  M1=10↑R1
920  M2=10↑R2
930 PRINT USING100,P,J(P),M,M1,M2
940  P=P+1
950 GOTO 820
960 PRINT
970 PRINT USING 110
975 W1=W1+2
980 FOR I=1 TO (P-1)
990 IF J(I)<W1 THEN 1010
1000 PRINT "SAMPLE ";I;" MUST BE DILUTED FOR VALID ASSAY"
1010 NEXT I
1020 PRINT USING 110
1030 GOTO 220
```

The standard dose-response curve can be calculated by a linear regression analysis using the equation: $\log_{10}$ (dose) $= a$ response $+ b$. When the constants a and b have been obtained from this standard line, it is then possible to calculate the dose of Ang. II in an unknown sample from the response measured.

A program (called assay 1) written in Dartmouth Basic for this calculation, is given in Table 1. A printout from this program is given in Table 2. In this printout, the data for standards is repeated so the assayist can confirm that the correct data was given to the machine. Then the correlation coefficient for the regression line, the slope and intercept are given. The dose intercept represents the theoretic maximum amount of Ang. II which would not produce a response in this animal. It is a rough index of the sensitivity of the animal.

A table is printed giving the unknown response found for verification purposes, the calculated amount of Ang. II for this response and the 95% confidence limits

Table 2. *Example of printout from the program Assay 1*

```
THE DATA FOR STANDARDS
DOSE            RESPONSE (MM)
 1.8              31.5
 3.6              38.5
 5.5              45
 1.8              32.5
 3.6              42
 1.8              34.5
 .9               25
 5.5              45
 5.5              45.5

CORR. COEF. FOR STD. LINE= .986866
SLOPE= .038213
INTERCEPT =-.991062            INTERCEPT (DOSE) = .102079 NG.

UNKNOWN NO.     RESPONSE(MM.)    NG ANGIOTENSIN    95 PERCENT PRED. LIMITS
                                  PER 0.1 ML.         LOWER          UPPER

     1       *       38.0     *       2.89      *    2.11     *      3.97
     2       *       25.0     *        .92      *     .64     *      1.33
     3       *       20.5     *        .62      *     .41     *       .93
     4       *       49.0     *       7.61      *    5.32     *     10.88
     5       *       26.0     *       1.01      *     .70     *      1.44
     6       *       37.0     *       2.65      *    1.93     *      3.64
     7       *       52.0     *       9.91      *    6.78     *     14.48

*******************************************
SAMPLE  4  MUST BE DILUTED FOR VALID ASSAY
SAMPLE  7  MUST BE DILUTED FOR VALID ASSAY
*******************************************
```

Table 3. *Example of printout obtained with an animal that gave poor responses to Ang. II*

```
THE DATA FOR STANDARDS
DOSE            RESPONSE (MM)
 1.8              21
 .9               16
 3.6              25
 5.5              29
 1.8              20
 5.5              30
 .9               15

CORR. COEF. FOR STD. LINE= .993677

********************************************

CAUTION: ASSAY MAY NOT BE VALID
RAT TOO INSENSITIVE--IF THE RAT HAS JUST BEEN SET UP
WAIT ABOUT 45 MINUTES AND TRY AGAIN.  IF IT IS NECESSARY
TO GIVE NEM.  DO THIS AT LEAST 15 MINUTES BEFORE
RE-RUNNING THE STANDARD
********************************************


SLOPE= 5.62916E-02
INTERCEPT =-.903633               INTERCEPT (DOSE) = .124844 NG.

UNKNOWN NO.        RESPONSE(MM.)    NG ANGIOTENSIN   95 PERCENT PRED. LIMITS
                                     PER 0.1 ML.        LOWER          UPPER

     1        *       15.0      *        .87      *       .63     *   1.20
     2        *       25.0      *       3.19      *      2.38     *   4.28
     3        *       31.0      *       6.94      *      4.98     *   9.67

********************************************
********************************************
```

for this individual result. Since this represents a single assay for this sample these limits are rather broad. It is generally considered good practice to average at least three assay results and, of course, these limits would then not be valid. However, these confidence limits can sometimes be useful in the evaluation of a single assay result. Finally, if the response of an unknown sample has exceeded the highest standard response by more than 2 mmHg, the operator is warned that this sample should be diluted for a more accurate assay.

In addition the program will print a warning to the operator if the standard results are too scattered (correlation coefficient less than 0.97) or if the rat is too insensitive (slope greater than 0.055). Examples of these printed warnings are given in Tables 3 and 4. The use of this program has not only increased the productivity of our assay work but, because of the built-in quality control devices, it has reduced the average standard deviation of our results from 0.96 ng/sample to 0.74 ng/sample.

Table 4. *Example of printout obtained with an assay animal giving highly variable blood pressure responses*

```
THE DATA FOR STANDARDS
DOSE            RESPONSE (MM)
 1.8               31
 3.6               32
 5.5               45
 1.8               30
 1.8               32
 .9                20
 5.5               43
 5.5               45

CORR. COEF. FOR STD. LINE= .951149

*******************************************
CAUTION: ASSAY MAY NOT BE VALID
CORRELATION COEFF. TOO LOW
*******************************************

SLOPE= 3.20707E-02
INTERCEPT =-.677275                INTERCEPT (DOSE) = .210245 NG.

UNKNOWN NO.      RESPONSE(MM.)     NG ANGIOTENSIN    95 PERCENT PRED. LIMITS
                                    PER 0.1 ML.          LOWER         UPPER

     1      *       30.0      *       1.93      *      .98     *      3.81
     2      *       35.0      *       2.79      *     1.43     *      5.44
     3      *       34.0      *       2.59      *     1.33     *      5.05
     4      *       27.0      *       1.54      *      .77     *      3.11

********************************************
********************************************
```

Myotropic Assay

A similar program has been developed to avoid graphic, manual evaluation of these assays. The results are calculated using both the level and the time of response according to the following equations:

$$\text{Level} = a \log_{10} (\text{dose}) + b$$

$$\frac{1}{\text{Time}} = a\,(\text{dose}) + b$$

Table 5. *Program for evaluation of myotropic assays*

```
1: DOSE    TIME(SEC)    RESP(MM)
2: ##.#     ###          ###
3: SAMP * TIME * HEIGHT * CALCD. ANGIOTENSIN IN SAMP.
4:  NO. * (SEC)*  (MM)  *  TIME    *   HEIGHT
5:  ##  * ###  *   ###  *  ##.##   *   ##.##
6::::::::::::::::::::
100 DIM T(30),X(30),Y(30),Z(30)
110 PRINT "DATA FOR STANDARDS:"
120 PRINT USING 1
130 READ A1,A2,A3
135 IF A1=0 THEN 310
140 REM A1=DOSE,A2=TIME,A3=HT. RESP
150 PRINT USING 2,A1,A2,A3
160 N=N+1
170 X(N)=A3
180 T(N)=1/A2
190 Y(N)=LOG(A1)/LOG(10)
200 Z(N)=A1
210 REM X=RESP,T-1/TIME,Y=LOG DOSE,Z=DOSE
220 B=B+X(N)
230 B1=B1+Y(N)
240 B2=B2+X(N)*Y(N)
250 B3=B3+(Y(N))↑2
260 C=C +T(N)
270 C1=C1+Z(N)
280 C2=C2+T(N)*Z(N)
290 C3=C3+(Z(N))↑2
300 GOTO 130
310 E=(N*B2-B*B1)/(N*B3-B1↑2)
320 E1=(N*C2-C*C1)/(N*C3-C1↑2)
330 F=(B/N)-(E*(B1/N))
340 F1=(C/N)-(E1*(C1/N))
350 FOR I=1 TO N
360 G=G+(X(I)-(B/N))↑2
370 G1=G1+(T(I)-(C/N))↑2
380 H=H+(X(I)-(F+(E*Y(I))))↑2
390 H1=H1+(T(I)-(F1+(E1*Z(I))))↑2
400 NEXT I
410 K=1-H/G
420 K1=1-H1/G1
430 L=SGN(E)*SQR(K)
440 L1=SGN(E1)*SQR(K1)
450 PRINT
460 PRINT "FOR HEIGHT OF RESPONSE:"
470 PRINT "CORR. COEFF.=";L,"SLOPE=";E
480 PRINT "INTERCEPT =";F;" MM"
490 PRINT
500 PRINT "FOR TIME OF RESPONSE:"
510 PRINT "CORR. COEFF.=";L1,"SLOPE=";E1
520 PRINT "INTERCEPT =";F1
```

Table V (continued)

```
530 PRINT
540 PRINT USING 3
550 PRINT USING 4
560 READ M1,M2
565 IF M1=0 THEN 620
570 REM M1=HT. RESP,M2=TIME RESP
580 R=(M1-F)/E
590 R1=((1/M2)-F1)/E1
600 P=P+1
610 PRINT USING 5,P,M2,M1,R1,10↑R
615 GOTO 560
620 PRINT
630 PRINT USING 6
640 B=B1=B2=B3=C=C1=C2=C3=G=G1=H=H1=P=0
650 FOR I=I TO N
660 X(I)=T(I)=Y(I)=Z(I)=0
670 NEXT I
680 N=0
690 READ O
700 IF O=0 THEN 9999
710 GOTO 110
9999 END
```

Table 6. *Example of printout from the program Assay 2*

```
DATA FOR STANDARDS:
 DOSE      TIME(SEC)     RESP(MM)
  3.0          64            61
  3.0          75            69
  3.0          65            68
  6.0          57            69
  9.0          41            74
  6.0          58            72

FOR HEIGHT OF RESPONSE:
CORR. COEFF.= .752841              SLOPE= 16.1495
INTERCEPT = 58.2233 MM

FOR TIME OF RESPONSE:
CORR. COEFF.= .935982              SLOPE= 1.45534E-03
INTERCEPT = 9.97635E-03

  SAMP * TIME  * HEIGHT * CALCD. ANGIOTENSIN IN SAMP.
   NO. * (SEC) *  (MM)  *  TIME    *   HEIGHT
    1  * 66    *   71   *  3.56    *   6.18
    2  * 63    *   72   *  4.05    *   7.13
    3  * 58    *   75   *  4.99    *   10.94

::::::::::::::::::
```

The program for this evaluation, called Assay 2, is given in Table 5 and a printout from this program is given in Table 6.

General Information on Programs

Data are entered into these programs by using data statements added at the end of the program. The linear regression analysis is conducted using the following equations:

1. $\text{Slope} = a = \dfrac{n\,\Sigma XY - \Sigma X \Sigma Y}{n\,\Sigma X^2 - (\Sigma X)^2}$
2. $\text{Intercept} = b = \overline{Y} - \overline{X}$
3. $G = (Yi - \overline{Y})^2$
4. $H = (Yi - Ye)^2$
5. $\text{Correlation coefficient} = r = 1 - H/G\,.$

Adrenal Medulla

Both Ang. I and II have been reported to stimulate release of catecholamines from the medulla of perfused cat adrenal (PEACH, 1971; PEACH et al., 1971). Isolated cat adrenals perfused retrogradely at a flow rate of 1 ml/min with a phosphate-buffered salt solution responded repearedly to doses as low as 0.001 ng Ang. I or II (PEACH, 1971) with no evidence of tachyphylaxis until doses at least 10^5 times higher were used. The catecholamines released were measured continuously using an automated trihydroxyindole procedure (ROBINSON and WATTS, 1965).

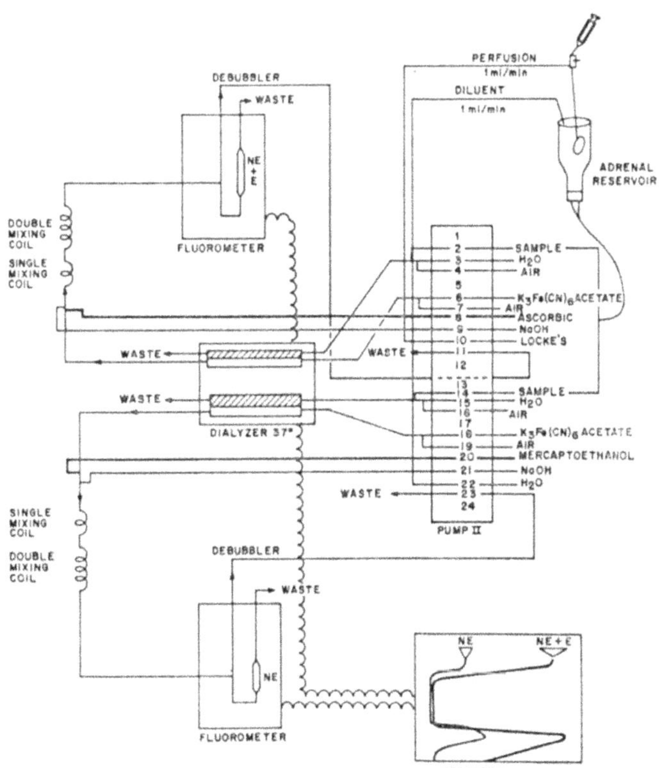

Fig. 1

Isolated perfused cat adrenal gland can be used for the assay of angiotensins if a Technicon Autoanalyzer II Proportioning Pump is used. One half of the effluent is pumped through a fluorometer set to measure norepinephrine, while the other half is used to measure norepinephrine plus epinephrine. Fig. 1 is a flow diagram of the system. The proportioning pump perfuses the isolated adrenal gland at the rate of 1 ml/min with Locke's solution. The same pump adds reagents to the effluent and passes it through the fluorometer. The peptides, dissolved in Locke's solution, are added to the perfusion fluid in volumes of 0.05 to 0.1 ml, and repeated every 20 to 30 min.

Although this method will most probably not be used for routine bioassays of angiotensin it may prove useful in certain circumstances. Responses to Ang. I and II are identical, thus the assay system could be used to assay total peptides, when the samples contain varying proportions of the two. The method is also the most sensitive of the bioassay systems, since responses to doses as low as 0.001 ng can be measured. The method is also specific at these low levels, since none of the other secreting agents act at such low doses. The method can be used for the measurement of circulating plasma or serum angiotensin levels. Plasma proteins are precipitated and washed, and the supernatant assayed for Ang. I and II together. It could be used in combination with radioimmunoassay, since the initial preparation of the plasma sample is the same. Ang. I can be measured by immunoassay, while the total peptide content, Ang. I and II can be measured by the adrenal medulla.

References

ARIENS, E. S., DE GROOT, W. M.: Affinity and intrinsic activity in the theory of competitive inhibition. III. Homologous decamethonium derivatives and succinyl-choline esters. Arch. int. Pharmacodyn. **99**, 193 (1954).

ARMITAGE, A. K., VANE, J. R.: A sensitive method for the assay of catecholamines. Brit. J. Pharmacol. **22**, 204 (1964).

BOUCHER, R., BIRON, P., GENEST, J.: Procedure for isolation and determination of human blood angiotensin. Canad. J. Biochem. **39**, 581 (1961).

BOUCHER, R., VEYRAT, R., DE CHAMPLAIN, J., GENEST, J.: New procedures for measurement of human plasma angiotensin and renin activity levels. Canad. med. Ass. J. **90**, 194 (1964).

BRAUN-MENEDEZ, E., FASCIOLO, J. C., LELOIR, L. F., MUÑOZ, J. M.: The substance causing renal hypertension. J. Physiol. **98**, 283 (1940).

DEKANSKI, J.: Quantitative assay of vasopressin. Brit. J. Pharmacol. **7**, 567 (1952).

DEKANSKI, J.: The quantitative assay of angiotensin. Brit. J. Pharmacol. **9**, 187 (1954).

DEXTER, L., HAYNES, F. W., BRIDGES, W. C.: Renal humoral pressor mechanism in man; preparation and assay of human renin, human hypertensinogen and hypertensin. J. clin. Invest. **24**, 62 (1945).

FINKELMAN, B.: On nature of inhibition in intestines. J. Physiol. **70**, 145 (1930).

GADDUM, J. H.: The technique of superfusion. Brit. J. Pharmacol. **8**, 321 (1953).

HODGE, R. L., LOWE, R. D., VANE, J. R.: The effects of alteration of blood volume in the concentration of circulating angiotensin in anaesthetized dogs. J. Physiol. **185**, 613 (1966).

HODGE, R. L., NG, K. K. G., VANE, J. R.: Disappearance of angiotensin from the circulation of the dog. Nature (Lond.) **215**, 138 (1967).

HOLTON, P.: A modification of the method of Dale and Laidlau for standardization of posterior pituitary extracts. Brit. J. Pharmacol. **3**, 328 (1948).

HOUSSAY, B. A., TAQUINI, A. C.: Action vaso-constrictrice du sang veineux du renin ischémié. C. R. Soc. Biol. (Paris) **128**, 1125 (1938).

ING, T. S., ANDERSON, R. N., PASSOVOY, M., LUCIS, O. J.: Dose-response relationship in angiotensin bioassay. Cardiovasc. Res. **2**, 39 (1968).

KHAIRALLAH, P. A., PAGE, I. H.: A vasopressor lipid in incubated plasma. Amer. J. Physiol. **199**, 341 (1960).

KWIATKOWSKI, H.: Observations on relation of histamine to reactive hyperaemia. J. Physiol. **100**, 147 (1941).

LUDUEÑA, F. P.: Acción de los preparados de hipertensina sobre los musculos lisas. Rev. Soc. argent. Biol. **16**, 1358 (1940).

MASSON, G. M. C., HELMCKE, G., CORCORAN, A. C., PAGE, I. H.: Pressor and myotrophic activities of incubated plasma. Proc. Soc. exp. Biol. (N. Y.) **94**, 544 (1957).

McCubbin, J. W., Page, I. H.: Renal inhibition of pressor responses to drugs. Circulat. Res. **2**, 35 (1954).

Page, I. H.: Method for perfusion of rabbit ears, and its application to study of renin-angiotonin vasopressor system, with a note on angiotonin tachyphylaxis. Amer. Heart J. **23**, 336 (1942).

Page, I. H., Helmer, O. M.: (1) A crystalline pressor substance (angiotonin) resulting from the reaction between renin and renin activator. J. exp. Med. **71**, 29 (1940).

Page, I. H., Helmer, O. M.: (2) Angiotonin-activator, renin- and angiotensin-inhibitor, and the mechanism of angiotonin tachyphylaxis in normal hypertensive and nephrectomized animals. J. exp. Med. **71**, 495 (1940).

Page, I. H., McCubbin, J. W.: Buffer reflexes, tolerance to ganglioplegics and their relationship to enhanced pressor responsiveness. Amer. J. Physiol. **197**, 217 (1959).

Page, I. H., McCubbin, J. W.: Mechanisms by which ganglioplegics and atropine enhance cardiovascular responsiveness. Amer. J. Physioi. **205**, 1 (1963).

Peach, M. J.: Adrenal medullary stimulation induced by angiotensin I, angiotensin II and analogues. Circulat. Res. **28** (Suppl. II), II—107 (1971).

Peach, M. J., Bumpus, F. M., Khairallah, P. A.: Release of adrenal catecholamines by angiotensin I. J. Pharmacol. exp. Ther. **176**, 366 (1971).

Peart, W. S.: A new method of large scale preparation of hypertensin, with a note on its assay. Biochem. J. **59**, 300 (1955).

Pickens, P. T., Bumpus, F. M., Lloyd, A. M., Smeby, R. R., Page, I. H.: Measurement of renin activity in human plasma. Circulat. Res. **17**, 438 (1965).

Regoli, D., Vane, J. R.: A sensitive method for the assay of angiotensin. Brit. J. Pharmacol. **23**, 351 (1964).

Robinson, R. L., Watts, D. T.: An automated trihydroxy indole procedure for the differential analysis of catecholamines. Clin. Chem. **11**, 986 (1965).

Rudinger, J., Krejčí, I.: Dose-response relations for some synthetic analogues of oxytocin, and the mode of action of oxytocin on the isolated uterus. Experientia (Basel) **18**, 585 (1962).

Schwarz, H., Masson, G. M. C., Page, I. H.: A method of assay of the oxytocic activity of angiotonin preparations on the rat's uterus. J. Pharmacol. exp. Therap. **114**, 418 (1955).

Türker, R. K., Yamamoto, M., Bumpus, F. M., Khairallah, P. A.: (1) Loss of activity of angiotensins I and II by superfusion over rabbit aorta and rat colon. Pharmacologist **13**, 214 (1971).

Türker, R. K., Yamamoto, M., Khairallah, P. A., Bumpus, F. M.: (2) Competitive antagonism of 8-ala-angiotensin II to angiotensin II on isolated rabbit aorta and rat ascending colon. Europ. J. Pharmacol. **15**, 285 (1971).

Vane, J. R.: A sensitive method for the assay of 5-hydroxy tryptamine. Brit. J. Pharmacol. **12**, 344 (1957).

Vane, J. R.: The use of isolated organs for detecting active substances in the circulating blood. Brit. J. Pharmacol. **23**, 360 (1964).

Vane, J. R.: The release and fate of vaso-active hormones in the circulation. Brit. J. Pharmacol. **35**, 209 (1969).

Yamamoto, M., Türker, R. K., Bumpus, F. M., Khairallah, P. A.: Loss of activity of angiotensins I and II in isolated superfused rat aorta and in perfused heart and kidney. Amer. J. Physiol. (1972) (in press).

Plasma of Serum Vasopressor Peptides Other than Angiotensins

H. R. CROXATTO

With 8 Figures

In 1942 the uncertainty about the enzymatic character of renin promoted investigations to establish whether typical proteolytic enzymes, such as those elaborated by digestive glands, could reproduce the action of renin upon the same blood substrates. The first experiments [CROXATTO and CROXATTO, 1941 (2)] not only showed that pepsin reproduced the typical action of renin, giving rise to a peptide similar to angiotensin, but also opened a new exploratory technique that strengthened the view that blood proteins are a rich potential source of vasoactive peptides. In fact, the well-known proteolytic enzymes of the digestive tract can produce vasoactive peptides similar or identical to those released by endogenous enzymatic systems (renin, kallikrein). However, the activity of the latter enzymes is far more restricted. Renin acts exclusively upon renin-substrate or its synthetic homologue, but it does not liberate kinins from kininogens and, in contrast, plasma kallikreins are unable to produce angiotensin from blood substrates. On the other hand, endopeptidases such as pepsin, trypsin and chymotrypsin can hydrolyze both renin-substrate and kininogen. In the terminal products of the hydrolyzate, it is possible to characterize angiotensin- and bradykinin-like peptides among the other pharmacologically active substances which are less known.

Both plasma and serum are complex and unstable systems. After blood shedding, they undergo slow and progressive changes, even at low temperatures shown by the occurrence of substances active on smooth muscle in relatively low concentrations. It has been shown that a progressive accumulation of vasopressor substances (the so-called vasoactive protein, VA) is a feature common to plasma or sera from different animal species. The VA appears slowly when preparations are left to stand for several hours or days at 37 °C. It forms with minimal manipulation and even if coagulation is prevented. Moreover, the procedure of altering the pH equilibrium of plasma by acid addition initiates reactions which accumulate peptides split from proteins.

This article deals with vasoactive substances other than angiotensins which induce predominantly vasoconstrictor effects, and, at the same time, raise blood pressure in most animal species. In addition, these vasopressor substances do not require renin for their formation.

Other peptides, which are not vasoconstrictors but occur in plasma or serum in the globulin fractions subjected to pepsin hydrolysis or acidification, will be reviewed only exceptionally. A description of these peptides is necessary to the understanding of the pharmacological differences observed under various experimental conditions.

A. Peptides formed by the action of pepsin.

I. Vasopressor peptide: pepsitensin.

II. Oxytocic peptide: pepsitocin.

III. Antidiuretic peptide: pepsanurin.

B. Vasopressor peptides formed by the action of proteolytic enzymes other than pepsin.

I. Effect of proteinase contained in alpha-amylase preparation. Nagarse.

II. Effect of chymotrypsin.

C. Vasopressor peptides formed in plasma or serum by mere acidification: anephrotensin.

D. Vasopressor albumin (VA) formed in plasma or serum incubated at 37 °C (at a normal pH for several hours [5 to 96], under sterile conditions).

E. Other unidentified components of plasma having vasopressor activities.

In paragraph E brief mention will be made of other substances reported in the last few years as occurring in normal plasma or in plasma obtained from the renal vein of infarcted kidneys. Some properties of these substances are somewhat similar to the active material that accumulates during plasma incubation, at either normal or acid pH.

A. Peptides Formed by the Action of Pepsin

I. Pepsitensin

The addition of pepsin to acidified human or other vertebrate plasma liberates a vasoconstrictor substance. It was observed that this plasma, or its peptidic fraction, quickly interrupts the circulation when neutralized and infused in the hind legs of the frog (Lowen Trendelenburg test) (Fig. 1) [Croxatto and Croxatto, 1941 (1, 2); Croxatto and Croxatto, 1942]. It increases blood pressure of several different animals (Fig. 2). Often, the sharp rise in blood pressure is preceded by a depression. Its effects are similar to angiotensin on the isolated uterus, intestine and urinary bladder (Fig. 2) (Alonso et al., 1943). These results were confirmed by the use of crystallized pepsin at optimal incubation conditions (Helmer and Page, 1942; Weber et al., 1942; Braun-Menendez et al., 1943; Blair, 1962). As the purification of peptides liberated by pepsin progressed it became clear that pepsitensin and angiotensin were similar. The initial hypotensive component in purified fractions disappears, suggesting that this fall in pressure is caused by a different peptide (Rioseco, 1945; Blair, 1962). This is not surprising, since simple acidification of plasma activates kallikrein (Rocha e Silva et al., 1960), and inhibits kininases, thus favoring kinin accumulation (Horton, 1959). The vasopressor component liberated by pepsin is formed from renin-substrate since if the latter is previously incubated with renin, the formation of pepsitensin is insignificant (Braun-Menendez et al., 1943). Furthermore, a study of the yield of pepsitensin from different fractions of plasma obtained by precipitation with ammonium sulfate demonstrates that the fraction containing renin-substrate has the highest yield of the vasopressor (Rioseco, 1945). Moreover, renin-substrate acidified at pH 3 for several hours without pepsin slowly liberates a peptide similar to angiotensin (Alonso et al., 1943). Equivalent yields of angiotensin and pepsitensin can be obtained by treating equivalent amounts of renin-substrate with renin or pepsin (Braun-Menendez and Paladini, 1958). However, vasopressor peptides of unknown chemical composition can be obtained by treating albumin and fibrinogen, separated by fractionating the plasma with ammonium-sulfate with pepsin, but the yield is 5 to 6 times lower than the yield with renin-substrate [Croxatto et al., 1951 (1)]. No data were provided about substrate purity. The peptides obtained by hydrolyzing different animal proteins with

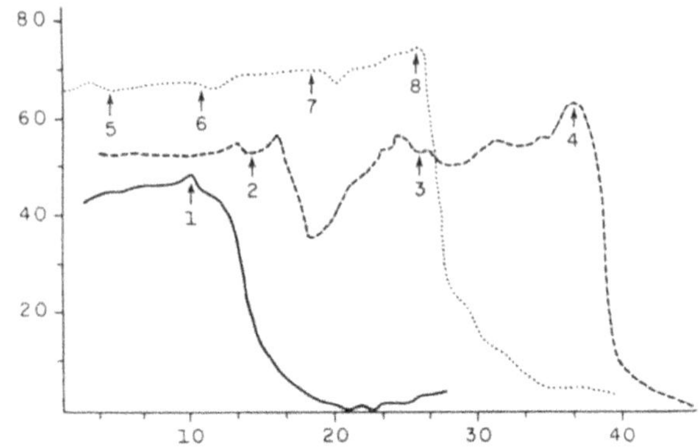

Fig. 1. Perfusion of hind legs of the Chilean giant frog (Löwen-Trendelenburg preparation). Ordinate, number of drops per min. Abscissa, time in min. Arrow indicate addition of different solutions. 1. dialyzate of a mixture of 3 ml renin-substrate (human), incubated for 10 min with pepsin, pH 3.5, 38 °C. 2. dialyzate of a similar mixture but without renin-substrate. 3. dialyzate of a mixture of renin-substrate plus trypsin (pH 7.8). 4. dialyzate of a mixture of 1 ml renin-substrate and pepsin (pH 3.5). 5. same as in 3. 6. dialyzate of a mixture of 3 ml renin-substrate, trypsin and pig renin incubated at 7.8 for 10 min. 7. non-dialyzed mixture of 2 ml renin-substrate and trypsin incubated for 15 min at pH 7.8; 8. mixture of 0.5 ml renin-substrate and pig renin, 10 min incubation. [Croxatto, H. R., Croxatto, R., 1941 (3)]

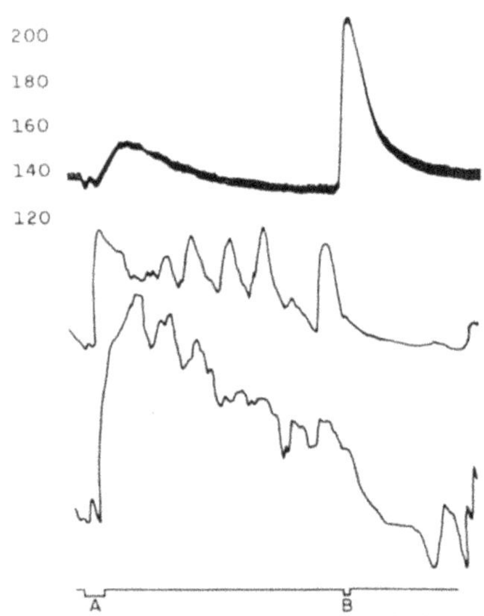

Fig. 2. Effect of pepsitensin on cat systemic blood pressure, uterine contractions and bladder contractions. A. 2 ml purified solution of pepsitensin i. v. B. 25 μg epinephrine i. v. Upper tracing: arterial pressure (mm Hg). Middle tracing: uterine contractions. Lower tracing: bladder contractions. (Alonso, O., Croxatto, R., Croxatto, H. R., 1943)

pepsin, such as ovo-albumin, lactalbumin, fibrin, and especially casein, induce intense and long-lasting vasopressor effects. In contrast, gelatin hydrolyzate lacks this property (Croxatto and Croxatto, 1942). McGlory et al. (1956) obtained a peptide similar to pepsitensin with no vasodepressor properties from casein.

Pharmacological action of pepsitensin: Normal, adrenalectomized, nephrectomized, pithed and spinal rats, and rats treated with hexamethonium or pentapyrrolidinium tartrate show exactly the same arterial blood-pressure response to purified pepsitensin and angiotensin (ALONSO et al., 1942; BLAIR, 1962). The vasopressor response to both substances is reduced after phenoxybenzamine. A less pronounced decrease in the vasoconstrictor response is observed after dihydroergotamine sulfate (2 mg/kg) even though this dose abolishes adrenaline (BLAIR, 1962). Atropine does not alter the intensity of the hypertensive effect of both peptides, but in contrast, p-(2-aminopropyl phenol) (Veritol) (80 mcg/kg) increases it (ALONSO, 1943). The hind leg of the frog *(Caliptocephalella Gayi)* is remarkably sensitive to the vasoconstrictor action of both substances. Minimum quantities of plasma, incubated with pepsin, produce a total and long-lasting arrest of the flow [CROXATTO and CROXATTO, 1941 (2)]. The hypotensive action recorded with non-purified pepsitensin preparations can be accounted for by the presence of kinins (or more likely prokinin) that can be formed either by activation of kallikrein by plasma acidification or through a partial hydrolysis of kinogen by pepsin (WERLE and HOCHSTRASSER, 1963; HABERMANN and SCHUCK, 1964). The smooth muscle in various organs (uterus, intestine and bladder) or intact animals contracts to pepsitensin administered intravenously (Fig. 2) much as it does to angiotensin. However, equipressor doses of both peptides produce variable responses on *in-vitro* smooth-muscle preparations. Crude pepsitensin is far more active than angiotensin (LUDUEÑA, 1940). This has been explained by the existence of an oxytocic peptide, designated pepsitocin, in the crude pepsitensin preparation formed during peptidic digestion [CROXATTO et al., 1951 (2)]. The stronger activity of crude pepsitensin as compared to 5-valine angiotensin II may be partly explained by the presence of bradykinin or kallidin as contaminants, which are potent stimulating peptides of uterine muscle (ROCHA E SILVA, 1959). However, carboxypeptidase B, which destroys kinins, does not significantly impair the oxytocic activity of crude pepsitensin, which is in keeping with the finding that a peptide other than pepsitensin (pepsitocin) and plasmakinins is formed by pepsin digestion (CROXATTO, unpublished).

Purification and chemical structure of pepsitensin: The low yield of the vasoactive peptide, and the large amount of other peptides formed during pepsin hydrolysis has delayed the isolation and identification of pepsitensin. There have been many attempts to decide whether pepsitensin is identical to angiotensin. PAIVA [1954 (1, 2)] showed that pepsitensin and angiotensin have identical actions on isolated smooth muscle organs, and could not be separated by paper chromatography in acetic butanol systems. It was, however, possible to separate the two substances by zone electrophoresis technique at pH 2.5 since pepsitensin had a greater mobility than angiotensin. DENGLER (1956) reported isolation of a pepsitensin containing 13 amino acids, but phenylalanine was not in the amino-acid sequence. BLAIR (1962), working with an impure material, used the method of PAGE and BUMPUS (1962) to purify angiotensin and established that pepsitensin and synthetic are quite similar, although some minor differences were found on isolated smooth muscle. FRANCE DE FERNANDEZ et al. (1965) demonstrated that the structure of pepsitensin from ox plasma was identical with that established by ELLIOT and PEART (1956) for ox Ang. I. The starting material was 500 l of ox plasma. The incubation conditions with pepsin are briefly described in Table 1. Table 1 shows the successive steps of the purification procedure. The major peaks in the countercurrent distribution system were analyzed by paper chromatography. The material eluted from the chromatograms gave values of specific activity and amino acid composition that could not be distinguished from those obtained with synthetic 5-valine Ang. I. C-terminal and N-terminal amino acid studies on the intact polypeptide and on the products of chymotrypsin digestion were similar to those with decapeptide Ang. I. A minor active component was also found in the counter current-distribution systems at pH 7.5, but it was not identified. However, its partition coefficients in two different solvents were identical to those of 5-valine Ang. II. These results are in contrast with those described by Werle et al. (1966). They used the Cohn fraction IV as a substrate, which was treated with perchloric acid to destroy interfering enzymes. Digestion was performed at pH 2.5 with 1 mg

Table 1. *Biological activity of the product at successive stages of purification during the isolation of a pepsitensin*

	Activity	
	(10^{-6} × rat units)	(rat units/ mg. of N)
Incubation mixture (500 l of ox plasma)	6·4	6·4
↓		
Ethanol precipitation and ether extraction	6·0	12·0
↓		
Butan-1-ol extraction; 0·01„-HCi extraction	4·0	23·0
↓		
Preparative countercurrent distribution	2·5	138
↓		
Salt precipitation; acetic acid extraction	2·4	235
↓		
CM-cellulose chromatography	2·2	3 900
↓		
Countercurrent distributions		
↓		
(System 1)		
↙ ↘		
Minor peak Major peak	1·5	43 000
↙		
(System 2)		
↓		
Fractions I and II	0·68	—
↓		
Paper chromatography		
↓		
Pepsitensin	0·62	280 000

of pepsin per 1 g substrate, at 37 °C, over 40 h; then the same amount of pepsin was added again for a second digestion. The pH was adjusted to 6 and pepsitensin was separated in the neutral fraction and pepsitocin in the basic fraction by means of a Dowex 1X2 ion-exchange column. After several purification steps and paper chromatography, an endecapeptide exhibiting 9 to 11% of the activity of 5-valine Ang. II was obtained on various biological tests. The amino-acid composition and the position of lysine in amino terminal group exhibited by the isolated vaso-active material are quite different from those of Ang. I or II. Hochstrasser et al. (1969), using the purification procedure outlined in Table 2, described a vaso-pressor peptide from a peptic hydrolyzate of bovine plasma (Cohn fraction IV). The peptide contained an N-terminal aspartic acid and the remaining amino acids were in the same proportion as Ang. I, except for leucine which occurred twice.

The additional leucine was probably C-terminal, therefore pepsitensin obtained from the denatured substrate at pH 3, according to HOCHSTRASSER et al. (1969), should correspond to an endecapeptide. The occurrence of an additional leucine residue may account for its *in-vitro* stability in the presence of converting enzyme. The pressor effect on dogs' blood pressure has been explained by assuming that in blood, the combined action of carboxypeptidase and converting enzyme transforms the decapeptide pepsitensin into Ang. II.

Pepsitensin inactivation: All proteolytic enzymes studied so far, including pepsin, inactivate pepsitensin [CROXATTO and CROXATTO, 1941 (2); CROXATTO, 1943; CROXATTO et al., 1942, 1945]. The sensitivity of pepsitensin to proteolytic enzymes is comparable to that of angiotensin (CROXATTO, 1943; PLENTL and PAGE, 1944), and these peptides have proven valuable in detection of proteolytic enzymes. Endo- and exopeptidases from different tissues inactivate pepsitensin. Moreover, these enzymes constitute part of the angiotensinase responsible for the short duration of angiotensin in the presence of blood or tissue extracts (CROXATTO, 1943; PLENTL and PAGE, 1944). Nonetheless, crude pepsitensin is more resistant than angiotensin to the peptidase activity of the plasma, hemolyzed erythrocytes and tissue extracts. This greater resistance has been attributed to the presence of other peptides that are present as impurities in crude pepsitensin (CROXATTO and RIOSECO, 1947).

These peptides added to angiotensin partially protect it from the action of angiotensinase obtained from erythrocytes. Purified tyrosinase inactivates angiotensin and pepsitensin. These results suggested tyrosine could be present in both molecules years before their chemical structure was known [ALONSO, 1942; CROXATTO and CROXATTO, 1941 (1, 2)]. Pepsitensin and angiotensin are inactivated by snake venoms obtained from *Crotalus terrifucus*, *Bothrops newidii* and *Bothrops alternatus*. This action can be attributed to proteolytic enzymes present in such poisons. These enzymes cannot inactivate pepsitocin (CROXATTO et al., 1944).

The identification of pepsitensin was facilitated by the observation that pepsitensin, like angiotensin, was resistant to thioglycollate, thiosorbitol and other SH compounds. In contrast, the neurohypophyseal hormones were easily inactivated (CROXATTO, 1943; BLAIR, 1962). Pepsitensin and angiotensin are relatively thermostable, even though boiling with 0.15 N NaOH inactivates them (BLAIR, 1962).

II. Oxytocic Peptide: Pepsitocin

Pepsitensin obtained by direct digestion of the serum produced a more intense contraction of the uterus (rat, guinea pig) than did equipressor concentrations of angiotensin (CROXATTO et al., 1950). This pharmacological observation suggested that either pepsitensin was not the same as angiotensin or that there was another smooth muscle-stimulating substance in the extract. Another peptide, distinct from pepsitensin, is present in the hydrolyzates. This peptide has been designated pepsitocin. Like angiotensin, pepsitocin is inactivated by pepsin, but if the hydrolyzate of renin-substrate or plasma, obtained by incubation with pepsin at pH 3.5 for 3 to 4 h, is further digested with pepsin (at pH 2.5) it loses all its vasopressor effects but retains most of its oxytocic effects [CROXATTO et al., 1951 (1)]. In addition, the peptides formed during the second digestion elicited a striking antidiuretic activity in the rat. This activity is apparently due to a peptide other than pepsitocin and is designated pepsanurin (see below). The evidence that a substance other than pepsitensin was responsible for activity was obtained by studying the actions of different proteolytic enzymes on the peptides accumulated during peptic hydrolysis of serum or angiotensin (human, ox or horse). The observation that there was no parallelism between the vasoconstrictor and oxytocic effects of different hydrolyzates suggested that there were two substances [CROXATTO et al., 1950, 1953 (2); CROXATTO, 1955, 1957, 1966]. The contractile effect of pepsitocin on the uterine muscle of rat or guinea pig is a nonspecific property shared by a number of natural peptides such as the blood kinins and prokinins (WERLE and HOCHSTRASSER, 1963) angiotensin (octapeptide) and the neurohypophyseal hormones. Moreover, pepsanurin has a moderate oxytocic effect. This makes it rather difficult to characterize pepsitocin in the peptic digestion. Oxytocic peptides accumulate after prolonged hydrolysis of plasma with pepsin at pH 2.5. These peptides are resistant to thioglycollate and increases the blood pressure of the rat. This suggests that the oxytocic peptide is not pepsitensin or a hormone from the neurohypophysis (CROXATTO, 1957).

Pepsitocin and neurohypophyseal hormones: Thioglycollate inactivates oxytocin and vasopressin but does not alter the oxytocic action of the product obtained as described above (ROBLERO, 1956; BLAIR, 1962). Moreover, incubation of pepsitocin with serum of pregnant women, which is rich in oxytocinase, does not affect its contractile effect on the rat uterus. It does not produce milk-ejection in the female rabbit and is therefore not identified with the neurohypophyseal hormones (CROXATTO, 1957). It does not increase arterial blood pressure like vasopressin or pepsitensin, but produces hypotension which is much less intense than when bradykinin is administered in equivalent oxytocic doses. However, pepsitocin preparations have a moderate hypotensive effect on arterial blood pressure of the chick, which is not modified by bradykinin (ROBLERO, 1956).

Pepsitocin inactivation: Pepsitocin has the same behavior as oxytocin and bradykinin in the presence of several proteolytic enzymes. Pepsitocin is inactivated by chymotrypsin but not by pepsin and trypsin (CROXATTO, 1957). The effect of carboxypeptidase B, which specifically inactivates bradykinin, has not been examined.

Pepsitocin precursor: The main source of pepsitocin from all sera assayed was the globulin fraction precipitated by half-saturation ammonium sulfate. Hydrolysis of renin-substrate previously treated with renin showed less oxytocic activity than the untreated renin-substrate (CROXATTO, 1957), but the precursor molecule which generates pepsitocin is not renin-substrate. Purified renin-substrate (supplied by BUMPUS) obtained from pig plasma, has a low yield (CROXATTO, 1955). WERLE and HOCHSTRASSER (1963) and HABERMANN (1966) reported that pepsitocin is derived from a globulin molecule identified as kininogen.

Pepsitocin chemical structure: Several attempts have been undertaken to purify pepsitocin (TUPPY, 1956, 1961). TURBA and HETZEL (1954) obtained an oxytocic peptide approximately 200 times less active than oxytocin (1 mg = 2.5 U oxytocin) from serum hydrolyzate. Their pepsitocin had three basic amino acids, arginine, histidine and lysine, which are not found in oxytocin. Proline, an amino acid present in the kinin molecule, was absent. WERLE (1963) and HABERMANN and SCHUCK (1964), HABERMANN (1966), HABERMANN and MÜLLER, 1966; HABERMANN et al., 1966) demonstrated that both pepsitensin and kininogen are present in the peptic hydrolyzate of plasma. This could account for most of the pharmacological differences displayed when the terminal products accumulate in plasma or globulin fractions, in one case by renin and by pepsin in the other. Part of the pharmacological activities described by CROXATTO for plasma incubated at low pH with pepsin, is the result of the simultaneous enzymatic breakdown of kininogen and renin-substrate. WERLE et al. (1963) demonstrated that in the presence of pepsin, kininogen is degraded to dialyzable products which still possess kinin-forming activity when treated with trypsin. The products of pepsin digestion are hypotensive in the rabbit and can contract the guinea-pig ileum. Furthermore, pepsin sets free peptides from ox kininogen which in the presence of kallikrein or *Crotalus-adamanteus* venom, release peptides similar to plasma kinins (HABERMANN and SCHUCK, 1964). The basic peptide formed following pepsin digestion of partially purified kininogen possesses bradykinin-like activity following subsequent trypsin hydrolysis (GREENBAUM et al., 1965). Finally, HABERMANN (1966), HABERMANN et al. (1966) and HABERMANN and MÜLLER (1966) digested purified ox serum kininogen with crystalline pepsin (20 to 100 μg/ml) under optimal conditions (37 °C, pH 1.8, 4 h), and obtained three fractions: a chromatographically and electrophoretically homogeneous peptide (PKL); a second peptide (PKFS) of unknown purity, and a third minor fraction separable by electrophoresis. All these fractions can be labeled pepsitocin. They act like kinins but are much weaker than bradykinin on several biological tests. The first two isolated peptides yield fragments which form kinins in the presence of kininogenases such as plasma and pancreatic kallikreins, trypsin, Crotalus venom, and also under carboxypeptidase A (HABERMANN and MÜLLER, 1966). The product formed when pepsin acts on kininogen contracts the guinea-pig ileum. This activity represents only 0.25 to 2% of the total activity if the same amount of substrate is incubated with trypsin or Crotalus venom. In one experiment 6.4 mg of the fragment PKFL and 1.4 mg of the fragment PKFS were obtained from the kininogen collected from 3 l ox serum. One mg of these peptides will contract the rat uterus to the same extent as 2 mcg of bradykinin. Both peptides contain met-lys-bradykinin, but they differ in the composition of the C-terminal chains. PKLF possesses Ser-Val-Glu. In addition to met-lys-bradykinin, PKFS contains met-lys-bradykinin, one valine, and probably one methionine residue attached to the C-terminal (HABERMANN, 1966).

III. Antidiuretic Peptide: Pepsanurin

Plasma, serum, or the globulin fraction hydrolyzed by pepsin, generates a peptide which has antidiuretic activity in the rat [CROXATTO et al., 1953 (2, 3)] (Fig. 3). Pepsanurin was coined to differentiate this peptide from pepsitensin and pepsitocin, the two other peptide components which accumulate during pepsin hydrolysis.

The substrate usually employed was the globulin fraction obtained by precipitating human or horse citrated plasma with half-saturated ammonium sulfate. The precipitate (globulins) is dialyzed in order to eliminate salts and fibrin. Dialysis also eliminates most of the antidiuretic effects of plasma or serum [HELLER, 1951; CROXATTO et al., 1953 (1, 2, 4)].

The pH adopted for the incubation has a decisive influence on the pharmacological properties of the globulin digest [CROXATTO et al., 1951 (1, 2); BLAIR, 1962]. Prolonged incubation of horse globulin with pepsin (10 to 200 mg per 100 ml globulin) produces extracts with intense antidiuretic activity but with a relatively weak hypertensive action [CROXATTO et al., 1951 (1, 2)]. After incubation at pH 3.5 to 4, the deproteinized extract (with 2 to 3 volumes ethanol) shows pressor response typical of pepsitensin and an intense oxytocic activity on rat and guinea-pig uterus, but no antidiuretic activity in the rat (CROXATTO et al., 1951 (1, 2); BLAIR, 1962]. The reverse occurs if the deproteinized extract is submitted to a second digestion with pepsin (pH 2.5 to 3.5) per 24 h. An intense antidiuretic activity takes place and the extract loses its vasopressor action, but the oxytocic activity does not change. If the first incubation is carried out at pH 2.5 or lower for 18 to 24 h, the vasopressor activity is lower than in incubations carried out at pH 3.5, but the antidiuretic action is striking [BLAIR, 1962; CROXATTO et al.,

1951 (2)]. A reciprocal relation between pressor and antidiuretic effects can be found in diverse globulin hydrolyzates. Similar treatments of plasma, albumin fraction, produced products with neglegible antidiuretic activity at pH 2.5 or 3.5. Negative results were obtained by incubating renin substrate without pepsin at pH 2.5 for 24 h or with inactivated pepsin (BLAIR, 1962).

According to these data, the optimum pH for pepsanurin formation is about 2.5. Higher pH favors pepsitensin formation but hinders pepsanurin accumulation

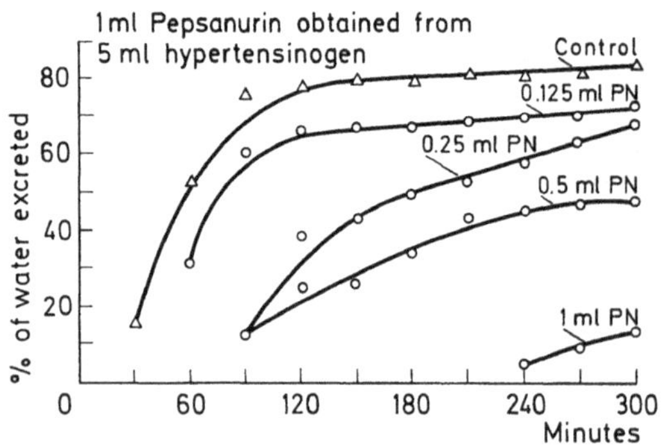

Fig. 3. Antidiuretic effect of different doses of an extract from horse serum renin-substrate incubated with pepsin (CROXATTO, H. R., 1956)

Table 2.

Period of incubation (h)	Pressor activity m-u. Pitressin equivalent with s.e. ($P = 0.95$)	Antidiuretic activity m-u. Pitressin equivalent with s.e. ($P = 0.95$)	Ratio pressor: antidiuretic activities
4	435 (3)	24.1 (± 2.6) (6)	18
8	765 (± 18) (5)	51.9 (± 2.7) (5)	15
8	3,476 (± 81) (4)	120 (± 11) (6)	29
11	1,000 (± 41) (4)	30.9 (± 1.5) (11)	32
14	421 (± 20) (5)	31.1 (± 2.6) (4)	14
20	Nil (3) (< 40)	31.9 (± 2.2) (10)	<1
20	152 (± 11) (4)	21.6 (± 1.1) (14)	7
4 h at pH 4 (pepsitensin)	2,970 (± 106) (5)	Nil (4) (< 2.5)	—

(Table 2). At optimum pH, the antidiuretic factor rises almost to its maximum after 10 h, and thereafter increases very slowly. The vasopressor peptide begins to decline during the second hour and reaches a minimum after 10 h. Renin substrate previously treated with renin and dialyzed to remove angiotensin retains its capacity to form pepsanurin when incubated with pepsin in a second stage [CROXATTO et al., 1954 (1)]. This result indicates that pepsanurin derives neither from the renin substrate fragment which contains pepsitensin nor from angiotensin [CROXATTO, 1957; CROXATTO et al., 1951 (2)]. It is also possible that pepsanurin is split from a globulin chain other than renin substrate. At the same time, pepsitensin derived from renin substrate accumulates under pepsin hydrolysis. The accumulation of pepsitensin counteracts the antidiuretic effect of pepsanurin, but following a second pepsin hydrolysis full antidiuretic activity is present.

Pepsanurin pharmacological actions: In normal hydrated and hyperhydrated rats pepsanurin inhibits urine excretion. The antidiuretic effect observed in the rat overloaded with water according to the procedures of BURN (1931) or JEFFERS et al. (1942) is particularly striking. The inhibition in water excretion can be reproduced in hypophysectomized rats and in animals with insipidus polyuria. In hypophysectomized hyperhydrated rats treated with cortisone, pepsanurin obtained from 0.5 ml of horse serum abolishes urine excretion for 40 to 70 min,

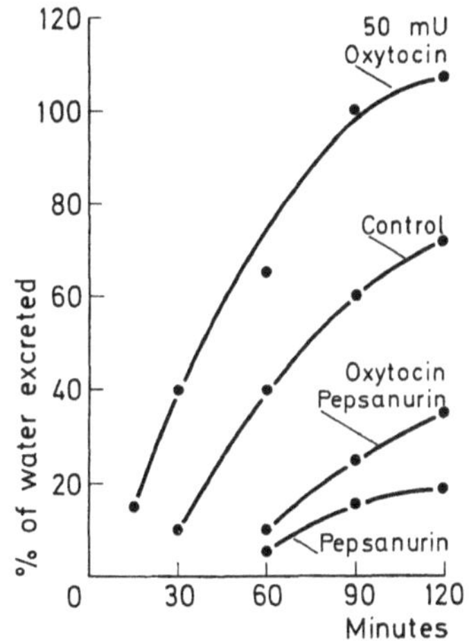

Fig. 4

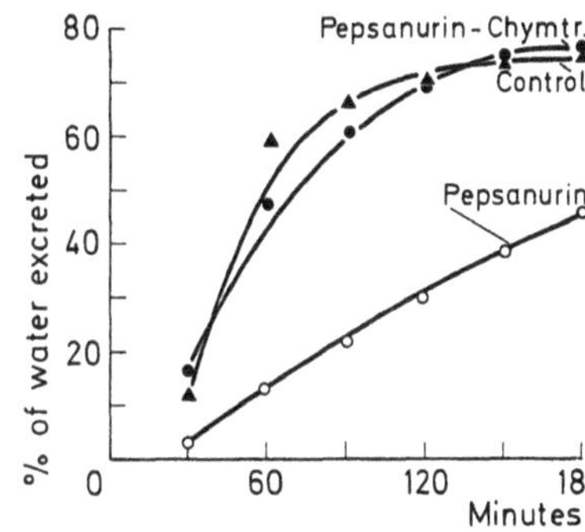

Fig. 5

Fig. 4. Effect obtained upon diuresis in water-loaded rats with injections of: a) 50 mU oxytocin. b) 0.9% NaCl solution, s. c. c) 50 mU oxytocin subcutaneously plus 0.1 pepsanurin extract solution i. p. d) 0.1 pepsanurin extract solution i. p. (CROXATTO, H. R., 1957)

Fig. 5. Antidiuretic effect (Burn's test) of 0.2 ml of an extract containing pepsanurin and of 0.2 ml of the same extract incubated with chymotrypsin. The preparation was obtained from horse serum renin-substrate. (CROXATTO, H. R., 1951)

during which control animals excrete 50% of the administered water (REYES, 1952). The antidiuretic effect of intravenous pepsanurin has been demonstrated in hydrated rats anesthetized with alcohol. The effect is intense although of shorter duration than the one observed in animals following intraperitoneal injections. Since the injection of pepsanurin in hypophysectomized rats produces pronounced inhibition of diuresis, the antidiuretic effect cannot be explained by stimulation of the neurohypophysis and release of vasopressin. The experiments in alcohol-anesthetized rats confirm this assumption (CROXATTO, 1957). Pepsanurin and vasopressin antagonize the augmented diuresis induced by renin or oxytocin (CROXATTO, 1957) (Fig. 4). The inhibition of diuresis in water-loaded rats (conscious or under ethanol anesthesia) is not the result of a delayed water absorption in the digestive tract. The antidiuretic effect of pepsanurin seems to be due to increased water absorption by the renal tubules. In moderate reduction of diuresis, creatinine clearance is not significantly altered (CROXATTO, 1955). Hydrogenated ergot alkaloids and dibenamine, which inhibit the antidiuretic effect of serotonin do not modify antidiuresis produced by pepsanurin or vasopressin. The most active fractions of pepsanurin obtained through two successive pepsin digestions of blood globulin have very little effect on blood pressure in rat (Blair, 1962). The small rise sometimes observed can be attributed to residual amounts of pepsin still present in the hydrolyzate. The pepsanurin obtained from purified renin substrate, previously incubated with renin, does not increase, but decreases blood pressure. Venezian (1955) obtained a peptide hydrolyzate from 5 to 10 mg of purified renin substrate with no pressor activity, but which possessed antidiuretic activity equivalent to 10 mU of vasopressin.

Pepsanurin enzymatic inactivation: Chymotrypsin abolishes the antidiuretic action of pepsanurin (Fig. 5), but trypsin only reduces it. However, neither pepsin or carboxypeptidase modifies its action. Vasopressin shows similar behavior, although trypsin acts more deeply on the hormone, which rapidly loses its vasopressor activity. The serum from pregnant women does not affect the activity of pepsanurin although it readily destroys vasopressin [Croxatto et al., 1954 (2)]. Thioglycollate does not modify the typical effect of the peptide under conditions which rapidly abolish the vasopressin activity [Croxatto and Barnafi, 1960 (1)]. The formation of pepsanurin by the hydrolytic action of pepsin might be regarded as an artifact or a pharmacological curiosity. However, there is a substrate in blood which following enzymatic cleavage liberates a substance which reversibly inhibits kidney excretion.

B. Vasopressor Peptides Formed by the Action of Protoeolytic Enzymes Other than Pepsin

I. Effect of Proteinase in Alpha-Amylase Preparation

Nagarse, Huggins and Walaszek (1959); Walaszek and Huggins (1959), and Walaszek et al. (1962) showed that a vasopressor polypeptide could be produced when fraction IV-4 of human plasma protein was incubated with a crude alpha-amylase preparation. This enzyme, prepared from the growth medium of *Bacillus subtilis*, has a high level of proteolytic activity (Huggins et al., 1964). The vasopressor substance, termed substance A, is a polypeptide closely related to angiotensin. A crystalline proteinase, obtained from the same organism (commercially available as Nagarse) proved very effective in the formation of the same vasoactive material. This stimulates the isolated rat uterus and guinea-pig ileum, and produces a pressor response on dog, cat and rat blood pressure. It is destroyed by chymotrypsin, trypsin, and pepsin and can be inactivated by Nagarse. Results obtained with subtilisin and a natural proteinase from *Bacillus subtilis* were practically identical (Tsuru et al., 1964). Prado et al. (1965) used the same crystalline proteinase, and formed a hypotensive material, provisionally designated substance N. When Nagarse is incubated for 10 min at 37 °C with heat-treated horse plasma substance N accumulates in the incubation mixture. This substance, like bradykinin, lowers blood pressure in the dog and relaxes the cat duodenum. Substance N is inactivated by chymotrypsin but not trypsin, and is slowly inactivated by Nagarse. Since substance N cannot be separated from bradykinin by paper electrophoresis, Prado et al. (1964) suggested that Nagarse was a kininogenase which releases the vasoactive bradykinin-like peptide. In contrast, Huggins and Thampi (1967) used horse-serum protein as a substrate, and under the same experimental conditions, found that the active material released by Nagarse has only pressor properties. Pepsin can split the peptide bonds from renin substrate forming pepsitensin, and form kinin-type or prokinin substances, from kininogens; it seems likely that angiotensin-like substances and bradykinin-like substances can be split from different blood globulins by Nagarse. Differences in protease concentrations, relative amounts of renin-substrate and bradykininogen in plasma or serum, the time elapsing after blood withdrawal and incubation time, could account for the divergence in results.

II. Effect of Chymotrypsin

NOLLY et al. (1971) described formation of an angiotensin-like substance when human plasma was incubated with alpha-chymotrypsin. It was thermostable, dialyzable and acid- and alkali-resistant. Trypsin inactivates it, but thioglycolate does not alter its pharmacological effects. If the plasma is previously incubated with renin, and the angiotensin formed is removed by dialysis, alpha-chymotrypsin is unable to release a vasoconstrictor substance. NOLLY et al. (1971) described a substance which increased blood pressure in the rat, contracted the isolated rat uterus and constricted vessels of the hind leg of the frog. Equipressor amounts (15 μg) of angiotensin and of this vasopressor substance produce similar vasoconstriction in the frog. A vasopressor substance with a single peak located between peaks corresponding to Ang. I and Ang. II can be obtained from a column of Sephadex G-25. Plasma can generate a vasoconstrictor substance if it is first acidified to pH 4 and incubated for 30 min at 37 °C, then readjusted to pH 5.6 with phosphate-citrate buffer and incubated for 15 min with chymotrypsin. The vasopressor activity is greater (1:2 or 1:4) than that obtained using homologous renin, particularly when blood plasma from mammals is employed (CABRERA et al., 1971). The liberation of a vasopressor peptide by the action of Padutin (kallikrein preparation) upon the plasma of the snake *Bothrops jararaca* has been attributed to a chymotrypsin contaminating the kallikrein. A similar vasoactive substance was obtained using pure chymotrypsin (LAVRAS et al., 1971).

C. Vasopressor Peptides Formed in Plasma or Serum by Acidification

Anephrotensin: CROXATTO et al. (1959) reported the formation of a peptide similar to the peptides formed by incubation of plasma with pepsin when dog serum was incubated at pH 3.5 to 4.5 at 37 °C for several hours. The peptide(s) formed mimic some of the pharmacological effects of angiotensin and bradykinin [CROXATTO et al., 1959, 1960 (2), 1961, 1963; CROXATTO and BARNAFI, 1960 (1)]. The formation of anephrotensin following a sudden change of pH is not rapid; it takes place progressively and requires several hours to reach a maximum. Its formation is also temperature-dependent and there is a species difference. 0.1 ml acidified dog plasma incubated for 70 h at 38 °C and given intravenously to a nephrectomized rat (200 g) under a sympathetic blockade, produces a vasopressor potency equipotent to 15 to 25 μg of 5-valine-Ang. II. This effect has been attributed to an angiotensin-like peptide which was provisionally designated anephrotensin. This name was proposed because the pressor effect of the acidified plasma is more striking in nephrectomized animals than in normal animals. In addition, the yield of pressor material obtained from the plasma or serum of nephrectomized animals is greater that that of intact animals. The difference observed in the pressor response between normal and nephrectomized sera is greater if the arterial blood pressure of the nephrectomized recipient animal is substantially lowered by the administration of sympathetic blocking agents. The increase in blood pressure of the rat following administration of plasma from nephrectomized dogs is 6 times greater than that caused by plasma from control dogs (CROXATTO et al., 1963). In addition, the acidified plasma from nephrectomized rats is 3 times more active than the corresponding acidified plasma of the non-operated control rats (CROXATTO, 1963). The pressor effect produced by the acidified serum in normal animals is slight, and is often preceded by transient hypotension. Thus, the blood pressure response is biphasic, but the hypotension decreases or disappears if the pressure level of the recipient rat has been reduced either by hemorrhage or by ganglionic blocking agents [CROXATTO et al., 1960 (2), 1963].

Anephrotensin pharmacological properties: The sera of various diverse species display common pharmacological properties when incubated at acid pH, but differ in certain respects. The serum of the Chilean giant frog *(Caliptocephalella Gayi)*, of Brazilian snakes *(Bothrops jararaca* and *Driadophis bifossatus bifossatus)* and of fishes, teleosts *(Sebastodes oculatus oculatus* and *Graus nigra)* elicits an angiotensin-like pressor response in the normal and nephrectomized rat or dog. The rise in blood pressure is dose-dependent and not preceded by a transient fall. Animals, including man, and particularly rat and guinea pig furnish sera which after acidification and incubation elicit hypotension in the normal rat or often biphasic responses, but increase blood pressure of the nephrectomized rat. Dog serum or its peptide fraction raises pressure which is sometimes preceded by a negligible fall in pressure regardless of the level of the blood pressure prior to injection. In nephrectomized dogs and rats only pressor response is observed following the administration of "acidified" sera obtained from frog and chicken. Animals treated with ganglionic blocking agents are particularly sensitive to the hypertensive effect of anephrotensin regardless of the origin of the plasma [CROXATTO et al., 1960 (2), 1963].

The hypertensive response is not significantly reduced if the recipient rat is adrenalectomized or pretreated with atropine or dibenamine. Peripheral resistance accounts for most of the increase in blood pressure. However, following ganglionic blockade, incubated rat serum increases cardiac output similar to bradykinin and angiotensin (ROSAS et al., 1965).

Serum obtained from different animals incubated at low pH produces (a) substance(s) which will contract isolated smooth muscle (Fig. 6). Rat serum, incubated at pH 4 for 24 to 36 h (optimum time) has an oxytocic activity assayed on the rat uterus equal to that of 30 to 100 mμ of oxytocin (CROXATTO et al., 1961). The oxytocic activity of anephrotensin from human, dog, frog, (Fig. 6) reptile and fish is lower than its vascular activity when compared to Ang. II or bradykinin (CROXATTO et al., 1963). Isolated rat duodenum relaxes to purified dog anephrotensin (An_2), free of bradykinin or kallidin, whereas angiotensin contracts the duodenum. Chicken and frog anephrotensin contracts the rat duodenum and chick caecum provided they are stored at low temperatures for several hours before the experiments are performed. Dog anephrotensin relaxes the chick caecum whereas Ang. II contracts it and bradykinin has no effect [CROXATTO and BARNAFI, 1960 (1)].

Anephrotensin, enzymatic system involved in its formation: Because of the temperature and pH relationships, it may be assumed that the release of active substance(s) is the result of an enzymatic action. Only preliminary studies have been undertaken to determine the enzymes involved. Renin and pepsin (enzymes present in plasma) have been ruled out with nephrectomized and gastrectomized animals [CROXATTO et al., 1960 (2)]. Acidification is very effective in preventing the inactivation of peptides in the plasma. Angiotensinase, vasopressinase, oxytocinase and kininases can be irreversibly inhibited by a drastic acidification. In addition, the change of plasma pH to acid facilitates some biochemical process favorable to protein cleavage. It is not known whether an enzyme-inhibitor complex is broken by acidification, dissociating the enzyme from an inhibitor moiety, ore some inactive enzyme precursor is directly activated. Since acidification furnishes favorable conditions for kallikrein activation (HORTON, 1959), this enzyme was postulated as one of the systems participating in the accumulation of active peptides. In fact, in purified material obtained from the peptide fraction of acidified serum, bradykinin and kallidin have been identified and separated from a vasopressor peptide (CROXATTO, 1966; CROXATTO et al., 1964). Although bradykinin elicits a dose-related lowering of blood pressure in the normotensive rat,

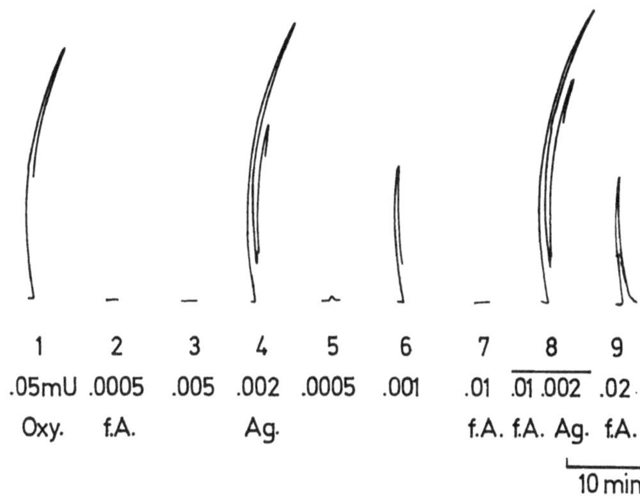

Fig. 6. Contractions of isolated rat uterus in Tyrode solution. The figures express the concentration of the substances per ml in the bath solution. 1. 0.05 ml of oxytocin. 2. 0.005 ml of anephrotensin obtained from intact frog. 3. 0.005 ml frog anephrotensin. 4. 2 ng of [5-valyl]-angiotensin II. 5. 0.5 ng of the same as 4. 6. 1 ng of the same as 4. 7. 0.01 ml of frog anephrotensin. 8. 0.01 ml of frog anephrotensin plus 2 ng [5-valyl]-angiotensin II mixed on adding to the bath. 9. 0.02 ml of frog anephrotensin. (CROXATTO, H. R., LABARCA, E., 1962)

it frequently increases blood pressure in the hypotensive rat (CROXATTO and BELMAR, 1961; CROXATTO et al., 1962).

The formation of the vasopressor peptide is not hindered by soya bean-trypsin inhibitor, and yield is the same whether or not it is exposed to pancreatic kallikrein for 12 to 24 h before acidification. This enzyme, under these conditions, exhausts kininogen and prevents bradykinin accumulation. The formation of the vasopressor peptide is not altered by heparin, sodium oxalate, silicone-coated glassware, or by centrifugation at low temperature (CROXATTO et al., 1964). The yield of anephrotensin is not modified in the blood of recently hypophysectomized or adrenalectomized rats (CROXATTO et al., 1964); but the kidneys have a considerable influence on the amount of vasopressor substances formed in the plasma during acidification. Higher yields of vasopressor peptides are obtained in nephrectomized animals than in intact animals. For example, the yield of anephrotensin from the blood of dogs nephrectomized 36 to 72 h before is 4 to 5 times greater than the yield of anephrotensin obtained from blood of control dogs. There is a progressive increase in anephrotensin in serum after nephrectomy (CROXATTO, 1963). These experiments exclude the participation of renin in the greater yield of anephrotensin, which is in keeping with the results of ROSAS (1963) which demonstrated that antirenin does not interfere with anephrotensin formation. The increase in renin substrate in the blood of nephrectomized animals (LELOIR et al., 1940; PAGE and HELMER, 1940) may account for the greater amount of anephrotensin or another substrate (anephrotensinogen) could be increased, forming the pressor peptide (ROSAS, 1963).

The greater yield of anephrotensin from serum of nephrectomized animals is not the result of the loss of excretory functions of the kidney nor of the accumulation of metabolic waste products, since the ligation of the ureters is not followed by similar increases in the peptides. In the dog, normal or slightly increased amounts were obtained 48 h after clamping both ureters (CROXATTO et al., 1963).

Inactivation of anephrotensin: All pharmacological properties of incubated serum or its active purified fractions are destroyed by chymotrypsin (pH 6 to 7.8). Fresh serum from different species inactivates the vasopressor and oxytocic activities of acidified incubated serum. Rat serum inactivates the oxytocic activity of anephrotensin more rapidly than the neurohypophyseal hormones. Unlike oxytocin and vasopressin, anephrotensin withstands thioglycollate treatment. Trypsin and pepsin inactivate chicken and frog anephrotensin (CROXATTO and LABARCA, 1962) and partially destroy the pharmacological effects of acidified serum and purified anephrotensin of other species such as man and rat. Purified dog anephrotensin, after treatment with carboxypeptidase, will relax the rat duodenum and increase blood pressure [CROXATTO and BARNAFI, 1960 (1)].

Anephrotensin purification. The observation that acidification of plasma or serum promoted the accumulation of both angiotensin and bradykinin-like peptides was confirmed (CROXATTO et al., 1964; CROXATTO, 1966). Using gel filtration (Sephadex G-25), gradient elution on a carboxymethyl-cellulose column with ammonium acetate (0.01 M, pH 5 to 0.3 M pH 7.5) from acidified incubated dog serum, 3 or 4 vasoactive fractions were separated. These were successively designated An1, An2, AnB and AnK. An1 and An2 are vasopressors in all the animals tested so far and AnB and AnK lower blood pressure of the rat. An2 is similar to Ang. I in many respects, but unlike the angiotensins it relaxes the rat duodenum. Its purification has been slow because of low yields. The purest substance has activity per mg equivalent to 1.7 mcg of Ang. II in the nephrectomized rat. An2 shows two separated spots on paper chromatography, but only one has biological activity. The effect of proteolytic enzymes: pepsin, trypsin, chymotrypsin and carboxypeptidase B is similar to that observed for the angiotensins. An1 is less active than An2 but raises blood pressure in normal and nephrectomized animals, contracts the rat uterus, and is inactivated by all the proteolytic enzymes previously mentioned except carboxypeptidase B. AnB is identical to bradykinin; it lowers pressure in the rat and produces biphasic changes in the blood pressure of nephrectomized hypotensive rats. It has no effect on blood pressure of the chicken, but relaxes the rat duodenum and contracts the rat uterus. It resists pepsin and trypsin but is rapidly inactivated by carboxypeptidase B. AnB has the same R_f value as bradykinin on paper chromatography and only a single spot is found when both substances are mixed. AnK appears inconstantly in very small amounts in gradient elution procedures. Pharmacologically and chromatographically it behaves like kallidin. Although the chemical identifications of these different components has been unsuccessful, the main vasopressor peptide An1 is similar to angiotensin but differs its effect on rat duodenum. While the chemical identification is still pending, this difference justifies the provisional use of the term anephrotensin. The formation of anephrotensin demonstrates that the amount of the protein precursor circulating in the blood is controlled by a renal function non-excretory in type (CROXATTO, 1963).

The peptides excreted in the urine of normal and DCA hypertensive rats are similar to the peptides which appear in acidified-circulated serum (ROSAS, 1960, 1963; ROSAS and CROXATTO, 1962; ROSAS et al., 1963) and may represent the renal clearance of similar substances present in the plasma. There is also an increase in uterotonic activity of extracts prepared from urine of DCA hypertensive rats (ROSAS and CROXATTO, 1962). Acid incubation (48 h) of blood serum from rats made hypertensive by the method of PAGE (1950) releases significantly larger amounts of peptides which can contract the isolated rat uterus and increase blood pressure of the nephrectomized rat (CROXATTO et al., 1964).

D. Vasopressor Albumin (VA) Formed in Plasma or Serum Incubated at 37° C at Normal pH for Several Hours (5 - 96) under Sterile Conditions

Several groups of investigators have found that plasma from different species incubated for several hours forms a pressor substance which is unlike any of the natural polypeptides or amines isolated so far from the body. ARNEIL and DEKANSKI (1954) reported the presence of a vasopressor material in normal plasma and plasma from children with a glomerulonephritis and hypertension. The vasopressor response was greater with the plasma incubated at 37 °C for 12 h. MASSON et al. (1957) demonstrated that incubated plasma from normotensive or hypertensive subjects had myotropic and pressor activity. The study included patients with malignant hypertension, renal hypertension, and chronic glomerulonephritis. Freshly frozen plasma produced irregular and insignificant pressor responses similar to those elicited by saline. All incubated samples (24 to 29 h) were pressor, approximately to the same degree and without reference to the presence of hypertension. Serum from monkeys immunized against renin and plasma from rats made tachyphylatic to renin by repeated daily injections of renin yielded full pressor activity on incubation. The effect has been attributed to a phospholipid, most probably a lysophosphatide, which results from the activity of an enzyme present in the plasma "heavy-density lipoprotein" fraction (KHAIRALLAH and PAGE, 1960). CROXATTO (1961) observed that the plasma incubated for many hours under similar conditions as acidified plasma (pH 3.8) also exhibited vasopressor activity, although with different pharmacological characteristics. The time required to attain the maximum vasopressor activity with the incubated plasma or serum varied according to the species used: it was 80 to 90 h for man and dog, and 30 h for rat (ROBLERO and CROXATTO, 1967). KENNER and WALDHÄUSL (1964) reported that serum incubated without acid or proteolytic enzyme produced a pressor substance; 0.25 ml of the incubated serum increased blood pressure by about 35 mmHg due to a non-dialyzable and heat-stable substance. This observation was confirmed by PETERLIK and WALDHÄUSL (1967), who demonstrated that most of the plasma-pressor activity was due to a macromolecule similar to albumin. Its activity appears in the elution volumes of the albumin through gel filtration in Sephadex G-100 (CROXATTO and DIAZ, 1969). The pressor activity is not modified by the use of carefully siliconized syringes and glassware, the presence of heparin or sodium oxalate (KHAIRALLAH and PAGE, 1960), the addition of fibrinolysin or soya bean-trypsin inhibitor (CROXATTO et al., 1965). Heparin administered in large doses to small animals before bleeding reduces the pressor activity by 50% (CROXATTO et al., 1965). Ethylenediaminetetraacetic acid also inhibits its formation (KHAIRALLAH and PAGE, 1960; CROXATTO et al., 1965), and both calcium and phosphate ions are required (KHAIRALLAH and PAGE, 1960) (Fig. 7).

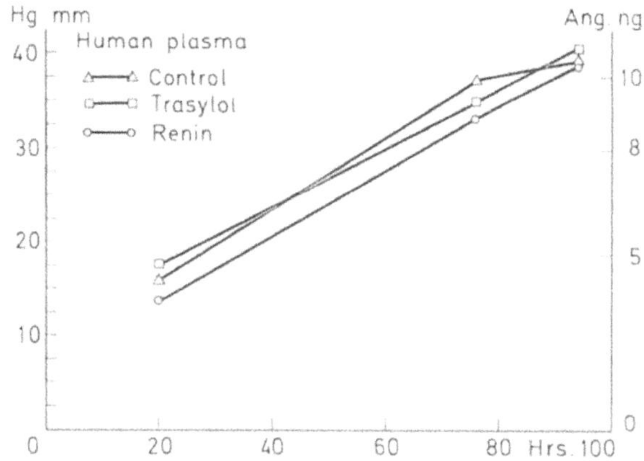

Fig. 7. Vasopressor substance (VA) formation in three separate samples of 40 ml of the same human plasma incubated for 92 h at 38 °C with: 1. 5000 U of Trasylol; 2. 20 Goldblatt units of human renin; 3. 9% NaCl solution (control). The activity is expressed by the extent of the blood pressure increase in mm Hg and in relation to that of angiotensin II valyl 5, obtained by 0.1 ml of plasma injected intravenously in the rat. (CROXATTO, H. R., ROBLERO, J., 1970)

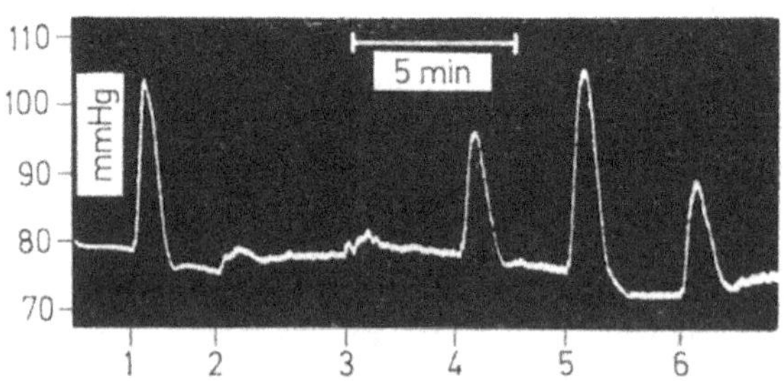

Fig. 8. Blood pressure response to 0.3 ml serum. 1. Incubated serum. 2. serum containing 2 mM EDTA, then incubated. 3. serum containing 5 mM pyrophosphate, and then incubated. 4. serum containing EDTA, then dialyzed. Before incubation, 3.0 mEq phosphate was added. 5. same as in 3 with both calcium and phosphate added. 6. same as 3 with 5.0 mEq calcium added. (KHAIRALLAH, P. A., PAGE, I. H., 1960)

The rate of formation of the vasopressor substance is not changed by kallikrein, kallikrein inhibitor (Trasylol), or renin added to the plasma (CROXATTO and ROBLERO, 1970) (Fig. 8). The optimum pH for the best yield of the vasopressor principle is 8-9 (KHAIRALLAH and PAGE, 1960; GORDON and RIESKE, 1967; and ROBLERO, unpublished). In contrast to anephrotensin formation, a smaller yield of hypertensive albumin (VA) is found in the blood of rats nephrectomized 24 to 28 h previously than in that of normal rats (CROXATTO et al., 1965). WALDHÄUSL and KENNER (1965) found that the pressor substance of the incubated plasma is protein-like or a protein-bound molecule. This pressor protein has also been found in the plasma and lymph of nephrectomized rabbits. In contrast with other work (MASSON et al., 1957; KHAIRALLAH and PAGE, 1960), trypsin, pepsin and chymotrypsin inactivated the vasopressor principle (KENNER and WALDHÄUSL, 1965). GORDON and RIESKE (1967) found that prolonged incubation with chymotrypsin destroyed the activity of the incubated plasma. ROBLERO and CROXATTO (1967, 1968) reported the endopeptidases greatly modified the effect of the active substance formed by incubation of dog, rat and human serum at a neutral pH. These findings suggest that the vasopressor principle is a large protein molecule and not a lipid as suggested by KHAIRALLAH and PAGE (1960). Moreover, identification with a protein molecule or a protein-bound molecule is not consistent with its solubility and stability in 50% ethanol (MASSON et al., 1957; ROBLERO and CROXATTO, 1967, 1968). Gel filtration through Sephadex G-100 of plasma of different species, collected in siliconized glassware, centrifuged at low temperature and incubated under sterile conditions at 37 °C enabled ROBLERO and CROXATTO (1967) to separate two different non-dialyzable proteins which increased the blood pressure of nephrectomized hypotensive rats. These fractions appeared in two different peaks in the effluent solution from the column. One fraction lowers blood pressure in the normal rat and the other increases pressure. Both are inactivated by chymotrypsin, but the former becomes more active under pepsin and trypsin hydrolysis. These changes are due to the release of dialyzable peptides. The peptides derived from peak 1 have bradykinin-like properties while the peptides released from peak 2 have vasopressor activity in intact and nephrectomized rats and show several pharmacological features similar to angiotensin.

Pharmacological actions. The pressor activity of plasma is not due to adrenergic amines or serotonin (ARNEIL and DEKANSKI, 1954; CROXATTO and DIAZ, 1969), since the pressor action is not blocked by dibenamine (ARNEIL and DEKANSKI, 1954) or by bromolysergic diethylamine. It is not vasopressin, since it survives treatment with 0.01 M thioglycollate (MASSON et al., 1957). ARNEIL and DEKANSKI (1954) suggested that the pressor substance is angiotensin or an angiotensin-like peptide. However, this possibility has been ruled out since: 1) angiotensin is rapidly inactivated by the plasma; 2) the addition of renin substrate does not enhance the yield; 3) the presence of antirenin does not prevent a full pressor activity on incubation, and 4) plasma retains this activity under the action of proteolytic enzymes which inactivate angiotensin (MASSON et al., 1957). The addition of homologous renin to plasma did not modify the rate of formation of the vasopressor substance (CROXATTO and ROBLERO, 1969), although nephrectomized rats and dogs provide plasma which generates smaller yields of pressor substance following incubation than normal ones. Incubated plasma contracted the rabbit aorta, guinea-pig ileum, rat and rabbit uterus (MASSON et al., 1957). The purified vasopressor principle obtained after gel filtration corresponds to albumin and has a negligible myotropic effect on isolated rat uterus (ROBLERO and CROXATTO, 1967). Nephrectomy or adrenalectomy does not alter the pressor response (CROXATTO et al., 1965). Azamethonium increases the effect of the incubated plasma or its active fraction (VA). Since alpha- or beta-adrenergic receptor-blocking agents did not inhibit the pressor response, the liberation of catecholamines was ruled out (CROXATTO and DIAZ, 1969). Previous injection of carboxypeptidase B in doses sufficient to produce a long-lasting inhibition of plasma kinins did not inhibit the pressor response to incubated plasma or its active albumin fraction (CROXATTO and CRUZATT, 1969). Intravenous injection of the incubated plasma increases blood pressure in the rat but decreases blood pressure in the cat (CROXATTO and CRUZATT, 1969).

Enzymatic system involved. The mechanism of formation of the vasopressor substance is still unexplained. The temperature- and pH-dependence and the effect of heating indicate that an enzyme is involved in its formation (KHAIRALLAH and PAGE, 1960; ROBLERO and CROXATTO, 1966; GORDON and RIESKE, 1967). Ethylenediaminetetracetic acid and pyrophosphate completely inhibit development of the active substance, which is restored by the addition of calcium and phosphate ions. The enzyme is not inhibited by diisopropylfluorophosphate or cyanide (MASSON et al., 1957). An active material containing phospholipids can be obtained by purification. The R_f values of lysophosphatides prepared from impure lecithin were similar to those of plasma fractions. Lecithin added to plasma before incubation increases the amount of the vasopressor material obtained 24 h after incubation (KHAIRALLAH and PAGE, 1960). The plasma enzyme could act like a phospholipase A, a calcium-dependent enzyme similar to snake-venom phospholipase. The pressor substance is not a lysophosphatide but probably an albumin or albumin-bound molecule since it is inactivated by chymotrypsin (ROBLERO and CROXATTO, 1966; KENNER and WALDHÄUSL, 1965; CROXATTO et al., 1965; GORDON and RIESKE, 1967). Pepsin and trypsin increases the vasopressor activity suggesting that the pressor agent is a peptide.

The biological change observed in the incubated plasma is a widely distributed property of mammalian blood but its biological significance is still unknown and the kidney has the most influence in the formation of the VA principle. Substrates and enzymes which generate vasoactive substances are partly handled by this organ.

E. Other Unidentified Components of Plasma with Vasopressor Activity

BOHR and JOHANSSON (1966) demonstrated that plasma contains vasoactive substance(s) which increase tension of strips of vascular smooth muscle. The component is present in the protein-free filtrate of plasma and is different from the known vasoactive agents. The active component is a cationic, heat-stable, inactivated by boiling for 1 h in 0.1 N HCl and not inactivated by trypsin or aminopeptidase (BOHR and SOBIEZKI, 1968). The active fraction (0.1 ml) elicits a greater response in the perfused vascular bed than 0.1 mcg norepinephrine. The response is not affected by blocking doses of phentolamine and methysergide. The addition of the vasoactive fraction to the physiological salt solution (PSS) perfusing an isolated rat kidney, increases renal vascular resistance. The response is not like that produced by epinephrine, angiotensin, vasopressin serotonin and KCl. The response produced by the plasma factor was greater during perfusion with "high-calcium" PSS, and the ability of vessels to respond to plasma factor was lost during perfusion with "calcium-free" PSS. HYSSEL and BOHR (1970) suggested that this factor might be a determinant of vascular tone "in situ" and could play a role in autoregulation of the kidney.

NAYLER and MCCULLOCH (1960), and LOWE and NAYLER (1965) reported that the effect of 1 mcg of a fraction of human plasma which contained a low molecular weight (5000 to 8000) substance with positive inotropic activity on the isolated toad heart was equivalent to the effect of 0.3 mcg adrenaline. The substance was called kinekard. The addition of this substance to the perfusion fluid of isolated toad-heart preparation produces, in addition to the positive inotropic response, augmentation of oxidative metabolism, increased efficiency of energy conversion and a greatly reduced response to cardiac glycosides. Intravenous injection of the active plasma fraction elevates systemic arterial pressure, increases cardiac output and ventricular pressures, and accelerates heart rate (NAYLER et al., 1965). Intra-arterial injection of this cardioactive substance increases hind limb perfusion pressure in the dog. It also increases in coronary blood flow (NAYLER et al., 1966).

The physiological significance of this cardioactive substance remains obscure, but NAYLER et al. have suggested that it may play a role in regulation of the activity of cardiac muscle.

HADJU et al. (1957); HADJU and LEONARD (1958) isolated from mammalian plasma a protein system which increases the contractile force of isolated frog hearts. This protein system consists of three globulins, termed cardioglobulins A, B and C, which are apparently necessary for the maintenance of inotropic activity. The question of whether cardioactive plasma described by NAYLER et al. (1965), has some relationship with the globulins isolated by HADJU and LEONARD (1958) requires further investigation.

GROLLMAN and EBIHARA (1968) described a pressor agent in the renal venous blood of patients with surgically remediable hypertension following severe constriction of the renal artery or infarction of the kidney. This pressor agent was neither renin or angiotensin. GROLLMAN and KRISHNAMURTI (1970) provided additional data that this newly described pressor agent, designated by them "nephrotensin", manifests a number of properties which differentiate it from any known vasopressor substance. The dose-response curve for nephrotensin resembles that for Ang. II, but unlike the latter, it is not dialyzable through cellophane membrane, nor is it adsorbed by Dowex 50WX2. Unlike Ang. I and II, this pressor agent does not contract the rat or rabbit aortic strip. It relaxes rat ascending colon and potentiates norepinephrine on several smooth-muscle preparations. It differs from renin in that it is not precipitated by ammonium sulfate and not adsorbed onto DEAE Sephadex. It also differs from renin in its pressor response, and its stability at 80 °C (10 min), and unlike renin it does not produce tachyphylaxis. SCHWEIKERT et al. (1971) measured this pressor substance by simultaneous bioassay and radio-immunoassay and concluded that the Grollman renal pressor substance is either Ang. I or an immunologically similar substance. Recently, it has been suggested that it is identical with Ang. II.

References

ALONSO, O., CROXATTO, R., CROXATTO, H. R.: A comparative study of pepsitensin and hypertensin. Proc. Soc. exp. Biol. (N. Y.) **52**, 61 (1943).

ARNEIL, G. C., DEKANSKI, J. B.: Excess of vasopressor activity in plasma of nephritic children with hypertension. Lancet **1954 II**, 1204.

BLAIR, A. M. J. N.: Pharmacological actions of pepsitensin. Brit. J. Pharmacol. **18**, 255 (1962).

BOHR, D. F., JOHANSSON, B.: Contraction of vascular smooth muscle. Comparison with response to known vasoactive agents. Circulat. Res. **19**, 593 (1966).

BOHR, D. F., SOBIEZKI, J.: An unidentified plasma component that causes constriction of perfused vascular bed. Fed. Proc. **27**, 1396 (1968).

BRAUN-MENENDEZ, E., FASCIOLO, J. C., LELOIR, L. F., MUÑOZ, J. M., TAQUINI, C.: Relaciones entre hipertensina y pepsitensina. Rev. Soc. argent. Biol. **19**, 304 (1943).

BRAUN-MENENDEZ, E., PALADINI, A. C.: Pressor polypeptides formed in vivo and in vitro as mediators of renal hypertension. Circulation **17**, 668 (1958).

BURN, D. H.: Estimation of the antidiuretic potency of pituitary (posterior lobe) extract. Quart. J. Pharmacol. **4**, 517 (1931).

CABRERA, R. R., NOLLY, H. L., FASCIOLO, J. C.: Acción de la quimotripsina sobre plasmas de diferentes especies. Resúmenes de Comunicaciones de la XVI reunión de la Soc. Argentina de Investigacion Clinica **1**, 71 (1971).

CROXATTO, H. B.: Estudio de la anefrotensina en la sangre humana. Tesis de Grado, Facultad de Medicina, Universidad Catolica de Chile (1961).

CROXATTO, H. R.: La acción hipertensinásica. Inactivación de la hipertensina y de los principios presor y acitócico de la posthipófisis en el organismo. Rev. Med. Aliment. (Santiago) 5, 259 (1943).

CROXATTO, H. R.: Active polypeptides formed by pepsin. In: Polypeptides which stimulate plain muscle (GADDUM, J. H., Ed.). Edinburgh-London: Livingstone 1955.

CROXATTO, H. R.: Polypeptides with posterior pituitary-like activities. London: Butterworth 1956.

CROXATTO, H. R.: Polypeptides with posterior pituitary-like activities. In: The Neurohypophysis 51 (1957) (HELLER, H., Ed.). Colston Papers 8,.

CROXATTO, H. R.: Active polypeptides obtained from the blood and arterial hypertension. In: Perspectives in Biology (CORI, C. F., FOGLIA, V. G., LELOIR, L. F., OCHOA, S., Eds.). Amsterdam: Elsevier Publishing 1963.

CROXATTO, H. R.: Polipéptidos vasoactivos derivados de substratos sanguineos. Ann. Ist Superiore di Sanità (Rome) **2**, 575 (1966).

CROXATTO, H. R., ANDRADE, F., BARNAFI, L.: (1) Acción antidiurética de plasma y suero sanguineos. Bol. Soc. Biol. (Santiago) **10**, 5 (1953).

CROXATTO, H. R., BARNAFI, L.: (3) Antidiuretic substances of the blood. Nature (Lond.) **172**, 304 (1953).

CROXATTO, H. R., BARNAFI, L.: (1) Hormone and hormone-like activity of active polypeptides. Recent Prog. Hormone Res. **16**, 263 (1960).

CROXATTO, H. R., BARNAFI, L., FERRER, R.: (2) The antidiuretic potency of pregnant women serum. Acta Physiol. lat.-amer. **4**, 166 (1954).

CROXATTO, H. R., BARNAFI, L., ROJAS, G., REYES, A., INFANTE, A.: (2) Antidiuretic and oxytocic substances liberated by the digestion of plasmatic proteins with pepsin. Nature (Lond.) **171**, 82 (1953).

CROXATTO, H. R., BARNAFI, L., VILLALOBOS, S.: (1) Influencia de la renina en la reacción hipertensinógeno-pepsina y liberación de un principio antidiurético. Bol. Soc. Biol. (Santiago) **9**, 47 (1954).

CROXATTO, H. R., BELMAR, J.: Hypertensive effects of bradykinin in rats. Nature (Lond.) **192**, 879 (1961).

CROXATTO, H. R., BELMAR, J., PEREDA, T., LABARCA, E.: Hypertensive effects of bradykinin and anephrotensin in normal and nephrectomized animals. Acta Physiol. lat.-amer. **12**, 19 (1962).

CROXATTO, H. R., CROXATTO, R.: (1) Inhibitory action of amino-oxydase and tyrosinase upon the vasoconstrictor effect of hypertensin. Proc. Soc. exp. Biol. (N. Y.) **48**, 392 (1941).

CROXATTO, H. R., CROXATTO, R.: (2) Naturaleza química de la hipertensina. Rev. Soc. argent. Biol. **17**, 439 (1941).

CROXATTO, H. R., CROXATTO, R.: (3) Rev. Méd. Chile **59**, 793 (1941).

CROXATTO, H. R., CROXATTO, R.: Pepsitensin — A hypertensin-like substance produced by peptic digestion of proteins. Science **95**, 101 (1942).

CROXATTO, H. R., CROXATTO, R., MANRIQUEZ, H., VALENZUELA, B.: Destruccion de la hipertensina y de la pepsitensina por la aminopeptidasa. Bol. Soc. Biol. (Santiago) **1**, 137 (1942).

CROXATTO, H. R., CROXATTO, R., RIOSECO, M.: Acción de la carboxipeptidasa sobre la pepsitensina, vasopresina y ocitocina. Rev. Soc. argent. Biol. **21**, 23 (1945).

CROXATTO, H. R., CRUZATT, H.: Ineffectiveness of carboxypeptidase B in inhibiting the pressor effect of incubated human plasma. Experientia (Basel) **25**, 59 (1969).

CROXATTO, H. R., DIAZ, G.: Adrenergic receptor blockers on pressor activity of incubated human plasma. Proc. Soc. exp. Biol. (N. Y.) **130**, 465 (1969).

CROXATTO, H. R., LABARCA, E.: Vasopressor polypeptide (anephrotensin) obtained from the serum of the amphibian Calyptocephalella gayi. Acta Physiol. lat.-amer. **12**, 251 (1962).

CROXATTO, H. R., MARSANO, A., CROXATTO, R.: Acción hipertensinogena y coagulante de venenos de serpientes. An. Soc. Biol. Bogota **1**, 147 (1944).

CROXATTO, H. R., PEREDA, T., BELMAR, J., LABARCA, E.: Polypeptides formed by acidification of blood serum. Ann. N. Y. Acad. Sci. **104**, 146 (1963).

CROXATTO, H. R., PEREDA, T., MELLADO, R.: Peptides with oxytocic and pressor activity obtained from acidified serum. Nature (Lond.) **184**, 1496 (1959).

CROXATTO, H. R., PEREDA, T., MELLADO, R., ZAMORANO, B.: (2) Anefrotensina un nuevo péptido de acción vascular. En: Péptidos activos (CROXATTO, H., Ed.). Santiago: Centro de Publicaciones Biologicas, Universidad de Chile 1960.

CROXATTO, H. R., PEREDA, T., ZAMORANO, B.: Oxytocic substances in blood serum. In: Oxytocin (CALDEYRO BARCIA, R., HELLER, H., Eds.). Oxford: Pergamon Press 1961.

CROXATTO, H. R., REYES, A., BARNAFI, L.: (4) Características del principio antidiurético liberado del suero sanguineo por la acción de la pepsina. Bol. Soc. Biol. (Santiago) **7**, 1 (1953).

CROXATTO, H. R., RIOSECO, M.: Hipertensinasa de glóbulos rojos y pepsitensina. Bol. Soc. Biol. (Santiago) **4**, 1 (1947).

CROXATTO, H. R., ROBLERO, J.: Enzymatic system and the formation of a vasopressor albumin in the incubated plasma. In: Bradykinin and related kinins: cardiovascular, biochemical and neural actions (SICUTERI, F., ROCHA DE SILVA, M., BECK, N., Eds.). New York: Plenum Press 1970.

CROXATTO, H. R., ROBLERO, J., OSSIO, M.: Substancias vasopresoras formadas en el suero sanguíneo por incubación a 38 °C a pH normal. Arch. Biol. Med. exp. **2**, 55 (1965).

CROXATTO, H. R., ROJAS, G., BARNAFI, L.: Acciones ocitocica y presora separables de la pepsitensina. Bol. Soc. Biol. (Santiago) 8, 84 (1950).

CROXATTO, H. R., ROJAS, G., BARNAFI, L.: (1) An antidiuretic substance obtained by digestion of globulin with pepsin. Science **113**, 494 (1951).

CROXATTO, H. R., ROJAS, G., BARNAFI, L.: (2) The liberation of an antidiuretic factor by the hypertensinogen-pepsin reaction. Acta Physiol. lat.-amer. **2**, 178 (1951).

CROXATTO, H. R., VERA, R., ROBLERO, J., BELMAR, J.: Polypeptides formed by acidification of blood serum of normal and hypertensive rats. Canad. med. Ass. J. **90**, 313 (1964).

DENGLER, H.: Untersuchungen über Pepsitensin. Z. ges. exp. Med. **41**, 378 (1956).

ELLIOT, D. F., PEART, W. S.: Aminoacid sequence in hypertensin. Nature (Lond.) **177**, 527 (1956).

FRANZE DE FERNANDEZ, M. T., PALADINI, A. C., DELIUS, A. E.: Isolation and identification of a pepsitensin. Biochem. J. **97**, 540 (1965).

GORDON, D. B., RIESKE, C. L.: Arneil factor: a pressor substance, probably a protein, in incubated plasma. Fed. Proc. **26**, 368 (1967).

GREENBAUM, L. M., YAMAFUJI, K., HOSODA, T.: Studies on the peptic degradation of bovine bradykininogen. Biochem. Pharmacol. **14**, 411 (1965).

GROLLMAN, A., EBIHARA, A.: Comparison of the pressor activity and the renin content of the renal venous effluent in patients suspected of suffering surgically remediable hypertension. Texas Rep. Biol. Med. **26**, 313 (1968).

GROLLMAN, A., KRISHNAMURTY, V. S. R.: A new pressor agent of renal origin; its differentiation from renin and angiotensin. Amer. J. Physiol. **221**, 1499 (1971).

HABERMANN, E.: Strukturaufklärung kininliefernder Peptide aus Rinderserumkininogen. Naunyn-Schmiedebergs Arch. Pharmak. exp. Path. **253**, 474 (1966).

HABERMANN, E., BLENNEMANN, G., MÜLLER, B.: Charakterisierung und Reinigung peptischer kininliefernder Fragmente (PKF) sowie von "Pepsitocin" aus Rinderserum-Kininogen. Naunyn-Schmiedebergs Arch. exp. Path. Pharmak. **253**, **444** (1966).

HABERMANN, E., MÜLLER, B.: Zur enzymatischen Spaltung peptischer kininliefernder Fragmente (PKF) sowie von Rinderserum-Kininogen. Naunyn-Schmiedebergs Arch. Pharmak. exp. Path. **253**, 464 (1966).

HABERMANN, E., SCHUCK, S.: Einige Beziehungen zwischen Pepsitocin und Plasmakininen. Naturwissenschaften **51**, 61 (1964).

HADJU, S., LEONARD, E.: A serum protein system affecting contractility of the frog heart present in increased amounts in patients with essential hypertension. Circulat. Res. **6**, 740 (1958).

HADJU, S., WEISS, H., TITUS, E.: The isolation of cardio-active principle from mammalian tissue. J. Pharmacol. exp. Ther. **120**, 99 (1957).

HELLER, H.: Antidiuretic substances. J. Pharm. Pharmacol. **3**, 609 (1951).

HELMER, O. M., PAGE, I. H.: Formation of angiotensin-like pressor substance from action of crystalline pepsin on renin-activator. Proc. Soc. exp. Biol. (N. Y.) **49**, 389 (1942).

HOCHSTRASSER, K., BACHHUBER, F., WERLE, E.: Zur Frage der Identität von Pepsitensin. Hoppe-Seylers Z. physiol. Chem. **350**, 1225 (1969).

HORTON, E. W.: The estimation of urinary kallikrein. J. Physiol. (Lond.) **148**, 267 (1959).

HUGGINS, C. G., PAVESI, G., ARIAS, L.: The enzymatic formation of the vasopressor polypeptide substance A by a crystalline enzyme of *Bacillus subtilis*. Biochem. Pharmacol. **13**, 697 (1964).

HUGGINS, C. G., THAMPI, S. N.: Vasopressor principle liberated by a crystalline enzyme of "Bacillus subtilis" (Nagarse) from heart treated plasma. In: International Symposium of vasoactive polypeptides: bradykinin and related kinins (ROCHA E SILVA, M., ROTHSCHILD, H. A., Eds.). Sao Paulo (Brasil): 1967.

HUGGINS, C. G., WALASZEK, E. J.: Formation of a pharmacologically active substance from plasma proteins. Proc. Soc. exp. Biol. (N. Y.) **100**, 100 (1959).

HYSSEL, J. W., BOHR, D. F.: Renal vascular response to plasma and to known vasoactive substances. Proc. Soc. exp. Biol. (N. Y.) **135**, 930 (1970).

JEFFERS, W. A., LIVEZEY, M. M., AUSTIN, J. H.: A method for demonstrating an antidiuretic action of minute amounts of Pitressin: statistical analysis of results. Proc. Soc. exp. Biol. (N. Y.) **50**, 184 (1942).

KENNER, Th., WALDHÄUSL, W.: A non-dialysable, heat-stable hypertensive substance in the serum of rats. Nature (Lond.) **204**, 581 (1964).

KENNER, T., WALDHÄUSL, W.: Zur biologischen Bedeutung des nach mehrstündiger Erwärmung in Serum und Plasma nachweisbaren pressorischen Prinzips. Z. Kreisl.-Forsch. **54**, 1143 (1965).

KHAIRALLAH, PH. A., PAGE, I. H.: Vasopressor lipid to incubated plasma. Amer. J. Physiol. **199**, 341 (1960).

LAVRAS, A. A. C., FICHMAN, M., HIRSICHI, E., SCHMUTZIGER, P., TOBO, T., BOUCAULT, M. A.: Acao da Quimotripsina sobre o plasma de Bothrops jararaca. Acta Cientifica Venezolana. X Congreso Latinoamericano de Ciencias Fisiologicas **22**, 39 (1971).

LELOIR, L. F., MUÑOZ, J. M., BRAUN-MENENDEZ, E., FASCIOLO, J. C.: La secreción de renina y formación de hipertensina. Rev. Soc. argent. Biol. **16**, 75 (1940).

LOWE, T. E., NAYLER, W. G.: Kinekard: A blood-plasma fraction with notable cardiovascular activity. Lancet **1965 II**, 218.

LUDUEÑA, F. P.: Acción de los preparados de hipertensina sobre los músculos lisos. Rev. Soc. argent. Biol. **16**, 358 (1940).

MASSON, G. M. C., HELMCKE, G., CORCORAN, A. C., PAGE, I. H.: Pressor and myotrophic activities of incubated plasma. Proc. Soc. exp. Biol. (N. Y.) **94**, 544 (1957).

MCGLORY, D. H., OLSEN, S., FIELD, L.: A pressor material produced by the action of pepsin and casein. J. biol. Chem. **219**, 299 (1956).

NAYLER, W. G., MCCULLOGH, M.: The action of anions on cardiac muscle. Australian J. exp. Biol. med. Sci. **38**, 117 (1960).

NAYLER, W. G., RACE, D., PRICE, J. M., LOWE, T. E.: Some effects of a cardioactive fraction isolated from human blood plasma on the peripheral circulation of the dog. Circulat. Res. **18**, 1 (1966).

NAYLER, W. G., ROBERTSON, P. G. C., PRICE, J. M., LOWE, T. E.: Some properties of a cardioactive substance isolated from human plasma. Circulat. Res. **16**, 553 (1965).

NOLLY, H. L., CABRERA, R. R., FASCIOLO, J. C.: Formación en plasma humano de una substancia presora angiotensin-like "in vitro". Resúmenes de Com. de la XVI Reunión de la Soc. Argentina de Invest. Clin. (1971).

PAGE, I. H.: Circulatory system: Hypertension, experimental compression capsules. In: Medical Physics, Vol. 2. Chicago: The Year Book Publishers 1950.

PAGE, I. H., BUMPUS, F. M.: A new hormone, angiotensin. Clin. Phar. exp. Ther. **3**, 758 (1962).

PAGE, I. H., HELMER, O. M.: Angiotonin-activator, renin and angiotonin-inhibitor, and the mechanism of angi-tonin tachyphylaxis in normal, hypertensive and nephrectomized animals. J. exp. Med. **71**, 495 (1940).

PAIVA, A. C. M.: (1) Estudio comparativo entre a pepsitensina e a hipertensina. Tese, Scola Paulista de Medicina, Sao Paulo, Brasil (1954).

PAIVA, A. C. M., BANDIERA, T., PRADO, J. L.: (2) Nonidentity between pepsitensin and hypertensin revealed by paper electrophoresis. Science **120**, 611 (1954).

PETERLIK, M., WALDHÄUSL, W.: Isolation of a non-dialysable active vasopressor peptide from pig serum. Nature (Lond.) **214**, 279 (1967).

PLENTL, A. A., PAGE, I. H.: The action of crystalline proteolytic enzymes on angiotensin. J. exp. Med. **79**, 205 (1944).

PRADO, J. L., PRADO, E. S., JURKIEWICS, A.: Crystalline bacterial proteinase from B. subtilis (Nagarse) as a new kininogenase. Arch. int. Pharmacodyn. **147**, 53 (1964).

REYES, A.: Características del principio antidiurético liberado del suero sanguíneo por la acción de la pepsina. Tesis de Grado, Facultad de Medicina, Universidad de Chile (1952).

RIOSECO, M.: Nueva contribución al estudio de la pepsitensina. Tesis de Grado, Facultad de Medicina, Universidad de Chile (1945).

ROBLERO, J.: Estudio comparativo entre ocitócina y el principio ocitocico obtenido por la digestión del suero humano. Tesis de Grado, Facultad de Filosofia y Educación, Universidad Católica de Chile (1956).

ROBLERO, J., CROXATTO, H. R.: Vasoactive substances formed in blood serum by incubation at 37 °C at normal pH. International Symposium on vasoactive polypeptides: bradykinin and related kinins (ROCHA E SILVA, M., ROTSCHILD, H. A., Eds.). Sao Paulo: Brasil 1967.

ROBLERO, J., CROXATTO, H. R.: Vasoactive substances formed in blood serum by incubation. N. Y. St. J. Med. **15**, 235 (1968).,

ROCHA E SILVA, M.: Bradykinin, its occurrence and physiological significance. XXI International Congress of Physiological Sciences, Buenos Aires. **1**, 50 (1959).

ROCHA E SILVA, M.: Biochemistry and Pharmacology of bradykinin. In: Polypeptides which affect smooth muscles and blood vessels. Oxford: Pergamon Press 1960.

ROSAS, R.: Anefrotensina en ratas tratadas con DCA. In: Peptidos Activos (CROXATTO, H., Ed.). Santiago: Universidad de Chile 1960.

ROSAS, R.: Vasoactive peptides and substrates and their relation to protein handling by the kidney. Circulat. Res. **12**, 573 (1963).

ROSAS, R., CROXATTO, H. R.: Vasoactive substance in blood and urine of DCA hypertensive rats. Circulat. Res. **10**, 880 (1962).
ROSAS, R., MIYATA, T., HOOBLER, S. W., BOHR, D. F.: Peptides in urine of DCA-treated and Figure-og-8 rats. Proc. Soc. exp. Biol. (N. Y.) **113**, 456 (1963).
ROSAS, R., MONTAGUE, D., GROES, M., BOHR, F. D.: Cardiac action of vasoactive polypeptides in the rat. I. Bradykinin. Circulat. Res. **16**, 150 (1965).
SCHWEIKERT, J. R., CAREY, R. M., LIDDLE, G. W.: Evidence that the "renal pressor substance" of Grollman is related to angiotensin I. Clin. Res. **19**, 32 (1971).
TSURU, D., MCCONN, J. D., YASUNOBU, K. T.: *Bacillus subtilis* neutral proteinase. II. Some physicochemical properties. J. biol. Chem. **240**, 2415 (1965).
TUPPY, H.: Natürliche oxytocische Substanzen. Naunyn-Schmiedebergs Arch. Pharmak. Exp. Path. **228**, 94 (1956).
TUPPY, H.: Biochemical studies on oxytocinase. In: Oxytocin (CALDEYRO-BARCIA, R., HELLER, H., Eds.). Oxford: Pergamon Press 1961.
TURBA, F., HETZEL, H.: Über ein oxytocisch wirkendes Peptid aus Serumprotein. Biochem. Z. **325**, 524 (1954)
VENEZIAN, S.: Polipéptidos activos derivados del hipertensinógeno purificado. Tesis de Grado, Facultad de Medicina, Universidad Católica de Chile (1955).
WALASZEK, E. J., HUGGINS, C. G.: Substance A: A hypertensive polypeptide from fraction IV-4 plasma protein. J. Pharmacol. exp. Ther. **126**, 258 (1959).
WALASZEK, E. J., BUNAG, R. D., HUGGINS, C. G.: The characterization of the hypertensive polypeptide substance. J. Pharmacol. exp. Ther. **138**, 139 (1962).
WALDHÄUSL, W., KENNER, TH.: Über die Entstehung einer nichtdialysierbaren vasopressorischen Aktivität der Erwärmung von Serum. Pharmacol. Exp. (Basel) **12**, 388 (1965).
WEBER, C. J., MAJOR, R. H., LOBB, D.: The production of a pressor substance from serum globulin by action of pepsin. Science **96**, 44 (1942).
WERLE, E., HOCHSTRASSER, K.: Versuche zur Isolierung eines niedermolekularen Kininogens. Hoppe-Seyler Z. physiol. Chem. **332**, 322 (1963).
WERLE, E., HOCHSTRASSER, K., TRAUTSCHOLD, I.: Studies of bovine plasma, kininogen, ornitho-kallikrein and ornithokinin. Symposium on hypotensive peptides. Berlin-Heidelberg-New York: Springer 1966.

Primary Aldosteronism: Importance of the Level of Plasma Renin as an Adjunct in Diagnosis*

J. W. CONN and E. L. COHEN

With 3 Figures

Background

The first description of the syndrome of primary aldosteronism (CONN, 1954) and its cure by surgical removal of an aldosterone-producing adreno-cortical tumor [CONN, 1955 (1, 2)] followed, by only a few months, the actual isolation and identification of the potent mineralocorticoid, aldosterone. At that time little was known of the physiological mechanisms controlling the secretion of aldosterone but we [CONN et al., 1948; CONN, 1949 (1, 2); CONN and LOUIS, 1950] had reported 5 years earlier that the need to conserve sodium stimulated the production of a 'salt-saving, desoxycorticosterone-like steroid' which was reflected in a precipitous lowering of the concentration of sodium in sweat; that this mechanism appeared to be independent of the pituitary-adrenal axis; that injections of desoxycorticosterone itself mimicked the changes induced by negative sodium balance; and that the concentration of sodium in sweat could be used as an index of the activity of the 'endogenous salt-active steroid'. The subsequent description of the renin-angiotensin-aldosterone system in 1959 extended and explained our earlier findings.

By 1959 many patients with primary aldosteronism had already been studied but the newly recognized renin-aldosterone relationship led to the demonstration that aldosteronism could also be secondary to lesions involving the renal arterial tree (LAIDLAW et al., 1960; GOWENLOCK and WRONG, 1962). In this situation adreno-cortical hyperplasia was often found. Thus, the differential diagnosis between primary and secondary aldosteronism in a hypertensive hypokalemic patient soon became critical (CONN and CONN, 1961). In 1962, we recommended that a hypertensive patient who exhibited, 1) consistently low serum potassium levels (usually below 3 mEq/L), 2) elevated aldosterone secretion or excretion rates, 3) normal cortisol secretion, 4) negative renal arteriograms and, 5) absence of hemorrhagic retinopathy with papilledema, had met the preoperative criteria for bilateral adrenal exploration. It was evident at that time that certain patients with borderline or even normal serum potassium levels were also harboring aldosterone-producing tumors since some of them were observed to progress to persistent hypokalemia with time [CONN, 1968; CONN et al., 1964 (2)]. However, we were unwilling at that time to recommend adrenal exploration in such patients as long as serum potassium levels were not consistently low. We therefore recommended that sodium loading be tried in order to augment renal potassium loss in patients with borderline levels of potassium, the objective being to induce

* Supported by United States Public Health Service Grants Nos. AM-10257 and HE-14520, and by a grant (RR-42) from the General Clinical Research Centers Program of the Division of Research Resources, National Institutes of Health.

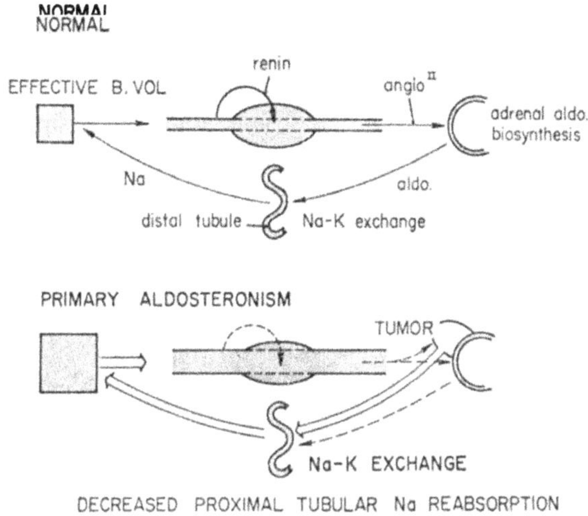

Fig. 1. This schematic representation of the renin-angiotensin-aldosterone system compares normal conditions with those found in primary aldosteronism

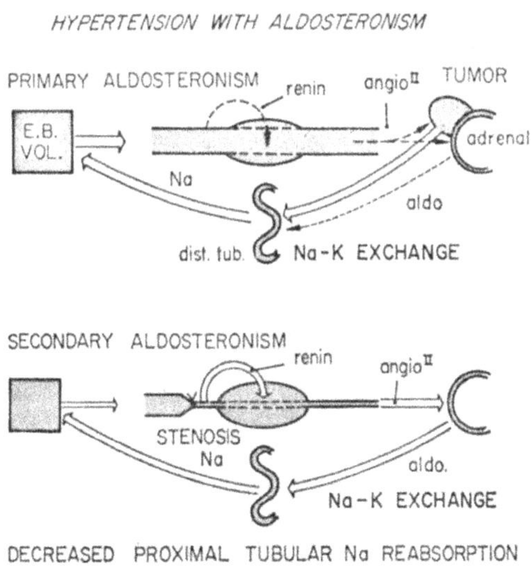

Fig. 2. This schematic representation of the renin-angiotensin-aldosterone system compares the supression of renin found in primary aldosteronism with the elevation of renin found in secondary aldosteronism due to renal artery stenosis

distinct hypokalemia [Conn et al., 1964 (2)]. We also warned, conversely, that a low sodium intake could result in diminished renal potassium loss, and a resultant normalization of serum potassium in such patients. Although sodium loading was helpful in many cases, it was, unfortunately, not consistently useful in clarifying the diagnosis. We therefore sought a more sensitive and specific diagnostic tool.

In 1963 [Conn et al., 1964 (2)], we suggested that the principles of the renin-angiotensin-aldosterone system should be applied in the diagnosis of primary aldosteronism. If the concept of the servomechanism between plasma volume expansion and renin production were correct, then aldosteronism associated with an adreno-cortical tumor should be associated with suppressed renin and angiotensin II levels (Fig. 1). Conversely, aldosteronism secondary to renal arterial disease should be associated with elevated renin and Ang. II levels (Fig. 2). Initial attempts to measure circulating plasma levels of Ang. II in patients with primary aldosteronism were not satisfactory. This was due to lack of sensitivity of the biological assay method, particularly at the low end of the scale. It was not possible to obtain consistent measurements of Ang. II levels in the plasma of normal people (GENEST et al., 1964). The subsequent development of improved biological assay systems for measuring plasma-renin activity (BOUCHER et al., 1964) or plasma-renin concentration [HELMER and JUDSON, 1963; BROWN et al., 1964 (2)] by enzyme kinetic techniques revolutionized the field. In 1964, we first utilized the plasma-renin activity method in our laboratory to estimate renin concentration in the plasma of normal people (COHEN et al., 1964, 1967). Subsequently we were able to demonstrate that plasma-renin activity is subnormal in patients with primary aldosteronism [CONN et al., 1964 (1)]. This technique provided the additional diagnostic criterion which we had been seeking, namely *suppressed plasma renin*. Furthermore, it offered, for the first time, a biochemical method which could effectively differentiate primary from secondary aldosteronism in the hypertensive patient.

Methods which have been Employed for Estimating Renin Concentration in Primary Aldosteronism

Although there has been considerable variability in methods for the estimation of the concentration of renin in plasma or serum, there has been no disagreement with the original demonstration that renin levels are low in the plasma of patients with primary aldosteronism. We initially used a modification (COHEN et al., 1967) of the biological assay of BOUCHER et al. (1964), which measures renin activity, i.e., the generation rate of angiotensin utilizing endogenous substrate. Other methods for renin activity (PICKENS et al., 1965; GUNNELS et al., 1967), similar in principle, have been developed, and along with the original method of BOUCHER, have been widely used to confirm our original observations (DE CHAMPLAIN et al., 1966; LARAGH et al., 1966; KUCHEL et al., 1967; CHANNICK et al., 1969; JOSE and KAPLAN, 1969; GUNNELS et al., 1970). These methods all run the theoretical risks of inaccuracies caused by wide changes in renin-substrate concentration and the possible presence of plasma inhibitors or accelerators of renin activity. In order to avoid these potential variables, LEVER et al. (1964), developed a method for renin concentration utilizing a plasma-renin purification step and the incubation of this plasma extract with excess heterologous substrate. BROWN et al. (1965), using this method, confirmed that renin concentration is low in patients with primary aldosteronism. Recently, the development of radioimmunoassay techniques for Ang. I (BOYD et al., 1969; HABER et al., 1969; HOLLEMANS et al., 1969; GIESE et al., 1970; COHEN et al., 1971; STOCKIGT et al., 1971; COHEN et al., 1972), have eliminated the need for cumbersome extraction and biological assay steps, and have been successfully applied to the measurement of plasma-renin activity (BOYD et al., 1969; HABER et al., 1969 COHEN et al., 1971, 1972) and plasma renin concentration (STOCKIGT et al., 1971; MCDONALD et al., 1971) in patients with primary aldosteronism. As expected, these methods confirm the earlier findings obtained with the biological assay methods. Radioimmunoassay methods can be made sensitive enough to measure circulating Ang. II and Ang. I; and low levels of both polypeptides have been found in the plasma of patients with primary aldosteronism (CATT et al., 1971; COHEN and CONN, 1971).

Hypokalemic Primary Aldosteronism

Early in the course of our work, we confirmed the findings of others that plasma-renin activity is elevated by dietary sodium restriction in normal people. We also found that the upright posture is a potent stimulus for renin elevation in normal people (COHEN et al., 1964, 1967). Table 1 reviews values for plasma-renin activity in normal people ingesting diets which are average (120 to 180 mEq) and very low (10 mEq) in sodium, and demonstrates the wide range of renin activity that can be

Table 1. *Plasma renin activity in normal people*

	Plasma-renin activity, bioassay, ng-% Ang. II equivalent/3 h			
Diet	120—180 mEq Na		10 mEq Na	
Posture	Recumbent	Upright (2—4 h)	Recumbent	Upright
Mean	153	365	417	1043
Range	<50—468	60—718	126—884	344—2371
S. D.	104	168	190	438
SEM	20	26	35	58
n	28	42	30	58

	Plasma-renin activity, radioimmunoassay Ang. I, ng Ang. I/ml/h			
Diet	120 mEq Na		10 mEq Na	
Posture	Recumbent	Upright (2—4 h)	Recumbent	Upright
Mean	2.5	7.7	7.1	17.2
Range	1.5—3.0	1.6—17.2	4.9—10.8	6.8—45.8
S. D.	1.4	4.6	2.0	10.1
SEM	0.5	1.0	0.8	2.2
n	6	20	6	20

induced by changes in diet and posture. GORDON et al. (1966), demonstrated that there is a normal circadian rhythm for renin activity, independent of posture, the values falling as the day progresses, and rising again in the early morning hours. This circadian rhythm can influence the values obtained during dietary and postural manipulations. It is thus evident that the interpretation of a particular measurement of plasma renin depends greatly upon the conditions of diet, posture, and time of day.

The first measurements of plasma renin activity in primary aldosteronism were performed upon patients with the florid disease characterized by severe hypokalemia. The values obtained were below the sensitivity of the bioassay method. As we began to study patients with less severe degrees of aldosteronism, we found that many demonstrated measureable, albeit subnormal, values for plasma-renin activity. Frequently it required the stimuli of sodium restriction and upright posture to bring the values into the measureable range of the assay. However, when these values were compared with those obtained in normal people under the same testing conditions, they were found to fall below the range of the normals. These findings are demonstrated in Table 2 in which we have reviewed

Table 2. *Hypokalemic primary aldosteronism, (tumor) plasma-renin activity (bioassay), (PRA) aldosterone excretion rate (AER)*

Diet Posture	PRA (ng Ang. II %/3 h)				AER μg/24 h
	120—180 mEq Na		10 mEq Na		120—180 mEq Na
	Recumbent	Upright	Recumbent	Upright	
				'0'[a]	64
				'0'	69
		'0'	'0'	'0'	109
	'0'	'0'	'0'	'0'	95
	'0'	'0'	'0'	'0'	88
			'0'	'0'	39
			'0'	'0'	24
			'0'	'0'	37
			'0'	'0'	19
	'0'	'0'	'0'	'0'	24
	'0'	'0'	'0'	'0'	35
		'0'		'0'	146
			'0'	'0'	24
				'0'	25
			'0'	'0'	48
			'0'	'0'	34
		'0'		'0'	40
				'0'	50
				'0'	52
				'0'	525
		'0'		'0'	41
		'0'		'0'	33
		'0'		'0'	35
		'0'		'0'	43
		'0'		'0'	72
		'0'		'0'	31
		'0'		'0'	21
		'0'		'0'	22
		'0'		'0'	67
		'0'		'0'	37
		'0'		'0'	26
		'0'		'0'	29
	'0'	65	83	197	27
	'0'	'0'	'0'	108	20
	'0'	'0'	'0'	164	17
	'0'	'0'	82	204	25
			57	95	70
	'0'	'0'	58	111	114
	'0'	'0'	108	124	28
	119	241	137	394	33
	'0'	177	120	124	40
		304		117	49
				142	72
		'0'		115	198
		144		135	48
		96		121	29
		94		311	44
		372		263	29
		'0'		117	28
		'0'		219	36
		145		133	37
		74		138	52
			Mean	79 ± 12 (SEM)	58 ± 10
			Normals Mean	1043 ± 58	11.4 ± 0.6

[a] '0' = <50 ng-% Ang. II/3 h
'0' = 25 ng-%/3 h for calculation of mean ± SEM

our *biological* assay data in patients with hypokalemic primary aldosteronism, and compared them with the values for normal people. Suppression of plasma-renin activity was most intense when aldosterone excretion exceeded 55 μg per 24 h. Table 3 reviews our more recent data obtained with the use of our sensitive *radio-immunoassay* system (Cohen et al., 1971). This new method is sufficiently sensitive to measure plasma-renin in all patients with primary aldosteronism. These data indicate that the upright posture is a distinct stimulus to plasma-renin activity in patients with primary aldosteronism and that dietary sodium restriction has

Table 3. *Primary aldosteronism (tumor) plasma-renin activity, radioimmunoassay, ng Ang. I/ml/h*[c]

Diet Posture	120 mEq Na Recumbent	 Upright	10 mEq Na Recumbent	 Upright
	0.09	1.01		
	0.19	0.99	0.22	0.61
	0.22	0.25		0.43
	0.30	0.34	0.18	0.46
	0.23	0.49		
	0.45	1.10		
	0.16	0.46	0.19	0.52
	0.37	0.40		0.75
		0.50		
		0.40		
		1.00		1.20
		0.12		0.50
		0.20		0.28
		0.28		0.28
		0.30		
		0.15		
		1.00		1.40
		2.00		
		0.50		0.40
Mean	0.25[a]	0.59[a]	0.20[b]	0.62[b]
S. D.	0.12	0.46	0.02	0.36
SEM	0.04	0.10	0.01	0.11

[a] $p < 0.05$.
[b] $p < 0.05$.
[c] see normal values in Table 1.

a less consistent effect. Similar findings have been reported by Brown et al. (1968) and Stockigt et al. (1971). It is important to note that the absolute rise in plasma-renin activity is very small in patients with primary aldosteronism (Table 3), whereas the same conditions of upright posture (2 to 4 h, 8 am to 12 noon) after 3 days of a low sodium (10 mEq) intake raises renin activity in normal people to much higher levels (Table 1). In our experience, overlapping between the two groups is very infrequent when these conditions are imposed.

Plasma-renin concentration has been measured in a large group of patients with primary aldosteronism by Brown et al. (1968). As a group, these values were also distinctly lower than those of normal people, although a greater degree of overlapping occurred than in our series using the plasma-renin activity immuno-assay. Since conditions of diet and posture had not been carefully controlled, such overlapping should be expected. STOCKIGT et al. (1971), have measured plasma-renin concentration using a modification of the method of SKINNER (1967) and a radioimmunoassay for Ang. I. They find consistently subnormal values in patients with primary aldosteronism, when measurements are performed in the "basal", i.e., recumbent state. As increasingly sensitive methods for the measurement of plasma-renin activity and plasma-renin concentration become available, it may become possible to distinguish patients with primary aldosteronism from normal

Table 4. *Plasma renin activity (PRA) and concentration (PRC) in anephric people: comparison with patients with primary aldosteronism*

	Anephric	Primary aldosteronism (recumbent)
PRA (ng Ang. I/ml/h)		
	0.14	0.09
	0.15	0.19
	0.07	0.22
	0.40	0.30
	0.11	0.23
	0.29	0.45
	0.04	0.16
	0.07	0.37
	0.03	
	0.12	
	0.19	
	0.13	
Mean ± SEM	0.14 ± 0.03[a]	0.25 ± 0.04[a]
PRC (Goldblatt units × 10^{-4}/ml)		
	0.018	0.022
	0.049	0.030
	0.012	0.045
	0.043	0.064
	0.006	0.030
	0.006	0.080
	0.039	0.020
		0.050
Mean ± SEM	0.025 ± 0.007[b]	0.043 ± 0.008[b]

[a] $p = < 0.05$.
[b] $p = 0.1 > 0.05$.

people at the lower range of the assay spectrum, without the necessity of using the stimuli of sodium restriction and upright posture to separate them.

Basal plasma-renin activity and basal plasma-renin concentration are very greatly suppressed in patients with primary aldosteronism. This is clearly demonstrated when measurements from these patients are compared with values obtained from bilaterally nephrectomized people (Table 4). This does not imply, however, that plasma renin cannot be stimulated to significantly higher levels while the tumor is still present. Renin levels can be elevated in patients harboring tumors if a significant natriuresis can be induced. This is demonstrated in Fig. 3. The subject, with classical hypokalemic primary aldosteronism and very low levels of plasma-renin activity, received 100 mg of hydrochlorothiazide and supplemental potassium for 3 days while ingesting only 10 mEq of sodium per day. Plasma-renin activity rose greatly and approached values seen in normal people studied under similar conditions (FISHMAN et al., 1968). STOCKIGT has reported similar findings using a low-sodium diet and diuretics in patients with proven

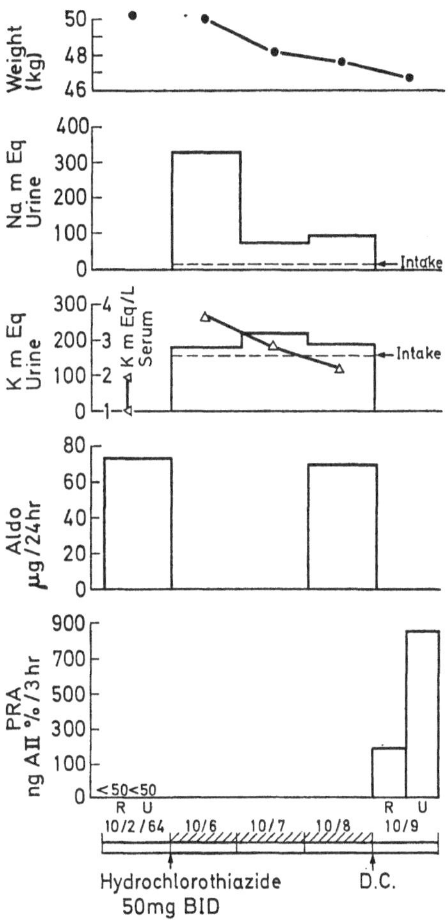

Fig. 3. This patient harbored an aldosterone-producing tumor and her plasma-renin activity was greatly suppressed. Natriuresis, produced by hydrochlorothiazide, induced a striking rise in plasma-renin activity in three days

primary aldosteronism (STOCKIGT et al., 1971). We have previously cautioned against this type of over-stimulation during attempts to employ plasma-renin activity values in the diagnosis of primary aldosteronism (CONN et al., 1969). Not only can severe hypokalemia be induced, but the diagnostic usefulness of the measurement of plasma renin may be lost, particularly in patients with the milder forms of the disease.

Spironolactone induces a gradual natriuresis in patients with primary aldosteronism. The effect is similar to that which follows partial or complete removal of the tumor, i.e., it depends upon the relationship between the degree of aldosteronism and the dose of spironolactone. A gradual rise in plasma-renin concentration or plasma-renin activity usually occurs. Table 5 reviews data obtained when spironolactone was given to a patient preoperatively. Natriuresis clearly preceded the rise in plasma-renin activity, and further elevation of aldosterone excretion occurred only after plasma-renin activity remained above the level which would have been appropriate for the level of sodium intake.

Table 5. *Primary aldosteronism, treatment with aldactone*
(Na intake — 120 mEq/day)

Date	Weight kg	Serum Na mEq/L	K	PRA ng/ml/h recumbent	ALDO µg/24 h	
24. 11.	59.3	153	4.0	0.32[a]	17.2	
25. 11.	—	144	3.6	0.17	23.8	
26. 11.	61.4	143	3.7	0.12	24.2	
27. 11.	61.1	—	—	0.09	19.4	
28. 11.	61.3	145	3.6	0.04	—	Aldactone
29. 11.	61.0	149	3.6	0.38[a]	15.4	400 mg/day
30. 11.	61.3	149	3.9	0.12	16.1	↓
1. 12.	61.1	143	3.5	0.35	—	
2. 12.	61.0	143	4.3	0.18	20.9	300 mg/day
3. 12.	60.0	—	—	0.12	21.7	
4. 12.	61.2	143	3.9	0.43	24.0	
5. 12.	59.8	—	—	2.10	22.9	
6. 12.	59.5	142	4.0	1.13	27.3	
7. 12.	60.0	—	—	1.89	24.9	
8. 12.	59.7	141	4.6	8.25	32.2	
9. 12.	60.0	—	—	8.11	34.8	
10. 12.	—	141	4.6	6.34	37.7	
11. 12.	58.1	—	—	10.22	—	
12. 12.	59.2	—	—	14.20	47.4	
13. 12.	59.0	—	—	12.50	46.3	
14. 12.	59.0	141	5.0	12.96	37.7	
15. 12.	59.0	—	—	7.06	28.8	
16. 12.	59.0	145	4.8	12.92	32.1	
17. 12.	58.4	—	—	8.68	37.2	↓
						Removal of tumor

[a] Upright.

When an aldosterone-producing tumor is surgically removed, aldosterone excretion falls rapidly within 24 h to levels below the normal range. This is followed by natriuresis and a subsequent rise in plasma-renin activity. Aldosterone secretion subsequently returns to normal but this may be delayed for many months. The time interval for return of plasma-renin activity also varies considerably from patient to patient and is probably influenced by the degree of initial renin suppression as well as by the level of sodium intake allowed postoperatively. We have previously reported that an intake of 40 mEq of sodium accelerates the postoperative rise in plasma-renin activity [Conn et al., 1965 (1)], but warned that the associated sodium depletion in an aldosterone-deficient patient could be dangerous. We therefore avoid postoperative dietary sodium restriction, and have observed that our patients gradually recover a normal renin-aldosterone system without untoward intervening effects. Table 6 reviews data obtained in the immediate 10 to 21 postoperative days from patients who underwent resection of aldosterone-producing tumors and adjacent adrenal tissue. Glucocorticoid deficiency did not develop in any of these patients. The degree of aldosteronopenia is severe, and in some patients the anticipated hyperreninemia is evident, but in others it is quite slow in its appearance. This abrupt change in the activity of the renin-aldosterone system, associated with normal levels of urinary 17-hydroxysteroids, indicates (1) that the source of excessive production of aldosterone has been removed, (2) that suppressed production of aldosterone by the normal

Table 6. *Primary aldosteronism, preoperative and postoperative plasma-renin activity and aldosterone excretion rates*

	PRA (bioassay) ng-%/3 h			AER μg/24 h		
	preop.	postop.	days postop.	preop.	postop.	days postop.
Mean	88	485	12 (3—21)	48	2.2	9.1 (3—20)
S. D.	82	453		34	1.8	
SEM	12	65		5	0.3	
n	48	48		48	48	
p	<0.001			<0.001		

	PRA (radioimmunoassay) ng Ang. I/ml/h			AER μg/24 h		
	preop.	postop.	days postop.	preop.	postop.	days postop.
Mean	0.63	8.66	11.7 (9—15)	47	2.8	11 (3—25)
S. D.	0.49	11.0		37	2.5	
SEM	0.15	2.8		10	0.8	
n	11	11		11	11	
p	<0.001			<0.001		

adrenal tissue has been unmasked, and (3) that a slow recovery of the renin-aldosterone system toward normal has begun.

Normokalemic Primary Aldosteronism

The demonstration that plasma renin was suppressed in hypertensive hypokalemic patients who harbored aldosterone-producing tumors, led us to postulate that in the presence of overproduction of aldosterone, renin suppression might be a more sensitive index of primary aldosteronism than the level of serum potassium (Conn, 1964). We had observed cases of primary aldosteronism whose serum potassium levels had been normal or borderline for several years prior to the development of clear hypokalemia. We therefore awaited the opportunity to test this hypothesis on normokalemic hypertensive patients. In 1965, we evaluated a young man with hypertension, an abnormal glucose-tolerance test, and consistently normal levels of serum potassium. Table 7 reviews the important preoperative data on this patient. Plasma-renin activity was persistently low despite low-sodium diet and upright posture, and aldosterone production was abnormally high. Tota

Table 7. *Normokalemic primary aldosteronism*
(First patient with 'essential hypertension' so diagnosed and cured)[b]

1. Range of B. P. (n = 72) $\frac{210}{130} - \frac{150}{90} \left(\text{Mean } \frac{167}{109}\right)$
2. Serum K (mEq/L 3.8—4.8 (Mean 4.2)
3. Serum Na (mEq/L) 142—145 (Mean 142.2)
4. NA_e — 38.6 mEq/kg } $NA_e/K_e = 0.97$
5. K_e — 39.6 mEq/kg }
6. *17 OHCS excretion* (mg/day) 4.0—4.8 (3.5—8.0)[a]
7. *Aldosterone excretion* (high Na diet) 24.5 μg/day (1.6—21.9)[a]
8. *Aldosterone secretion* (high Na diet) 278 μg/day (65—170)[a]
9. *Renin activity* (3 days — 10 mEq Na diet) (4th day — upright 4 h) } 191 ng/100 ml (446—2371)[a]

[a] Normal range.
[b] B. P. $\frac{118}{76}$ — 20 mo. post-op.

Table 8. *Normokalemic primary aldosteronism*[a]

Diet Posture	PRA (ng-%/3 h) 120—180 mEq Na Recumbent	 Upright	 10 mEq Na Recumbent	 Upright	AER (μg/24 h) 120—180 mEq Na
		'0'[b]	'0'	'0'	33
	'0'	'0'	'0'	'0'	46
		50		'0'	45
		59		68	29
		'0'		99	23
	'0'	'0'	'0'	63	24
	'0'	'0'	'0'	85	31
	'0'	'0'	'0'	131	32
	'0'	'0'	'0'	155	35
		'0'	'0'	191	25
			'0'	58	23
	'0'	'0'	'0'	106	23
		165	93	224	30
	'0'	98	84	118	34
				'0'	33
		'0'		64	32
		'0'		60	40
		84		140	55
		270		367	24
		'0'		175	22
		'0'		'0'	33
			Mean ± SEM	110 ± 19	32 ± 1.9

[a] See normal values in Table 1.
[b] '0' = < 50 ng-% Ang. II/3 h.

exchangeable potassium was borderline low, and serum potassium was consistently normal. The patient was cured of his aldosteronism and his hypertension by removal of the left adrenal gland which contained two 5-mm tumors. Postoperatively, he became aldosteronopenic and it took 5 months for the underproduction of aldosterone to rise into the normal range.

Table 8 reviews data obtained since 1965 from 21 patients with normokalemic primary aldosteronism. Although the aldosterone excretion is often less elevated than it is in patients with classical hypokalemic primary aldosteronism, the *plasma-renin activity is similarly suppressed.*

Thus our criteria for the diagnosis of primary aldosteronism have undergone a significant change over the years (Table 9). Originally the "sine qua non" for the diagnosis was hypokalemia. Our demonstration that plasma renin is always subnormal in primary aldosteronism made this a most valuable adjunct in the diagnosis when we were faced with a hypertensive patient whose production of aldosterone was excessive; and it facilitated recognition of the normokalemic cases. In addition, it greatly simplified the differential diagnosis between primary aldosteronism and the secondary form of aldosteronism which often accompanies renovascular hypertension. The demonstration that plasma renin is suppressed *prior to the development of hypokalemia* permits the diagnosis of primary aldosteronism in an earlier and milder form [Conn et al., 1965 (2), 1966]. It thus opens the way for a new search for this disease in the hypertensive population with the use of newer, more sensitive immunoassay techniques for renin and aldosterone.

Table 9. *Evolution of diagnostic criteria for primary aldosteronism*

1954—1964	I	Hypokalemia — below 3.0 mEq/L
	II	Overproduction of aldosterone
	III	Normal 17 OHCS and 17 KS
To help rule out renal hypertension	IV	Absence of hyponatremia
	V	Absence of papilledema
	VI	Normal renal arteriograms
1964—1965	VII	Suppression of renin activity (low Na — ↑)
	I	Hypokalemia — below 3.8 mEq/L
	II	Overproduction of aldosterone
	III	Normal 17 OHCS and 17 KS
1965—1967	VII	Suppression of renin activity (low Na — ↑)
	II	Overproduction of aldosterone
	III	Normal 17 OHCS and 17 KS

„Idiopathic" Aldosteronism

Laragh et al. (1967) described a hypertensive patient who had met all the preoperative criteria for the diagnosis of hypokalemic primary aldosteronism and whose adrenal glands demonstrated bilateral cortical hyperplasia. Earlier cases of bilateral hyperplasia had been reported, but since plasma renin had not been measured, secondary aldosteronism had not been ruled out. Since plasma renin was low in Laragh's case, he suggested that this form of bilateral adreno-cortical hyperplasia was caused by an unknown stimulus, and should therefore be regarded as another type of secondary aldosteronism. In the discussion that followed it was suggested that the term "idiopathic" aldosteronism be used since the etiology was unknown. Since that time the term "pseudo-primary aldosteronism" has also been used (Baer et al., 1970). We believe that the term "idiopathic" aldosteronism is preferable, until it can be shown that the genesis of this form of hyperplasia is either extra-adrenal or intra-adrenal in origin.

The incidence of idiopathic aldosteronism in patients meeting the diagnostic criteria for primary aldosteronism varies among clinics, being relatively high in some, and lower in others. In our experience with 95 cases operated upon since we began to employ plasma-renin activity values in the diagnosis, 14% have proven to have idiopathic aldosteronism. In a similarly large group of cases (102) BIGLIERI (1971) finds an incidence of 16%. BAER et al. (1970) find a much higher incidence (48%). The possibility of making a preoperative distinction between tumor and hyperplasia has become an important problem for researchers. The prospect of a subtotal or total adrenalectomy when bilateral hyperplasia is encountered in

Table 10. *'Idiopathic' aldosteronism, plasma-renin activity (PRA) and aldosterone excretion rates (AER)*[a]

	PRA (ng %/3 h) (10 mEq Na, upright)	AER (μg/24 h) (120—180 mEq Na)
	'0'[b]	23
	386	33
	270	24
	179	25
	366	20
	97	33
	376	23
	250	44
	161	26
Mean ± SEM	234 ± 43	
	PRA (radioimmuno-assay) (ng/ml/h)	
	5.1	30
	3.2	43
	0.6	19
	2.3	36
Mean ± SEM	2.8 ± 0.9	29 ± 2.3 n = 13

[a] See normal values in Table 1.
[b] '0' = < 50 ng-% Ang. II/3 h.

the operating room does not meet with enthusiasm, since the etiology of this hyperplasia is not yet known, and since medical therapy with spironolactone may prove beneficial in many cases. But it should be appreciated that these patients *are* explored because the preoperative diagnosis has been tumor. To date, the diagnosis of bilateral hyperplasia has been made in the operating room when a tumor fails to materialize. The surgeons' choice is between removing the hyperplastic adrenal tissue already exposed or allowing it to remain in the patient. The former procedure is usually followed. Reports of distinctly less favorable postoperative control of blood pressure in these cases have been made (BAER et al., 1970; BIGLIERI et al., 1970) but the last word has not yet been said in this area. Our own results in such cases and those of BARTTER (1971) and GUNNELLS et al. (1970) indicate that postoperative improvement approaches that obtained in the group with primary aldosteronism.

FERRISS et al. (1970), BIGLIERI et al. (1970), BAER et al. (1970), and their respective coworkers have suggested that the biochemical aberrations in those patients with bilateral adreno-cortical hyperplasia are less severe than in those with tumors, and have pointed to a lesser degree of suppression of plasma renin. We, too, have found that patients with idiopathic aldosteronism exhibit, as a group, higher values for plasma renin activity than do patients with tumors, though their values are still subnormal (Table 10 and 11) (COHEN et al., 1971). Thus, although overlapping values for plasma renin does occur between the two groups, mild suppression of plasma renin should alert one to the possibility of bilateral adreno-cortical hyperplasia.

However, because the degree of suppression of plasma renin cannot be depended upon to distinguish between the two groups, tumor versus hyperplasia, other attempts have been made. FERRIS et al. (1970) have put a large amount of data into a computer program (quadric analysis), and believe that this multiple-variable approach effectively separates primary from idiopathic aldosteronism. WOTMAN et al. (1970) have suggested that submaxillary salivary potassium concentration can differentiate these cases, the tumor cases secreting the greater amount of potassium. STOCKIGT et al. (1971) have recommended a comparison of basal plasma renin and urinary aldosterone excretion following desoxycorticosterone administration, patients with hyperplasia demonstrating higher renin concentration and lower aldosterone excretion. MELBY et al. (1967) and HORTON and FINCH (1971) have used bilateral adrenal venous aldosterone levels to locate tumors. We have examined the morphology of the adrenal glands directly by the use of bilateral selective adrenal venography (CONN et al., 1969), or more recently by bilateral adrenal gland photoscanning after administration of I^{131}-19-iodocholesterol [CONN et al., 1971, 1972 (1, 2)]. While it is not within the scope of this discussion to evaluate and compare all the approaches to this important problem, we believe that greater experience and considerably more data are needed for each one. It will be particularly important to apply these techniques to cases of normokalemic primary aldosteronism, in which the aldosteronism is also mild, to determine whether a clear distinction from "idiopathic" hyperplasia can be accomplished.

Table 11. *Summary of plasma renin activity and aldosterone excretion rate in hypokalemic primary aldosteronism, normokalemic primary aldosteronism, and 'idiopathic' aldosteronism*

	PRA (ng-% 3 h)	AER (μg/24 h)
Hypokalemic	79 ± 12[a]	58 ± 10[a]
Normokalemic	110 ± 19[a]	32 ± 1.9[a]
'Idiopathic'	234 ± 43[b]	29 ± 2.3[a]

[a] N. S.
[b] $p < 0.001$ (hypokalemic)
$p < 0.005$ (normokalemic).

There exists a rare form of familial adreno-cortical hyperplasia originally reported by SUTHERLAND et al. (1966), and described in further detail by SALTI et al. (1969). In this disorder, our criteria for the diagnosis of primary aldosteronism are satisfied (and plasma-renin values are *very* low), but the aldosteronism, the suppressed plasma-renin activity and the hypertension are reversed by treatment with 1 to 2 mg of dexamethasone daily. Since ACTH levels are not elevated in these cases and there is no clear evidence of any abnormalities in cortisol production, the mechanism for the effect of dexamethasone is unclear. This "cortisol-suppressible" aldosteronism differs from the cases of idiopathic aldosteronism described above, in that the latter group fails to reverse the syndrome upon treatment with cortisol.

Mention should also be made of the equally rare form of adreno-cortical hyperactivity associated with hypertension and hypokalemia, and caused by a probable deficiency in the 17-hydroxylation step in the biosynthesis of steroid hormones (Biglieri et al., 1966). This interesting disorder can be differentiated from other forms of adreno-cortical hyperplasia with suppressed plasma renin since 1) aldosteronopenia rather than overproduction of aldosterone exists, the mineralocorticoid excess being caused by increased production of desoxycorticosterone and corticosterone, and 2) the gonads share in the enzyme deficiency, producing hypogonadism.

Low Renin in Essential Hypertension

Following our original report [Conn et al., 1964 (1)] that suppression of plasma-renin activity is an effective adjunctive criterion in the diagnosis of primary aldosteronism, we suggested that the incidence of primary aldosteronism in the hypertensive population might be greater than we had previously expected (Conn, 1964). In suggesting that a figure of 20% would not be an unreasonable expectation, we (Conn, 1964) had analyzed the then published values [Brown et al., 1964 (1)] for plasma-renin concentration in groups of hypertensive people and pointed out that among a group classified as having essential hypertension, 21% exhibited subnormal values, a fact not commented upon by the authors. We suggested that aldosterone-secretion rates were needed in such patients. In another group of hypertensives characterized as having serum-potassium values of 3.1 mEq per liter or below, with normal renal arteriograms [Brown et al., 1964 (1)], we observed that plasma-renin concentration was subnormal in 38% and suggested that these patients very probably had primary aldosteronism but that the demonstration of overproduction of aldosterone was needed to confirm the diagnosis. At the very least, we had directed attention to the fact that *subnormal* levels of plasma renin could have important clinical significance; and that they occurred in a large segment (20%) of the hypertensive population.

Our own studies in essential hypertension failed to sustain our earlier prediction that as many as 20% might prove to have normokalemic primary aldosteronism. We found instead a surgically proven incidence of 7.6% (Conn et al., 1967) in patients who preoperatively had exhibited overproduction of aldosterone, normal cortisol production and subnormal plasma renin. An additional 18% showed subnormal plasma renin but their aldosterone excretion values fell within the normal range.

Following our suggestion that low renin values might help to separate out some patients with remediable hypertension, many groups have screened essential hypertensives, using plasma renin as an index, and have uniformly found large numbers of patients with subnormal values. The incidence of low plasma renin in the hypertensive population ranges from approximately 10 to 40%, averaging 28% (Jose et al., 1970). But most of these patients have failed to satisfy the criteria for the diagnosis of primary aldosteronism. In some clinics (Laragh et al., 1966), the incidence of increased aldosterone production in patients with 'essential' hypertension has been exceedingly low. Others (Gunnells et al., 1970; Harris et al., 1967) have found a higher incidence and have discovered cases of normokalemic primary aldosteronism. It is fair to say that, at present, the true incidence of normokalemic primary aldosteronism remains unknown. The number of hypertensives studied to date has been limited by the labor and expense involved in carrying out multiple determinations for renin and aldosterone. Recently developed radioimmunoassays for Ang. I and II as well as for aldosterone will help to remedy this limitation.

Since it appears now that only about one third of the hypertensives with low plasma renin have normokalemic primary aldosteronism, what is the mechanism of the low plasma renin in the other two-thirds? The answer is not yet known, but there are several lines of evidence to suggest that excessive mineralocorticoid activity, probably of adrenal origin, may be involved. Patients with normal aldosterone excretion rates and subnormal plasma-renin activity have undergone adrenal exploration, and bilateral cortical hyperplasia has been described (GUNNELLS et al., 1970; GRIM and PETERS, 1971). WOODS et al. (1969) reported that aminoglutethimide, a blocker of adreno-cortical hormone biosynthesis could ameliorate hypertension in patients with suppressed renin activity who had normal production of aldosterone and desoxycorticosterone. MELBY et al. (1970) reported that 18-OH-desoxycorticosterone production was elevated in some of these patients, and that the hypertension was alleviated by suppression of ACTH production with dexamethasone. However, since the mineralocorticoid action of 18-OH-desoxycorticosterone may be relatively weak, serious doubts have been raised as to whether it is solely responsible for the syndrome. We (ROVNER et al., 1971) have described the case of a normokalemic hypertensive patient with low plasma renin, normal aldosterone production, and high excretion of 18-OH-desoxycorticosterone from whom an adrenal adenoma was removed which, in vitro, produced increased quantities of 18-OH-desoxycorticosterone. CRANE and HARRIS (1970), SPARK and MELBY (1971), and CAREY et al. (1972), and their associates have recently reported that hypertensive patients with suppressed plasma-renin activity and normal aldosterone production respond much more favorably to treatment with spironolactone than do essential hypertensives with normal plasma-renin activity. COLLINS et al. (1970) have reported that patients with low plasma-renin activity and normal aldosterone production fail to suppress their aldosterone production rates in the normal way during salt loading.

All these findings together suggest that in such patients there is increased production of unidentified adrenal mineralocorticoid or that certain people are excessively sensitive to normal quantities of aldosterone. This is a fertile field for further study.

We must be alert to the possibility that exogenous factors with known mild sodium-retaining activities, such as licorice (glycyrrhizic acid) (CONN et al., 1968), or other foods and food additives not yet known to have such properties, may be the cause not only of the low renin but also of the hypertension in some of these patients. In such cases, as well as in the congenital anomaly described by LIDDLE et al. (1964) low plasma renin and low aldosterone production would be expected. Finally, certain drugs, particularly those used in the treatment of hypertension, such as alpha-methyldopa (MOHAMMED et al., 1969) and propanolol (WINER et al., 1969), which may block renin production or release, and others (diuretics) which may increase them (COHEN et al., 1968; TERAZI et al., 1970), must be discontinued prior to evaluation of the hypertensive patient. The influence of estrogens and birth control pills on plasma-renin activity should also be mentioned in this connection but further discussion will be found elsewhere in this volume.

Comment

A major breakthrough in the preoperative diagnosis of primary aldosteronism occurred when subnormal plasma renin was made one of the necessary diagnostic criteria. The currently available methods for estimating renin in extremely minute amounts indicate that in this disease the plasma contains only about 10% of that found in healthy people under the same standard conditions. In the presence of overproduction of aldosterone, suppression of plasma renin was found to be a more sensitive index of the presence of an aldosterone-producing tumor than was the existence of hypokalemia. It soon became evident that this disorder exists as a continuum, with classical hypokalemic primary aldosteronism at one end of the spectrum and normokalemic primary aldosteronism at the other.

Early in the evolution of our criteria for diagnosis we believed that the combination of suppression of plasma renin, elevation of aldosterone production, and normal cortisol production was singularly diagnostic of an aldosterone-producing tumor. However, about 15% of patients with these findings are now known to disclose adrenal hyperplasia at operation rather than tumor. The application of newer radioimmunoassay techniques to this problem indicates that plasma renin, although subnormal, is usually less suppressed in the cases with idiopathic hyperplasia. But other, more reliable, methods of distinction are needed. Adrenal photoscanning with radiocholesterol would appear, at present, to hold out the greatest possibility of success.

The usefulness of plasma renin values in determination of the etiology of surgically correctable hypertensive disease is now accepted in most major medical centers and will no doubt be used with increasing frequency as use of the radioimmunoassay techniques becomes widespread. Increasing numbers of normokalemic cases of primary aldosteronism and of intermittently hypokalemic cases are being detected with the use of this technique as an adjunct in diagnosis. Normal values for serum potassium do not rule out primary aldosteronism. The incidence of normokalemic primary aldosteronism in the population of essential hypertensives remains controversial and unsettled, but continued interest and the use of newer techniques should hasten clarification.

The ability to classify hypertensive patients according to plasma renin and aldosterone levels is an important first step in investigating other subgroups in the large "wastebasket' of patients now said to have 'essential' hypertension. That the metabolism and distribution of sodium in the body will be found to be key factors seems a safe prediction.

References

BAER, L., SOMMERS, S. C., KRAKOFF, L. R., NEWTON, M. A., LARAGH, J. H.: Pseudo-primary aldosteronism. Circulat. Res. **26** and **27**, I-203 (1970).

BARTTER, F.: International Symposium on the Renin-Angiotensin. Aldosterone-Sodium System in Hypertension, Mt. Gabriel Lodge, Quebec, Canada, September 30—October 4, 1971.

BIGLIERI, E. G.: Third Annual Searle Aldosterone Symposium. San Francisco, California, June 23, 1971.

BIGLIERI, E. G., HERRON, M. A., BRUST, N.: 17-hydroxylation deficiency in man. J. clin. Invest. **45**, 1946 (1966).

BIGLIERI, E. G., SCHAMBELAN, M., SLATON, P. E., STOCKIGT, J. R.: The intercurrent hypertension of primary aldosteronism. Circulat. Res. **26** and **27**, I—195 (1970).

BOUCHER, R., VEYRATT, R., DE CHAMPLAIN, J., GENEST, J.: New procedures for measurement of human plasma angiotensin and renin activity levels. Canad. med. Ass. J. **90**, 194 (1964).

BOYD, G. W., ADAMSON, A. R., FITZ, A. E., PEART, W. S.: Radioimmunoassay determination of plasma renin activity. Lancet **1969 I**, 213.

BROWN, J. J., DAVIES, D. L., FRASER, R., ROBERTSON, J. I. S., CHINN, R. H., DÜSTERDIECK, G., LEVER, A. F., TREE, M.: Plasma electrolytes, renin, and aldosterone in the diagnosis of primary hyperaldosteronism. Lancet **1968 II**, 55.

BROWN, J. J., DAVIES, D. L., LEVER, A. F., PEART, W. S., ROBERTSON, J. I. S.: Plasma concentration of renin in a patient with Conn's syndrome with fibrinoid lesions of the renal arterioles: the effect of treatment with spironolactone. J. Endocr. **33**, 279 (1965).

BROWN, J. J., DAVIES, D. L., LEVER, A. F., ROBERTSON, J. I. S.: (1) Variations in plasma renin concentration in several physiologic and pathological states. Canad. med. Ass. J. **90**, 210 (1964).

BROWN, J. J., DAVIES, D. L., LEVER, A. F., ROBERTSON, J. I. S., TREE, M.: (2) The estimation of renin in human plasma. Biochem. J. **93**, 594 (1964).

CAREY, R. M., DOUGLAS, J. G., LIDDLE, G. W.: Spironolactone in patients with essential hypertension and suppressed plasma renin activity. Clin. Res. **20**, 72 (1972).

CATT, K., CRAN, E., ZIMMET, P. Z., BEST, J. B., CAIN, M. D., COGHEAN, J. P.: Angiotensin II blood-levels in human hypertension. Lancet **1971 I**, 459.

CHANNICK, B. J., ADLIN, E. V., MARKS, A. D.: Suppressed plasma renin activity in hypertension. Arch. intern. Med. **123**, 131 (1961).

COHEN, E. L., CONN, J. W.: Personal observations (1971).

COHEN, E. L., CONN, J. W., LUCAS, C. P., MCDONALD, W. J., GRIM, C. E., MAYOR, G. H., SALTMAN, S. E., CLADWELL, J. M.: Radioimmunoassay for angiotensin I: Measurement of plasma renin activity, plasma renin concentration, renin substrate concentration, and angiotensin I, in normal and hypertensive people. Proceedings Int'l. Symposium on Renin-Angiotensin-Aldosterone-Sodium System in Hypertension. Berlin-Heidelberg-New York: Springer 1972 (in press).

COHEN, E. L., CONN, J. W., ROVNER, D. R.: Postural augmentation of plasma renin activity and aldosterone excretion in normal people. J. clin. Invest. **46**, 418 (1967).

COHEN, E. L., GRIM, C. E., CONN, J. W., BLOUGH, W. M., Jr., GUYER, R. B., KEM, D. C., LUCAS, C. P.: Accurate and rapid measurement of plasma renin activity by radioimmunoassay. Results in normal and hypertensive people. J. Lab. clin. Med. **77**, 1025 (1971).

COHEN, E. L., ROVNER, D. R., CONN, J. W., BLOUGH, W. M., Jr.: The effects of position, exercise and sodium intake on plasma renin activity in normal people. Clin. Res. **12**, 362 (1964).

COHEN, E. L., ROVNER, D. R., CONN, J. W., MCNAMARA, J. A., GUSSIN, D. A., KLOOT, L.: The effects of chronic benzothiadiazine therapy upon the renin-angiotensin-aldosterone system. Clin. Res. **16**, 440 (1968).

COLLINS, R. D., WEINBERGER, M. H., DOWDY, A. J., NOKES, G. W., GONZALES, C. M., LUETSCHER, J. A.: Abnormally sustained aldosterone secretion during salt loading in patients with various forms of benign hypertension, relation to plasma renin activity. J. clin. Invest. **49**, 1415 (1970).

CONN, J. W.: (1) Electrolyte composition of sweat: Clinical implications as an index of adrenal cortical function. Arch. intern. Med. **83**, 416 (1949).

CONN, J. W.: (2) The mechanism of acclimatization to heat. Advanc. intern. Med. **3**, 373 (1949).

CONN, J. W.: Potassium-losing nephritis. Brit. med. J. **1954 II**, 1415.

CONN, J. W.: (1) Presidential address. Part I. Painting background. Part II. Primary aldosteronism, a new clinical syndrome. J. Lab. clin. Med. **45**, 3 (1955).

CONN, J. W.: (2) Primary aldosteronism. J. Lab. clin. Med. **45**, 661 (1955).

CONN, J. W.: Plasma renin activity in primary aldosteronism. Importance in differential diagnosis and in research of "essential" hypertension. J. Amer. med. Ass. **190**, 222 (1964).

CONN, J. W.: The evolution of primary aldosteronism — 1954—1967. In: The Harvey Lectures, Series 62, New York: Academic Press 1968.

CONN, J. W., BEIERWALTES, W. H., LIEBERMAN, L. M., ANSARI, A. N., COHEN, E. L., BOOKSTEIN, J. J., HERWIG, K. R.: Primary aldosteronism: Preoperative tumor visualization by scintillation scanning. J. clin. Endocr. **33**, 713 (1971).

CONN, J. W., COHEN, E. L., ROVNER, D. R.: (1) Suppression of plasma renin activity in primary aldosteronism. Distinguishing primary from secondary aldosteronism in hypertensive disease. J. Amer. med. Ass. **190**, 213 (1964).

CONN, J. W., COHEN, E. L., ROVNER, D. R., NESBIT, R. M.: (2) Normokalemic primary aldosteronism. A detectable cause of curable "essential" hypertension. J. Amer. med. Ass. **193**, 200 (1965).

CONN, J. W., CONN, E. S.: Primary aldosteronism versus hypertensive disease with secondary aldosteronism. Rec. Prog. Hormone Res. **17**, 389 (1961).

CONN, J. W., KNOPF, R. F., NESBIT, R. M.: (2) Primary aldosteronism: Present evaluation of its clinical characteristics and of the results of surgery. In: Aldosterone, A Symposium. Oxford: Blackwell Scientific Publications 1964.

CONN, J. W., LOUIS, L. H.: Production of endogenous "salt-active" corticoids as reflected in the concentrations of sodium and chloride of thermal sweat. J. clin. Endocr. **10**, 12 (1950).

CONN, J. W., LOUIS, L. H., JOHNSTON, M. W., JOHNSON, B. J.: The electrolyte content of thermal sweat as an index of adrenal cortical function. J. clin. Invest. **27**, 529 (1948).

Conn, J. W., Morita, R., Cohen, E. L., Beierwaltes, W. H., McDonald, W. J., Herwig, K. R.: (1) Primary aldosteronism: Photoscanning of tumors after ^{131}I-Iodocholesterol. Arch. intern. Med. 1972 (in press).

Conn, J. W., Morita, R., Cohen, E. L., Beierwaltes, W. J., McDonald, W. H., Herwig, K. R.: (2) Photoscanning of tumors in primary aldosteronism: Possible distinction from 'idiopathic' aldosteronism. Proceedings Int'l. Symposium on Renin-Angiotensin-Aldosterone-Sodium System in Hypertension. Berlin-Heidelberg-New York: Springer 1972 (in press).

Conn, J. W., Rovner, D. R., Cohen, E. L.: (1) Natural history of recovery of the renin-angiotensin-aldosterone system following long term suppression by aldosterone secreting tumors. Prog. 47th Meet. Endo. Soc., p. 60 (1965).

Conn, J. W., Rovner, D. R., Cohen, E. L., Nesbit, R. M.: Normokalemic primary aldosteronism. Its masquerade as 'essential' hypertension. J. Amer. med. Ass. **195**, 21 (1966).

Conn, J. W., Rovner, D. R., Cohen, E. L.: Newer knowledge of primary aldosteronism. Proceedings of the Third Asia and Oceania Cong. of Endo., 158 (1967).

Conn, J. W., Rovner, D. R., Cohen, E. L.: Licorice-induced pseudo-aldosteronism. Hypertension, hypokalemia, aldosteronopenia, and suppressed plasma renin activity. J. Amer. med. Ass. **205**, 492 (1968).

Conn, J. W., Rovner, D. R., Cohen, E. L., Bookstein, J. J., Cerny, J. C., Lucas, C. P.: The preoperative diagnosis of primary aldosteronism. Including a comparison of operative findings and preoperative tumor localization by adrenal phlebography. Arch. intern. Med. **123**, 113 (1969).

Crane, M. G., Harris, J. J.: Effect of spironolactone in hypertensive patients. Amer. J. med. Sci. **260**, 311 (1970).

DeChamplain, J., Genest, J., Veyratt, R., Boucher, R.: Factors controlling renin in man. Arch. intern. Med. **117**, 355 (1966).

Ferriss, J. B., Brown, J. J., Fraser, R., Kay, A. W., Neville, A. M., O'Muircheartaigh, I. G., Robertson, J. I. S., Symington, T., Lever, A. F.: Hypertension with aldosterone excess and low plasma renin: Preoperative distinction between patients with and without adrenocortical tumor. Lancet **1970 II**, 995.

Fishman, L. M., Kuchel, O., Liddle, G. W., Michelakis, A. M., Gordon, R. D., Chick, W. T.: Incidence of primary aldosteronism in "essential hypertension". J. Amer. med. Ass. **205**, 497 (1968).

Genest, J., Boucher, R., DeChamplain, J., Veyratt, R., Chretien, M., Brion, P., Tremb-ley, G., Roy, P., Cartier, P.: Studies on the renin-angiotensin system in hypertensive patients. Canad. med. Ass. J. **90**, 263 (1964).

Giese, J., Jörguensen, M., Nielsen, M. D., Lund, O., Munch, O.: Plasma renin concentration measured by use of radioimmunoassay for angiotensin I. Scand. J. clin. Lab. Invest. **26**, 355 (1970).

Gordon, R. D., Wolfe, L. K., Island, D. P., Liddle, G. W.: A diurnal rhythm in plasma renin activity in man. J. clin. Invest. **45**, 1587 (1966).

Gowenlock, A. H., Wrong, O.: Hyperaldosteronism secondary to renal ischemia. Quart. J. Med. **31**, 323 (1962).

Grim, C. E., Peters, T. J.: Low renin hypertension: A state of inappropriate secretion of aldosterone. Proceedings of the Central Society for Clinical Research **44**, 36 (1971).

Gunnels, J. C., Jr., Grim, C. E., Robinson, R. R., Wildermann, N. M.: Plasma renin activity in healthy subjects and patients with hypertension. Preliminary experience with a rapid and quantitative bio-assay. Arch. intern. Med. **119**, 232 (1967).

Gunnells, J. C., Jr., McGuffin, W. L., Robinson, R. R., Grim, C. E., Wells, S., Silver, D., Glenn, J. F.: Hypertension, adrenal abnormalities, and alterations in plasma renin activity. Ann. intern. Med. **73**, 901 (1970).

Haber, E., Koerner, T., Page, L. B., Kliman, B., Purnode, A.: Application of a radioimmunoassay for angiotensin I to the physiological measurements of plasma renin activity in normal subjects. J. clin. Endocr. **29**, 1349 (1969).

Harris, J. J., Crane, M. G., Johns, V. J., Jr.: Plasma renin activity in hypertension. 48th Annual Session, Proc. Amer. College Physicians, p. 86 (1967).

Helmer, O. M., Judson, W. E.: The quantitative determination of renin in the plasma of patients with arterial hypertension. Circulation **27**, 1050 (1963).

Hollemans, H. J. G., van der Meer, J., Kloosterziel, W.: Measurement of renin activity in plasma by a radioimmunoassay for angiotensin I. Clin. chim. Acta **24**, 353 (1969).

Horton, J. C., Finch, E.: Diagnosis and localization of an aldosteronoma. Clin. Res. **19**, 159 (1971).

Jose, A., Crout, J. R., Kaplan, N. M.: Suppressed plasma renin activity in essential hypertension. Ann. intern. Med. **72**, 9 (1970).

JOSE, A., KAPLAN, N. M.: Plasma renin activity in the diagnosis of primary aldosteronism. Arch. intern. Med. **123**, 141 (1969).

KUCHEL, O., FISHMAN, L. M., LIDDLE, G. W., MICHELAKIS, A.: Effect of diazoxide on plasma renin activity in hypertensive patients. Ann. intern. Med. **67**, 791 (1967).

LAIDLAW, J. C., YENDT, E. R., GORNALL, A. G.: Hypertension caused by renal artery occlusion simulating primary aldosteronism. Metabolism **9**, 612 (1960).

LARAGH, J. H., LEDINGHAM, J. L. G., SOMMERS, S. C.: Secondary aldosteronism and reduced plasma renin in hypertensive disease. Trans. Ass. Amer. Phycns. **80**, 168 (1967).

LARAGH, J. H., SEALEY, J. E., SOMMERS, S. C.: Patterns of adrenal secretion and urinary excretion of aldosterone and plasma renin activity in normal and hypertensive subjects. Circulat. Res. **18** and **19**, I—158 (1966).

LEVER, A. F., ROBERTSON, J. I. S., TREE, M.: The estimation of renin in plasma by an enzyme kinetic technic. Biochem. J. **91**, 346 (1964).

LIDDLE, G. W., BLEDSOE, T., COPPAGE, W. S., Jr.: A familial renal disorder simulating primary aldosteronism but with negligible aldosterone production. Aldosterone, A Symposium. Oxford: Blackwell Scientific Publications 1964.

MCDONALD, W. J., CONN, J. W., COHEN, E. L., LUCAS, C. P.: Increased generation velocity of angiotensin I (AI) in plasma of patients with primary aldosteronism (PA). Clin. Res. **19**, 652 (1971).

MELBY, J. C., DALE, S. L., WILSON, T. E.: 18-hydroxy-desoxycorticosterone in human hypertension. Circulat. Res. **28**, II—153 (1970).

MELBY, J. C., SPARK, R. F., DALE, S. L., EGDAHL, R. H., KAHN, P. C.: Diagnosis and localization of aldosterone producing adenomas by adrenal vein catheterization. New Engl. J. Med. **277**, 1050 (1967).

MOHAMMED, S., FASOLA, A. F., PRIVITERA, P. J., LIPICKY, R. J., MARTZ, B. L., GAFFNEY, T. E.: Effect of methydopa on plasma renin activity in man. Circulat. Res. **25**, 543 (1969).

PICKENS, P. T., BUMPUS, F. M., LLOYD, A. M., SMEBY, R. R., PAGE, I. H.: Measurement of renin activity in human plasma. Circulat. Res. **17**, 438 (1965).

ROVNER, D. R., CONN, J. W. VADER, S. D.: Rapid production of 18-OH, 11-desoxycorticosterone (18OH DOC) by a "non-functioning" adrenal adenoma ('NF'AA). Prog. 53rd Meet. of the Endocr. Soc.' p. 94 (1971).

SALTI, I. S., STIEFEL, M., RUSE, J. L., LAIDLAW, J. C.: Non-tumorous "primary" aldosteronism: Type relieved by glucocorticoid. Canad. med. Ass. J. **101**, 1 (1969).

SKINNER, S. L.: Improved assay methods for renin "concentration" and "activity" in human plasma. Circulat. Res. **20**, 391 (1967).

SPARK, R. F., MELBY, J. C.: Hypertension and low plasma renin activity. Presumptive evidence for mineralocorticoid excess. Ann. intern. Med. **75**, 831 (1971).

STOCKIGT, J. R., COLLINS, R. D., BIGLIERI, E. G.: Determination of plasma renin concentration by angiotensin I radioimmunoassay. Circulat. Res. **28** and **29**, II—175 (1971).

SUTHERLAND, D. J., RUSE, J. L., LAIDLAW, J. C.: Hypertension, increased aldosterone secretion and low plasma renin activity relieved by dexamethasone. Canad. med. Ass. J. **95**, 1109 (1966).

TERAZI, R. C., DUSTAN, H. P., FROHLICH, E. D.: Long-term thiazide therapy in essential hypertension. Circulation **41**, 709 (1970).

WINER, N., CHOKSKI, D. S., YOON, M. S., FREEDMAN, A. D.: Adrenergic receptor mediation of renin secretion. J. Clin. Endocr. **29**, 1168 (1969).

WOODS, J. C., LIDDLE, G. W., STAUT, E. C., MICHELAKIS, A. M., BRILL, A. B.: Effect of an adrenal inhibitor in hypertensive patients with suppressed renin. Archives intern. Med. **123**, 366 (1969).

WOTMAN, S., BAER, L., MANDEL, I. D., LARAGH, J. H.: Submaxillary potassium concentration in true and pseudoprimary aldosteronism. Arch. intern. Med. **126**, 248 (1970).

Secondary Hyperaldosteronism*

E. G. Biglieri, J. R. Stockigt, M. Schambelan, and R. D. Collins

Secondary hyperaldosteronism implies that increased aldosterone production results from extra-adrenal stimulation of the zona glomerulosa of the adrenal gland. The stimulus can be a single factor or the interplay of a number of regulatory influences. The events that activate these factors are of primary concern, and the resultant increase in aldosterone production must be viewed as a physiologic response appropriate to the stimulus, which may have pathophysiologic implications in the course of the primary disease. In considering the various types of secondary hyperaldosteronism we will examine the circumstances under which these stimuli are abnormal. It is sometimes difficult to find a clear-cut association between hyperaldosteronism and one of the major extra-adrenal factors. However, the renin-angiotensin system is implicated as the causal mechanism of the increased secretion of aldosterone in the vast majority of cases.

There are several singularly important cases that suggest that factors, as yet unidentified, other than the renin-angiotensin system may be responsible for clinically significant hyperaldosteronism. These are the cases of glucocorticoid-remediable hypertension (Sutherland et al., 1966; New and Peterson, 1967; Salti et al., 1969): In a setting of severely reduced plasma-renin activity (PRA) and hyperaldosteronism, treatment with dexamethasone effects remission of the hypertension and hyperaldosteronism and normalization of PRA levels.

There is substantial and mounting evidence that variations in the levels of angiotensin II cannot explain all clinical and experimental conditions of hyperaldosteronism. Possibly our definition of primary aldosteronism must be reconsidered (Coghlan et al., 1971; Blair-West et al., 1971). Aldosterone has little direct influence on adrenal production of aldosterone (Blair-West et al., 1962) or on renin release (Geelhoed and Vander, 1967). Instead, "feedback" control results from the physiologic effects of aldosterone. The unique feature of secondary hyperaldosteronism is that either the effects of aldosterone excess have little feedback influence on the initiating stimulatory factor or the response to the effects of aldosterone is modified by clinical conditions or experimental designs.

We shall not attempt to enumerate the conditions of secondary hyperaldosteronism, but rather we shall examine three major areas in which aldosterone regulation is clearly related to a specific factor and consider the clinical circumstances in which these abnormalities occur. In this context the following questions will be subjected to critical consideration: Is there any disease in which hyperaldosteronism is a constant finding? Can secondary hyperaldosteronism contribute to the symptomatology and course of a disease? Will the disorder modify aldosterone production as well as its effects? Is the presence of hyperaldosteronism

* Supported in part by U.S. Public Health Service Research Grants HE-11046 from the National Heart Institute and AM-06415 from the National Institute of Arthritis and Metabolic Diseases. The studies were carried out in part in the General Clinical Research Center, RR-83, at San Francisco General Hospital, supported by Division of Research Resources, National Institutes of Health.

Table 1. *Secondary hyperaldosteronism*

I. Abnormalities of the renin-angiotensin system
- *Hypertension*
  - Malignant
  - Essential
  - Renal or renovascular
  - Indeterminate hyperaldosteronism
  - Renin-secreting tumors
- *Hypertension not present*
  - Bartter's syndrome
  - Renal disorders
    - Chronic renal insufficiency
    - Nephrotic syndrome
    - Renal tubular acidosis (RTA)
  - Pregnancy
  - Estrogen therapy

II. Abnormalities of ACTH secretion

III. Abnormalities of potassium metabolism

useful in diagnosis and choice of therapy? Can prolonged chronic stimulation result in irreversible adrenal steroid overproduction?

Abnormalities of the Renin-Angiotensin System

Hypertension

Malignant Hypertension

The almost consistent concomitant occurrence of hyperaldosteronism and hyperreninemia in patients with malignant hypertension has been well documented and suggests that overproduction of renin is secondary to accelerating renal ischemia (Laragh et al., 1960; Brown et al., 1966; Hollenberg et al., 1969; Sambhi et al., 1963; Creditor and Loschky, 1967). Correction of hyperaldosteronism and renal sodium loss by vigorous antihypertensive treatment was observed initially by Gill et al. (1964).

The studies of McAllister et al. (1971) provide new insight into the relationships between renin and aldosterone in this type of hypertension: Their observations during the acute and recovery phases challenge the close relationships observed previously and suggest that the group of patients was heterogeneous, that renin secretion is variable and that our definition of malignant hypertension is inadequate. In the acute stage of the disorder aldosterone secretion was increased in 19 of 22 patients, whereas PRA was above normal limits in only 8, and during treatment aldosterone production frequently remained elevated for several months after PRA had returned to normal levels. Thus, aldosterone and renin production may not be causally related in all patients with malignant hypertension. These studies suggest that a non-angiotensin aldosterone-stimulating factor might be present or that excessive chronic stimulation of aldosterone secretion might lead to "relative" autonomous over-production. The observations of McAllister's group as well as those of Brown et al. (1970) in patients with renal ischemia and of Baer et al. (1970) in patients with renal parenchymal disease support the latter possibility. However, classification of malignant hypertension as "tertiary" hyperaldosteronism (Baer et al., 1970) must await further examination of aldosterone regulation.

The combined effects of hyperaldosteronism and frequent hyperreninemia may well contribute to the relatively low serum sodium and potassium concentrations observed in patients with this type of secondary hyperaldosteronism.

Essential Hypertension

Secretion of aldosterone is within the normal range in patients with essential hypertension (LARAGH et al., 1960; KAPLAN, 1967; FISHMAN et al., 1968; BIGLIERI et al., 1968), but a state of relative secondary hyperaldosteronism may be present in hypertensive patients with low renin levels. However, recently NOWACZYNSKI et al. (1971) found elevated plasma levels associated with reduction of the metabolic clearance rate of aldosterone. Even more intriguing is the observation of low PRA or plasma renin concentration (PRC) in up to 30% of patients with essential hypertension who had "normal" aldosterone levels (CHANNICK et al., 1969; JOSE and KAPLAN, 1969; JOSE et al., 1970; KOTCHEN et al., 1971). The significance of normal aldosterone levels in the face of low PRA or PRC has been challenged by several maneuvers. After salt deprivation the renin levels tend to remain low and often the aldosterone responses tend to be subnormal. However, the two low-renin hypertensive patients reported by CHRISTLIEB et al. (1969) had a limited aldosterone response and a normal increase in PRA. Furthermore, salt loading did not depress plasma aldosterone levels in such patients (COLLINS et al., 1970). The negligible influence of salt intake on aldosterone production suggests some degree of adrenal autonomy.

Essential hypertension is clearly *not* associated with hyperaldosteronism resulting from renin excess. In some of the instances just described aldosterone production appears to be little influenced by known aldosterone-regulating factors. Whether this represents adrenal autonomy or not is not certain. In patients with either normal or low PRA levels, aldosterone production is readily suppressed by the administration of deoxycorticosterone acetate (DOCA) [BIGLIERI et al., 1972 (1)]. Relative secondary hyperaldosteronism may be present since the level of aldosterone is disproportionately high for the renin level or maintained at a new level by an unknown stimulating factor. Essential hypertension could be categorized into three groups according to levels of renin secretion, and the groups may or may not be interrelated: Type 1, essential hypertension with normal renin levels and normal aldosterone production that is readily suppressible by either salt loading or DOCA; Type 2, essential hypertension with subnormal renin levels and normal aldosterone production that is readily suppressible by either salt loading or DOCA; and Type 3, indeterminate hyperaldosteronism with mild but persistent elevation of aldosterone production suppressible by DOCA, subnormal PRA levels in most cases, and normal to slightly low serum potassium concentrations [BIGLIERI et al., 1972 (2)]. Since patients with Type 3 differ from hypertensive patients with primary adrenal disease in the extent to which aldosterone production can be suppressed by DOCA, this group may represent either a variant of essential hypertension or a transitional phase between Type 2 and primary adrenal disease. This transitional stage may develop into either primary aldosteronism due to an adenoma or idiopathic hyperaldosteronism (nodular hyperplasia).

Renal Hypertension

Hyperaldosteronism has been observed in patients with benign and with malignant renovascular hypertension. Plasma-renin activity [BROWN et al., 1965 (2); BARRACLOUGH et al., 1965; GUNNELLS et al., 1969], aldosterone [LAIDLAW et al., 1960; COPE et al., 1962 GEORGE et al., 1968 KOTCHEN et al., 1970 (2); SLATON and BIGLIERI, 1965], and Ang. II (MASSANI et al., 1966 BLAIR-WEST et al., 1968) may all be elevated although usually the levels are within the normal range. KOTCHEN et al. (1971) observed elevated aldosterone secretion in only 4 of the 14 patients with benign renovascular hypertension but in all 5 patients with malignant renovascular hypertension [KOTCHEN et al., 1970 (2)]. In the patients studied by BROWN et al. [1965 (2)] PRC was usually elevated in patients with malignant renovascular hypertension and frequently within the normal range in patients with the benign form. It has been suggested by SLATON and BIGLIERI (1965) and KOTCHEN et al. [1970 (2)] that increased aldosterone production is indicative of a good response to surgery in renal artery stenosis; possibly hyperaldosteronism is an early manifestation of this disease. However, direct interpretation of aldosterone values at any one time may be difficult because both the severity and the duration of hypertension can influence the activity of the renin-angiotensin-aldosterone system in man and experimental animals. When hypertension follows acute constriction of the renal artery in dogs and sheep, the increase in both renin and aldosterone is usually brief, normal levels being regained within 1 to 4 days despite persistence of hypertension (BLAIR-WEST et al., 1968; BIANCHI et al., 1970). However, in some sheep with renal hypertension, rapid progression of hypertension was associated with severe urinary sodium loss and progressive increases in renin and aldosterone (BLAIR-WEST et al., 1968). This could possibly be the experimental counterpart of the "hyponatremic hypertensive syndrome" [BROWN et al., 1965 (1); BARRACLOUGH, 1966] in which malignant hypertension, often renal artery stenosis, is associated with hyponatremia, hypokalemia, weight loss, polyuria, and high levels of renin and aldosterone. We have found that peripheral levels of PRA are elevated in only about one half the patients with renal artery stenosis, and that hyperaldosteronism is related to hyperreninemia. In patients with renal hypertension, elevated levels of aldosterone appear to be normally suppressible by either DOCA [BIGLIERI et al., 1972 (1)] or saline infusion (KEM et al., 1971). Although WARREN and FERRIS (1970) suggested that secretion of renin may not be normally suppressible, certainly aldosterone can be suppressed into the normal range. Hyperaldosteronism does not appear to be an essential factor in the pathogenesis of renal hypertension. MCCAA et al. (1965) found that aldosterone secretion remains at normal levels during the onset of experimental renal hypertension in dogs, and BLAIR-WEST et al. (1968) showed that renal hypertension can be induced and maintained in adrenalectomized sheep receiving a maintenance dosage of steroids. In contrast to the situation in primary hyperaldosteronism a clear relationship between hyperaldosteronism and hyperreninemia can frequently be established. Under these circumstances suppressive tests clearly separate primary from secondary adrenal disease one of the most effective tests is the DOCA maneuver [BIGLIERI et al., 1972 (1)].

Indeterminate Hyperaldosteronism

[Biglieri et al., 1972 (2)]

This type of hyperaldosteronism further emphasizes the importance of a suppressive test in the hypertensive patient with hyperaldosteronism. It is still extremely difficult to distinguish between primary aldosteronism due to an adenoma and primary aldosteronism due to nodular hyperplasia. The two approaches that show considerable promise are quadric analysis of multiple variables (AITCHISON et al., 1971) and plotting of the basal recumbent PRC against the level of aldosterone after DOCA [BIGLIERI et al., 1972 (2)]. Identification of the adrenal pathology is crucial because adrenalectomy successfully corrects hypertension in patients with an adenoma (Conn, 1966, 1967; Biglieri et al., 1970) but not in those with nodular hyperplasia (Baer et al., 1970; Biglieri et al., 1970), which is an unusual finding in primary adrenal disease. The presence of reduced PRA provides only corroborative evidence of a possible aldosterone-producing adenoma. The susceptibility of elevated aldosterone levels to suppression by DOCA or other techniques raises the question of whether or not this group genuinely does represent primary adrenal disease. Fortunately the mild hypertension can usually be effectively treated medically until a more precise diagnosis can be established. The high incidence of nodular hyperplasia in patients with the syndrome of primary aldosteronism in some reported series (Gunnells et al., 1970; George et al., 1970) may be due, in part, to the fact that the authors included many patients with indeterminate hyperaldosteronism since suppressive studies were not performed.

Renin-Secreting Tumor

At the time of this report only four cases of renin-secreting tumor of the kidney arising from the juxtaglomerular cells have been reported (Kihara et al., 1968; Eddy and Sanchez, 1971; Robertson et al., 1967; Lee, 1971). Severe hypertension, hyperaldosteronism, and increased PRA are present. This is a rare form of curable hypertension occurring predominantly in young persons. Until recently preoperative diagnosis involved considerable difficulties. Arteriography does not always allow diagnosis of a renal lesion. Aldosterone production reaches extremely high levels with subsequent severe hypokalemia and it is not possible to suppress the hyperaldosteronism with DOCA (Schambelan and Biglieri, 1972), which is rare in patients with secondary hyperaldosteronism. However, the extremely high levels of renin show little response to large doses of DOCA, which probably accounts for the absence of a fall in aldosterone. Thus, failure to suppress elevated levels of PRA and aldosterone with DOCA may be indicative of a renin-secreting tumor. Bilateral renal vein PRA studies identify the side where excessive renin is produced, and in one patient we were able to locate the tumor exactly by venous sampling from various areas of the involved kidney (Schambelan and Biglieri, 1972). In our patient the lesion was a hemangiopericytoma, which responded to certain stimulating maneuvers such as upright posture and spironolactone treatment with an increase in PRA before surgery. Renin from the contralateral kidney produced no renin at all before unilateral nephrectomy because PRA levels fell to zero for several days before gradually returning to normal levels after nephrectomy. Hypertension was completely corrected postoperatively.

Chauvel et al. reported a child with increased PRA levels, secondary hyperaldosteronism, and hypertension who may well have this disease but it is still uncertain whether the source of excess renin is unilateral or bilateral (Chauvel et al., 1970).

There is a significant incidence of hypertension in patients with Wilms' tumors (Bradley and Drake, 1949). Voûte et al. (1971) and Mitchell et al. (1970) observed that elevated PRA levels fall after removal of the tumor. It is uncertain whether or not secondary hyperaldosteronism is consistently present with such tumors. The possibility of renin secretion by an oat-cell carcinoma was suggested by Hauger-Klevene (1970) when hyperaldosteronism responsive to salt changes and increased PRA were observed in patients with such a malignancy.

Hypertension not Present

Bartter's Syndrome

In this syndrome, which is characterized by hyperplasia of the juxtaglomerular complex and hypokalemic alkalosis (BARTTER et al., 1962), hyperaldosteronism and hyperreninemia occur without associated hypertension or edema. The pathogenesis of this disorder remains uncertain and has been variously attributed to vascular insensitivity to the pressor effect of Ang. II (BARTTER et al., 1962), to relatively autonomous secretion of renin (BRACKETT et al., 1968), and to excessive loss of sodium from the proximal renal tubule (GOODMAN et al., 1969). Reduced sensitivity to the pressor effect of Ang. II is not a unique feature of this syndrome as it also occurs in patients with cirrhosis of the liver (AMES et al., 1965) or renal hypertension (KAPLAN and SILAH, 1964). In the case reported by GOODMAN et al. (1969) pressor sensitivity was restorted to normal after volume expansion by albumin infusion. Aldosterone production can be suppressed into the normal range by sodium loading or albumin infusion in most cases, but renin levels, while significantly reduced, remain well above the normal range (BRYAN et al., 1966; BEILIN et al., 1967; BRACKETT et al., 1968; GOODMAN et al., 1969). However, these studies were performed, in most instances, in the presence of severe long-standing hypokalemia, making the renin responses difficult to evaluate because potassium depletion augments renin secretion (BRUNNER et al., 1970) while reducing aldosterone production (CANNON et al., 1966).

Impairment of proximal tubular sodium reabsorption has been postulated as the primary abnormality leading to the hypersecretion of renin and aldosterone and to the increased distal exchange of sodium for potassium and hydrogen ions (CANNON et al., 1968; GOODMAN et al., 1969). The finding of glomerulo-distal-tubular shunts (BIAVA et al., 1969) suggests that in some cases the proximal tubule may be bypassed with the same functional result. While sodium conservation is adequate in most cases, inappropriate sodium loss has been observed (CANNON et al., 1968).

Aldosterone excess may not be the sole mechanism responsible for the hypokalemia because potassium loss may persist after aldosterone excess is corrected by subtotal adrenalectomy (BRYAN et al., 1966) or albumin infusion (GOODMAN et al., 1969; BRACKETT et al., 1968). While sodium restriction can correct hypokalemia in patients with primary aldosteronism, it is rarely effective in patients with BARTTER's syndrome where potassium is required in large doses (BARTTER, 1969). While spironolactone may be effective in short-term studies, "escape" occurs with long-term treatment (BRACKETT et al., 1968).

Renal Disorders

Chronic renal insufficiency: Aldosterone levels may be either subnormal or supranormal in patients with chronic renal insufficiency, and there are few studies that directly relate these changes to renin secretion. Increased aldosterone secretion has been observed in patients with chronic azotemic renal failure (COPE and PEARSON, 1963; VECSEI et al., 1969), and GOLD et al. (1965) found that aldosterone secretion is little influenced by changes in sodium balance. About half the patients with chronic renal insufficiency studied by KOTCHEN et al. [1970 (1)] had elevated levels of PRA prior to dialysis, which rose further after dialysis, whereas the PRA levels in TU's (1965) patients were within normal limits.

Patients who have persistent severe hypertension after hemodialysis often have markedly elevated levels of PRA (VERTES et al., 1969), but at present it is uncertain whether or not hyperaldosteronism is present in these patients. Clear-cut secondary hyperaldosteronism has been described in cases of renal disease with sodium loss (FRASER et al., 1966), but it may only represent a normal physiologic response to sodium loss.

Aldosterone deficiency has also been reported in patients with chronic renal failure (GERSTEIN et al., 1968; VAGNUCCI, 1970) and may aggravate hyperkalemia. The expected elevation of renin in the presence of hypoaldosteronism does not always occur (GERSTEIN et al., 1968). SCHAMBELAN et al. (1972) reported a group of patients with moderate diminution of renal function in whom hypoaldosteronism and hyperkalemia were associated with subnormal levels of PRA and PRC. In these patients the renin and aldosterone levels were refractory to stimulation by salt depletion while the production of deoxycorticosterone, corticosterone, and cortisol was normal and responded normally to intravenous administration of adrenocorticotropin (ACTH), ruling out an adrenal enzymatic defect. Correction of hyperkalemia with exchange resins had no effect on aldosterone or renin levels.

Nephrotic syndrome: The finding of a highly potent mineralocorticoid in the urine of children with nephrotic syndrome was one of the original observations leading to the isolation of aldosterone (LUETSCHER et al., 1954), followed by demonstration of increased aldosterone secretion (VECSEI et al., 1969) and hyperreninemia in these patients (VEYRAT et al., 1964). While normal subjects and hypertensive patients escape the sodium-retaining effect of excess aldosterone, this may not occur in patients with nephrosis with refractory sodium retention (NELSON and AUGUST, 1959). The formation of edema is probably a result of the reduced serum-albumin concentration and the increased escape of intravascular fluid into the extravascular compartment, triggering the renin-angiotensin-aldosterone system.

Renal tubular acidosis: The hyperaldosteronism in patients with classic renal tubular acidosis may be reduced by sustained correction of the acidosis and retardation of urinary potassium wasting (GILL et al., 1967). However, in the patients reported by SEBASTIAN et al. (1971) hyperaldosteronism and renal potassium loss persisted despite sustained correction of acidosis, normal sodium intake, and maintenance of the measured plasma volume. There appears to be a spectrum of disorders in which hyperaldosteronism participates in sustaining potassium wasting. BARTTER (1969) pointed out several similarities between renal tubular acidosis and Bartter's syndrome and suggested that proximal tubular sodium loss might result in hyperaldosteronism and increased distal exchange of sodium for potassium in both disorders.

Increased levels of PRA inappropriate to the state of sodium balance have been observed in patients with renal tubular acidosis, but the mechanism leading to the increase in renin and aldosterone remains obscure (SEBASTIAN et al., 1971). It is possible that a state of chronic hyperaldosteronism might be sustained by the need for continued potassium supplementation or a form of tertiary aldosteronism might have resulted from prolonged sodium depletion before therapy.

Pregnancy

Hyperaldosteronism can develop during pregnancy and progress during the second trimester, reaching levels of $\geq$ 1,000 μg/day during the last trimester (SIMS et al., 1964). The hyperaldosteronism is most probably effected by the ncrease in renin production that normally occurs during pregnancy (BROWN et al., 1963). The PRA level is usually elevated throughout normal pregnancy and is most probably the cause of secondary hyperaldosteronism (BROWN et al., 1963).

Despite the excessive secretion of aldosterone and the associated positive sodium balance, little potassium depletion occurs. This is probably due to the increased production of progesterone during pregnancy, which inhibits the potassium-losing activity of aldosterone but does not interfere with the sodium-retaining action of aldosterone. The plasma level of aldosterone is elevated during pregnancy and it is not clear why hypertension and profound potassium depletion do not occur.

Estrogen Treatment

The frequency of hypertension in women taking oral estrogen-containing contraceptive drugs and in patients taking estrogen for osteoporosis, cancer of the prostate, and breast cancer is uncertain but this obviously does occur, as described by a number of workers (SWAAB, 1966; LARAGH et al., 1967; WOODS, 1967; TYSON, 1968; WEINBERGER et al., 1969; NEWTON et al., 1968; CRANE and HARRIS, 1969). Of all the drugs studied, the effects of estrogen on the renin-angiotensin-aldosterone system are the best documented (CRANE and HARRIS, 1969). LARAGH and co-workers (1967) demonstrated that after the initiation of regular treatment with estrogenic compounds PRA approximately doubles and a three- to five-fold increase occurs in the concentration of circulating renin substrate. When renin substrate is greatly increased, the generation of Ang. II is enhanced at physiologic levels of renin both *in vivo* and *in vitro*. CATT et al. (1971) observed high circulating levels of Ang. II within days after initiation of oral contraceptive or estrogen therapy. A high circulating level of Ang. II may be the stimulus for an increase in blood pressure when combined with genetic, environmental, and renal factors. Ang. II is one of the factors that regulates the amount of renin excreted by the kidneys. When Ang. II generation is increased by estrogens, PRC is correspondingly suppressed (CAIN et al., 1971). It has been suggested that PRC is not reduced to the same degree in hypertensive persons on estrogen therapy as in those who are normotensive (SARUTA et al., 1970). In almost every circumstance in which estrogen therapy is administered a secondary increase in aldosterone occurs that is related to the increased production of Ang. II. Further supporting evidence that the hyperaldosteronism is secondary is that aldosterone production is readily suppressed by DOCA (BIGLIERI et al., 1972).

Abnormalities of ACTH Secretion

The exact nature of the role of ACTH in the normal regulation of aldosterone production remains controversial and uncertain. It is clear that ACTH, when administered in large doses, can stimulate an increase in aldosterone production. However, continued administration of ACTH fails to maintain the high level of aldosterone achieved initially, although the levels of other adrenal steroids remain high (NEWTON and LARAGH, 1968; BIGLIERI et al., 1969): aldosterone decreases to control or basal levels usually within 3 days. Another interesting facet is that when ACTH is discontinued, aldosterone becomes subnormal and remains so for up to a week (BIGLIERI et al., 1969). The initial increase and the subsequent decrease in aldosterone production in response to ACTH occur in normal subjects during both salt-restricted and normal salt diets and in patients with primary aldosteronism. It seems unlikely that the response is due to the suppression of renin. However, the question of the effect of ACTH on renin production is not completely settled although studies by NEWTON and LARAGH have demonstrated that PRA levels are unchanged in patients given exogenous ACTH (NEWTON and LARAGH, 1968). The possibility that ACTH might lead to intra-adrenal accumulation of aldosterone precursors effecting substrate inhibition is supported by the fact that addition of corticosterone (Vecsei et al., 1965), cortisol (Burrow et al., 1966), or even deoxycorticosterone (Kaplan and Bartter, 1962) can suppress aldosterone production *in vitro*.

In disorders in which excessive ACTH is continually produced (as in Cushing's syndrome due to adrenal hyperplasia, aldosterone levels are uniformly within normal limits (Christy and Laragh, 1961; Biglieri et al., 1963). In the ectopic ACTH syndrome, in which even higher levels of ACTH are observed, the mineralocorticoid in excess is deoxycorticosterone rather than aldosterone, and aldosterone production is normal or reduced (Schambelan et al., 1971).

Since continued oversecretion of ACTH does not affect aldosterone levels significantly it would only transiently effect hyperaldosteronism in the acute situations of trauma or stress. A sustained effect would not be observed unless the glucocorticoid hormones were affected with the subsequent consequence of excessive production of cortisol.

Abnormalities of Potassium Metabolism

Potassium is an extremely potent stimulus to aldosterone excretion. The narrow confines to which it is maintained in the circulating blood make it difficult to alter its concentration substantially. Its effect seems to be direct rather than mediated through any other mechanism. The mechanism of action may vary from a direct effect on adrenocortical cells to an increase in the intra-adrenal potassium concentration or the local alteration of the concentration in the adrenal blood supply. Potassium loading in man produces increases in aldosterone secretion that are as great or even greater than those produced by ACTH or angiotensin (Cannon et al., 1966). In a reverse maneuver, potassium depletion decreases aldosterone production. It does not block the increased aldosterone response to sodium depletion. The most pronounced effects of potassium on aldosterone production are observed in patients with primary aldosteronism who have profound depletions of potassium. In these patients, a change of 2 to 3 mEq/L in the serum-potassium concentration can produce profound increases in aldosterone secretion (Slaton et al., 1969). The production of aldosterone by tumors is exquisitely sensitive to the potassium concentration.

A more important role ascribed to potassium is the regulation of aldosterone concentration in anephric man. The rise in the plasma concentration of aldosterone appears to result from an increase in the serum potassium concentration between dialyses despite the expected suppressant effects of salt and water accumulation. Aldosterone fails to increase if an increase in potassium concentration is prevented (Bayard et al., 1971). It is intriguing to note the independence of potassium from the renin-angiotensin system. While potassium loading increases aldosterone production it tends to suppress PRA and, conversely, potassium depletion increases PRA and decreases aldosterone production (Sealey et al., 1970).

In most situations in which chronic hyperkalemia occurs in the absence of renal failure, aldosterone production is usually reduced or absent as in patients with Addison's disease or adrenal insufficiency. An isolated deficiency of aldosterone appears to be secondary to renin deficiency. PRA and PRC are extremely low in these patients and fail to respond to any of the known stimuli even after the reduction of the serum potassium level to the normal range by resin therapy. Treatment with small doses of 9-α-fluorohydrocortisone is an effective way of managing hyperkalemia in these patients (Schambelan et al., 1972).

References

AITCHISON, J., BROWN, J. J., FERRISS, J. B., FRASER, R., KAY, A. W., LEVER, A. F., NEVILLE, A. M., SYMINGTON, T., ROBERTSON, J. I. S.: Quadric analysis in the preoperative distinction between patients with and without adrenocortical tumors in hypertension with aldosterone excess and low plasma renin. Amer. Heart J. **82**, 660 (1971).

AMES, R. P., BORKOWSKI, A. J., SICINSKI, A. M., LARAGH, J. H.: Prolonged infusions of angiotensin II and norepinephrine and blood pressure, electrolyte balance and aldosterone and cortisol secretion in normal man and in cirrhosis with ascites. J. clin. Invest. **44**, 1171 (1965).

BAER, L., SOMMERS, S. C., KRAKOFF, L. R., NEWTON, M. A., LARAGH, J. H.: Pseudoprimary aldosteronism: An entity distinct from true primary aldosteronism. Circulat. Res. **26** and **27** (Suppl. I), I—203 (1970).

BARRACLOUGH, M. A.: Sodium and water depletion with acute malignant hypertension. Amer. J. Med. **40**, 265 (1966).

BARRACLOUGH, M. A., BACCHUS, B., BROWN, J. J., DAVIES, D. L., LEVER, A. F., ROBERTSON, J. I. S.: Plasma-renin and aldosterone secretion in hypertensive patients with renal or renal artery lesions. Lancet **1965 II**, 1310.

BARTTER, F. C.: So-called Bartter's Syndrome. New Engl. J. Med. **281**, 1483 (1969).

BARTTER, F. C., PRONOVE, P., GILL, J. R., Jr., MAC CARDLE, R. C.: Hyperplasia of the juxtaglomerular complex with hyperaldosteronism and hypokalemic alkalosis: A new syndrome. Amer. J. Med. **33**, 811 (1962).

BAYARD, F., COOKE, C. R., TILLER, D. J., BEITINS, I. Z., KOWARSKI, A., WALKER, W. G., MIGEON, C. J.: The regulation of aldosterone secretion in anephric man. J. clin. Invest. **50**, 1585 (1971).

BEILIN, L. J., SCHIFFMAN, N., CRANE, M., NELSON, D. H.: Hypokalaemic alkalosis and hyperplasia of the juxtaglomerular apparatus without hypertension or oedema. Brit. med. J. **1967 IV**, 327.

BIANCHI, G., TILDE-TENCONI, L., LUCCA, R.: Effect in the conscious dog of constriction o the renal artery to a sole remaining kidney on haemodynamics, sodium balance, body fluid volumes, plasma renin concentration and pressor responsiveness to angiotensin. Clin. Sci. **38**, 741 (1970).

BIAVA, C., DESJARDINS, R., BRAVO, E., BARTTER, F.: Glomerular changes with glomerulo-distotubular shunts in patients with Bartter's Syndrome. Lab. Invest. **20**, 575 (1969).

BIGLIERI, E. G., HANE, S., SLATON, P. E., Jr., FORSHAM, P. H.: *In vivo* and *in vitro* studies of adrenal secretions in Cushing's Syndrome and primary aldosteronism. J. clin. Invest. **42**, 516 (1963).

BIGLIERI, E. G., SCHAMBELAN, M., SLATON, P. E., Jr.: Effect of adrenocorticotropin on deoxycorticosterone, corticosterone and aldosterone excretion. J. clin. Endocr. **29**, 1090 (1969).

BIGLIERI, E. G., SCHAMBELAN, M., SLATON, P. E., Jr., STOCKIGT, J. R.: The intercurrent hypertension of primary aldosteronism. Circulat. Res. **26** and **27** (Suppl. I), I—195 (1970).

BIGLIERI, E. G., SCHAMBELAN, M., STOCKIGT, J. R.: (1) Hypertension and hyperaldosteronism: Discriminating value of deoxycorticosterone acetate (DOCA) testing. Clin. Res. **20**, 163 (1972).

BIGLIERI, E. G., SLATON, P. E., Jr., SCHAMBELAN, M., KRONFIELD, S. J.: Hypermineralocorticoidism. Amer. J. Med. **45**, 170 (1968).

BIGLIERI, E. G., STOCKIGT, J. R., SCHAMBELAN, M.: (2) Adrenal mineralocorticoids causing hypertension. Amer. J. Med. **52**, 623 (1972).

BLAIR-WEST, J. R., CAIN, M. D., CATT, K. J., COGHLAN, J. P., DENTON, D. A., FUNDER, J. W., SCOGGINS, B. A., WRIGHT, R. D.: The dissociation of aldosterone secretion and systemic renin and angiotensin II levels during the correction of sodium deficiency. Acta endocr. (Kbh.) **66**, 229 (1971).

BLAIR-WEST, J. R., COGHLAN, J. P., DENTON, D. A.: Evidence against an aldosterone feedback mechanism within the adrenal gland. Acta endocr. (Kbh.) **41**, 61 (1962).

BLAIR-WEST, J. R., COGHLAN, J. P., DENTON, D. A., ORCHARD, E., SCOGGINS, B. A., WRIGHT, R. D.: Renin-angiotensin-aldosterone system and sodium balance in experimental renal hypertension. Endocrinology **83**, 1199 (1968).

BRACKETT, N. C., KOPPEL, M., RANDALL, R. E., Jr., NIXON, W. P.: Hyperplasia of the juxtaglomerular complex with secondary aldosteronism without hypertension (Bartter's Syndrome). Amer. J. Med. **44**, 803 (1968).

BRADLEY, J. E., DRAKE, M. E.: The effect of preoperative roentgen-ray therapy on arterial hypertension in embryoma (kidney). J. Pediat. **35**, 710 (1949).

BROWN, J. J., DAVIES, D. L., DOAK, P. B., LEVER, A. F., ROBERTSON, J. I. S.: Plasma renin in normal pregnancy. Lancet **1963 II**, 900.

BROWN, J. J., DAVIES, D. L., LEVER, A. F., ROBERTSON, J. I. S.: Variations in plasma renin concentration in several physiological and pathological states. Canad. med. Ass. J. **90**, 201 (1964).
BROWN, J. J., DAVIES, D. L., LEVER, A. F., ROBERTSON, J. I. S.: (1) Plasma renin concentration in human hypertension. I. Relationship between renin, sodium, and potassium. Brit. med. J. **1965 II**, 144.
BROWN, J. J., DAVIES, D. L., LEVER, A. F., ROBERTSON, J. I. S.: (2) Plasma renin concentration in human hypertension. II. Renin in relation to aetiology. Brit. med. J. **1965 II**, 1215.
BROWN, J. J., DAVIES, D. L., LEVER, A. F., ROBERTSON, J. I. S.: Plasma renin concentration in human hypertension. III. Renin in relation to complications of hypertension. Brit. med. J. **1966 I**, 505.
BRUNNER, H. R., BAER, L., SEALEY, J. E., LEDINGHAM, J. G. G., LARAGH, J. H.: The influence of potassium administration and potassium deprivation on plasma renin in normal and hypertensive subjects. J. clin. Invest. **49**, 2128 (1970).
BRYAN, G. T., MAC CARDLE, R. C., BARTTER, F. C.: Hyperaldosteronism, hyperplasia of the juxtaglomerular complex, normal blood pressure and dwarfism: Report of a case. Pediatrics **37**, 43 (1966).
BURROW, G. W., MULROW, P. J., BONDY, P. K.: Protein synthesis and aldosterone production. Endocrinology **79**, 955 (1966).
CAIN, M. D., WALTERS, W. A., CATT, K. J.: Effects of oral contraceptive therapy on the renin-angiotensin system. J. clin. Endocr. **33**, 671 (1971).
CANNON, P. J., AMES, R. P., LARAGH, J. H.: Relation between potassium balance and aldosterone secretion in normal subjects and in patients with hypertensive or renal tubular disease. J. clin. Invest. **45**, 865 (1966).
CANNON, P. J., LEEMING, J. M., SOMMERS, S. C., WINTERS, R. W., LARAGH, J. H.: Juxtaglomerular cell hyperplasia and secondary hyperaldosteronism (Bartter's Syndrome): A reevaluation of the pathophysiology. Medicine (Baltimore) **47**, 107 (1968).
CATT, K. J., ZIMMET, P. Z., CAIN, M. D., CRAN, E., BEST, J. B., COGHLAN, J. P.: Angiotensin II blood-levels in human hypertension. Lancet **1971 I**, 459.
CHANNICK, B. J., ADLIN, E. V., MARKS, A. D.: Suppressed plasma renin activity in hypertension. Arch. intern. Med. **123**, 131 (1969).
CHAUVEL, P. J., BEVERIDGE, J., STOKES, G. S.: Increased plasma renin activity, secondary aldosteronism, and hypertension. Amer. J. Dis. Child. **119**, 159 (1970).
CHRISTLIEB, A. R., HICKLER, R. B., LAULER, D. P., WILLIAMS, G. H.: Hypertension with inappropriate aldosterone stimulation: A syndrome. New Engl. J. Med. **281**, 128 (1969).
CHRISTY, N. P., LARAGH, J. H.: Pathogenesis of hypokalemic alkalosis in Cushing's Syndrome. New Engl. J. Med. **265**, 1083 (1961).
COGHLAN, J. P., BLAIR-WEST, J. R., DENTON, D. A., SCOGGINS, B. A., WRIGHT, R. D.: Perspectives in aldosterone and renin control. Aust. N. Z. J. Med. **2**, 178 (1971).
COLLINS, R. D., WEINBERGER, M. H., DOWDY, A. J., NOKES, G. W., GONZALES, C. M., LUETSCHER, J. A.: Abnormally sustained aldosterone secretion during salt loading in patients with various forms of benign hypertension; relation to plasma renin activity. J. clin. Invest. **49**, 1415 (1970).
CONN, J. W.: The evolution of primary aldosteronism: 1954—1967. Harvey Lect. **62**, 257 (1966—1967).
COPE, C. L., HARWOOD, M., PEARSON, J.: Aldosterone secretion in hypertensive diseases. Brit. med. J. **1**, 659 (1962).
COPE, C. L., PEARSON, J.: Aldosterone secretion in severe renal failure. Clin. Sci. **25**, 331 (1963.)
CRANE, M. G., HARRIS, J. J.: Plasma renin activity and aldosterone excretion rate in normal subjects. I. Effect of ethinyl estradiol and medroxyprogesterone acetate. J. clin. Endocr. **29**, 550 (1969).
CREDITOR, M. C., LOSCHKY, U. K.: Plasma renin activity in hypertension. Amer. J. Med. **43**, 371 (1967).
EDDY, R. L., SANCHEZ, S. A.: Renin-secreting renal neoplasm and hypertension with hypokalemia. Ann. intern. Med. **75**, 725 (1971).
FISHMAN, L. M., KÜCHEL, O., LIDDLE, G. W., MICHELAKIS, A. M., GORDON, R. D., CHICK, W. T.: Incidence of primary aldosteronism in uncomplicated "essential" hypertension: A prospective study with elevated aldosterone secretion and suppressed plasma renin activity used as diagnostic criteria. J. Amer. med. Ass. **205**, 497 (1968).
FRASER, R., JAMES, V. T., BROWN, J. J., DAVIES, D. L., LEVER, A. F., ROBERTSON, J. I. S.: Changes in plasma aldosterone, cortisol, corticosterone and renin concentration in a patient with sodium-losing renal disease. J. Endocr. **35**, 311 (1966).
GEELHOED, G. W., VANDER, A. J.: The role of aldosterone in renin secretion. Life Sci. **6**, 525 (1967).

GEORGE, J. M., GILLESPIE, L., BARTTER, F. C.: Aldosterone secretion in hypertension. Ann. intern. Med. **69**, 693 (1968).

GEORGE, J. M., WRIGHT, L., BELL, N. H., BARTTER, F. C.: The syndrome of primary aldosteronism. Amer. J. Med. **48**, 343 (1970).

GERSTEIN, A. R., KLEEMAN, C. R., GOLD, E. M., FRANKLIN, S. S., MAXWELL, M. H., GONICK, H. C., FEFFER, M. L., STEINMAN, T. I.: Aldosterone deficiency in chronic renal failure. Nephron **5**, 90, (1968).

GILL, J. R., Jr,. GEORGE, J. M., SOLOMON, A., BARTTER, F. C.: Hyperaldosteronism and renal sodium loss reversed by drug treatment for malignant hypertension. New Engl. J. Med. **270**, 1088 (1964).

GILL, J. R., Jr., BELL, N. H., BARTTER, F. C.: Impaired conservation of sodium and potassium in renal tubular acidosis and its correction by buffer anions. Clin. Sci. **33**, 577 (1967).

GOLD, E. M., KLEEMAN, C. R., LING, S., YAWATA, M., MAXWELL, M.: Sustained aldosterone secretion in chronic renal failure. Clin. Res. **13**, 135 (1965).

GOODMAN, A. D., VAGNUCCI, A. H., HARTROFT, P. M.: Pathogenesis of Bartter's Syndrome. New Engl. J. Med. **281**, 1435 (1969).

GUNNELLS, J. C., Jr., MCGUFFIN, W. L., JOHNSRUDE, I., ROBINSON, R. R.: Peripheral and renal venous plasma renin activity in hypertension. Ann. intern. Med. **71**, 555 (1969).

GUNNELLS, J. C., Jr., MCGUFFIN, W. L., Jr., ROBINSON, R. R., GRIM, C. E., WELLS, S., SILVER, D., GLENN, J. F.: Hypertension, adrenal abnormalities and alterations in plasma renin activity. Ann. intern. Med. **73**, 901 (1970).

HAUGER-KLEVENE, J. H.: High plasma renin activity in an oat cell carcinoma: A renin-secreting carcinoma? Cancer **26**, 1112 (1970).

HOLLENBERG, N. K., EPSTEIN, M., BASCH, R. I., COUCH, N. P., HICKLER, R. B., MERRILL, J. P.: Renin secretion in essential and accelerated hypertension. Amer. J. Med. **47**, 855 (1969).

JOSE, A., CROUT, J. R., KAPLAN, N. M.: Suppressed plasma renin activity in essential hypertension. Roles of plasma volume, blood pressure, and sympathetic nervous system. Ann. intern. Med. **72**, 9 (1970).

JOSE, A., KAPLAN, N. M.: Plasma renin activity in diagnosis of primary aldosteronism: Failure to distinguish primary aldosteronism from essential hypertension. Arch. intern. Med. **123**, 141 (1969).

KAPLAN, N. M.: The steroid content of adrenal adenomas and measurements of aldosterone production in patients with essential and primary aldosteronism. J. clin. Invest. **46**, 728 (1967).

KAPLAN, N. M., BARTTER, F. C.: The effect of ACTH, renin, angiotensin II, and various precursors on biosynthesis of aldosterone by adrenal slices. J. clin. Invest. **41**, 715 (1962).

KAPLAN, N. M., SILAH, J. G.: The effect of angiotensin II on the blood pressure in humans with hypertensive disease. J. clin. Invest. **43**, 659 (1964).

KEM, D. C., WEINBERGER, M. H., MAYES, D. M., NUGENT, C. A.: Saline suppression of plasma aldosterone in hypertension. Arch. intern. Med. **128**, 380 (1971).

KIHARA, I., KITAMURA, S., HOSHINO, T., SEIDA, H.: A hitherto unreported vascular tumor of the kidney: A proposal of "juxtaglomerular cell tumor". Acta path. jap. **18**, 197 (1968).

KOTCHEN, T. A., KNIGHT, E. L., KASHGARIAN, M., MULROW, P. J.: (1) A study of the renin-angiotensin system in patients with severe chronic renal insufficiency. Nephron **7**, 317 (1970).

KOTCHEN, T. A., LYTTON, B., MORROW, L. B., MULROW, P. J., SHUTKIN, P. M., STANSEL, H. C.: (2) Angiotensin and aldosterone in renovascular hypertension. Arch. intern. Med. **125**, 265 (1970).

KOTCHEN, T. A., MULROW, P. J., MORROW, L. B., SHUTKIN, P. M., MARIEB, N.: Renin and aldosterone in essential hypertension. Clin. Sci. **41**, 321 (1971).

LAIDLAW, J. C., YENDT, E. R., GORNALL, A. G.: Hypertension caused by renal artery occlusion simulating primary aldosteronism. Metabolism **9**, 612 (1960).

LARAGH, J. H., SEALEY, J. E., LEDINGHAM, J. G. G., NEWTON, M. A.: Oral contraceptives: Renin, aldosterone, and high blood pressure. J. Amer. med. Ass. **201**, 918 (1967).

LARAGH, J. H., ULICK, S., JANUSZEWICZ, V., DEMING, Q. B., KELLY, W. G., LIEBERMAN, S.: Aldosterone secretion and primary and malignant hypertension. J. clin. Invest. **39**, 1091 (1960).

LEE, M. R.: Renin secreting kidney tumours. Lancet **1971 II**, 254.

LUETSCHER, J. A., Jr., JOHNSON, B. B., DOWDY, A., HARVEY, J., LEW, W., POO, L. J.: Observations on the sodium-retaining corticoid (aldosterone) in the urine of children and adults in relation to sodium balance and edema. J. clin. Invest. **33**, 1441 (1954).

MASSANI, Z. M., FINKIELMAN, S., WORCEL, M., AGREST, A., PALADINI, A. C.: Angiotensin blood levels in hypertensive and non-hypertensive diseases. Clin. Sci. **30**, 473 (1966).

McAllister, R. G., Jr., Van Way III., C. W., Dayani, K., Anderson, W. J., Temple, E., Michelakis, A. M., Coppage, W. S., Jr., Oates, J. A.: Malignant hypertension: Effect of therapy on renin and aldosterone. Circulat. Res. 28 (Suppl. II), II—160 (1971).

McCaa, C. S., Richardson, T. Q., McCaa, R. E., Sulya, L. L., Guyton, A. C.: Aldosterone secretion by dogs during the developmental phase of Goldblatt hypertension. J. Endocr. **33**, 97 (1965).

Mitchell, J. D., Baxter, T. J., Blair-West, J. R., McCredie, D. A.: Renin levels in nephroblastoma (Wilms' tumour): Report of a renin secreting tumour. Arch. Dis. Childh. **45**, 376 (1970).

Nelson, D. H., August, J. T.: Abnormal response of oedematous patients to aldosterone or deoxycortone. Lancet **1959 II**, 883.

New, M. I., Peterson, R. E.: A new form of congenital adrenal hyperplasia. J. clin. Endocr. **27**, 300 (1967).

Newton, M. A., Laragh, J. H.: Effect of corticotropin on aldosterone excretion and plasma renin in normal subjects, in essential hypertension and in primary aldosteronism. J. clin. Endocr. **28**, 1006 (1968).

Newton, M. A., Sealey, J. E., Ledingham, J. G. G., Laragh, J. H.: High blood pressure and oral contraceptives. Amer. J. Obstet. Gynec. **101**, 1037 (1968).

Nowaczynski, W., Küchel, O., Genest, J.: A decreased metabolic clearance rate of aldosterone in benign essential hypertension. J. clin. Invest. **50**, 2184 (1971).

Robertson, P. W., Klidjian, A., Harding, L. K., Walters, G., Lee, M. R., Robb-Smith, A. H. T.: Hypertension due to a renin secreting renal tumor. Amer. J. Med. **43**, 963 (1967).

Salti, I. S., Ruse, J. L., Stiefel, M., De Larue, N. C., Laidlaw, J. C.: Non-tumorous "primary aldosteronism". I. Type relieved by glucocorticoid (glucocorticoid-remediable hypertension). Canad. med. Ass. J. **101**, 11 (1969).

Sambhi, M. P., Beck, J. C., Venning, E. H.: Malignant hypertension and aldosterone secretion: Influence of reversal and progression of the syndrome in two cases. Amer. J. Med. **35**, 251 (1963).

Saruta, T., Saade, G. A., Kaplan, N. M.: A possible mechanism for hypertension induced by oral contraceptives: Diminished feedback suppression of renin release. Arch. intern. Med. **126**, 621 (1970).

Schambelan, M., Biglieri, E. G.: Regulation and significance of hyper-reninemia from renin-secreting tumor (RST). Clin. Res. **20, 439** (1972).

Schambelan, M., Slaton, P. E., Jr., Biglieri, E. G.: Mineralocorticoid production in hyperadrenocorticism: Role in pathogenesis of hypokalemic alkalosis. Amer. J. Med. **51**, 299 (1971).

Schambelan, M., Stockigt, J. R., Collins, R. D., Biglieri, E. G.: Aldosterone deficiency secondary to hyporeninemia. Clin. Res. **20**, 220 (1972).

Sealey, J. E., Clark, I., Bull, M. B., Laragh, J. H.: Potassium balance and the control of renin secretion. J. clin. Invest. **49**, 2119 (1970).

Sebastian, A., McSherry, E., Biglieri, E. G., Morris, R. C., Jr.: Persistence of hyperaldosteronism during sustained correction of acidosis in patients with renal tubular acidosis (RTA). Clin. Res. **19**, 547 (1971).

Sebastian, A., McSherry, E., Morris, R. C., Jr.: Renal potassium wasting in renal tubular acidosis (RTA). J. clin. Invest. **50**, 667 (1971).

Sims, E. A. H., Meeker, C. I., Gray, M. J., Watanabe, M., Solomon, S.: The secretion of aldosterone in normal pregnancy and in pre-eclampsia. In: Aldosterone: A symposium, pp. 499—508 (Baulieu, E. E., Robel, P., Eds.). Philadelphia: F. A. Davis Company 1964.

Slaton, P. E., Jr., Biglieri, E. G.: Hypertension and hyperaldosteronism of renal and adrenal origin. Amer. J. Med. **38**, 324 (1965).

Slaton, P. E., Jr., Schambelan, M., Biglieri, E. G.: Stimulation and suppression of aldosterone secretion in patients with an aldosterone-producing adenoma. J. clin. Endocr. **29**, 239 (1969).

Sutherland, D. J. A., Ruse, J. L., Laidlaw, J. C.: Hypertension, increased aldosterone secretion and low plasma renin activity relieved by dexamethasone. Canad. med. Ass. J. **95**, 1109 (1966).

Swaab, L. I.: Blood pressure and oral contraception. Excerpta med. int. Congr. Series No. **111**, 198 (1966).

Tu, W. H.: Plasma renin activity in acute tubular necrosis and other renal diseases associated with hypertension. Circulation **31**, 686 (1965).

Tyson, J. E. A.: Oral contraception and elevated blood pressure. Amer. J. Obstet. Gynec. **100**, 875 (1968).

Vagnucci, A. H.: Selective aldosterone deficiency in chronic pyelonephritis. Nephron **7**, 524 (1970).

VECSEI, P., DÜSTERDIECK, G., JAHNECKE, J., LOMMER, D., WOLFF, H. P.: Secretion and turnover of aldosterone in various pathological states. Clin. Sci. **36**, 241 (1969).
VECSEI, P., FARKAS, K., KEMENY, V., HARANGOZO, M.: Investigations on the mechanism of reduced aldosterone production caused by administration of hydrocortisone. Steroids **5**, 415 (1965).
VERTES, V., CANGIANO, J. L., BERMAN, L. B., GOULD, A.: Hypertension in end-stage renal disease. New Engl. J. Med. **280**, 978 (1969).
VEYRAT, R., DE CHAMPLAIN, J., BOUCHER, R., GENEST, J.: Measurement of human arterial renin activity in some physiological and pathological states. Canad. med. Ass. J. **90**, 215 (1964).
VOÛTE, P. A., Jr., VAN DER MEER, J., STAUGAARD-KLOOSTERZIEL, W.: Plasma renin activity in Wilms' tumor. Acta endocr. (Kbh.) **67**, 197 (1971).
WARREN, D. J., FERRIS, T. F.: Renin secretion in renal hypertension. Lancet **1970 I**, 159.
WEINBERGER, M. H., COLLINS, R. D., DOWDY, A. J., NOKES, G. W., LUETSCHER, J. A.: Hypertension induced by oral contraceptives containing estrogen and gestagen: Effects on plasma renin activity and aldosterone excretion. Ann. intern. Med. **71**, 891 (1969).
WOODS, J. W.: Oral contraceptives and hypertension. Lancet **1967 II**, 653.

Intermediary Metabolism of Aldosterone

J. C. MELBY

With 4 Figures

Introduction

Since the isolation of aldosterone by SIMPSON et al. (1953), the principal biosynthetic reactions involved in its production, the important factors which activate its secretion and the nature of its distribution and metabolic fate have been partially or wholly elucidated. Several extensive reviews have been written on these topics though the recent monograph by MÜLLER (1971) and papers by COGHLAN and BLAIR-WEST (1967), BOYD and PEART (1971), COGHLAN et al. (1971), and MULROW (1966) are among the more complete dealing with biosynthesis and its regulation. The chapters by COGHLAN and BLAIR-WEST (1967) and PETERSON (1971) provide excellent reviews of the distribution and metabolic fate of secreted aldosterone. In the discussion to follow, the biogenesis of aldosterone will be considered in a biochemical context, though factors with a direct influence on the biosynthesis of aldosterone will be discussed briefly. Discussion of the distribution and metabolic disposal of secreted aldosterone, while more limited in scope and less fraught with controversy, will include quantitative aspects of the metabolic fate of aldosterone as well as a qualitative assessment.

A. Biogenesis of Aldosterone

1. Functional Zonation of the Adrenal Cortex: Aldosterone Secretion by the Zona Glomerulosa

Evidence that aldosterone is specifically and exclusively elaborated by the cells of the zona glomerulosa of the adrenal cortex in most mammalian species derives from *in vitro* studies in which the zona glomerulosa is removed with the adrenal capsule by dissection and incubated separately from the zona fasciculata-reticularis decapsulated adrenal [AYRES et al., 1956; GIROUD et al., 1956 (1); BANIUKIEWICZ et al., 1968; SHEPPARD et al., 1963]. The most convincing evidence for the specificity of the zona glomerulosa cells for the production of aldosterone was obtained by HANING et al. (1970) in a study on the secretory behavior of suspensions of glomerulosa versus fasciculata-reticularis cells. They found the secretion of aldosterone by the fasciculata-reticularis cells was negligible. In the rat, the zona glomerulosa and the zona fasciculata-reticularis both possess the biosynthetic capability of producing all of the known precursors of aldosterone. The rat adrenal cortex is devoid of 17 α-hydroxylase activity, and thus is not as functionally unique as the human adrenal cortex in which 17 α-hydroxylase activity is limited to the zona fasciculata and zona reticularis. Aldosterone-producing adenomas of the human adrenal cortex apparently possess a variation in functional cell types with multipotential cells in terms of steroid production since they are capable of producing significant quantities of cortisol in addition to aldosterone (KAPLAN, 1967).

2. Aldosterone Biosynthetic Sequence

The principal pathway of aldosterone biosynthesis depicted in Fig. 1 is well established and has survived serious and repeated biochemical scrutiny for the past several years. It is generally accepted that in all steroid-bearing tissues cholesterol is the most important sterol precursor of the steroids. Cholesterol may

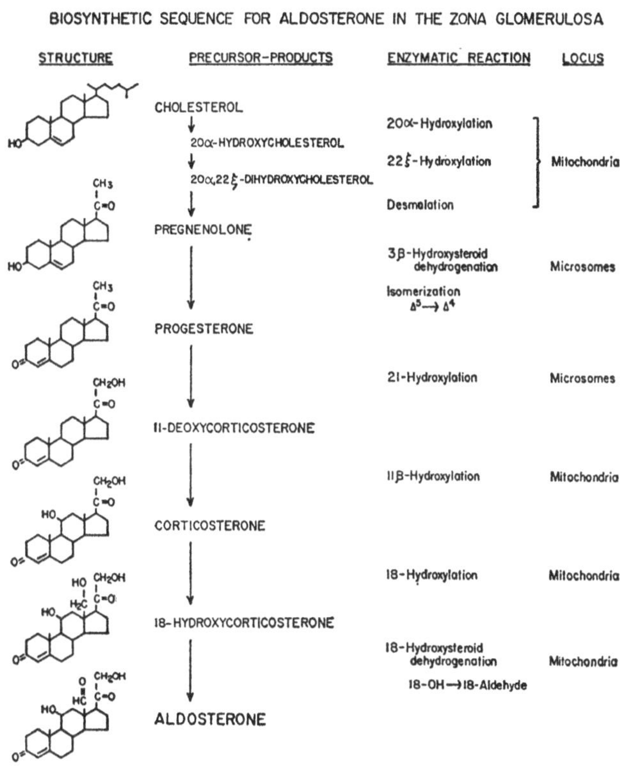

Fig. 1. Biosynthetic sequence for aldosterone in the zona glomerulosa

be synthesized *in situ* or it may be extracted by the adrenal cortex from the circulation. In most species, plasma cholesterol is by far the major component of the substrate for steroidogenesis (MORRIS et al., 1967). Evidence that plasma cholesterol is the most important source of cholesterol for steroid synthesis derives from a number of experiments in animals and man in which radioactively labeled cholesterol is infused intravenously and comparison made between the specific activities of plasma cholesterol fraction and circulating adrenocortical steroid hormones (BORKOWSKI et al., 1967). MELBY et al. (1966) injected radioactive cholesterol into control and dexamethasone-suppressed dogs with permanent adrenal vein cannulas. Isotopic equilibrium among plasma-free and esterified cholesterol and adrenal-free and esterified cholesterol was achieved within 5 to 7 days after injection in the control dogs. Specific activity of adrenal venous cortisol was 80% of cholesterol in the basal state. After ACTH stimulation specific activity of cortisol equalled that of cholesterol. In dexamethasone-suppressed dogs isotopic equilibrium was not achieved until after ACTH stimulation. It can be concluded that plasma-free cholesterol contributes most of the substrate for steroidogenesis in the unstimulated state and all of the substrate for steroidogenesis in the stimulated state.

The transformation of cholesterol to pregnenolone results from the activation of an enzymatic cholesterol side chain cleavage system involving hydroxylations at C-20 and C-22 of the cholesterol molecule, and cleavage of the six carbon isocaproaldehyde side chain (CONSTANTOPOULOS et al., 1966). The system is intramitochondrial and the rate limiting step is 20 α-hydroxylation. This step is the locus for the action of trophic hormones on steroidogenesis (HALL and YOUNG, 1968).

Table 1. *Principal steroid/sterol biosynthetic precursors of aldosterone*

Substrate	Preparation	References
Cholesterol	Bovine adrenal capsule strippings	AYRES et al. (1957)
Pregnenolone	Domestic duck adrenal slices	SANDOR et al. (1963)
	Human adrenal adenoma slices	RAMAN et al. (1965)
Progesterone (P)	Bovine adrenal capsule strippings	AYRES et al. (1957/1960)
	Bullfrog adrenal slices	ULICK and SOLOMON (1960)
	Human adrenal slices	SANDOR and LANTHIER (1963)
11-Deoxycorticosterone (DOC)	Bovine adrenal homogenates	KAHNT et al. (1955)
	Human adrenal adenoma slices	RAMAN et al. (1965)
Corticosterone (B)	Bullfrog adrenal slices and homogenates	AYRES et al. (1960)
	Human adrenal slices	MULROW and COHN (1959)
18-Hydroxycorticosterone (18-OH-B)	Bullfrog adrenal homogenate	NICOLIS and ULICK (1965)
	Human adrenal slices	PASQUALINI (1964)

NADPH is required and the system conforms to a mixed function oxidase system in which one atom of molecular oxygen is incorporated into the substrate and the other is reduced to water. Cytochrome P-450 serves as the terminal oxidase in the steroid hydroxylation reactions (SIMPSON et al., 1969).

The conversion of pregnenolone to progesterone is catalyzed by the enzyme system 3 β-hydroxysteroid dehydrogenase/isomerase. This enzyme system resides in an extramitochondrial locus and is essential to the production of aldosterone though its substrate need not be pregnenolone nor its product, progesterone. 21-Hydroxypregnenolone can be transformed into aldosterone quite efficiently (PASQUALINI, 1964; STACHENKO and GIROUD, 1962). The principal precursors of aldosterone are listed in Table 1 along with the experimental work which demonstrated their role in the biosynthesis. AYRES et al. (1957) among others, demonstrated the efficiency of the conversion of progesterone, 11-deoxycorticosterone and corticosterone. Later studies by AYRES et al. (1960) in which bovine adrenal capsule strippings were incubated with labeled corticosterone suggested that over 90% of aldosterone formed was derived from corticosterone.

The pathway from corticosterone to aldosterone is less securely established. It has been proposed by NICOLIS and ULICK (1965) that 18-hydroxycorticosterone is the intermediate between corticosterone and aldosterone. The efficiency of corticosterone as a precursor of aldosterone is so much greater than that of 18-hydroxycorticosterone that there is some doubt as to whether 18-hydroxycorticosterone is an obligatory intermediate in the biogenesis of aldosterone. The efficiency of the conversion of 18-hydroxycorticosterone to aldosterone was significant in incubations with ovine adrenal mitochondria (RAMAN et al., 1966) and slices of an aldosterone-producing adenoma of the adrenal cortex (PASQUALINI, 1964). The fact that GREENGARD et al. (1967), demonstrated that cytochrome P-450 participates in the biosynthesis of aldosterone from corticosterone is an important proof that a hydroxylation reaction occurs on the C-18 methyl group of corticosterone and that 18-hydroxycorticosterone is the immediate precursor of aldosterone. GREENGARD et al. (1967) proposed that an enzyme-18-hydroxycorticosterone complex is the intermediate in aldosterone formation, and explained the poor conversion of free 18-hydroxycorticosterone to aldosterone *in vitro* on the basis of equilibrium being strongly in favor of dissociation of this complex. NICOLIS and ULICK (1965) have suggested that the inefficient conversion of 18-hydroxycorticosterone to aldosterone may reside in the fact that 18-hydroxylated compounds exist in solution as 18 → 20 cyclic hemiketals. In this state they are resistant to enzymatic dehydrogenation. The existence of a clinical disorder involving a specific 18-hydroxysteroid dehydrogenase deficiency, a rare familial syndrome in which hypoaldosteronism and hypersecretion of 18-hydroxycorticosterone exist (DAVID et al., 1968; TOUITOU et al., 1970) constitutes indirect evidence for he obligatory intermediate role of 18-hydroxycorticosterone.

3. Alternative Pathways of Aldosterone Biosynthesis

A variety of other steroids have served as precursors of aldosterone and these are listed in Table 2. Fig. 2 shows a hypothetical pathway for aldosterone biosynthesis from progesterone in which 11 β-hydroxylation precedes 21-hydroxylation. GIROUD et al. (1958) demonstrated that 11 β-hydroxyprogesterone was an efficient precursor of aldosterone, and 21-deoxyaldosterone was shown by KAHNT and NEHER (1965) to have the same function. One need only postulate the existence of the compound 11 β, 18-dihydroxyprogesterone to complete this hypothetical pathway. Indirect evidence for the existence of this steroid has been presented by ULICK (1966) in which the metabolite 3 α, 18, 20 α-trihydroxy-5 β-pregnane-11-one was found in the urine of a patient with congenital adrenal hyperplasia. This compound could be the reduced urinary metabolite of 11 β, 18-dihydroxyprogesterone. The biological significance of this hypothetical pathway is unknown.

When 18-hydroxylase activity occurs prior to 11 β-hydroxylation and 21-hydroxylation, two hypothetical pathways for the biosynthesis of aldosterone exist as depicted in Fig. 3. If 11-deoxycorticosterone undergoes 18-hydroxylation prior to 11 β-hydroxylation, 18-hydroxy-11-deoxycorticosterone is synthesized, which may then undergo 11 β-hydroxylation to 18-hydroxycorticosterone and thence to aldosterone or be converted to 18-aldehyde-11-deoxycorticosterone then 11 β-hydroxylated to aldosterone. 18-hydroxy-11-deoxycorticosterone was a slightly more efficient precursor of aldosterone than was 18-hydroxycorticosterone when incubated in the bullfrog adrenal homogenate system of NICOLIS and ULICK (1965).

No evidence has been evinced that 18-hydroxy-11-deoxycorticosterone can be converted to 11-deoxyaldosterone. MELBY et al. (1972) incubated ^{3}H-18-hydroxy-11-deoxycorticosterone with human and rat adrenal slices and were able to demonstrate 1% conversion to aldosterone and 1 to 5% conversion to 18-hydroxycortico-

Table 2. *Steroid precursors of aldosterone (? Non-obligatory intermediates)*

Substrate	Preparation	References
11 β-Hydroxyprogesterone (11-OH-P)	Bovine adrenal glomerulosa slices	Giroud et al. (1958)
18-Hydroxyprogesterone (18-OH-P)	Bullfrog adrenal homogenate	Nicolis and Ulick (1965)
11-Dehydrocorticosterone	Bovine adrenal slices	Stachenko and Giroud (1964)
18-Hydroxy-11-deoxycorticosterone (18-OH-DOC)	Bullfrog adrenal homogenate	Nicolis and Ulick (1965)
	Human adrenal slices	Melby et al. (1972)
21-Hydroxypregnenolone	Bovine glomerulosa slices	Stachenko and Giroud (1962)
21-Deoxyaldosterone	Bovine adrenal slices	Kahnt and Neher (1965)
11-Dehydroaldosterone	Bovine adrenal slices	Kahnt and Neher (1965)

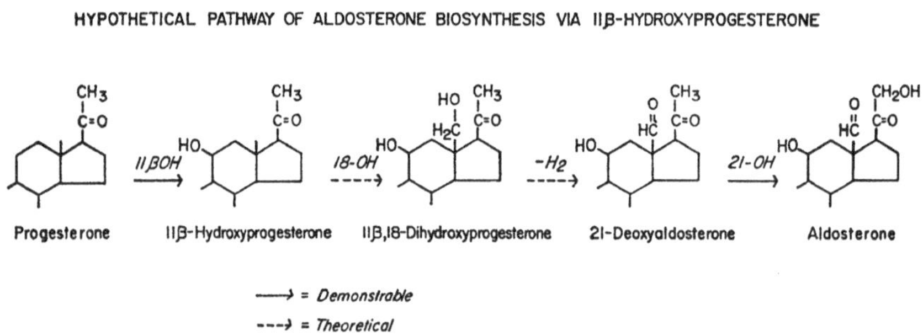

Fig. 2. Hypothetical pathway of aldosterone biosynthesis via 11 β-hydroxyprogesterone

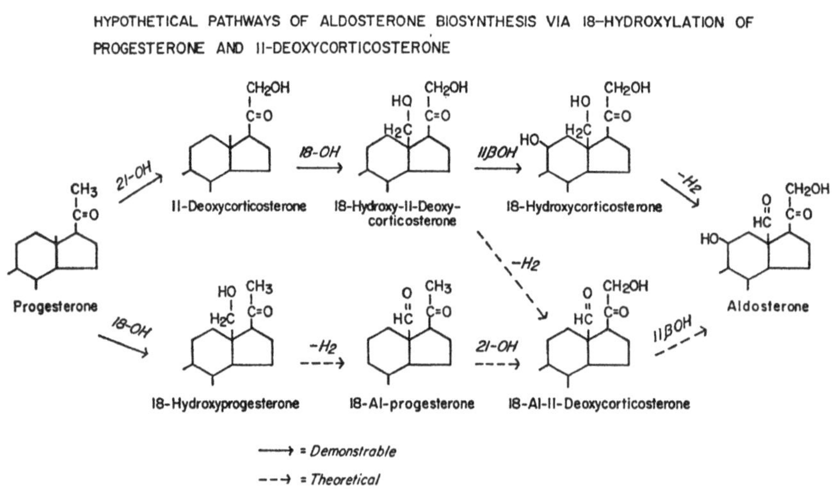

Fig. 3. Hypothetical pathways of aldosterone biosynthesis via 18-hydroxylation of progesterone and 11-deoxycorticosterone

sterone. The conversion to aldosterone and 18-hydroxycorticosterone was greater by rat than by human adrenal slices. 18-Hydroxy-11-deoxycorticosterone was also converted to a more polar material in addition to aldosterone and 18-hydroxycorticosterone in incubations of human adrenal glands. When subjected to, mass spectral analysis this product appeared to have an additional hydroxyl group, but its position is unknown. Though 18-hydroxy-11-deoxycorticosterone may serve as a precursor of aldosterone, it is likely that most of the 18-hydroxy-11-deoxycorticosterone produced arises from the zona fasciculata and is not available to serve as substrate for aldosterone biosynthesis (MELBY et al., 1972).

WETTSTEIN (1961) was able to demonstrate the conversion of progesterone to 18-aldehyde-progesterone. Subsequent 21-hydroxylation and 11 β-hydroxylation of this precursor could yield aldosterone. The significance of this hypothetical pathway is unknown.

4. Activation of Aldosterone Biosynthesis

A group of widely disparate compounds directly stimulate aldosterone biosynthesis *in vitro*. A list of these substances may be found in Table 3. By contrast, the stimulation of cortisol formation appears to be a much simpler process involving ACTH as the sole trophic substance and cyclic AMP as the intracellular mediator of ACTH action. It would appear that the stimulators of aldosterone biosynthesis act by controlling the cleavage of the cholesterol side chain to form pregnenolone. This is the same general locus as the action of ACTH and/or cyclic

Table 3. *Compounds which directly stimulate aldosterone formation by mammalian adrenal tissue (in vitro)*

Stimulus	Species	Preparation	References
Ang. II	Ox	Slices of outer adrenal cortex	KAPLAN and BARTTER (1962)
	Rat	Slices of adrenal cortex	MULLER (1965)
	Rat	Superfusion of capsular gland	TAIT et al. (1970)
	Rat	Isolated capsular (glomerulosa (cells	HANING et al. (1970)
	Human	Aldosteronoma slices	SPARK et al. (1969)
ACTH	Rat	Adrenal slices	GIROUD et al. (1956)
	Rat	Superfused capsular adrenals	TAIT et al. (1970)
	Ox	Outer adrenal slices	KAPLAN and BARTTER (1962)
	Human	Adrenal slices	DYRENFURTH et al. (1960)
Cyclic AMP	Rat	Capsular adrenals	MULLER (1971)
	Ox	Outer adrenal slices	KAPLAN (1965)
Prostaglandins	Ox	Outer adrenal slices	SARUTA and KAPLAN (1971)
Potassium	Rat	Adrenal slices	GIROUD (1956)
	Rat	Adrenal slices (augmentation of other stimuli)	MULLER (1971)
	Rat	Isolated (glomerulosa) capsular cells	HANING et al. (1970)
	Ox	Adrenal slices	KAPLAN (1962)
Monovalent cations Ammonium Rubidium Cesium	Rat	Adrenal slices	MÜLLER (1971)
NADPH	Rat	Adrenal slices	MÜLLER (1966)
Serotonin	Rat	Adrenal slices	JOUAN (1967)
	Rat	Adrenal slices	MULLER and WEICK (1965)
	Rat	Isolated capsular (glomerulosa) cells	HANING et al. (1970)

AMP for the stimulation of cortisol secretion. This discussion will treat only those substances which have been shown to directly stimulate aldosterone biogenesis in an *in-vitro* preparation. Most of the studies alluded to have utilized labeled precursors of aldosterone to identify the locus of action of these stimuli.

a) Angiotensin II

Ang. II stimulates the formation of aldosterone in a wide variety of animal species. The effect of Ang. II on mammalian adrenal tissue *in vitro* in a variety of species has been demonstrated (Table 3). Stimulation of aldosterone formation by Ang. II in rat adrenal slices, capsular glands, and isolated glomerulosa cells has been amply demonstrated (KAPLAN and BARTTER, 1962; MÜLLER, 1965; TAIT et al., 1970; HANING et al., 1970). The fact that other investigators have failed to demonstrate an *in vitro* effect on aldosterone production must be explained by differences in experimental design (SPÄT et al., 1969). The larger doses of angiotensin required for stimulation of aldosterone formation in rat adrenal slices and the failure of a large number of investigators (EILERS and PETERSON, 1964; MARIEB and MULROW, 1965) to demonstrate effects of angiotensin *in vivo* suggest that Ang. II may not have a significant physiologic regulatory effect on aldosterone secretion in the rat (HANING et al., 1970). Ang. II stimulated aldosterone production by human aldosterone-producing adenoma slices intensely *in vitro* (SPARK et al., 1969).

Ang. II regularly stimulates the conversion of labeled cholesterol to aldosterone but does not increase the rate of incorporation of other precursors such as deoxycorticosterone, pregnenolone, progesterone or corticosterone into aldosterone in adrenal-slice preparation *in vitro*. These observations were made both by KAPLAN and BARTTER (1962) using ox adrenal outer layers, and by MÜLLER (1966) using quartered rat adrenals. HANING et al. (1970) demonstrated that labeled corticosterone added during the incubation of isolated rat adrenal glomerulosa cells was markedly enhanced in its incorporation into aldosterone by angiotensin, suggesting an effect on a late stage in aldosterone biosynthesis between corticosterone and aldosterone. The studies of AGUILERA and MARUSIC (1971) demonstrated that acute administration of Ang. II or dog renin to hypophysectomized nephrectomized dogs by injection had no effect on the conversion of corticosterone to aldosterone in isolated mitochondrial fractions. Increased conversion was demonstrated when they injected homologous dog renin for 4 days and then incubated the mitochondrial fractions.

HANING et al. (1971) have offered an alternative interpretation of these data on the basis of a series of experiments. Endogenous cold corticosterone in the adrenal glomerulosa cell preparation induced a two-fold increment in the conversion of tritium-labeled corticosterone to aldosterone which suggested that the concentration of corticosterone substrate itself was inducing intensified conversion of labeled corticosterone to aldosterone. These experiments by HANING et al. (1971) seem to explain the intensified conversion of labeled corticosterone to aldosterone caused by a number of stimulatory substances in this *in vitro* isolated adrenal glomerulosa-cell system. If the stimulants acted at an early stage in the synthesis of aldosterone, then more corticosterone would be available as substrate and, hence, the conversion of labeled corticosterone to aldosterone would be increased. They believe this is due to the mechanism proposed by BURSTEIN (1970), in which corticosterone activates its own enzymatic conversion by increasing co-enzyme concentrations or by an allosteric effect. This same explanation could be applied to the studies in which prolonged sodium deprivation *in vivo* increased the conversion of labeled corticosterone to aldosterone *in vitro* (MARUSIC and MULROW, 1967).

b) ACTH

Short-term studies in which ACTH is given *in vivo* and the adrenals examined *in vitro* clearly show a marked effect of ACTH on the production of aldosterone. MÜLLER (1971), in studying the effect of ACTH on the production of aldosterone by capsular rat adrenals *in vitro*, was able to demonstrate no effect of sodium deficiency on the response in aldosterone production to ACTH. On the other hand potassium deficiency markedly impaired the *in vitro* response to ACTH.

It seems reasonably certain that the action of ACTH is at an early stage in the pathway of aldosterone biosynthesis, specifically on the conversion of cholesterol to pregnenolone, perhaps more specifically at the stage of 20 α-hydroxylation. MÜLLER (1966) showed that ACTH did not stimulate the conversion of any precursor of aldosterone except labeled cholesterol *in vitro*. These same observations were made on outer bovine adrenal slices by KAPLAN and BARTTER (1962). Again, HANING et al. (1970) showed that in their isolated glomerulosa cell preparation, the incorporation of labeled corticosterone into aldosterone was enhanced by the presence of ACTH in the medium. They offered the explanation that these observations may be due to the mechanism described above with increased substrate availability stimulating conversion of the labeled substrate.

c) Cyclic AMP

MÜLLER (1971) demonstrated a seven-fold increment in the production of aldosterone by capsular rat adrenal glands incubated with cyclic AMP. KAPLAN (1965) demonstrated no enhancement of the effect of ACTH by cyclic AMP on the secretion of aldosterone by ox outer adrenal slices. The assumption that ACTH stimulates aldosterone secretion through cyclic AMP generation by activation of adenyl cyclase with cyclic AMP acting as a second messenger cannot be made from any of the experiments on aldosterone secretion to date. The hypothesis of GARREN et al. (1965), that new protein synthesis is involved in the action of ACTH and cyclic AMP on the cleavage of the cholesterol side chain, is confirmed by the effect of protein-synthesis inhibitors on the production of aldosterone *in vitro* by BURROW et al. (1966). They showed a marked decline (more than 50%) in aldosterone production by rat adrenal incubates after the addition of cyclohexamide, an inhibitor of protein synthesis. The site of inhibition of aldosterone biosynthesis by cyclohexamide is probably at a stage between cholesterol and pregnenolone (DAVIS and GARREN, 1968).

d) Prostaglandins

SARUTA and KAPLAN (1972) reported that prostaglandin PGE_1 and PGE_2 markedly stimulated aldosterone biosynthesis, whereas prostaglandins PGA, $PGF_{1\alpha}$ and $PGF_{2\alpha}$ had no effect on the formation of aldosterone. One curious observation made by these investigators is that PGE_1 increased stimulation of aldosterone biosynthesis by Ang. II but not the stimulation of aldosterone biosynthesis by ACTH, cyclic AMP or potassium. The role of prostaglandins in the stimulation of aldosterone biosynthesis is unclear at present. The locus of stimulation of aldosterone biosynthesis by prostaglandins was not examined in the studies by SARUTA and KAPLAN (1972).

e) Potassium and other Monovalent Cations

BOYD et al. [1971 (1)] demonstrated that increments of as little as 0.3 mEq/l of potassium in the incubation medium of quartered rat adrenals could significantly increase aldosterone production. Although the ability of potassium ions to stimulate aldosterone biosynthesis directly has been well known since the observations of GIROUD et al. [1956 (2)], it was not appreciated that such small alterations in concentration could modify aldosterone secretion *in vitro*. Potassium ions stimulate only the formation of aldosterone, with no effect on the extraglomerulosa adrenal cortex (FUNDER et al., 1969). MÜLLER (1971) also found potassium ions increased the production of aldosterone precursors in the zona glomerulosa, including corticosterone and deoxycorticosterone, without affecting the zona fasciculata. *In vivo*, potassium deprivation results in the marked diminution of the secretion of aldosterone.

BAUMBER et al. (1971) suggested that potassium is the final common pathway of the stimulators of aldosterone biosynthesis. They based this on the findings of increased potassium content in the adrenal cortex following stimulation by ACTH, Ang. II, sodium depletion, hyperkalemia induced by infusion, etc. KAPLAN (1965) found potassium ions potentiated the aldosterone stimulating effect of Ang. II. This could be explained if potassium were involved in the action of Ang. II on the conversion of cholesterol to pregnenolone.

MÜLLER (1971) has shown that potassium stimulates the formation of aldosterone at an early stage between cholesterol and its conversion products by using labeled precursors of aldosterone in the incubation of quartered rat adrenals. In addition to stimulating conversion of cholesterol to pregnenolone, there is some evidence that potassium ions are effective at a later stage in aldosterone biosynthesis. BAUMANN and MÜLLER (1972) incubated capsular adrenal glands from potassium-deficient rats and found a marked reduction in the conversion of tritium-labeled corticosterone to aldosterone and to 18-hydroxycorticosterone as compared with the adrenal production from animals in potassium balance. They found that only the 18-hydroxylase activity of the zona glomerulosa was involved, while production of 18-hydroxy-11-deoxycorticosterone and 18-hydroxycorticosterone by the decapsulated portion of the gland (zona fasciculata) was unchanged by potassium depletion. The hypothesis that changes in potassium ion affect 18-hydroxylation in the zona glomerulosa is supported by the studies of BOYD et al. [1971 (2)], in which oral potassium given to rats increased conversion of corticosterone to aldosterone with a sustained rise in aldosterone secretion but no change in corticosterone secretion. The work of HANING et al. (1971) may account for these findings. That is, if changes in potassium ion markedly alter the amount of corticosterone produced as substrate, changes in the amount of substrate-enzyme complex should also occur, to effect a similar alteration in the conversion of trace amounts of labeled corticosterone to aldosterone.

f) NADPH

MÜLLER (1966) found NADPH (reduced nicotinamide adenine dinucleotide phosphate) stimulated aldosterone biosynthesis when rat adrenal capsules were quartered and incubated with ^{3}H-labeled cholesterol. The stimulation was found to occur between cholesterol and pregnenolone because tritiated cholesterol was the only precursor of aldosterone to be incorporated into aldosterone significantly with stimulation by NADPH and glucose-6-phosphate in the bathing medium. NADPH participates in all steroid hydroxylations within the adrenal cortex. The introduction of an oxygen atom into the steroid molecule is associated with the oxidation of NADPH to NADP. NADPH is required for the hydroxylations of cholesterol prior to enzymatic cleavage of the side chain. Although NADPH appears to have its effect in the early stage of biogenesis, the effect is not at the same point or in the same pool as ACTH and the other stimulators of aldosterone production. Furthermore NADPH, when incubated with ACTH, has a cumulative effect on steroidogenesis, suggesting a qualitatively different action of NADPH. NADPH has a relatively weaker stimulatory effect on aldosterone biosynthesis than do the other stimulators such as ACTH, potassium ions, ammonium ions, angiotensin and serotonin (MÜLLER, 1966). NADPH's stimulatory effect on aldosterone biosynthesis probably results from the availability of NADPH for the hydroxylations at C-20 and 22 of the cholesterol molecule and as such it may be necessary for cyclic AMP to be active. NADPH of course is required for 18-hydroxylase activity converting corticosterone to 18-hydroxycorticosterone, and therefore, NADPH may act at several sites, once it has stimulated cholesterol conversion to pregnenolone. This may account for some of the differences observed between NADPH and other stimulating substances.

g) Serotonin

Although serotonin is inactive in stimulating aldosterone production *in vivo* (BLAIR-WEST et al., 1962), JOUAN (1967) and MULLER and ZIEGLER (1968) determined that serotonin was one of the most potent aldosterone-stimulating substances studied using *in vitro* techniques. Serotonin also increased deoxycorticosterone production, but not corticosterone production. MÜLLER and ZIEGLER (1968) found the incorporation of ^{3}H-cholesterol into aldosterone much greater than that of any other precursor of aldosterone under the influence of serotonin. However, they did show a measurable effect on the conversion of ^{3}H-pregnenolone to aldosterone. In more recent studies MÜLLER (1971) failed to demonstrate a stimulatory effect of serotonin on the conversion of ^{3}H-pregnenolone to aldosterone when unlabeled pregnenolone was added to the medium in substrate amounts.

Compounds related to serotonin such as bufotenine, 5-methoxytryptamine and 5-hydroxytryptophan share the ability of serotonin to stimulate aldosterone biogenesis (MÜLLER, 1971). Serotonin antagonists such as methysergide completely abolish the effect of serotonin on the stimulation of aldosterone synthesis, and actually significantly reduce basal aldosterone secretion in the absence of serotonin (MÜLLER and ZIEGLER, 1968). HANING et al. (1970) also found that serotonin exhibited aldosterone-stimulating activity in isolated glomerulosa (capsular) cells from the rat adrenal gland. The effect of serotonin on aldosterone production was much less efficient than that of ACTH. HANING et al. (1970) also demonstrated that serotonin stimulated the conversion of tritium-labeled corticosterone to aldosterone in the isolated capsular cells of rat adrenals. HANING et al. (1971), in explaining the effect of serotonin on the conversion of labeled corticosterone to aldosterone again suggested that stimulation was related to the increase in corticosterone substrate due to an effect on the conversion of cholesterol to pregnenolone. MÜLLER (1971) observed that serotonin did not increase the production of corticosterone from quartered whole rat adrenals, and HANING et al. (1970) were able to demonstrate only a small increase in production of corticosterone by adding serotonin to the medium bathing the isolated capsular cells.

Ang. II, potassium ions, ACTH, cyclic AMP and serotonin are among the substances which will significantly increase aldosterone biogenesis *in vitro*. No conclusion as to the relative importance of these stimuli is justified at this time. All these stimulants of aldosterone secretion appear to act in the adrenal glomerulosa cells at some point between cholesterol and pregnenolone. However, experiments showing the stimulation of conversion of labeled corticosterone to aldosterone have been repeatedly cited. Prolonged sodium depletion in rats has similarly been shown by several investigators (Baniukiewicz et al., 1968; Müller and Huber, 1969) to cause increased conversion of labeled corticosterone to aldosterone by capsular adrenal glands and by rat adrenal slices. Marusic and Mulrow (1967) obtained adrenal mitochondria from rats on sodium-deficient and sodium-adequate diets and found that the adrenal mitochondria from rats on the sodium-deficient diet had markedly increased the conversion of corticosterone to aldosterone as compared with the sodium-replete rat adrenal mitochondria. Haning et al. (1970) were able to show the same stimulation of the conversion of labeled corticosterone to aldosterone by isolated adrenal glomerulosa cells obtained from rats on a low sodium diet. Again, Haning et al. (1971) have invoked the same interpretation of the results of sodium deficiency as with other stimulators of aldosterone secretion i.e., that increased amounts of corticosterone are generated as substrate for the production of aldosterone and this substrate apparently stimulates its own transformation. Haning et al. (1971) have provided an acceptable hypothesis for the prime locus of activity of all aldosterone stimulating substances being between cholesterol and pregnenolone, at the same time explaining the stimulation of conversion of labeled corticosterone to aldosterone observed for all the stimulating substances described. Reduction in corticosterone production *per se* by the adrenal glomerulosa cells in favor of aldosterone adds indirect substantation of the hypothesis of Haning et al. (1971).

B. Distribution and Metabolic Fate of Aldosterone

It is generally conceded that steroid hormones including aldosterone act by inducing specific proteins in target tissues and that induction of these proteins begins with the binding of the steroid to specific receptor proteins in the cytosol. In the instance of aldosterone, sterospecific binding to both cytosol and nuclear proteins has been demonstrated for several mammalian tissues including the rat kidney, duodenal mucosa, spleen, liver, salivary glands and brain (Swaneck et al., 1969). A specific protein is induced which is intimately related to the stimulation of active sodium transport by the target cells. No evidence exists that aldosterone undergoes biotransformation during this induction.

In order that aldosterone may reach the subcellular constituents of the target cells it is associated with plasma proteins and delivered to the target tissues (Meyer et al., 1961). In contrast to cortisol, aldosterone is not associated to any great extent with plasma proteins other than albumin. No more than 7% of circulating aldosterone is bound to corticosteroid-binding globulin, which possesses a much greater affinity for cortisol (Meyer et al., 1961). Binding of aldosterone to albumin is rather weak, which probably accounts in part for its prompt arrival at the target cells and association with receptor proteins in the cytosol.

Tait et al. (1962) suggested that ^{3}H-aldosterone distributed itself in two compartments in man, and Tait and Burstein (1964) interpreted the disappearance curve of ^{3}H-aldosterone as follows: the initial course of the curve reflects the equilibration of aldosterone in blood with an "inner" compartment giving an apparent volume of distribution of some 27 l. The half-life of radiolabeled aldosterone in plasma is 15 min as derived from the initial curve with rapid descent reflecting equilibration with the "inner" pool. After this, the curve becomes less steep at the point of equilibrium of the theoretical "inner" and "outer" compartments. The second portion of the curve, declining less steeply, allows an estimation of about 30 min for the biological half-life of the radiolabeled aldosterone in plasma

(PETERSON, 1965). This part of the curve is actually the net result of re-entry of labeled aldosterone from the outer compartment into the inner compartment and biotransformation of labeled aldosterone in the inner compartment. The volume of distribution during the slower portion of the curve can be estimated to be about 40 l which is approximately the same as the intracellular fluid volume (TAIT and BURSTEIN, 1964). HOLLANDER et al. (1966), confirmed the two-component disappearance curve of labeled aldosterone from plasma and demonstrated its existence in the tissues by single i.v. injections of ^{3}H-aldosterone into dogs. Maximum concentrations of ^{3}H-aldosterone were obtained in 5 to 15 min in the kidney, liver, heart, and aorta; kidney, liver and heart exhibited significantly higher concentrations of labeled aldosterone than the plasma.

PEARLMAN (1957) considered the relationship of the plasma concentration of a steroid to the secretion rate of that steroid could best reflect the overall rate of metabolism. TAIT (1963) and TAIT and BURSTEIN (1964) described the relationship between the concentration of aldosterone and its secretion rate using the concept which has evolved as the metabolic clearance rate (MCR). The MCR is a mathematical expression to describe overall metabolism of aldosterone. Aldosterone which is discharged into the circulation is cleared from the blood to a greater or lesser extent by each tissue the blood perfuses. The clearance rate of aldosterone by a specific tissue may be derived from the product of the blood flow of the specific tissue and the extraction of aldosterone by that tissue. Extraction represents the fraction of aldosterone irreversibly metabolized by the tissue. The clearance rate of aldosterone for a tissue may be expressed as the volume of blood or plasma cleared per unit time, and the overall MCR of aldosterone would be the volume of blood cleared of aldosterone by the whole body per unit time. The overall MCR of aldosterone can best be approximated by simulating the secretion of aldosterone by the adrenal into systemic venous circulation during a steady state by the constant intravenous infusion of radiolabeled aldosterone to give the general equation:

$$\text{MCR} = \frac{\text{R(infusion rate of radiolabeled aldosterone)}}{\text{X}_c\ \text{(constant concentration of radioactivity in aldosterone).}}$$

Constant-infusion technique requires a priming dose of radiolabeled aldosterone at time 0. After 30 min radiolabeled aldosterone is infused at a constant rate for 120 min. By this time concentration of radioactivity measured specifically as aldosterone is usually constant and three samples of blood are drawn at 15-min intervals over the last 30 min. The mean of the concentration in these samples is used to determine the MCR. Since the liver is the predominant organ irreversibly metabolizing aldosterone, marked reduction in hepatic blood flow or hepatic extraction of the steroid will tend to reduce the overall MCR of aldosterone. The single-injection technique for the determination of MCR requires additional assumptions and mathematical treatment to approximate the true MCR. Constant-infusion technique automatically integrates the plasma radioactivity providing the final concentrations are constant.

Because aldosterone is weakly bound to albumin and nearly all of it is extracted and metabolized from all of the arterial blood perfusing the liver, the MCR for aldosterone approximates hepatic blood flow. On the other hand, cortisol, which is bound with much higher affinity by corticosteroid-binding globulin, is only partially extracted from arterial blood by the liver during each circulation. Thus, the MCR for cortisol is considerably less than that of aldosterone. TAIT et al. (1961) estimated the MCR of aldosterone in healthy recumbent adults to average 1620 l/day of plasma, an amount approximating to human hepatic blood flow. BAIRD et al. (1969) compared the published data on several steroids in which the splanchic extraction was expressed as the percentage of the MCR estimated by direct analysis of peripheral and hepatic venous blood during continuous infusion of labeled steroids. Cortisol and testosterone, which are bound to corticosteroid binding globulin and testosterone binding globulin respectively, exhibited a substantially lower percentage of MCR as splanchnic extraction, whereas androstenedione, progesterone, and aldosterone, which are bound to albumin under normal conditions have splanchnic extractions which exceed 75% of MCR. BOUGAS et al. (1964) estimated that no more than 15% of the MCR of aldosterone could be accounted for by extra hepatic extraction of aldosterone. Pathological conditions and physiological alterations which change the rate of biotransformation of aldosterone by enzymes in the liver hepatic blood flow might be expected to produce alterations in the MCR of aldosterone and seem to do so predictably. LUETSCHER et al. (1963) and KONO et al. (1966) demonstrated that in hypothyroidism, in which enzymatic biotransformation of aldosterone is reduced, the MCR of aldosterone was similarly significantly reduced whereas in hyperthyroidism the opposite alterations in enzymatic metabolism of aldosterone exist and the MCR or aldosterone is significantly elevated.

COPPAGE et al. (1962) demonstrated low MCR of aldosterone in liver disease and suggested the high circulating levels of aldosterone in the plasma can be accounted for in part by the decreased MCR of aldosterone. In the case of cardiac failure, alterations in the MCR of aldosterone have been demonstrated but their significance is uncertain. TAIT et al. (1965) found the mean MCR of aldosterone in patients with severe cardiac disease to be less than 50% of that observed in normal subjects. Similarly the hepatic extraction of aldosterone was reduced more than 20%. CAMARGO et al. (1965) and CHEVILLO et al. (1966) also found a marked reduction in metabolic clearance, hepatic clearance, and hepatic extraction of aldosterone in patients with severe congestive heart failure. Less than a third of patients with congestive heart failure who have not received diuretic therapy exhibit increased secretion rates of aldosterone (HICKIE and LAZARUS, 1966; CAMARGO et al., 1965; SANDERS and MELBY, 1964). The relative importance of reduction of the MCR of aldosterone in congestive cardiac failure has not been adequately determined. If the MCR describes the relationship of the secretion rate of aldosterone and the plasma concentration of aldosterone, then it can be reasoned that a 50% reduction in the MCR should result in a substantial reduction in the secretion rate of aldosterone if the plasma level is to remain within the normal range. The fact that some patients with congestive heart failure have elevated aldosterone secretion rates in the face of diminished MCR's suggests the existence of a defect in the feed back control of aldosterone secretion which has not been sufficiently defined. The simultaneous determination of the MCR, plasma concentration of aldosterone, and 24-h secretion rate will have to be made in the variety of disorders in which the MCR of aldosterone appears to be altered in order to know whether the theoretical relationship between these three variables is in keeping with that observed. In the instance of liver disease, elevated plasma aldosterone has been demonstrated in association with both reduced MCR and increased aldosterone secretion rate. Relative contributions of reduction in MCR and accelerated aldosterone secretion to the elevated plasma aldosterone concentration have not been well studied. If the physiologic control systems for the activation and damping of aldosterone secretion are operative, plasma aldosterone levels ought not to rise as a consequence of reduced MCR of aldosterone.

C. The Biotransformation and Disposal of Aldosterone

A comprehensive discussion of the characteristics of the hepatic enzymes involved in the biotransformation and ultimate disposal of aldosterone and its metabolites is included in the discussion on the metabolism of adrenal corticosteroids by PETERSON (1971). Following the intravenous infusion of radiolabeled aldosterone into man, approximately 90% of the label can be recovered in urine passed in the 48 h after the injection. 80% or more of the radioactivity in urine is excreted during the first 24 h after injection. There is no evidence of significant biliary excretion of aldosterone in man. It is possible to account for up to 70 to 75% of the radioactivity recovered from urine after intravenous injection of labeled aldosterone as specific metabolites of aldosterone. Five urinary metabolites of aldosterone have been isolated and their structures elucidated (Fig. 4), and these five structures account for most of the identifiable steroidal radioactivity.

1. Aldosterone-18-Glucuronide

This is a unique steroidal metabolite since aldosterone retains its biological activity until conjugated without any prior reduction processes. It was recognized as early as 1955 by AXELRAD et al. that unaltered aldosterone could be retrieved from urine by extraction with reasonably non-polar solvents following prolonged acid hydrolysis (pH1-labile conjugate). Because the ring A portion of the aldosterone molecule was identifiable after acid hydrolysis, this metabolite of aldosterone was referred to by AYRES et al. (1958) as the 3-oxo-conjugate of aldosterone. It was estimated that the 3-oxo-conjugate of aldosterone accounted for somewhere between 5 and 15% of secreted aldosterone. UNDERWOOD and TAIT (1964) developed convincing evidence that the 3-oxo-conjugate of aldosterone was in fact aldosterone-18-monoglucuronide. The mode of linkage of glucuronic acid to the 18-position has not been elucidated but it is possible that glucuronide may link through the oxygen of the C-18 hydroxyl group when aldosterone forms the hemiacetal structure in solution as seen in Fig. 4.

After injection of radioactive aldosterone, incubation of urine at pH 1 for 24 h at 25° centigrade releases 10 to 20% of the radioactivity, which can then be extracted into dichloromethane (JONES et al., 1959). PETERSON (1965) estimated that half this material released after pH 1 hydrolysis is aldosterone, though UNDERWOOD and TAIT (1964) have deduced that more than twice this amount is actually formed as the aldosterone-18-glucuronide conjugate. SANDOR and LANTHIER (1962) incubated 4-^{14}C-aldosterone with human liver and kidney slices and were able to demonstrate conversion of aldosterone to the 3-oxo-conjugate (aldosterone-18-glucuronide) by both tissues. It is of interest that when tritium-labeled aldosterone-18-glucuronide is injected intravenously into man, practically all of it is excreted in urine unchanged within 4 to 6 h.

SIEGENTHALER et al. (1964) studied the renal clearance of free aldosterone, the 18-glucuronide, and the reduced metabolite, tetrahydroaldosterone. Tubular reabsorption of free aldosterone was 90% whereas the renal clearance of aldosterone-18-glucuronide was three times higher than the inulin clearance, suggesting that aldosterone-18-glucuronide is secreted by the renal tubules. They also noted that hepatectomized dogs excreted normal amounts of the 3-oxo-conjugate, suggesting probable renal production of this metabolite. LUETSCHER et al. (1965) provided similar evidence for the conversion of aldosterone to aldosterone-18-glucuronide by the kidney and its secretion into tubular urine. Thus, aldosterone-18-glucuronide is a unique steroidal substance in its structure, site of formation, and mode of excretion in the kidney. Speculation as to the relationship between the ability of the kidney to metabolize aldosterone and the pre-eminence of the distal convoluted tubulal of the kidney as a site of aldosterone action has yielded no plausible connection between these two activities.

Aldosterone-18-glucuronide excretion in the urine is the most commonly used clinical index of the magnitude of aldosterone secretion in man. It is the urinary metabolite most often quantified, and the most commonly isolated metabolite following the intravenous injection of radioactive aldosterone for the purpose of estimating the secretion rate of aldosterone (see below).

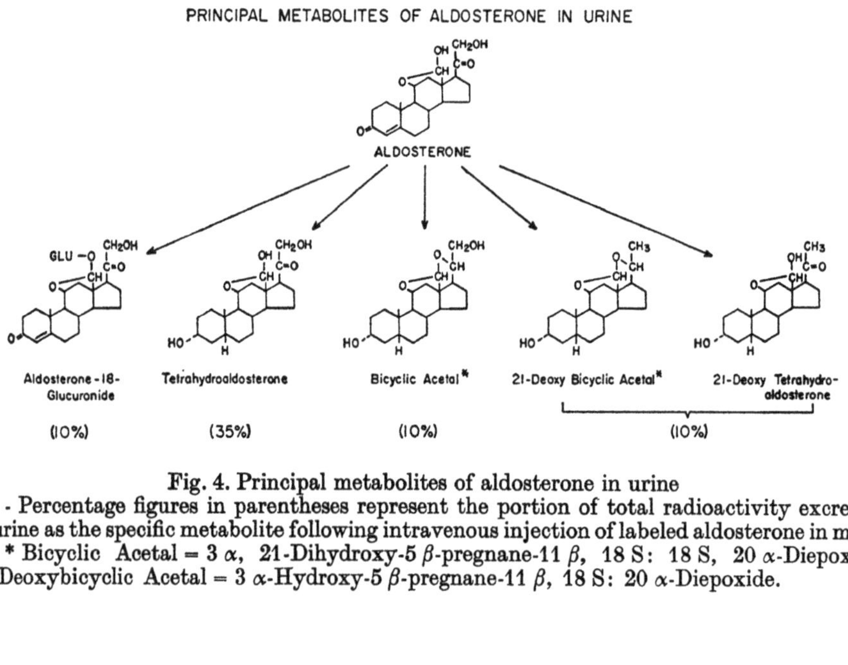

Fig. 4. Principal metabolites of aldosterone in urine
- Percentage figures in parentheses represent the portion of total radioactivity excreted in urine as the specific metabolite following intravenous injection of labeled aldosterone in man.
* Bicyclic Acetal = 3 α, 21-Dihydroxy-5 β-pregnane-11 β, 18 S: 18 S, 20 α-Diepoxide
21-Deoxybicyclic Acetal = 3 α-Hydroxy-5 β-pregnane-11 β, 18 S: 20 α-Diepoxide.

2. Tetrahydroaldosterone

Tetrahydroaldosterone-3-glucuronide was demonstrated by ULICK and LIEBERMAN (1957), and ULICK et al. (1958) first found this metabolite of aldosterone in human urine. ULICK et al. (1961) elucidated the structure of tetrahydroaldosterone as a 3 α, 5 β-steroid. Of the ring A reduced metabolites of aldosterone, only the 5 β-configuration exists in more than negligible quantities in urine. Glucuronide conjugation occurs at the 3 α-hydroxyl position of these steroids. Tetrahydroaldosterone is the most abundant metabolite of aldosterone found in human urine. It accounts for 35 to 40% of radioactivity excreted following intravenous injections of labeled aldosterone (FLOOD et al., 1961; PETERSON, 1965; MELBY et al., 1967).

SANDOR and LANTHIER (1962), when incubating labeled aldosterone with kidney and liver slices, found that in contrast to the aldosterone-18-glucuronide, tetrahydroaldosterone was formed exclusively by the liver slices. Metabolism of aldosterone to tetrahydroaldosterone involves Δ^4, 5 β-reductase which is found in the soluble fraction of liver homogenates. NADPH functions as a cofactor. It is of interest that the metabolites of aldosterone are the products of 5 β-enzyme reduction even though they possess the 11 β-hydroxyl group. KELLY et al. [1963 (1, 2)] characterized the 21-deoxytetrahydroaldosterone as a metabolite of aldosterone in conjunction with the isolation of a large number of other metabolites of aldosterone including a bicyclic acetal. These compounds are depicted in Fig. 4. KELLY et al. [1962, 1963 (1)] demonstrated the importance of the bicyclic acetal structure in the metabolism of aldosterone since one of the bicyclic acetals accounts for nearly 10% of radiolabeled aldosterone administered. These metabolites of aldosterone undergo reduction of the 20-keto group to the 20 α-hydroxy form, condensation with the hydroxyl of the C-18 hemi-acetal, dehydration, and formation of the bicyclic acetal rings. KELLY et al. [1963 (2)] also described 4, 5 β-dihydroaldosterone which is similar to dihydro derivatives of the other steroids.

D. Quantitative Aspects of the Intermediary Metabolism of Aldosterone

A brief description of the laboratory methods for the estimation of intermediary metabolism of aldosterone will be given. The quantitative indices of aldosterone biosynthesis and metabolism have relevance to clinical medicine and this discussion will concern current methodological approaches.

Metabolic clearance rate (MCR) of aldosterone has been described above. The MCR has significance only to the extent to which it alters the concentration of circulating aldosterone and thus, MCR will not be discussed in this section.

1. The Measurement of Aldosterone in Plasma

Plasma aldosterone was first quantitated by the double isotope-derivative assay. A comprehensive discussion of the usefulness of the double isotope-derivative assay for the measurement of aldosterone may be found in the paper by COGHLAN and BLAIR-WEST (1967). PETERSON (1964) developed one of the first useful double isotope-derivative assays for aldosterone. COGHLAN and SCOGGINS (1967) developed a sensitive, reproducible double isotope-derivative assay for plasma aldosterone and there are a few other published methods. Both BRODIE et al. (1967) and COGHLAN and SCOGGINS (1967) found the chief difficulty of the double isotope derivative assay was the problem of "background". The procedure depends upon double isotope-dilution technique using ^{3}H- or ^{14}C-labeled aldosterone. The mass of the steroid is determined by the use of labeled acetic anhydride of known specific activity. Aldosterone is extracted from plasma with dichloromethane, washed, partitioned, and esterified with the acetic anhydride. A minimum of three or four paper chromatograms are then used to purify the aldosterone-18, 21-diacetate. Aldosterone diacetate is then oxidized with chromium trioxide and purified in several more chromatographic systems. Mean plasma-aldosterone concentration in normal subjects regardless of posture varied in the three methods mentioned above from 0 to 17 ng/100 ml. The double isotope-derivative assay procedure for measurement of plasma aldosterone is tedious and time-consuming and therefore of limited value in the assessment of alterations in metabolism of aldosterone.

Development of a specific radioimmunoassay for plasma aldosterone has provided sensitivity and specificity without undue technical investment. Several radioimmunoassays of aldosterone have been developed (MAYES et al., 1970; BAYARD et al., 1970; ITO et al., 1972; ST. CYR et al., 1972). All these procedures involve the use of antibodies to aldosterone produced by injection of an aldosterone-beef serum albumin conjugate into rabbits, guinea-pigs, or sheep. HANING et al. (1972) developed an antibody to aldosterone in hyperimmunized sheep. This antibody, whose characteristics have been well described, has been distributed by the National Institute of Health and its availability is virtually unlimited because of its high titer. In general, antibodies to aldosterone are sufficiently specific to make it unnecessary to purify the aldosterone extracted from plasma so completely as in the double isotope-derivative assay. Most of the applied radioimmunoassays of aldosterone in plasma utilize a single paper or thin-layer chromatographic system and the immunoassay can be performed after elution from the system. The technique is described in detail by ST. CYR et al. (1972). The range of plasma aldosterone in the recumbent position in healthy adult subjects varies from 2 to 10 ng/ml with a mean of 7.6 ± 0.7 ng/ml. After 2 h in the upright position mean plasma aldosterone increased to 15.5 ± 1.7 ng/ml (ST. CYR et al., 1972). Comparison of the range of plasma aldosterone levels among the various radioimmunoassays published reveals remarkable consistency and similarity. The diagnostic value of plasma aldosterone determination is considerable, and when simultaneous measurement of plasma-renin activity is made, recognition of aldosterone-producing tumors of the adrenal cortex and secondary aldosteronism is possible. Indirect methods for the estimation of plasma aldosterone can be abandoned with the widespread availability of the radioimmunoassay of plasma aldosterone.

2. Urinary Aldosterone Metabolite Excretion per 24 h

a) Measurement of Aldosterone-18-Glucuronide Excretion

Both physicochemical and double isotope-derivative assay methods have been used for the measurement of this metabolite of aldosterone. Both types of analysis have also been used to determine the aldosterone secretion rate which will be mentioned below. Physicochemical methods and the double isotope-derivative assay involve the hydrolysis of urine at pH 1 with the release of free aldosterone. Following hydrolysis, extraction is carried out and a wide variety of methods have been used for subsequent chromatographic purification. The various methods used for the estimation of urinary aldosterone-18-glucuronide have been reviewed in detail by BRODIE and TAIT (1967). The excretion of the acid labile conjugate (aldosterone-18-glucuronide) in the urine of most healthy adults ranges from 2 to 19 μg/24 h.

The double isotope-derivative assay for urinary aldosterone-18-glucuronide has most commonly been based on the method of KLIMAN and PETERSON (1960). Several modifications of the original Kliman-Peterson procedure have been reviewed by BRODIE and TAIT (1967). All the methods involve acid hydrolysis, acetylation with ^{3}H-acetic anhydride, chromatographic purification, and oxidation with chromium trioxide to corticosterone-18-oic-18 > 11-lactone-^{3}H-acetate. This procedure continues to be the principal means of assessing aldosterone secretion.

b) Urinary Tetrahydroaldosterone-3-Glucuronide

Various methods for the measurement of this, the major metabolite of aldosterone in urine, are described by BRODIE and TAIT (1967). For reasons which are not clear, tetrahydroaldosterone has not been quantified as widely as the 18-glucuronide of aldosterone. After hydrolysis with β-glucuronidase, tetrahydroaldosterone is extracted into dichloromethane and separated in a wide variety of systems involving paper and thin-layer chromatography. Tetrahydroaldosterone must be separated from 18-hydroxytetrahydro-11-dehydrocorticosterone, the principle metabolite of 18-hydroxycorticosterone (DALE et al., 1972). In this procedure some three thin-layer chromatography systems are used and aldosterone is quantified by a modification of the Porter-Silber reaction in which aldosterone is oxidized by cupric acetate to a Porter-Silber positive chromogen and quantified spectrophotometrically (LEWBART and MATTOX, 1961). In thirty-two healthy adults urinary tetrahydroaldosterone ranged from 19 to 63 μg/24 h with a mean excretion of 38.4 μg/24 h. Normal ranges of tetrahydroaldosterone excretion found by DALE et al. (1972) are compatible with the excretion rates of tetrahydroaldosterone reported by FLOOD et al. (1967), NEW et al. (1966), SIEGENTHALER et al. (1962), and ULICK et al. (1964).

DALE et al. (1972) measured both tetrahydroaldosterone and aldosterone-18-glucuronide while measuring secretion rate of aldosterone in more than 40 non-hospitalized healthy adults on sodium intakes exceeding 110 mEq/day. They found tetrahydroaldosterone accounted for a more constant fraction of the secretion rate than did the 3-oxo-conjugate. These data suggest that urinary tetrahydroaldosterone excretion provides a more reliable index of aldosterone secretion than does urinary excretion of aldosterone-18-glucuronide. This procedure has been widely applied in diagnosis of alterations in adrenocortical function (MELBY et al., 1967).

3. Determination of the Aldosterone Secretion Rate for a 24 h Period

The secretion rate of aldosterone may be determined by isotope-dilution methodology, and has the advantage over the urinary excretion of specific metabolites that it is unaltered by changes in the ratio of aldosterone metabolized to aldosterone-18-glucuronide and tetrahydroaldosterone (DALE et al., 1972). Secretion rate procedure involves the intravenous injection of radiolabeled aldosterone in a tracer dose and collection of all urine passed over the next 24 h. One of the urinary metabolites of aldosterone is then isolated and its specific activity determined. When this quantity is divided into the administered dose of radioactivity an integrated dilution of radioactivity or secretion rate is obtained, that is;

$$\text{secretion rate} = \frac{\text{counts/min of isotope injected}}{\text{specific activity of urinary metabolite of aldosterone.}}$$

TAIT and BURSTEIN (1964) discussed the validity of the secretion rate measurement in terms of the following assumptions:

1. Labeled aldosterone is radiochemically homogeneous,
2. The ^{3}H- or ^{14}C-isotope is stable,
3. Labeled aldosterone is chemically indentical to endogenously secreted aldosterone,
4. Labeled aldosterone given is a tracer dose and has no biological significance,
5. The fraction of endogenous secreted aldosterone metabolized to the 18-glucuronide or to tetrahydroaldosterone is constant during the period of collection of urine,
6. Secretion of the labeled metabolite of aldosterone is complete within the time of collection of urine,
7. The metabolite has aldosterone as its exclusive precursor,
8. The metabolite of aldosterone is homogeneous.

The validity of the secretion-rate methodology may be undisputed if a strict routine is followed and radiochemical homogeneity of the isotope administered is assured. Specific activities of the two urinary metabolites of aldosterone, aldosterone-18-glucuronide and tetrahydroaldosterone, are usually identical in healthy subjects and in patients with disorders of aldosterone secretion. Table 4 shows data obtained from DALE et al. (1972), which demonstrate close agreement between the secretion rates determined from measurements of the specific activity of aldosterone-18-glucuronide and tetrahydroaldosterone in the same individual. BRODIE and TAIT, however, found secretion rates on unrestricted sodium diets were lower when derived from the excretion of aldosterone-18-glucuronide than those derived from the excretion of tetrahydroaldosterone.

The occasional presence of 17-isoaldosterone as a contaminant in commercial preparations of radioactive aldosterone has interfered with the accurate assessment of the aldosterone secretion rate (FLOOD et al., 1967). These two compounds are metabolized differently, resulting in an invalid estimation of the specific activity of the urinary metabolite.

Table 4. *Comparison of secretory rates by tetrahydroaldosterone and aldosterone-18-glucuronide*[a]

Subject	Diagnosis	μg/24 h	
		Aldosterone-18-glucuronide	TH Aldosterone
B. B. (1)	Secondary aldosteronism	543	523
(2)		530	536
J. H.	Secondary aldosteronism malignant hypertension	1,206	1,038
J. J.	Normal after < 50 mEq sodium intake	282	277
M. P.	Secondary aldosteronism	250	306
M. T.	Primary aldosteronism	2,530	2,570
V. S.	Primary aldosteronism	346	372

[a] From DALE et al. (1972).

Table 5. *Aldosterone secretion rates and tetrahydroaldosterone excretion in healthy subjects*[a]

	Sex	No.		μg/24 h	
				TH Aldo	ASR
Normals age 25 to 50 years	Male	19	mean	40.3	105.5
			range	(21—63)	(51—160)
	Female	13	mean	36.5	93.8
			range	(19—53)	(43—156)

[a] From DALE et al. (1972)

Table 5 shows data obtained from DALE et al. (1972) on aldosterone secretion rates and tetrahydroaldosterone excretion in healthy subjects. It can be seen that the mean secretion rate of aldosterone is approximately 100 μg/24 h. It should be noted that the oldest normal subject studied was 50 years of age. Since aldosterone secretion appears to be inversely related to advancing age (FLOOD et al., 1967), older subjects would be expected to have lower secretion rates.

Techniques for the quantification of aldosterone metabolism are widely available for testing almost every aspect of the intermediary metabolism of aldosterone. These techniques should provide the basis for an understanding of the nature of the physiologic regulation of aldosterone secretion.

Acknowledgements

This work was supported in part by Grants-in-Aid AM-12027-04, T01-AM 05446-06, 2-P02-AM08657-07 and HE-07299.

References

AGUILERA, G., MARUSIC, E. T.: Role of the renin-angiotensin system in the biosynthesis of aldosterone. Endocrinology **89**, 1524 (1971).

AXELRAD, B. J., CATES, J. E., JOHNSON, B. B., LUETSCHER, J. A.: Aldosterone in urine of normal man and of patients with oedema its increased recovery after hydrolysis with acid and with beta-glucuronidase. Brit. Med. J. **1955 I**, 196.

AYRES, P. J., EICHHORN, J., HECHTER, O., SABA, N., TAIT, J. F., TAIT, S. A. S.: Some studies on the biosynthesis of aldosterone and other adrenal steroids. Acta endocr. (Kbh.) **33**, 27 (1960).

AYRES, P. J., GARROD, O., TAIT, S. A. S., TAIT, J. F.: Primary aldosteronism (Conn's syndrome). In: An International Symposium on Aldosterone, 1st Ed., p. 143 (MULLER, A. F., O'CONNOR, C. M., Eds.). London: Churchill 1900.

AYRES, P. J., GOULD, R. P., SIMPSON, S. A., TAIT, J. F.: The *in vitro* demonstration of different corticosteroid production within the ox adrenal gland. Biochem. J. **63**, 19 (1956).

AYRES, P. J., HECHTER, O., SABA, N., SIMPSON, S. A., TAIT, J. F.: Intermediates in the biosynthesis of aldosterone by capsule strippings of ox adrenal gland. Biochem. J. (abstract) **65**, 22 (1957).

BAIRD, D. T., HORTON, R., LONGCOPE, C., TAIT, J. F.: Steroid dynamics under steady-state conditions. Recent Prog. Hormone Res. **25**, 611—664 (1969).

BANIUKIEWICZ, S., BRODIE, A., FLOOD, C., MOTTA, M., OKAMOTA, M., TAIT, J. F., TAIT, S. A. S., BLAIR-WEST, J. R., COGHLAN, J. P., DENTON, D. A., GODING, J. R., SCOGGINS, B. A., WINTOUR, E. M., WRIGHT, R. D.: Adrenal biosynthesis of steroids *in vitro* and *in vivo* using continuous superfusion and infusion procedures. In: Functions of the adrenal cortex, Vol. 1, p. 153 (MCKERNS, K. W., Ed.). New York: Appleton-Century-Crofts 1968.

BAUMANN, K., MÜLLER, J.: Effect of potassium intake on the final steps of aldosterone biosynthesis in the rat. Acta endocr. (Kbh.) **69**, 701 (1972).

BAUMBER, J. S., DAVIS, J. O., JOHNSON, J. A., WITTY, R. T.: Increased adrenocortical potassium in association with increased biosynthesis of aldosterone. Amer. J. Physiol. **220**, 1094 (1971).

BAYARD, F., BEITINS, I., KOWANSKI, A., MIGEON, C.: Measurements of plasma aldosterone by radioimmunoassay. J. clin. Endocr. **31**, 1 (1970).

BLAIR-WEST, J. R., COGHLAN, J. P., DENTON, D. A., GODING, J. R., MUNRO, J. A., PETERSON, R. E., WINTOUR, E. M.: Humoral stimulation of adrenal cortical secretion. J. clin. Invest. **41**, 1606 (1962).

BORKOWSKI, A. J., LEVIN, S., DELCROIX, C., MAHLER, A., VERHAS, V.: Blood cholesterol and hydrocortisone production in man: quantitative aspects of the utilization of circulating cholesterol by the adrenals at rest and under adrenocorticotropin stimulation. J. clin. Invest. **46**, 797 (1967).

BOUGAS, J., FLOOD, C., LITTLE, B., TAIT, J. F., TAIT, S. A. S., UNDERWOOD, R. H.: Dynamic aspects of aldosterone metabolism. In: Aldosterone, p. 25 (BAULIEN, E. E., ROBEL, P., Eds.). Oxford: Blackwell 1964.

BOYD, G. W., PEART, W. S.: The relationship between angiotensin and aldosterone. Advanc. metab. Disord. **5**, 77 (1971).

BOYD, J. E., PALMORE, W. P., MULROW, P. J.: (1) Potassium: Is it the adrenal glomerulotrophin? J. clin. Invest. **50** (abstract), 35 (1971).

BOYD, J. E., PALMORE, W. P., MULROW, P. J.: Role of potassium in the control of aldosterone secretion in the rat. Endocrinology **88**, 556 (1971).

BRODIE, A., TAIT, J. F.: Assays of aldosterone. In: Methods in Hormone Research, Vol. 1 ed. 2 (DORFMAN, R. I., Ed.). New York: Academic Press 1968.

BRODIE, A., SHIMIZU, N., TAIT, S. A. S., TAIT, J. F.: A method for the measurement of aldosterone in peripheral plasma using ^{3}H-acetic anhydride. J. clin. Endocr. **27**, 997 (1967).

BURROW, G. N., MULROW, P. J., BONDY, P. K.: Protein synthesis and aldosterone production Endocrinology **79**, 955 (1966).

BURSTEIN, S.: Genetic aspects of adrenal and hepatic cortisol 2 α- and 6 β-hydroxylation in guinea pigs: developmental pattern and effect of substrate concentration. Endocrinology **86**, 851 (1970).

CAMARGO, C. A., DOWDY, A. J., HANCOCK, E. W., LUETSCHER, J. A.: Decreased plasma clearance and hepatic extraction of aldosterone in patients with heart failure. J. clin. Invest. **44**, 356 (1965).

CHEVILLO, R. A., LUETSCHER, J. A., HANCOCK, E. W., DOWDY, A. J., NOKES, G. W.: Distribution, conjugation, and excretion of labeled aldosterone in congestive heart failure and in controls with normal circulation: development and testing of a model with an analog computer. J. clin. Invest. **45**, 1302 (1966).

Coghlan, J. P., Blair-West, J. R.: Aldosterone. In: Hormones in Blood, Vol. 2, p. 391 (Gray, C. H., Bacharach, A. L., Eds.). London, New York: Academic Press 1967.
Coghlan, J. P., Blair-West, J. R., Denton, D. A., Scoggins, B. A., Wright, R. D.: Perspectives in aldosterone and renin control. Aust. N. Z. J. Med. **2**, 178 (1971).
Coghlan, J. P., Scoggins, B. A.: Measurements of aldosterone in peripheral blood of man and sheep. J. clin. Endocr. **27**, 1470 (1967).
Constantopoulos, G., Carpenter, A., Satoh, P. S., Tchen, T. T.: Formation of isocaproaldehyde in the enzymatic cleavage of cholesterol side chain by adrenal extract. Biochemistry **5**, 1650 (1966).
Coppage, W. S., Island, D. P., Cooner, A. E., Liddle, G. W.: The metabolism of aldosterone in normal subjects and patients with hepatic cirrhosis. J. clin. Invest. **41**, 1672 (1962).
Dale, S. L., Wilson, T. E., Melby, J. C.: unpublished observations (1972).
David, R., Golan, S., Drucker, W.: Familial aldosterone deficiency: enzyme defect, diagnosis and clinical course. Pediatrics **41**, 403 (1968).
Davis, W. W., Garren, L. G.: On the mechanism of action of adrenocorticotropic hormone. The inhibitory site of cycloheximide in the pathway of steroid biosynthesis. J. biol. Chem. **243**, 5153 (1968).
Dyrenfurth, I., Lucis, O. J., Beck, J. C., Venning, E. H.: Studies in patients with adrenocortical hyperfunction. III. *In vitro* secretion of steroids by human adrenal glands. J. clin. Endocr. **20**, 765 (1960).
Eilers, E. A., Peterson, R. E.: Aldosterone secretion in the rat. In: Aldosterone, p. 251 (Baulien, E. E., Robel, P., Eds.). Oxford: Blackwell 1964.
Flood, C., Layne, D. S., Ramcharan, S., Rossipal, E., Tait, J. F., Tait, S. A. S.: An investigation of the urinary metabolites and secretion rates of aldosterone and cortisol in man and a description of methods for their measurement. Acta endocr. (Kbh.) **36**, 237 (1961).
Flood, C., Pincus, G., Tait, J. F., Tait, S. A. S., Willoughby, S.: A comparison of the metabolism of radioactive 17-isoaldosterone administered intravenously and orally to normal human subjects. J. clin. Invest. **46**, 717 (1967).
Funder, J. W., Blair-West, J. R., Coghlan, J. P., Denton, D. A., Scoggins, B. A., Wright, R. D.: Effect of plasma [K^+] on the secretion of aldosterone. Endocrinology **85**, 381 (1969).
Garren, L. G., Ney, R. L., Davis, W. W.: Studies on the role of protein synthesis in the regulation of corticosterone production by adrenocorticotropic hormone *in vivo*. Proc. Nat. Acad. Sci. (Wash.) **53**, 1443 (1965).
Giroud, C. J. P., Saffran, M., Schally, A. V., Stachenko, J., Venning, E. H.: (1) Production of aldosterone by rat adrenal glands *in vitro*. Proc. Soc. exp. Biol. (N. Y.) **92**, 855 (1956).
Giroud, C. J. P., Stachenko, J., Piletta, P.: *In vitro* studies of the functional zonation of the adrenal cortex and of the production of aldosterone. In: Aldosterone, p. 56 (Müller, A. F., O'Conner, C. M., Eds.). Boston: Little, Brown and Co. 1958.
Giroud, C. J. P., Stachenko, J., Venning, E. H.: (2) Secretion of aldosterone by the zona glomerulosa of rat adrenal glands incubated *in vitro*. Proc. Soc. Exp. Biol. (N. Y.) **92**, 154 (1956).
Greengard, P., Psychoyos, S., Tallan, H. H., Cooper, D. Y., Rosenthal, O., Estabrook, R.: Aldosterone synthesis by adrenal mitochondria. Arch. Biochem. **121**, 298 (1967).
Hall, P. F., Young, D. G.: Site of action of tropic hormones upon the biosynthesis pathways to steroid hormones. Endocrinology **82**, 559 (1968).
Haning, R., Tait, J. F., Tait, S. A. S., Williams, G. H.: Stimulation of the conversion of corticosterone to aldosterone by rat adrenal glomerulosa cells and tissue. Proc. Soc. Endocrinol. J. Endocrinol. **49**, xii (1971).
Haning, R., Tait, S. A. S., Tait, J. F.: *In vitro* effects of ACTH, angiotensins, serotonin and potassium on steroid output and conversion of corticosterone to aldosterone by isolated adrenal cells. Endocrinology **87**, 1147 (1971).
Hickie, J. B., Lazarus, L.: Aldosterone metabolism in cardiac failure. Aust. Ann. Med. **15**, 289 (1966).
Hollander, W., Kramsch, D. M., Chobanian, A. V., Melby, J. C.: Metabolism and distribution of intravenously administered d-aldosterone-1,2-^{3}H in the arteries, kidneys, and heart of dog. Circulat. Res. (Suppl. 1), **18**, 35 (1966).
Ito, T., Woo, J., Haning, R., Horton, R.: A radioimmunoassay for aldosterone in human peripheral plasma including a comparison of alternate techniques. J. clin. Endocr. **34**, 106 (1972).
Jones, K. M., Lloyd-Jones, R., Riondel, A., Tait, J. F., Tait, S. A. S., Bulbrook, R. D., Greenwood, F. C.: Aldosterone secretion and metabolism in normal man and women and in pregnancy. Acta endocr. (Kbh.) **30**, 321 (1951).

JOUAN, P.: Epiphyse, 5 hydroxytryptamine et corticoidogenèse *in vitro*. Path. et Biol. **15**, 1145 (1967).

KAHNT, F. W., NEHER, R.: Über die adrenale Steroid-Biosynthese *in vitro*. I. Umwandlung endogener und exogener Vorstufen im Nebennieren-Homogenat des Rindes. Helv. chim. Acta **48**, 1457 (1965).

KAHNT, F. W., NEHER, R., WETTSTEIN, A.: Umwandlung von radioaktiven Cortexon in Aldosteron durch Nebennieren-Enzyme. Experientia (Basel) **11**, 446 (1955).

KAPLAN, N. M.: The biosynthesis of adrenal steroids: effects of angiotensin II, adrenocorticotropin and potassium. J. clin. Invest. **44**, 2029 (1965).

KAPLAN, N. M.: The steroid content of adrenal adenomas and measurement of aldosterone production in patients with essential hypertension and primary aldosteronism. J. clin. Invest. **46**, 728 (1967).

KAPLAN, N. M., BARTTER, F. C.: The effect of ACTH, renin, angiotensin II, and various precursors on biosynthesis of aldosterone by adrenal slices. J. clin. Invest. **41**, 715 (1962).

KELLY, W. G., BANDI, L., LIEBERMAN, S.: (1) Isolation and characterization of human urinary metabolites of aldosterone. IV. The synthesis and stereochemistry of two bicyclic acetal metabolites. Biochemistry **2**, 1243 (1963).

KELLY, W. G., BANDI, L., LIEBERMAN, S.: (2) Isolation and characterization of human urinary metabolites of aldosterone. V. Dihydroaldosterone and 21-deoxytetrahydroaldosterone. Biochemistry **2**, 1249 (1963).

KELLY, W. G., BANDI, L., SHOOLERY, J., LIEBERMAN, S.: Isolation and characterization of aldosterone metabolites from human urine; two metabolites bearing a bicyclic acetal structure. Biochemistry **1**, 172 (1962).

KLIMAN, B., PETERSON, R. E.: Double isotope derivative assay of aldosterone in biological extracts. J. biol. Chem. **235**, 1639 (1960).

KONO, T., YOSHIMI, T., MIYAKE, T.: Metabolic clearance of aldosterone, cortisol and corticosterone in various clinical conditions. In: Steroid dynamics, p. 1429 (PINCUS, G., NAKAO, T., TAIT, J. F., Eds.). New York: Academic Press 1966.

LEWBART, M. L., MATTOX, V. R.: Extension of the Porter-Silber reaction to 17-deoxy-α-ketolic steroids. Analyt. Chem. **33**, 559 (1961).

LUETSCHER, J. A., COHN, A. O., CAMARGO, C. A., DOWDY, A. J., CALLAGHAN, A. M.: Aldosterone secretion and metabolism in hyperthyroidism and myxedema. J. clin. Endocr. **23**, 873 (1963).

LUETSCHER, J. A., HANCOCK, E. W., CAMARGO, C. A., DOWDY, A. J., NOKES, G. W.: Conjugation of 1,2-^{3}H aldosterone in human liver and kidneys and renal extraction of aldosterone and labeled conjugates from blood plasma. J. clin. Endocr. **25**, 628 (1965).

MARIEB, N. J., MULROW, P. J.: Role of the renin-angiotensin system in the regulation of aldosterone secretion in the rat. Endocrinology **76**, 657 (1965).

MARUSIC, E. T., MULROW, P. J.: (2) Stimulation of aldosterone biosynthesis in adrenal mitochondria by sodium depletion. J. clin. Invest. **46**, 2101 (1967).

MAYES, D., FURUYAMA, S., KEM, D., NUGENT, C.: A radioimmunoassay for plasma aldosterone. J. clin. Endocr. **30**, 682 (1970).

MELBY, J. C., DALE, S. L., GREKIN, R. J., GAUNT, R., WILSON, T. E.: 18-Hydroxy-11-deoxycorticosterone (18-OH-DOC) secretion in experimental and human hypertension. Rec. Prog. Hormone Res. **28**, 287 (1972).

MELBY, J. C., EGDAHL, R. H., DALE, S. L.: Role of circulating free cholesterol of plasma in adrenal steroidogenesis. Excerpta Medica, Intern'l Congress Series **111**, Abstract, 437 (May) (1966).

MELBY, J. C., SPARK, R. F., DALE, S. L., EGDAHL, R. H., KAHN, P. C.: Diagnosis and localization of aldosterone-producing adenoma by adrenal vein catheterization. New Engl. J. Med. **277**, 1050 (1967).

MEYER, C. J., LAYNE, D. S., TAIT, J. F., PINCUS, G.: The binding of aldosterone to plasma proteins in normal, pregnant and steroid-treated women. J. clin. Invest. **40**, 1663 (1961).

MORRIS, M. D., KRUM, A. A., LEE, J. A.: Relationship of plasma and adrenal gland sterols to corticosterone in the rabbit. Arch. Biochem. **121**, 331 (1967).

MÜLLER, J.: (1) Aldosterone stimulation *in vitro*. I. Evaluation of assay procedure and determination of aldosterone-stimulating activity in a human urine extract. Acta endocr. (Kbh.) **48**, 283 (1965).

MÜLLER, J.: Aldosterone stimulation *in vitro*. Acta endocr. (Kbh.) **52**, 515 (1966).

MÜLLER, J.: Regulation of aldosterone biosynthesis. Berlin-Heidelberg-New York: Springer 1971.

MÜLLER, J., HUBER, R.: Effects of sodium deficiency, potassium deficiency, and uremia upon the steroidogenic response of rat adrenal tissue to serotonin, potassium ions, and adrenocorticotropin. Endocrinology **85**, 43 (1969).

MÜLLER, J., WEICK, W. J.: Aldosterone stimulation *in vitro*. IV. Corticosteroid stimulating activity in rat serum. Acta endocr. (Kbh.) **54**, 63 (1967).
MÜLLER, J., ZIEGLER, W. H.: Stimulation of aldosterone biosynthesis *in vitro* by serotonin. Acta endocr. (Kbh.) **59**, 23 (1968).
MULROW, P. J.: Neural and other mechanisms regulating aldosterone secretion. In: Neuroendocrinology, Vol. **1**, p. 407. New York: Academic Press 1966.
MULROW, P. J., COHN, G. L.: Conversion of corticosterone 4-^{14}C to aldosterone by human adrenal slices. Proc. Soc. exp. Biol. (N. Y.) **101**, 731 (1959).
NEW, M. I., MILLER, B., PETERSON, R. E.: Aldosterone excretion in normal children and in children with adrenal hyperplasia. J. clin. Invest. **45**, 412 (1966).
NICOLIS, G. L., ULICK, S.: Role of 18-hydroxylation in the biosynthesis of aldosterone. Endocrinology **76**, 514 (1965).
PASQUALINI, J. R.: Conversion of tritiated 18-hydroxycorticosterone to aldosterone by slices of human cortico-adrenal gland and adrenal tumor. Nature (Lond.) **201**, 501 (1964).
PEARLMAN, W. H.: Circulating steroid hormone levels in relation to steroid hormone production. Ciba Foundation Colloq. Endocrinol. **II**, 233 (1957).
PETERSON, R. E.: Determination of peripheral plasma aldosterone. In: Aldosterone. Oxford: Blackwell 1964.
PETERSON, R. E.: The use of radioactive aldosterone in man. In: Isotopes in experimental pharmacology. Chicago: University of Chicago Press 1965.
PETERSON, R. E.: Metabolism of adrenal cortical steroids. In: The Human Adrenal Cortex. New York: Harper and Row 1971.
RAMAN, P. B., SHARMA, D. C., DORFMAN, R. I.: Studies on aldosterone biosynthesis *in vitro*. Biochemistry **5**, 1795 (1966).
RAMAN, P. B., SHARMA, D. C., DORFMAN, R. I., GABRILOVE, J. L.: Biosynthesis of C-18-oxygenated steroids by an aldosterone-secreting human adrenal tumor. Metabolism of [4-^{14}C]-progesterone, [1,2-^{3}H]-11-deoxycorticosterone and [4-^{14}C]-pregnenolone. Biochemistry **4**, 1376 (1965).
ST. CYR, M. J., SANCHO, J. M., DALE, S. L., MELBY, J. C.: Quantitation of plasma aldosterone by radioimmunoassay. Clin. Chem. (1972) (in press).
SANDERS, L. L., MELBY, J. C.: Aldosterone of the edema of congestive heart failure. Arch. intern. Med. **113**, 331 (1964).
SANDOR, T., LAMOUREUX, J., LANTHIER, A.: Adrenocortical function in birds: *in vitro* biosynthesis of radioactive corticosteroids from pregnenolone-7-^{3}H and progesterone-4-C^{14} by adrenal glands of the domestic duck (anas platyrhynchos) and the chicken (gallus domesticus,. Endocrinology **73**, 629 (1963).
SANDOR, T., LANTHIER, A.: The *in vitro* biosynthesis of 18-hydroxycorticosterone-4-^{14}C by slices of zona glomerulosa of beef adrenals and by human adrenals. Acta endocr. (Kbh.) **42**, 355 (1963).
SARUTA, T., KAPLAN, N. M.: Prostaglandins and other stimuli of beef adrenal steroidogenesis. J. clin. Invest. **51**, 2246 (1971).
SHEPPARD, H., SWENSON, R., MOWLES, T. F.: Steroid biosynthesis by rat adrenal: functional zonation. Endocrinology **73**, 819 (1963).
SIEGENTHALER, W. E., DOWDY, A., LUETSCHER, J. A.: Determination of the secretion rate of aldosterone in normal man by use of 7-^{3}H-d-aldosterone and acid hydrolysis of urine. J. clin. Endocr. **22**, 172 (1962).
SIEGENTHALER, W. E., PETERSON, R. E., FRIMPTER, G. W.: The renal clearance of aldosterone and its major metabolites. In: Aldosterone. Oxford: Blackwell 1964.
SIMPSON, E. R., COOPER, D. Y., ESTABROOK, R. W.: Metabolic events associated with steroid hydroxylation by the adrenal cortex. Rec. Progr. Hormon Res. **25**, 523 (1969).
SIMPSON, S. A., TAIT, J. F., WETTSTEIN, A., NEHER, R., VON EUW, J., REICHSTEIN, R.: Isolierung eines neuen kristallisierten Hormons aus Nebennieren mit besonders hoher Wirksamkeit auf den Mineralstoffwechsel. Experientia (Basel) **9**, 333 (1953).
SPARK, R. F., DALE, S. L., KAHN, P. C., MELBY, J. C.: Activation of aldosterone secretion in primary aldosteronism. J. clin. Invest. **48**, 96 (1969).
SPÄT, A., SOLYOM, J., STURCZ, J., MESZAROS, I., LUDWIG, E.: Effect of angiotensin superfusion on the rate of aldosterone production by incubated rat adrenals. Acta physiol. Acad. Sci. hung. **35**, 149 (1969).
STACHENKO, J., GIROUD, C. J. P.: Some aspects of steroidogenesis in the zona glomerulosa. In: The human adrenal cortex. Baltimore: Williams and Wilkins 1962.
STACHENKO, J., GIROUD, C. J. P.: Functional zonation of the adrenal cortex; site of ACTH action. Canad. J. Biochem. **42**, 1777 (1964).
SWANECK, G. E., HIGHLAND, E., EDELMAN, I. S.: Stereospecific nuclear and cytosol aldosterone-binding proteins of various tissues. Nephron **6**, 297 (1969).

TAIT, J. F.: Review: the use of isotopic steroids for the measurement of production rates *in vivo*. J. clin. Endocr. **23**, 1285 (1963).
TAIT, J. F., BOUGAS, J., LITTLE, B., TAIT, S. A. S., FLOOD, C.: Splanchnic extraction and clearance of aldosterone in subjects with minimal and marked cardiac dysfuction. J. clin. Endocr. **25**, 219 (1965).
TAIT, J. F., BURSTEIN, S.: *In vivo* studies of steroid dynamics in man. In: The hormones, Vol. V. New York: Academic Press 1964.
TAIT, J. F., LITTLE, B., TAIT, S. A. S., FLOOD, C.: The metabolic clearance rate of aldosterone in pregnant and non-pregnant subjects estimated by both single-injection and constant-infusion methods. J. clin. Invest. **41**, 2093 (1962).
TAIT, J. F., TAIT, S. A. S., LITTLE, B., LAUMAS, K.: The disappearance of 7-^{3}H-d-aldosterone in the plasma of normal subjects. J. clin. Invest. **40**, 72 (1961).
TAIT, S. A. S., SCHULSTER, D., OKAMOTO, M., FLOOD, C., TAIT, J. F.: Production of steroids by *in vitro* superfusion of endocrine tissue. II. Steroid output from bisected whole capsular and decapsulated adrenals of normal intact hypophysectomized and hypophysectomized-nephrectomized rats as a function of time of superfusion. Endocrinology **86**, 360 (1970).
TOUITOU, Y., MALMEJAC, A., AUPETIT, B., BIANCANI, J., LEGRAND, J.-C.: Taux de sécrétion de 18-hydroxycorticostérone. Application de la méthode d'Ulick modifiée à différents cas cliniques. Ann. Biol. clin. **28**, 49 (1970).
ULICK, S.: Aldosterone biosynthesis in congenital adrenal hyperplasia. Excerpta Medica Int. Congr. Sec. III, No. 315, **1**, 186 (1966).
ULICK, S., KUSCH, K., AUGUST, J. T.: Correction of the structure of a urinary metabolite of aldosterone. J. Amer. chem. Soc. **83**, 4482 (1961).
ULICK, S., LARAGH, J. H., LIEBERMAN, S.: The isolation of a urinary metabolite of aldosterone and its use to measure the rate of secretion of aldosterone by the adrenal cortex of man. Trans. Ass. Amer. Phycns. **71**, 225 (1958).
ULICK, S., LIEBERMAN, S.: Communications to Editor: Evidence for the occurrence of a metabolite of aldosterone in urine. J. Amer. chem. Soc. **79**, 6567 (1957).
ULICK, S., NICOLIS, G., L., VETTER, K. K.: Relationship of 18-hydroxycorticosterone to aldosterone. In: Aldosterone. Oxford: Blackwell 1964.
ULICK, S., SOLOMON, S.: Communications to the Editor: The synthesis of aldosterone from progesterone by the amphibian adrenal. J. Amer. chem. Soc. **82**, 249 (1960).
UNDERWOOD, R. H., TAIT, J. F.: Purification, partial characterization and metabolism of an acid-labile conjugate of aldosterone. J. clin. Endocr. **24**, 1110 (1964).
WETTSTEIN, A.: Biosynthèse des hormones steroides. Experientia (Basel) **17**, 329 (1961).

The Renin-Angiotensin System in the Control of Aldosterone Secretion

JAMES O. DAVIS

With 6 Figures

Introduction

In 1960, two new findings suggested that the renin-angiotensin system is important in the control of aldosterone secretion. First, it was discovered that a potent aldosterone-stimulating hormone was secreted by the kidney (DAVIS, 1960, 1961) and, second, it was reported that synthetic Ang. II increased the rate of aldosterone secretion (LARAGH et al., 1960) and excretion (GENEST et al., 1960) in man. These two observations led to the merging of two fields of research, namely, that concerned with the pathogenesis of arterial hypertension and that involved with the control of aldosterone secretion. It is the purpose of this chapter to present the evidence for the important role of the renin-angiotensin system in the regulation of aldosterone secretion and to describe how this control mechanism functions in both homeostasis and disease.

Evidence for an Aldosterone-Stimulating Hormone in the Control of Aldosterone Secretion

In the early studies, it was recognized that the immediate stimulus to aldosterone production might be nervous or humoral or both. The observations of LEVY and BLALOCK in 1939 demonstrated that neural connections to the adrenal gland are unnecessary for the control of aldosterone secretion. These workers transplanted one adrenal gland to the neck and removed the other adrenal in dogs; several of their animals lived for months in a normal healthy condition. Later, several different groups of investigators demonstrated that the nerves to the adrenal glands are not essential for increased aldosterone secretion to occur in response to several different stimuli in either the dog or the sheep. FLEMING and FARRELL (1956) were the first to show that an elevated rate of aldosterone secretion occurred from the acutely transplanted adrenal gland in the dog. Subsequently, in chronic studies in dogs with only one adrenal gland which was transplanted to the neck and thus denervated [CARPENTER et al., 1961 (2)], a striking increase in aldosterone secretion occurred following acute hemorrhage and after chronic thoracic inferior vena cava constriction. Similarly, in conscious sheep with only one adrenal which was transplanted to the neck, an increase in aldosterone secretion occurred in response to sodium depletion (DENTON et al., 1959). These findings provide important indirect evidence for a humoral mechanism in the control of aldosterone biosynthesis since they show that the nerves to the adrenals are unnecessary for hypersecretion of aldosterone to occur.

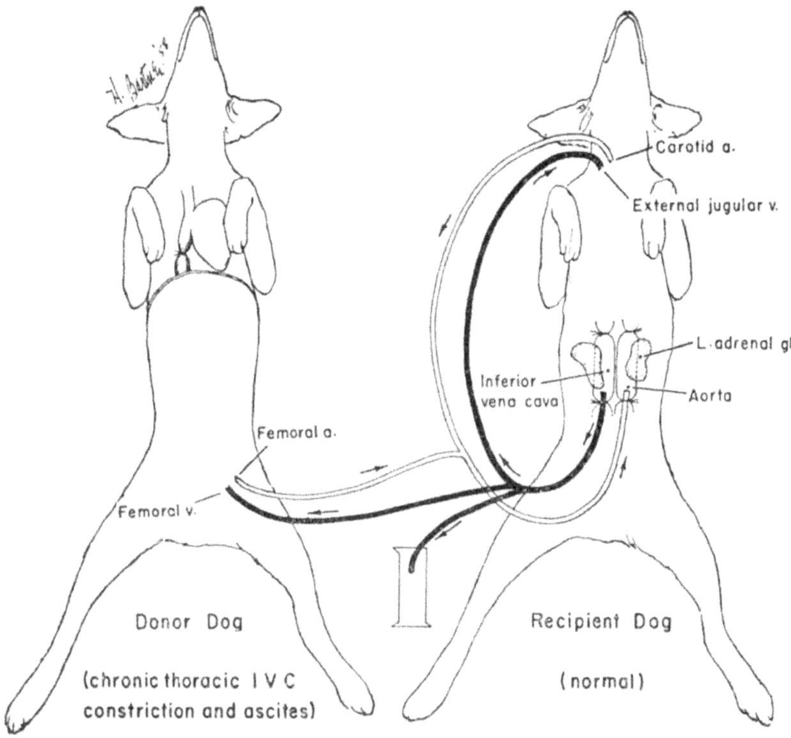

Fig. 1. Experimental arrangement for cross-circulation of blood from donor dogs with hyperaldosteronism secondary to chronic thoracic inferior vena cava constriction and ascites through the isolated adrenals of normal dogs. (From Yankopoulas et al., 1959)

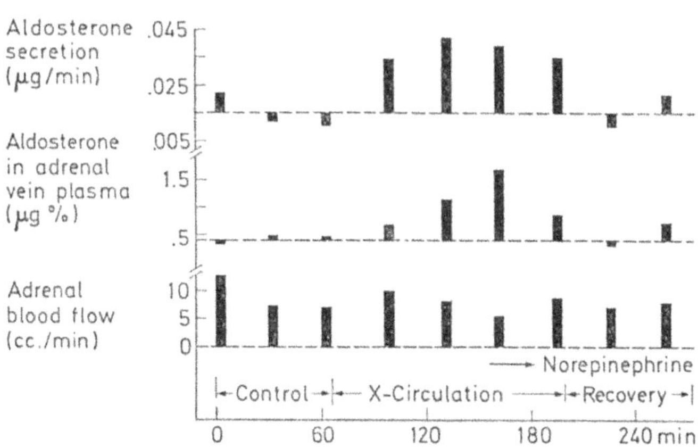

Fig. 2. Increased aldosterone secretion by the isolated adrenals of a normal recipient dog during cross-circulation of blood from a donor with hyperaldosteronism. (From Yankopoulas et al., 1959)

The first direct evidence for a humoral mechanism other than ACTH or altered plasma electrolyte concentrations in aldosterone control was attained from cross-circulation studies in dogs and sheep. Circulation of blood from donor dogs with hyperaldosteronism secondary to thoracic caval constriction through normal isolated adrenals of a recipient (Fig. 1) produced an increase in aldosterone secretion (Fig. 2) (Yankopoulas et al., 1959). When blood was cross-circulated from normal donor dogs through normal isolated adrenals, aldosterone secretion was unchanged. At essentially the same time, an Australian team (Denton et al., 1959) provided similar data from cross-circulation studies with conscious, sodium-depleted sheep as the donors. In the studies in both dogs and sheep, the findings clearly indicated that a new and as yet unidentified humoral agent stimulated aldosterone secretion. Plasma sodium and potassium concentrations were not altered and a causative role of ACTH was excluded. Thus, independently, it was concluded by both groups of workers who used different stimuli in different species that a humoral agent other than ACTH or plasma electrolyte concentrations provides a primary stimulus to the adrenals to increase aldosterone secretion. It was suggested that this humoral agent is a hormone and the term aldosterone-stimulating hormone (ASH) was proposed (Davis, 1959). In addition, at the Laurentian Hormone Conference in 1958, it was reported (Davis, 1959) that ASH is specific for stimulation of aldosterone secretion.

Early Evidence on the Relation of the Kidney and Adrenal Cortex

Many studies in the early fifties suggested a close functional relationship between the kidney and the adrenal cortex. In 1951, Deane and Masson reported that 1) injection of partially purified extracts of rat kidneys produced enlargement of the zona glomerulosa in rats, and 2) encapsulation of one kidney in the rat led to hypertrophy of the zona glomerulosa of the adrenal cortex. In 1953, Hartcroft and Hartroft fed rats a low-salt diet and observed increased granulation of the renal juxtaglomerular (JG) cells. Subsequently, Hartcroft and collaborators (1959) provided convincing evidence in both the rat and the dog that the JG cells are the principal source of renin and that renin has a potent trophic influence on the zona glomerulosa. In 1957, an inverse relationship between the dose of desoxycorticosterone acetate given and the degree of JG cell granulation was found by Dunihue and Robertson. In 1958, Pasqualino and Bourne reported that unilateral renal artery constriction in the rat led to the development of zona glomerulosa hypertrophy with a few days. Also in 1958, Gross postulated an inverse relationship between sodium balance and the secretion of aldosterone from studies of the renin content of the kidney in rats. By 1960, a large amount of evidence (Tobian, 1960) had accumulated on the close functional interrelationships of the degree of granulation of the JG cells, renin and the zona glomerulosa.

Discovery of the Renin-Angiotensin-Aldosterone System

With the realization that a humoral agent is a primary regulator of aldosterone production, researchers took the logical approach of determining the locus of secretion and the chemical nature of ASH. The methods used were classical endocrinological procedures of removal of an organ or ablation of a specific area of the body and observation of the effect on aldosterone secretion and subsequent study of the response to a stimulus adequate to increase aldosterone secretion. Also, extracts of various tissues were given in an effort to replace the deleted hormone. The several organs or regions of the body which were considered as the most likely loci for secretion of ASH included the hypothalamus, other brain stem regions, the pineal gland, the anterior pituitary, the liver and the kidneys. The stimuli used most extensively in an attempt to produce hypersecretion of aldosterone were acute hemorrhage, sodium depletion, and chronic thoracic caval constriction. In addition, several synthetic substances including Ang. II [Car-

PENTER et al., 1961 (1); GANONG et al., 1962], urine (ORTI et al., 1957; MULROW et al., 1959) and lymph (HIGGINS et al., 1964) were tested for aldosterone-stimulating activity.

At essentially the same time that it was discovered that a potent aldosterone-stimulating agent exists (DAVIS, 1959; DENTON et al., 1959), FARRELL (1959) proposed that the pineal gland or some closely associated structure secretes an aldosterone-stimulating substance. He suggested the name glomerulotrophin for the hormone, and later (1960) the term adrenoglomerulotrophin. Farrell (1959) reported that pineal gland extracts stimulated aldosterone secretion with little influence on cortisol production. An attempt (FARRELL and MCISAAC, 1961) at chemical identification of the active agent in these extracts led to the report that the agent had "colorimetric, chromatographic, and fluorometric characteristics" identical to those of 1-methyl-6-methoxy-1,2,3,4-tetrahydro-2-carboline. Others (BLAIR-WEST et al., 1963; MULROW et al., 1963) were unable to confirm their finding that this compound stimulated aldosterone secretion. Ablation studies (DAVIS, 1961) also failed to provide data in support of the FARRELL hypothesis. It seems unlikely from the subsequent studies of aldosterone secretion that either the pineal gland or an associated structure is involved in the regulation of aldosterone secretion. The response to pineal extracts reported by FARRELL in 1960 might have been more apparent than real, or the observed aldosterone-stimulating activity might have reflected the presence of a substance isolated from pineal tissue during the extraction process rather than a physiological substance which is secreted.

In a series of experiments by DAVIS (1960) and DAVIS et al. [1961 (2)], successive ablation of the anterior pituitary, the head, the liver, and the kidneys was performed; aldosterone secretion was measured after removal of the region and again following acute hemorrhage. Hypophysectomy decreased the rate of aldosterone secretion and acute hemorrhage of these animals produced a significant increase in aldosterone output [DAVIS, 1960; DAVIS et al., 1962 (2); MULROW and GANONG, 1961]. Several subsequent studies in hypophysectomized dogs revealed that hypersecretion of aldosterone occurred during superimposed sodium depletion (BINNION et al., 1965), thoracic caval constriction [DAVIS et al., 1961 (1)], low-output heart failure (DAVIS, 1962), or high-output heart failure [DAVIS et al., 1964 (2)]. All these observations suggest an extrapituitary origin of ASH.

The effects of decapitation, hepatectomy, or nephrectomy were studied in this order and all experiments were performed in hypophysectomized dogs. This experimental design was used because the stress of the surgical procedure for cannulation of the adrenal vein increases ACTH secretion and a high plasma level of ACTH could conceivably maintain a high rate of aldosterone secretion even after removal of the locus of secretion of ASH. Decapitation or hepatectomy of hypophysectomized dogs failed to decrease aldosterone secretion and aldosterone output increased in response to acute hemorrhage in both experiments [DAVIS et al., 1961 (2)]. In contrast, removal of the kidneys in hypophysectomized dogs produced a fall in aldosterone secretion and acute blood loss failed to increase aldosterone output [DAVIS et al., 1961 (2); MULROW and GANONG, 1961] (Fig. 3). Injection of saline extracts of kidneys into these hypophysectomized animals produced a striking increase in aldosterone secretion (Fig. 3) [DAVIS, 1960; DAVIS et al., 1961 (2); MULROW and GANONG, 1961]. In a control experiment, injections of similarly prepared saline extracts of liver were without effect [DAVIS et al., 1961 (2)]. It is important to emphasize that the negative evidence from ablation studies of the head, the anterior pituitary, the pineal area and the liver provided strong indirect supporting evidence for the renal origin of ASH.

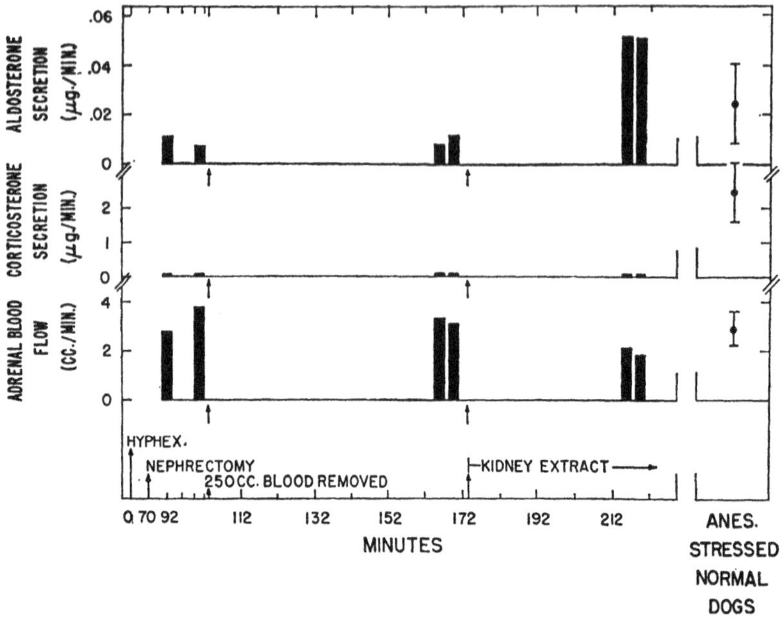

Fig. 3. Effects of hemorrhage and subsequent infusion of a saline extract of kidneys in a hypophysectomized-nephrectomized dog. For comparison, data are presented in the right panel on mean values ± SEM from anesthetized stressed normal dogs. [From DAVIS et al., 1961 (2)]

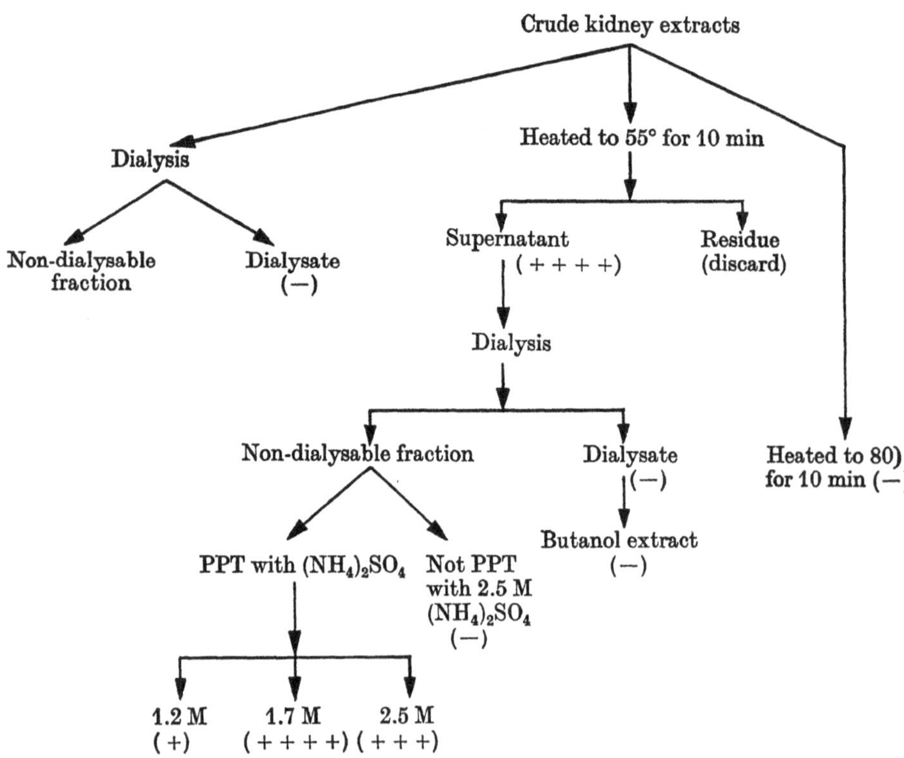

Fig. 4. Fractionation scheme for crude kidney extracts to separate fractions with aldosterone-stimulating and pressor activity. The fractions with (+ + + +) showed the most marked biological activity of both types. (From DAVIS et al., 1962)

At essentially the same time in 1960 that ASH was discovered, GENEST and associates (1960) reported that intravenous infusion of synthetic Ang. II augmented urinary aldosterone excretion in man, and LARAGH and co-workers (1960) found an increased rate of aldosterone secretion during Ang. II infusion to humans. These observations on the steroidogenic activity of Ang. II and the clear-cut evidence for a renal aldosterone-stimulating hormone [DAVIS, 1960; DAVIS et al., 1961 (2)] led to a search for the active agent in kidney extracts (DAVIS et al., 1962). Crude saline extracts of kidney were fractionated with ammonium sulfate and it was found that the two most active fractions for both aldosterone-stimulating and pressor activity were the 1.7 and 2.5 M ammonium sulfate fractions (Fig. 4).These two fractions are known to contain large amounts of renin. Also, heating these kidney extracts to 80 °C. for 10 min, which denatures renin, destroyed all steroidogenic and pressor activity. These findings strongly suggested that ASH and renin were identical. These fractionation studies in 1962 were followed by extensive observations from many laboratories and the findings have clearly demonstrated a fundamental role for the renin-angiotensin system in the control of aldosterone secretion. In retrospect, it is now evident that the humoral aldosterone-stimulating agent (ASH) detected in the early cross-circulation experiments (YANKOPOULAS et al., 1959; DENTON et al., 1959) was Ang. II.

Evidence for the Renin-Angiotensin System as a Primary Mechanism in the Control of Aldosterone Secretion

Pattern of Steroid Response to Ang. II. The pattern of response in adrenal steroid secretion to Ang. II is essentially the same [CARPENTER et al., 1961 (1)] as that observed [DAVIS et al., 1961 (2)] with crude preparations of kidney extracts. A striking increase in aldosterone secretion occurred with small amounts of crude renin preparations or with synthetic Ang. II whereas only slight increments in corticosterone or cortisol secretion were observed; such slight changes in glucocorticoid secretion are probably of no physiological significance. Indeed, in long-term infusion experiments with Ang. II in dogs (URQUHART, 1965), a selective increase in aldosterone secretion was observed with no change in cortisol or corticosterone production. Failure of glucocorticoid secretion to increase in these chronic experiments apparently reflects a negative corticosteroid feedback mechanism mediated by the anterior pituitary (BINNION et al., 1965). A selective steroidogenic action of renin on aldosterone secretion has also been observed in the primitive mammal, the American opossum and in a lower vertebrate, the American bullfrog [JOHNSTON et al., 1967 (1)]. Finally, it should be pointed out that the steroid response to Ang. II is distinctly different from that observed with ACTH; small amounts of ACTH produced a prominent response in 17-hydroxycorticoid output with considerably less effect on aldosterone secretion (Fig. 5, from MULROW and GANONG, 1961).

The observations that large doses of Ang. II increase the secretion of several adrenocortical steroids suggest that this peptide has a biosynthetic action at an early stage in steroidogenesis. *In-vitro* studies on the biosynthesis of aldosterone (cf. MÜLLER, 1971) also indicate that Ang. II acts early in steroidogenesis.

Direct Action of Ang. II on Adrenal Cortex. An important piece of evidence which links the renin-angiotensin system with the adrenal cortex was provided by studies on the metabolic fate of [H^3]-Ang. II (BUMPUS et al., 1964). Following the intravenous injection of this compound, [H^3]-Ang. II was taken up more extensively by the adrenals than by any other organ tested. The radioactive substance in the adrenals had the same electrophoretic mobility as Ang. II. Evidence for a direct action of Ang. II on the adrenal cortex to increase the biosynthesis of aldosterone was obtained by infusion of the octapeptide into the arterial supply of isolated adrenals (Davis, 1962; Ganong et al., 1962). As pointed out above, the direct biosynthetic action of Ang. II on adrenocortical tissue has been repeatedly demonstrated by *in-vitro* studies (cf. Müller, 1971).

Effects of Nephrectomy and Saline Extracts of Kidneys in Experimental Secondary Aldosteronism. The important role of the renin-angiotensin system in the pathogenesis of experimental hyperaldosteronism was obtained from studies of dogs with chronic sodium depletion, chronic thoracic caval constriction, experimental low-output failure, experimental high-output failure (Davis et al., 1961, 1962, 1964). Removal of the kidneys in hypophysectomized dogs with hyperaldosteronism secondary to these experimental manipulations produced a striking fall in

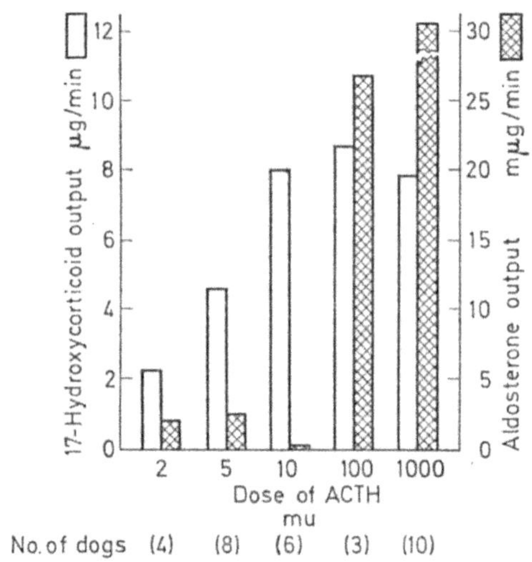

Fig. 5. Effects of ACTH on aldosterone and 17-hydroxycorticoid output in dogs. (From Mulrow and Ganong, 1961)

aldosterone secretion, and a selective increase in aldosterone secretion occurred in response to the saline extracts from the kidneys of the same nephrectomized dogs.

Effects of Prolonged Infusion of Ang. II. In sheep, Blair-West and associates [1962 (2)] reported that tachyphylaxis developed in response to aldosterone synthesis within 3 to 10 h. In contrast, in the dog Urquhart et al. (1963) found that Ang. II increased urinary aldosterone excretion for 11 days of infusion even with non-pressor doses. Also, in man, Laragh and associates (Laragh et al., 1962, 1964) have repeatedly demonstrated that infusions of Ang. II increased aldosterone secretion without evidence of tachyphylaxis for as long as 11 days. And, as mentioned earlier, Urquhart (1965) administered Ang. II to dogs by i.v. infusion and observed an increase in aldosterone secretion which lasted for 8 days. These results from chronic infusion studies in both dog and man are consistent with the view that the renin-angiotensin-aldosterone system is an important homeostatic mechanism in the control of salt and water metabolism and body-fluid volume.

Evidence from Renal Renin Content, JG Cells and the Pressor Response to Ang. II. A marked increase in the renin content of the kidneys was observed in dogs with hyperaldosteronism secondary to thoracic caval constriction, and the renal JG cells were hypergranulated and hyperplastic (DAVIS et al., 1962). In addition, in rats with nephrosis produced by amino-nucleoside, a high positive correlation was observed between the degree of JG-cell granulation and the extent of sodium retention (TOBIAN et al., 1962). The arterial pressure response to an intravenous injection or infusion of Ang. II was found to be markedly reduced in dogs with hyperaldosteronism secondary to thoracic caval constriction (DAVIS et al., 1962), sodium depletion (DAVIS et al., 1962), or high-output failure from an A-V fistula [DAVIS et al., 1964 (1)]. The blood pressure response to Ang. II was reduced in patients with cirrhosis of the liver (LARAGH et al., 1962). These observations have been interpreted as reflecting an increased plasma level of Ang. II, and in patients with hypertensive disease, a decreased pressor response to synthetic Ang. II has been used as a screening test for the presence of increased activity of the renin-angiotensin system.

Effects of Antibodies on Renin Preparations, on Aldosterone Secretion and Sodium Excretion. Studies with antisera and preparations of renin have provided evidence consistent with a role of the renin-angiotensin system in the control of aldosterone secretion. Passive transfer of antisera produced by injection of crude preparations of renin into sodium-depleted dogs was followed by an increase in sodium excretion (HARTCROFT, 1963). GANONG and associates (1963) found that both the aldosterone-stimulating and pressor activities of dog and hog renin preparations were inhibited by incubation with plasma from dogs immunized with hog renin. Also, the response in aldosterone secretion to suprarenal aortic constriction was partially blocked by immunization of dogs with hog renin (GANONG et al., 1963). One of the limitations of this type of evidence is that crude renin preparations were used and the specificity of the antigen is uncertain.

Plasma-Renin Activity and Plasma Ang. II in Secondary Aldosteronism. One of the most convincing lines of evidence for the pathogenic role of the renin-angiotensin system in hyperaldosteronism was provided by analysis of renal vein or peripheral venous plasma or lymph for renin or Ang. II. The first indication that increased secretion of renin occurs in heart failure was the report of MERRILL and associates in 1946 of a high renin concentration in renal vein blood. During the last decade, many reports of studies on patients and animals with different types of secondary aldosteronism have demonstrated increased plasma-renin activity or Ang. II. The situations include 1) decompensated hepatic cirrhosis, 2) thoracic caval constriction, 3) low sodium intake or sodium depletion, 4) low- and high-output cardiac failure, 5) the nephrotic syndrome, 6) pregnancy, 7) some cases with renal artery stenosis and hypertensive disease, 8) patients with parenchymatous kidney disease and hypertension, 9) acute experimental renal hypertension, 10) hypertension secondary to constriction of one renal artery but in the presence of both kidneys in rats, and 11) following acute hemorrhage (cf. DAVIS, 1967). Increased amounts of renin were found in renal lymph following acute renal artery stenosis in dogs (LEVER and PEART, 1962) and in thoracic duct lymph in dogs with chronic thoracic caval constriction (HIGGINS et al., 1964).

Comparative Physiology of the Renin-Angiotensin-Aldosterone System. It is abundantly clear that the renin-angiotensin system is very important in the pathogenesis of hyperaldosteronism in disease but it has been difficult to obtain evidence on the extent of its importance in homeostasis. During the past decade, the methodology has been inadequate to evaluate the renin-angiotensin-aldosterone system in homeostasis. With the development of the radioimmunoassay for aldosterone and Ang. II, data on this important problem may soon become available. In the meantime, extensive studies of the comparative physiology of the renin-angiotensin system and aldosterone secretion have been made to obtain evidence which has a bearing on the role of this system in homeostasis. It has been suggested [DAVIS, 1971 (1)] that if the renin-angiotensin system controls aldosterone secretion in primitive mammals and in lower vertebrates and, therefore, if this relationship is a fundamental one phylogenetically, then surely it is of importance in homeostasis in man.

The presence of renin or a renin-like substance has been reported in several species of marine teleosts [cf. DAVIS, 1971 (1)], and JG cells which contain intracellular granules similar to those observed in higher mammals have been described in fish (CONNEL and KALEY, 1964). There is convincing evidence for a renal-pressor system in the eel (CHESTER-JONES et al., 1966) and it resembles the renin-angiotensin system in mammals. Renin extracted from carp kidney produced a striking increasing in aldosterone and corticosterone secretion and pressor activity when injected into the American bullfrog (TAYLOR and DAVIS, 1971).

The most extensive studies of the renin-angiotensin-aldosterone system in lower vertebrates have been made in amphibia. Frog renin infused intravenously into the American bullfrog increased aldosterone, corticosterone and desoxycorticosterone secretion and arterial pressure [JOHNSTON et al., 1967 (1); TAYLOR, 1971]. The frog renin preparation had characteristics similar to mammalian renin. Evidence for a functional renin-angiotensin-aldosterone system was obtained from the observations that both chronic sodium depletion (ULICK and FEINHOLTZ, 1968; BRAVERMAN and DAVIS, 1972) and acute postcaval vein constriction (BRAVERMAN and DAVIS, 1972) increased aldosterone secretion in the bullfrog.

In the fresh-water turtle (Pseudyms sueanniensis) (NOTHSTINE et al., 1971) and in the chicken (Gallus domesticus) (TAYLOR et al ., 1970) there is evidence for a renal-pressor system with characteristics similar to the renin-angiotensin system in man. The concentrations of steroids in postcaval vein plasma were so low that only corticosterone was detected in the turtle; and in the chicken, although aldosterone was detected in the adrenal effluent, the concentration was too low for the studies with injected renin to be meaningful.

Finally, in the North American opossum, there is evidence for a renin-angiotensin-aldosterone system which appears similar in every way studied to that present in dog and man [JOHNSTON et al., 1967 (2)].

There is evidence, therefore, that the renin-angiotensin-aldosterone system is phylogenetically deep-seated and that it is functional in a lower vertebrate, the American bullfrog, and in a primitive mammal, the North American opossum. This indirect evidence supports the view that the renin-angiotensin system is important in homeostasis throughout the vertebrate kingdom. And, therefore, these studies of comparative physiology add evidence to the observations in humans during altered sodium intake, changes in posture and during pregnancy that the renin-angiotensin-aldosterone system is an important homeostatic mechanism.

A Negative-Feedback Mechanism in the Control of Aldosterone Secretion

Shortly after the discovery of the renin-angiotensin-aldosterone system in 1960, it was suggested that it functions as a negative-feedback mechanism. Evidence continues to accumulate to support this concept and the principal components of the renin-angiotensin-aldosterone system are presented in Fig. 6. Two intrarenal receptors, 1) the so-called baroreceptor in the renal afferent arterioles and 2) the macula densa, perceive signals which lead to renin release by the JG cells. It seems likely that the vascular receptor in the afferent arterioles responds to changes in wall tension (BLAINE and DAVIS, 1971). In this event, the receptor probably operates from a set point determined by several different inputs which influence afferent arteriolar wall tension. The possible inputs include 1) the transmural pressure gradient, 2) nervous influences which are mediated by the renal sympathetic nerves, 3) elastic components of the vessel wall, and 4) myogenic and autoregulatory mechanisms within the arterioles. It has been proposed that the macula densa responds to changes in sodium load or sodium concentration in renal tubule fluid [cf. DAVIS, 1971 (2)] or to a change in sodium transport by the macula densa cells (VANDER and CARLSON, 1969). It was suggested that decreased sodium load at the macula densa or decreased sodium transport increased renin release whereas THURAU and associates (1967) proposed that increased sodium concentration augmented renin secretion. Additional studies are needed to define what the macula densa does perceive and how this message is delivered to the JG cells.

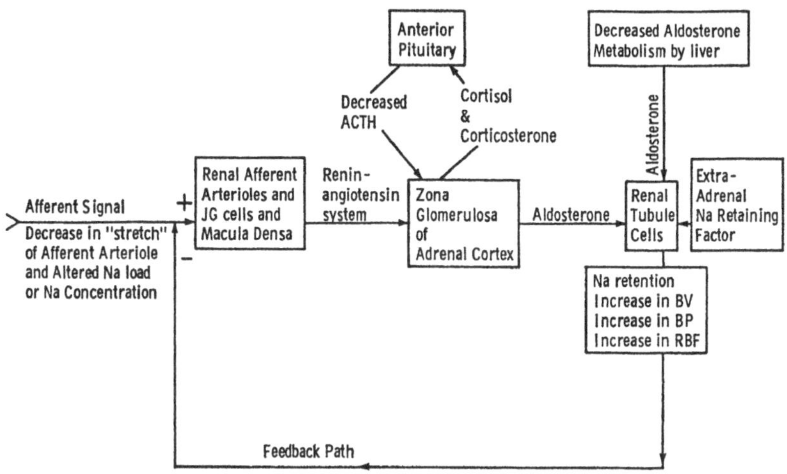

Fig. 6. Negative-feedback diagram to explain the renin-angiotensin-aldosterone system. (From Chapter in the Physiology Handbook on "The Regulation of Aldosterone Secretion", Amer. Physiol. Soc., 1972)

Furthermore, the role of each of these receptors in homeostasis and their relative dominance in pathophysiological situations remains to be defined. For simplicity the roles of the renal nerves and of certain humoral agents as epinephrine and norepinephrine on renin release have been omitted from the feedback diagram. The afferent signals to the vascular receptor in the renal afferent arterioles and to the macula densa which lead to renin release are provided by a decrease in renal arterial pressure and/or renal blood flow. Renin is secreted into the lumen of the renal afferent arterioles and into renal lymph. Increased amounts of renin have been found in renal (LEVER and PEART, 1962) and thoracic duct lymph (HIGGINS et al., 1964) in association with increased renin secretion in blood. In blood and lymph, renin acts on renin-substrate, a tetradecapeptide secreted by the liver, to produce Ang. I, a decapeptide. Ang. I is converted almost quantitatively to the octapeptide, Ang. II, by converting enzyme as blood passes through the lungs; there is also a slow rate of conversion throughout the circulation and in the lymphatic system. As pointed out earlier, Ang. II acts directly on the zona glomerulosa to stimulate the biosynthesis of aldosterone. Initially, an acute increase in cortisol and corticosterone secretion also occurs if the plasma level of

Ang. II is high (Binnion et al., 1965). It was proposed by Binnion et al. (1965) that the initial increase in glucocorticoid output is reduced by a negative corticosteroid feedback mechanism by way of the anterior pituitary so that the plasma level of these glucocorticoids returns to normal. According to this hypothesis, the mechanism controlling ACTH release is adjusted so that less circulating ACTH is present. Thus, in chronic secondary aldosteronism, the glucocorticoid output is normal and increased plasma aldosterone results from increased aldosterone secretion secondary to a high plasma level of Ang. II.

A decreased rate of aldosterone metabolism also contributes to the high plasma level of aldosterone in certain types of secondary aldosteronism (Davis et al., 1965). The liver is the principal site for metabolism of aldosterone and the rate of hepatic blood flow is the primary determinant of aldosterone metabolism. A change in posture from the supine to the upright position reduced hepatic blood flow by about 50% (Culbertson et al., 1951) and the rate of aldosterone metabolism was approximately halved (Bougas et al., 1964); as a result the plasma level of aldosterone doubled. In several clinical conditions and in certain experimental situations, the rate of aldosterone metabolism is reduced with a resultant increase in the plasma concentration of aldosterone. These conditions include acute hemorrhage (Davis et al., 1965), experimental low- and high-output heart failure (Davis et al., 1965), experimental hepatic venous congestion (Ayers et al., 1962), and low-output heart failure in man (Camargo et al., 1965). In all these situations, hepatic blood flow is reduced and the rate of aldosterone metabolism appears to be controlled by a flow-limited system (Bougas et al., 1964; Davis et al., 1965).

The mechanisms by which a high plasma level of aldosterone exerts a negative feedback action to decrease renin release or aldosterone secretion have been investigated extensively. Aldosterone does not act directly on either the adrenal cortex (Davis, 1962; Ganong et al., 1962) or on the JG cells (Geelhoed and Vander, 1967). Intravenous infusion of aldosterone with a substantial elevation in the plasma level of the hormone failed influence the rate of aldosterone secretion [Blair-West et al., 1962 (1)]. Instead, aldosterone acts on the distal tubule to promote sodium reabsorption which leads to a sequence of changes that indirectly decrease aldosterone biosynthesis.

Retention of salt and water by the kidneys is dependent upon the presence of an additional factor which acts in association with aldosterone. This factor has been called the extra-adrenal sodium-retaining factor [Davis et al., 1964 (2)]. In normal animals, including man, retained fluid increases the circulating blood volume, arterial pressure, renal blood flow and the rate of glomerular filtration. Both intrarenal receptors, the vascular receptor and the macula densa, might be stimulated. Thus, this increase in body-fluid volume and the changes secondary to it lead to decreased renin release by the negative feedback loop depicted in Fig. 6.

The Renin-Angiotensin System in Various Types of Secondary Aldosteronism

Hemorrhage. It is now clear that both the renin-angiotensin system and ACTH are important in the hypersecretion of aldosterone following hemorrhage. The early finding that acute hemorrhage increased aldosterone secretion in hypophysectomized dogs (Davis et al., 1961 (2); Mulrow and Ganong, 1961] was later recognized as a reflection of increased activity of the renin-angiotensin system. There are now many reports (cf. Blaine et al., 1971) on the striking increase in renin release following hemorrhage. Acute blood loss increases renal sympathetic nerve activity, releases epinephrine and norepinephrine from the adrenal medulla, decreases the filtered load of sodium and leads to renal arteriolar constriction as evidenced by decreased renal blood flow; all these changes are possible factors contributing to increased renin release. Also, hemorrhage decreases hepatic blood flow which in turn decreases the rates of metabolism of both renin (JOHNSON et al., 1971) and aldosterone (DAVIS et al., 1965) and increases the plasma levels of these hormones. In terms of the feedback diagram (Fig. 6), the feedback loop is not opened, so that compensation occurs as soon as adequate retention of salt and water is accomplished. As fluid is retained, blood volume, blood pressure and renal blood flow are restored to normal and renin secretion decreases.

Thoracic Caval Constriction. This intervention decreases cardiac output and, if severe enough, arterial pressure (DAVIS and HOWELL, 1953). Renal blood flow is consistently decreased and, occasionally, GFR is low (DAVIS and HOWELL, 1953). It appears, therefore, that both the renal vascular receptor and the macula densa are stimulated especially if the cardiovascular changes are marked. Renin secretion is increased, aldosterone production is augmented, salt and water are retained by the kidneys and expansion of the extracellular fluid volume occurs. Decreased hepatic blood flow is another consistent finding following thoracic caval constriction, and this leads to decreased aldosterone metabolism which contributes to the high plasma level of the hormone (DAVIS et al., 1965). This expansion of body fluid volume is distributed abnormally as ascites or edema rather than throughout the entire vascular system as in the normal state, and the retained fluid fails to provide the signal to the kidneys to reduce the rate of renin secretion. Therefore, the control system functions as an "open-loop" system, increased renin secretion continues and the extracellular fluid becomes increasingly large.

Congestive Heart Failure. In this syndrome, the heart fails to pump enough blood to the tissues for normal function to occur. The absolute level of cardiac output may be low, as in classical low-output failure, or high (above the normal cardiac index of 3.2 $l/min/M^2$), even though the amount perfusing the tissues is inadequate for normal functioning. In either low- or high-output failure, there is a marked reduction in renal blood flow. The subsequent changes and factors operative in congestive failure are very similar to those in thoracic caval constriction except that they vary with the degree of the myocardial failure. If cardiac failure is slight, instead of an "open-loop" system as in caval constriction, there is a reduction of gain in the functional components which lead to increased renin release. If the compensatory mechanisms become adequate, the signal perceived by the kidney to promote increased renin release ceases to occur and renin secretion declines toward or even to the normal rate. In this event, plasma aldosterone has been observed to be elevated in patients with a slight or moderate degree of failure as a result of only one mechanism, namely, decreased aldosterone metabolism by the liver (CAMARGO et al., 1965). Thus, in congestive heart failure the renin-angiotensin-aldosterone system is activated to different degrees dependent upon the severity of the failure.

Summary and Conclusions

The renin-angiotensin system is one of the primary mechanisms in the control of aldosterone secretion. The renin-angiotensin-aldosterone system is present in lower vertebrates and primitive mammals and appears to be important in both homeostasis and disease. There is evidence that the renin-angiotensin-aldosterone system functions as a negative feedback mechanism and the components of this system have been described. The changes in the renin-angiotensin system and aldosterone secretion during hemorrhage, caval constriction and congestive heart failure have been described in terms of the negative-feedback hypothesis.

References

AYERS, C. R., DAVIS, J. O., LIEBERMAN, F., CARPENTER, C. C. J., BERMAN, M.: The effects of chronic hepatic venous congestion on the metabolism of d,1-aldosterone and d-aldosterone. J. clin. Invest. **41**, 884 (1962).

BINNION, P. F., DAVIS, J. O., BROWN, T. C., OLICHNEY, M. J.: Mechanisms regulating aldosterone secretion during sodium depletion. Amer. J. Physiol. **208**, 655 (1965).

BLAINE, E. H., DAVIS, J. O.: Evidence for a renal vascular mechanism in renin release: New observations with graded stimulation by aortic constriction. Circulat. Res. **28** and **29**, II—118 (1971).

BLAIR-WEST, J., COGHLAN, J. P., DENTON, D. A.: (1) Evidence against an aldosterone feedback mechanism within the adrenal gland. Acta Endocr. (Kbh.) **41**, 61 (1962).

BLAIR-WEST, J., COGHLAN, J. P., DENTON, D. A., GODING, J. R., MUNROE, J. A., PETERSON, R. E., WINTOUR, M.: (2) Humoral stimulation of adrenal cortical secretion. J. clin. Invest. **41**, 1606 (1962).

BLAIR-WEST, J. R., COGHLAN, J. P., DENTON, D. A., GODING, J. R., WINTOUR, M., WRIGHT, R. D.: The control of aldosterone secretion. Recent Progr. Hormone Res. **19**, 311 (1963).

BOUGAS, J., FLOOD, C., LITTLE, B., TAIT, J. F., TAIT, S. A. S., UNDERWOOD, R.: Dynamic aspects of aldosterone metabolism. In: Aldosterone. Oxford: Blackwell Scientific Publications 1964.

BRAVERMAN, B., DAVIS, J. O.: Effects of sodium depletion and postcaval vein constriction on adrenal steroid secretion in the bullfrog (abstract). Fed. Proc. (1972) (in press).

BUMPUS, F. M., SMEBY, R. R., PAGE, I. H., KHAIRALLAH, P. A.: Distribution and metabolic fate of angiotensin II and various derivatives. Canad. med. Ass. J. **90**, 190 (1964).

CAMARGO, C. A., DOWDY, A. J., HANCOCK, E. W., LUETSCHER, J. A.: Decreased plasma clear. ance and hepatic extraction of aldosterone in patients with heart failure. J. clin. Invest- **44**, 356 (1965).

CARPENTER, C. C. J., DAVIS, J. O., AYERS, C. R.: (1) Relation of renin, angiotensin II and experimental renal hypertension to aldosterone secretion. J. clin. Invest. **40**, 2026 (1961).

CARPENTER, C. C. J., DAVIS, J. O., HOLMAN, J. E., AYERS, C. R., BAHN, R. C.: (2) Studies on the response of the transplanted kidney and the transplanted adrenal gland to thoracic inferior vena caval constriction. J. clin. Invest. **40**, 196 (1961).

CHESTER-JONES, I., HENDERSON, I. W., CHAN, D. K. O., RANKIN, J. C., MOSLEY, W., BROWN, J. J., LEVER, A. F., ROBERTSON, J. I. S., TREE, M.: Pressor activity in extracts of the corpuscles of Stannius from the European eel *(Anguilla anguilla L.)*. J. Endocr. **34**, 393 (1966).

CONNEL, G. M., KALEY, G.: Evidence for the presence of "renin" in the kidneys of marine fish and amphibia. Biol. Bull. **127**, 366 (1964).

CULBERTSON, J. W., WILKINS, R. W., INGELFINGER, F. J., BRADLEY, S. E.: The effect of the upright position upon hepatic blood flow in normotensive and hypertensive subjects. J. clin. Invest. **30**, 305 (1951).

DAVIS, J. O.: Discussion on pp. 298—304 to paper by G. FARRELL on Recent progress in hormone research, Vol. 15. New York: Academic Press 1959.

DAVIS, J. O.: Evidence for secretion of an aldosterone-stimulating hormone by the kidney. Presented at a Symposium at the First International Congress of Endocrinology, Copenhagen 1960.

DAVIS, J. O.: Mechanisms regulating the secretion and metabolism of aldosterone in experimental secondary hyperaldosteronism. Recent Progr. Hormone Res. **17**, 293 (1961).

DAVIS, J. O.: Adrenocortical and renal hormonal function in experimental cardiac failure. Circulation **25**, 1002 (1962).

DAVIS, J. O.: The regulation of aldosterone secretion. In: The Adrenal Cortex (EISENSTEIN, A., Ed.). Boston: Little, Brown and Company (Inc.) 1967.

DAVIS, J. O.: (1) The renin-angiotensin system in the control of aldosterone secretion. In: Kidney Hormones (FISHER, J. W., Ed.). New York: Academic Press 1971.

DAVIS, J. O.: (2) What signals the kidney to release renin? Circulat. Res. **28**, 301 (1971).

DAVIS, J. O., AYERS, C. R., CARPENTER, C. C. J.: (1) Renal origin of an aldosterone-stimulating hormone in dogs with thoracic caval constriction and in sodium-depleted dogs. J. clin. Invest. **40**, 1466 (1961).

DAVIS, J. O., CARPENTER, C. C. J., AYERS, C. R., HOLMAN, J. E., BAHN, R. C.: (2) Evidence for secretion of an aldosterone-stimulating hormone by the kidney. J. clin. Invest. **40**, 684 (1961).

DAVIS, J. O., HARTCROFT, P. M., TITUS, E. O., CARPENTER, C. C. J., AYERS, C. R., SPIEGEL, H. E.: The role of the renin-angiotensin system in the control of aldosterone secretion. J. clin. Invest. **41**, 378 (1962).

DAVIS, J. O., HOLMAN, J. E., CARPENTER, C. C. J., URQUHART, J., HIGGINS, J. T., Jr.: (2) An extra-adrenal factor essential for renal sodium retention in the presence of increased sodium-retaining hormone. Circulat. Res. **14**, 17 (1964).

DAVIS, J. O., HOWELL, D. S.: Comparative effect of ACTH, cortisone and DCA on renal function, electrolyte excretion and water exchange in normal dogs. Endocrinology **52**, 245 (1953).

DAVIS, J. O., OLICHNEY, M. J., BROWN, T. C., BINNION, P. F.: Metabolism of aldosterone in several experimental situations with altered aldosterone secretion. J. clin. Invest. **44**, 1433 (1965).

DAVIS, J. O., URQUHART, J., HIGGINS, J. T., RUBIN, E. C., HARTROFT, P. M.: (1) Hypersecretion of aldosterone in dogs with a chronic aortic-caval fistula and high output heart failure. Circulat. Res. **14**, 471 (1964).

DEANE, H. W., MASSON, G. M. C.: Adrenal cortical changes in rats with various types of experimental hypertension. J. clin. Endocr. **11**, 193 (1951).

DENTON, D. A., GODING, J. R., WRIGHT, R. D.: Control of adrenal secretion of electrolyte-active steroids. Brit. Med. J. **1959 II**, 447.

DUNIHUE, F. W., ROBERTSON, M. V. B.: The effect of desoxycorticosterone acetate and of sodium on the juxtaglomerular apparatus. Endocrinilogy **61**, 293 (1957).

FARRELL, G.: The physiological factors which influence the secretion of aldosterone. Recent Progr. Hormone Res. **15**, 275 (1959).

FARRELL, G.: Adrenoglomerulotropin. Circulation **21**, 1009 (1960).

FARRELL, G., MCISAAC, W. M.: Adrenoglomerulotropin. Arch. Biochem. **94**, 543 (1961).

FLEMING, R., FARRELL, G.: Aldosterone and hydrocortisone secretion by the denervated adrenal. Endocrinology **59**, 360 (1956).

GANONG, W. F., MULROW, P. J., BORYCZKA, A., CERA, A.: Evidence for a direct effect of angiotensin II on adrenal cortex of the dog. Proc. Soc. exp. Biol. (N. Y.) **109**, 381 (1962).

GANONG, W. F., VAN BRUNT, E. E., LEE, T. C., MULROW, P. J.: Inhibition of aldosterone-stimulating activity of hog and dog renin by the plasma of dogs immunized with hog renin. Proc. Soc. exp. Biol. (N. Y.) **112**, 1062 (1963).

GEELHOED, G. W., VANDER, A. J.: The role of aldosterone in renin secretion. Life Sci. **6**, 525 (1967).

GENEST, J. E., KOIW, E., NOWACZYNSKI, W., SANDOR, T.: Study of urinary adrenocortical hormones in human arterial hypertension (abstract). First International Congress of Endocrinology, Copenhagen 1960.

GROSS, F.: Renin und Hypertension, physiologische oder pathologische Wirkstoffe? Klin. Wschr. **36**, 693 (1958).

HARTROFT, P. M.: Histological and functional aspects of juxtaglomerular cells. In: Angiotensin systems and experimental renal diseases (METCOFF, J., Ed.). Boston: Little, Brown and Company (Inc.) 1963.

HARTROFT, P. M., HARTROFT, W. S.: Studies on renal juxtaglomerular cells: I. Variations produced by sodium chloride, and desoxycorticosterone acetate. J. exp. Med. **97**, 415 (1953).

HARTROFT, P. M., NEWMARK, L. N., PITCOCK, J. A.: Relationship of renal juxtaglomerular cells to sodium intake, adrenal cortex and hypertension. In: Hypertension (MOYER, J., Ed.). Philadelphia: W. B. Saunders 1959.

HIGGINS, J. T., Jr., DAVIS, J. O., URQUHART, J.: Demonstration by pressor and steroidogenic assays of increased renin in lymph of dogs with secondary hyperaldosteronism. Circulat. Res. **14**, 218 (1964).

JOHNSON, J. A., DAVIS, J. O., BAUMBER, J. S., SCHNEIDER, E. G.: Effects of hemorrhage and chronic sodium depletion on hepatic clearance of renin. Amer. J. Physiol. **220**, 1677 (1971).

JOHNSTON, C. I., DAVIS, J. O., HARTROFT, P. M.: (2) Renin-angiotensin system, adrenal steroids and sodium depletion in a primitive mammal, the American opossum. Endocrinology **81**, 633 (1967).

JOHNSTON, C. I., DAVIS, J. O., WRIGHT, F. W., HOWARDS, S. S.: (1) Effects of renin and ACTH on adrenal steroid secretion in the American bullfrog. Amer. J. Physiol. **213**, 393 (1967).

LARAGH, J. H.: Interrelationships between angiotensin, norepinephrine, epinephrine, aldosterone secretion, and electrolyte metabolism in man. Circulation **25**, 203 (1962).

LARAGH, J. H., ANGERS, M., KELLY, W. G., LIEBERMAN, S.: The effect of epinephrine, norepinephrine, angiotensin II, and others on the secretory rate of aldosterone in man. J. Amer. med. Ass. **174**, 234 (1960).

LARAGH, J. H., CANNON, P. J., AMES, R. P.: Interaction between aldosterone secretion, sodium and potassium balance, and angiotensin activity in man: Studies in hypertension and cirrhosis. Canad. med. Ass. J. **90**, 248 (1964).

LEVER, A. F., PEART, W. S.: Renin and angiotensin-like activity in renal lymph. J. Physiol. **160**, 548 (1962).

LEVY, L. E., BLALOCK, A.: A method for transplanting the adrenal gland of the dog with re-establishment of its blood supply. Ann. Surg. **109**, 84 (1939).
MERRILL, A. J., MORRISON, J. L., BRANNON, E. S.: Concentration of renin in renal venous blood in patients with chronic heart failure. Amer. J. Med. **1**, 468 (1946).
MULROW, P. J., GANONG, W. F.: The effect of hemorrhage upon aldosterone secretion in normal and hypophysectomized dogs. J. clin. Invest. **40**, 579 (1961).
MULROW, P. J., GANONG, W. F., BORYCZKA, A.: Further evidence for a role of the renin-angiotensin system in regulation of aldosterone secretion. Proc. Soc. exp. Biol. (N. Y.) **112**, 7 (1963).
MULROW, P. J., SHMAGRANOFF, G. L., LIEBERMAN, A. H., SLADE, C. I., LUETSCHER, J. A.: Stimulation of rat adrenocortical secretion by a factor present in human urine. Endocrinology **64**, 631 (1959).
NOTHSTINE, S. A., DAVIS, J. O., DEROOS, R. M.: Kidney extracts and ACTH on adrenal steroid secretion in a turtle and a crocodilian. Amer. J. Physiol. **221**, 726 (1971).
ORTI, E., RALLI, E. P., LAKEN, B., DUMM, M. E.: Presence of an aldosterone stimulating substance in the urine of rats deprived of salt. Amer. J. Physiol. **191**, 323 (1957).
PASQUALINO, A., BOURNE, G. H.: Chemical changes in kidneys and adrenals of rats made hypertensive by the Goldblatt method. Nature (Lond.) **182**, 1426 (1958).
TAYLOR, A. A.: Control of desoxycorticosterone secretion in the bullfrog and the dog. Ph. D. Dissertation, University of Missouri, 1971.
TAYLOR, A. A., DAVIS, J. O.: Effects of carp kidney extracts and angiotensin II on adrenal steroid secretion. Amer. J. Physiol. **221**, 652 (1971).
TAYLOR, A. A., DAVIS, J. O., BREITENBACH, R. P., HARTROFT, P. M.: Adrenal steroid secretion and a renal-pressor system in the chicken *(Gallus domesticus)*. Gen. and Comp. Endocrinology **14**, 321 (1970).
THURAU, K., SCHNERMANN, J., NAGEL, W., HORSTER, M., WOHL, M.: Composition of tubular fluid in the macula densa segment as a factor regulating the function of the juxtaglomerular apparatus. Circulat. Res. **21** (Suppl. II), 79 (1967).
TOBIAN, L.: Interrelationship of electrolytes, juxtaglomerular cells and hypertension. Physiol. Rev. **40**, 280 (1960).
TOBIAN, L., PERRY, S., MORK, J.: The relationship of the juxtaglomerular apparatus to sodium retention in experimental nephrosis. Ann. intern. Med. **57**, 382 (1962).
ULICK, S., FEINHOLTZ, E.: Metabolism and rate of secretion of aldosterone in the bullfrog. J. clin. Invest. **47**, 2523 (1968).
URQUHART, J.: Selective stimulation of aldosterone secretion by angiotensin II in intact dogs (abstract). Forty-seventh meeting of the Endocrine Society, p. 62 (1965).
URQUHART, J., DAVIS, J. O., HIGGINS, J. T., Jr.: Effects of prolonged infusion of angiotensin II in normal dogs. Amer. J. Physiol. **205**, 1241 (1963).
VANDER, A. J., CARLSON, J.: Mechanism of the effects of furosemide on renin secretion in anesthetized dogs. Circulat. Res. **25**, 145 (1969).
YANKOPOULAS, N. A., DAVIS, J. O., KLIMAN, B., PETERSON, R. E.: Evidence that a humoral agent stimulates the adrenal cortex to secrete aldosterone in experimental secondary hyperaldosteronism. J. clin. Invest. **38**, 1278 (1959).

Aldosterone Regulation in Sodium Deficiency: Role of Ionic Factors and Angiotensin II

J. R. Blair-West, J. P. Coghlan, D. A. Denton and B. A. Scoggins

With 7 Figures

A. Format

This section describes the biosynthetic control of aldosterone secretion by reference to studies of humoral factors which affect aldosterone production *in vivo* and *in vitro*. The model thus built up is concerned with the processes most likely to be involved during sodium depletion. For example, Ang. II and ionic factors are considered in detail whilst the action of ACTH is treated only briefly and serotonin is only mentioned. The biosynthetic summary is then used to examine the control of aldosterone during sodium deficiency with particular attention to the role of ionic factors and the question of whether the renin-angiotensin system is the major regulator of aldosterone secretion in sodium deficiency.

B. Introduction

Changes of body sodium or potassium balance, change of posture, pregnancy, blood loss and perhaps emotional stress are naturally occurring events that affect aldosterone secretion (Coghlan and Blair-West, 1967). Sodium deprivation, or sodium depletion by uncompensated loss of natural secretions or by the use of saliuretics, potassium loading, haemorrhage, constriction of the thoracic inferior vena cava, arterio-venous fistula and surgical trauma are some of the procedures used in experiments to investigate the mechanism of increased aldosterone secretion. High aldosterone is also seen in several pathological states, particularly those involving the kidney, e.g. "salt-wasting" diseases, nephrosis, malignant hypertension, some cases of renovascular hypertension and "Bartter's syndrome", as well as diseases of other organs such as hepatic cirrhosis. In addition there are the diseases of the adrenal cortex itself, notably primary hyperaldosteronism and bilateral hyperplasias of uncertain aetiology.

These subjects have been reviewed by Davis (1967, 1971), by Coghlan and Blair-West (1967) and Coghlan et al. (1971) and, more recently, by Muller (1971) in the form of a comparison with *in-vitro* studies of aldosterone production. It is important to keep in mind that detailed findings have been made in only four species, man, dog, sheep and rat. There are substantial inconsistencies in the data from the four species (see below), perhaps due as much to different methods of investigation as to any real interspecies differences. Studies of the North American and Australian marsupials suggest that aldosterone-secretion rate varies with sodium status and the presence of a renin-angiotensin system has also been demonstrated [Johnston et al., 1967; Blair-West et al., 1968 (1); Reid and McDonald, 1969; Scoggins et al., 1970]. However, investigation of mechanisms of sodium homeostasis by organ ablations, hormone infusions and measurements of hormones in blood under physiological conditions has only begun in marsupial species. The need to apply these approaches before any conclusions are drawn concerning the control system has been well demonstrated by the results of experimentation in the rat. It appears possible that the regulation of aldosterone in sodium deficiency in the rat (LEE and DE WIED, 1968; KINSON and SINGER, 1968; PALMORE et al., 1972) differs from the mechanism operative in other species. There may be substantial variation amongst eutherian mammals in the relative importance of the pituitary, renal and ionic pathways in the control of aldosterone secretion. Differences between species would raise the question of whether there is a simple system for aldosterone biosynthesis and, at the same time, emphasize the value of a comparative approach to unravel this complex system.

This chapter is primarily concerned with the control of aldosterone secretion in sodium deficiency.

C. Factors with Direct Action on Aldosterone Secretion

Four *humoral* changes have been shown to stimulate aldosterone secretion *in vivo* and the same factors affect aldosterone production *in vitro*, although there are large quantitative differences in different preparations and species. These changes are increased concentration of angiotensin II, ACTH, and potassium, and reduced concentration of sodium.

1. ACTH

The data on ACTH is extensive and it has been reviewed recently by MULLER (1971). In relation to its role in sodium deficiency the four points below are most relevant: I. Infusions of ACTH, or stresses causing ACTH release, may stimulate aldosterone secretion but usually glucocorticoid secretion is simultaneously elevated unless it is already maximal; II. The increase of aldosterone secretion caused by sodium deficiency is not associated with any substantial rise in glucocorticoid secretion or, presumably, ACTH release; III. The aldosterone response to the stimulus of sodium depletion may be reduced after hypophysectomy or when pituitary function is impaired. The effect may not be a rigorous test of the contribution of ACTH to aldosterone secretion in response to sodium deficiency. In the rat there is evidence for a pituitary factor, other than ACTH, which affects the response to sodium deficiency (PALMORE and MULROW, 1967; LEE and DE WIED, 1968); also GANONG et al. [1967 (1)] found that the reduced aldosterone responsiveness of hypophysectomized dogs was not seen in intact dogs when ACTH was suppressed for 4 days by treatment with glucocorticoids. A similar difference was found between patients with panhypopituitarism and patients with chronic suppression of ACTH (WILLIAMS et al., 1971). However, hypophysectomized sheep, maintained on ACTH for several weeks to prevent adrenal atrophy and then subjected to sodium depletion in the absence of ACTH support, showed the same aldosterone response as normal animals [BLAIR-WEST et al., 1968 (2)]; IV. Biosynthetic studies have shown that ACTH acts on the conversion of cholesterol to pregnenolone whereas sodium deficiency stimulates later steps (see below).

The general conclusion is that the effect of sodium depletion on aldosterone secretion is not mediated by ACTH.

2. Potassium

Increased intake of potassium stimulates aldosterone secretion and potassium depletion suppresses aldosterone secretion in several species including man (review

COGHLAN and BLAIR-WEST, 1967). *In-vivo* studies involving local infusion into the arterial supply of the adrenal autotransplant in the sheep (DENTON et al., 1959; BLAIR-WEST et al., 1962) and to the surgically isolated adrenal of the dog (DAVIS et al., 1963) showed the direct effect of increased plasma potassium concentration on aldosterone secretion. *In-vitro* studies with rat adrenal [MULLER, 1965 (1)] and with bovine adrenal (KAPLAN, 1965) showed a similar direct action. Therefore, at least part of the response to potassium loading is due to a direct action of potassium on aldosterone biosynthesis. Changes of potassium balance may affect aldosterone secretion through reciprocal changes of sodium status, but the response to potassium was observed when these changes were prevented (GANN et al., 1964). An additional complexity is that renin release is suppressed by potassium loading or stimulated by potassium depletion (VEYRAT et al., 1967; SEALEY et al., 1970), probably by a direct intrarenal action of potassium (VANDER, 1970; DAVIS et al., 1971).

Ovine adrenal glomerulosa has been shown to be exquisitely sensitive to local increase of potassium concentration (FUNDER et al., 1969) and similarly high sensitivity might hold in man (CANNON et al., 1966) and rat (BOYD and MULROW, 1972). A very important and as yet undecided question is whether the stimulation of aldosterone by an increased extracellular potassium level is due to a reaction at the cell membrane or to increase of potassium concentration at specific intracellular sites. BAUMBER et al. (1971) have suggested that the intraadrenal concentration of potassium may be the final common pathway for stimulation of aldosterone secretion during potassium loading, sodium depletion, infusion of ACTH or Ang. II. However, their observation that the potassium content of the adrenal cortex is increased in these states is not consistent with other results from the same laboratory. BINNION et al., (1965) reported that sodium deficiency did not increase adrenal potassium; nor was it increased by thoracic caval constriction (YANKOPOULOS et al., 1960) though aldosterone secretion was raised and so presumably was plasma renin.

Certainly severe potassium depletion and hypokalaemia may oppose these stimuli *in vivo* or *in vitro* (MULLER, 1971) and may reduce aldosterone production in primary hyperaldosteronism (BIGLIERI et al., 1967; SLATON et al., 1969). However, the treatments used by BAUMBER et al. (1971) are not identical in terms of biosynthetic response [KAPLAN, 1965; BANIUKIEWICZ et al., 1968; TAIT et al., 1970; BLAIR-WEST et al., 1970 (1); MULLER, 1971]. In the sheep, sodium depletion enhanced the aldosterone response to infused ACTH [BLAIR-WEST et al., 1963 (1)], reduced the response to infused Ang. II [BLAIR-WEST et al., 1970 (2)] and had little effect on responses to increased adrenal arterial potassium concentration (FUNDER et al., 1969). These findings are difficult to reconcile with a theory that each stimulus has the same mechanism of action on aldosterone production. Moreover it is not yet known whether the increased adrenal concentrations of potassium in the recent experiments of BAUMBER et al. (1971) are either appropriately sited, that is in the glomerulosa cells, or necessarily the cause of the rise of aldosterone secretion.

According to MULLER (1971) previous potassium deficiency in the rat decreased production of aldosterone by capsular adrenals incubated in media containing ACTH, Ang. II or high potassium concentration; production of DOC was increased but corticosterone production was unchanged. These findings suggest that potassium deficiency suppressed aldosterone biosynthesis at a site or sites later than DOC. This proposal is consistent with the observation that increased potassium concentration stimulated 11-hydroxylation in outer slices of adrenal gland (BURWELL et al., 1969), but this site may have minor importance according to BAUMANN and MULLER [1972 (1)]. In the rat, potassium loading stimulated conversion of corticosterone to aldosterone (BOYD et al., 1968, 1971) and potassium depletion suppressed it [BAUMANN and MULLER, 1972 (2)]. High potassium concentration *in vitro* also stimulated this conversion (HANING et al., 1970) but the effect was correlated with corticosterone production and addition of ACTH or corticosterone also stimulated this step. As stated earlier, potassium loading may act on aldosterone through several mechanisms and it is significant that altered potassium balance requires hours or days before taking effect on corticosterone to aldosterone conversion, suggesting that the stimulus may be mediated by extra-adrenal mechanisms. Other incubation studies have shown that increased potassium concentration, like ACTH, acts mainly before pregnenolone (MULLER, 1966, 1971). Although it is established that changes of extracellular potassium concentration may have considerable effect on aldosterone biosynthesis, the possibility that potassium stimulation may contribute to the increase of aldosterone in sodium deficiency is a relatively recent suggestion. BOYD et al. (1971) have proposed that the potassium ion is the major factor mediating the aldosterone response to sodium depletion in the rat. In a more recent study BOYD and MULROW (1972) showed that the rat adrenal is modestly sensitive *in vitro* to the small changes in external potassium concentration seen in plasma in sodium deficiency, but their major argument in favour of a potassium mechanism is that the aldosterone response to sodium depletion is not duplicated by Ang. II infusion and that it occurs in sodium-depleted, nephrectomized rats. It may be that the potassium change is a contributory cause of hypersecretion but that there is another effective mechanism; this is considered later. Certainly an increase of plasma potassium concentration is not necessary for the aldosterone response to sodium depletion in other species [BLAIR-WEST et al., 1963 (1)].

If neither increased levels of ACTH nor increased levels of potassium are necessary for the changes of aldosterone with sodium balance, although any changes that may occur can contribute to the secretion rate response, then the effective humoral signal should be Ang. II and/or change of plasma-sodium concentration, unless there is another effective stimulus. Evidence for the existence of hitherto undefined factors will be presented below.

3. Renin-Angiotensin II

Increase of blood concentrations of Ang. II or renin by infusion may stimulate aldosterone secretion (GENEST et al., 1960; LARAGH et al., 1960; CARPENTER et al., 1961; BLAIR-WEST et al., 1962). Ang. II was shown to have a direct effect on the adrenal glomerulosa in sheep and dog (BLAIR-WEST et al., 1962; GANONG et al., 1962) and at low rates of infusion the effect, in the sheep, was specifically on aldosterone secretion. It cannot be assumed that the effect of a raised blood level of renin on aldosterone secretion will be expressed entirely through Ang. II action on the adrenal cortex. Apart from possible extra-adrenal effects of Ang. II, e.g. on ACTH release (RAYYIS and HORTON, 1971) or renal excretion of sodium, the precursor and fragments of the octapeptide may also act on the adrenal cortex. The small aldosterone output observed during direct infusion of Ang. I into the adrenal arterial supply of the autotransplanted sheep adrenal gland [BLAIR-WEST et al., 1963 (1)] might result from local conversion of Ang. I to Ang. II, although rapid conversion at that site has not been shown. But, more recently it has been shown that the 2 to 8 heptapeptide of Ang. II is almost equipotent with Ang. II in aldosterone-stimulating activity [BLAIR-WEST et al., 1971 (1)]; negative results have been obtained with infusion of smaller fragments of the natural octapeptide.

Seemingly physiological concentrations of renin or Ang. II in blood, achieved by systemic infusions, may be adequate to elevate aldosterone secretion for a short time to the levels seen in sodium deficiency in the sheep [BLAIR-WEST et al., 1969 (1)]. There appears to be a substantial discrepancy in man (BOYD et al., 1969). Infusion of Ang. II caused an increase of plasma aldosterone concentration but sodium deficiency caused a much greater increase in aldosterone associated with an equal or smaller rise of plasma Ang. II concentration. The rat presents a more striking difference. High rates of infusion of renin preparations or Ang. II may have little or even no effect on aldosterone secretion in intact rats (EILERS and PETERSON, 1964; MARIEB and MULROW, 1965; BOJESEN, 1966) and only a slight effect in hypophysectomized, nephrectomized rats (MARIEB and MULROW, 1965; KINSON and SINGER, 1968). This low responsiveness *in vivo* has also been found for rat adrenal *in vitro* [KAPLAN and BARTTER, 1962; MULLER, 1965 (1); SPAT et al., 1969; BANIUKIEWICZ et al., 1968; TAIT et al., 1970].

Despite these findings of minimal effects of Ang. II *in vitro* and the evidence that the aldosterone response to sodium deficiency in the rat can occur in the absence of the kidney, much of the present knowledge concerning the action of Ang. II on aldosterone biosynthesis has been derived from *in-vitro* incubation and the rat preparation. The specificity of Ang. II action on the zona glomerulosa and aldosterone production vis-à-vis glucocorticoid production appears to depend on dosage of Ang. II, both *in vivo* (BLAIR-WEST et al., 1962; MULROW et al., 1962; AMES et al., 1965) and *in vitro* (KAPLAN, 1965). Although higher doses may stimulate secretion of 17-hydroxy corticosteroids when infused directly into the adrenal arterial blood supply of the dog (GANONG et al., 1962) the non-selective effect seen with high rates of systemic infusion of Ang. II seems likely to result from ACTH release.

4. Sodium

It is usually assumed that the effect of change of plasma sodium concentration on aldosterone secretion is small. Reduction of the sodium concentration of adrenal arterial plasma by 10 to 20 mEq/l increased aldosterone secretion in the sheep and the dog (BLAIR-WEST et al., 1962; DAVIS et al., 1963). Local increase of plasma sodium concentration by 7 to 15 mEq/l reduced aldosterone secretion by an average value of about 25% in sheep with established sodium deficiency, but the effect was usually transient (BLAIR-WEST et al., 1966). Increase of adrenal arterial plasma sodium concentration by 7 to 15 mEq/l appeared to delay the rise of aldosterone secretion during the onset of sodium depletion in the sheep [BLAIR-WEST et al., 1966 (1)]. More recent studies with adrenal arterial infusion of hypertonic $NaHCO_3$ solution in sodium-deficient sheep showed that aldosterone secretion was reduced by up to 20% when plasma sodium was increased by less than 10 mEq/l [BLAIR-WEST et al., 1971 (2)]. Such sensitivity has not been demonstrated *in vitro* (MULLER, 1971). It seems likely that the direct contribution to aldosterone secretion by plasma sodium change in sodium deficiency is a small one but the situation is not rigorously defined in species other than the sheep, nor is the possible effect of long-term changes of intracellular sodium concentration in the adrenal cortex defined.

For completeness in summarizing the humoral elements known to stimulate aldosterone secretion mention should be made of the other monovalent cations, caesium, rubidium and ammonium, all of which exert direct effects at very high and unphysiological concentrations [BARTTER et al., 1964; MULLER, 1965 (2); BLAIR-WEST et al., 1968 (3)]. Serotonin has a potent effect on aldosterone production by rat adrenal glands or isolated cells *in vitro* (MULLER and ZIEGLER, 1968;

HANING et al., 1970), but not significant effect in the sheep *in vivo* (BLAIR-WEST et al., 1962). Recently two compounds of the prostaglandin series have been shown to affect aldosterone secretion probably by a direct action on the adrenal cortex; PGE_1 inconsistently but often substantially reduced aldosterone and glucocorticoid secretion when infused directly into the adrenal arterial blood supply of sodium deficient sheep [BLAIR-WEST et al., 1971 (3)]; PGA_1 increased aldosterone and often glucocorticoid secretion when infused to the sheep adrenal (BLAIR-WEST et al., 1968) or systemically in human subjects (FICHMAN et al., 1971). The human aldosterone responses were not eliminated by treatment with dexamethazone and all responses were not attributable to change of concentration of Ang. II or ionic factors. The non-specific response of the sheep adrenal to PGE_1 suggests an early site of inhibition of corticosteroid biosynthesis; the effect found by FICHMAN et al. (1971) with PGA_1 indicates a relatively selective stimulation of zona glomerulosa cells; the physiological significance of these findings has yet to be determined.

D. Interaction Between Factors and Alteration of Adrenal Sensitivity

Consideration of the role of the known factors that affect aldosterone secretion in an analysis of sodium depletion should include the possibility that the regulatory process may be influenced by interaction between factors. Such interaction might be expressed physiologically by alterations in sensitivity of the adrenal glomerulosa to the specific actions of the four factors concerned. This prediction is reasonable theoretically and has been demonstrated by experiments, but the importance of interactions in aldosterone regulation during sodium depletion, and other conditions, is not fully explored or understood.

Rigorous analysis for interactions requires that the variables be controlled separately and quantitatively. These requirements can be met in the *in-vitro* procedures developed by KAPLAN and BARTTER (1962), MULLER [1965 (1)], MARUSIC and MULROW (1967), BANIUKIEWICZ et al. (1968), and HANING et al. (1970). However, the validity of these procedures depends on how closely they reproduce the physiological condition and, in most experiments, the required concentrations of the effective stimuli are considerably in excess of measured levels *in vivo*. Technically more difficult are the procedures using surgical preparation of whole animals to permit local administration of substances affecting aldosterone e.g. the adrenal autotransplant in the conscious sheep (McDONALD et al., 1958; DENTON et al., 1959) and the adrenal pouch preparation in the anaesthetized dog (HILTON et al., 1960). These methods almost eliminate the problem of extra-adrenal reactions to the infused substances and also the problem of recirculation to the adrenal, because adrenal blood flow is small (although the organs have a high blood flow: mass ratio) and therefore the amount of infused material required to achieve a high intra-adrenal blood concentration can be made small enough to avoid a significant rise in peripheral blood level. Experiments have also been carried out in animals, and even in man, after surgical ablations, e.g. nephrectomy and hypophysectomy or after treatment with blocking agents, e.g. dexamethazone or peptides from bothrops venom (converting-enzyme antagonist). These approaches may eliminate or may be used to control ACTH or Ang. II blood levels. In addition, experiments in intact animals and in man have been designed with measured or assumed values for the variables involved but without direct control of them. Such procedures require careful management because the factors known to affect aldosterone secretion interact at extra-adrenal sites, e.g. sodium and potassium balance may be inversely related, changes of potassium balance may affect renin release (VEYRAT et al., 1967), renin or Ang. II infusion may affect renal sodium excretion (PEART, 1965; GROSS et al., 1965).

Sodium deficiency has measurable but inconsistent effects on the sensitivity of the adrenal cortex to aldosterone-stimulating factors when tested in man or in intact or surgically-prepared animals or by *in-vitro* methods. Consistent with this observation is the fact that sodium deficiency causes changes in adrenal ionic composition [BLAIR-WEST et al., 1963 (1); BAUMBER et al., 1971] although it is not known whether these changes specifically involve the zona glomerulosa. Of primary concern is the impact of sodium deficiency on responses to Ang. II. In sodium-depleted man, Ang. II infusion caused a further increase of aldosterone secretion without any particular evidence for increased responsiveness (AMES et al., 1965). Sodium depletion increased the responsiveness of the adrenal glomerulosa to infused Ang. II in the hypophysectomized, nephrectomized dog (GANONG et al., 1966); the effect could be reproduced in sodium-replete dogs treated for 5 days with homologous renin [GANONG et al., 1967 (2)]. On the other hand, aldosterone responses to Ang. II infusion were almost negligible in moderately sodium-deficient sheep [BLAIR-WEST et al., 1970 (2)]. KINSON and SINGER (1968) found that the response to Ang. II was increased by sodium deficiency in rats that were hypophysectomized and nephrectomized.

The aldosterone response to ACTH infusion is enhanced by sodium deficiency in the hypophysectomized, nephrectomized dog [GANONG et al., 1965 (1), 1966] and in the conscious sheep [BLAIR-WEST et al., 1963 (1)]; a similar variation appears to occur in man (MULLER et al., 1956; VENNING et al., 1962). A similar sensitization was achieved by 5 days treatment with renin in the dog (GANONG et al., 1966). The significance of this alteration in sensitivity to ACTH is uncertain because the levels of ACTH required to stimulate aldosterone secretion also cause rises in glucocorticoid secretion which are not normally seen in sodium deficiency. However, in situations also involving trauma, this potentiation might have substantial additional impact on the aldosterone level. Recent studies in the rat (KINSON and SINGER, 1968; MULLER, 1971) indicate that sodium deficiency does not enhance the effect of ACTH on aldosterone secretion in this species. The aldosterone response to direct potassium stimulation in the sheep (FUNDER et al., 1969) or in incubated rat adrenal capsules (MULLER, 1971) is not substantially changed from normal by sodium deficiency.

Sodium loading reduces aldosterone secretion to lower levels than normal and it has been shown to suppress aldosterone biosynthesis in the rat adrenal *in vitro* (BANIUKIEWICZ et al., 1968). Positive sodium balance due to sodium loading or arising from sodium retention suppressed the aldosterone response to Ang. II infusion in dog (DAVIS et al., 1969) and sheep [BLAIR-WEST et al., 1970 (2)] but not in man (AMES et al., 1965). Concurrent infusion of Ang. II and hypertonic NaCl (to increase plasma sodium concentration by about 10 mEq/l) into the adrenal arterial supply of the sodium-replete sheep caused a lesser rise of aldosterone secretion than infusion of Ang. II alone at the same rate (BLAIR-WEST et al., 1965). This suggests that Ang. II action may be modulated by local concentration of sodium but there is no evidence that the aldosterone response to Ang. II is potentiated by low intra-adrenal concentration of sodium [BLAIR-WEST et al., 1970 (2)]. Sodium loading might also affect responses to Ang. II by effects on potassium balance and resulting changes of potassium concentration in blood or in the adrenal cortical cells. The role of potassium in aldosterone biosynthesis is more complex than the direct effect of plasma level on the adrenal glomerulosa. Hypokalaemia in patients with primary hyperaldosteronism may suppress aldosterone secretion towards normal values (SLATON et al., 1969); however, in normal sodium-depleted subjects the suppression of aldosterone secretion by potassium depletion is not so marked (BRUNNER et al., 1970) and this difference might be attributed to stimulation of renin production. This argument is based on the idea that one stimulus or another is adequate to promote aldosterone secretion through stimulation of the early steps of aldosterone biosynthesis. However, recent experiments in the sheep (BLAIR-WEST et al., unpublished) have shown that severe hypokalaemia may abolish the aldosterone response to sodium depletion although blood Ang. II concentration was very high. The potent inhibition by potassium deficiency of biosynthetic steps later than DOC (MULLER, 1971) indicates that a major cause of the reduction of aldosterone secretion by low potassium is the suppression of conversion at a step later than that common to potassium and Ang. II.

Continued treatment with high doses of ACTH in man [NEWTON and LARAGH, 1968 (1); BIGLIERI et al., 1969], rat (MULLER, 1972), dog (GANONG, 1971) and sheep (SCOGGINS et al., 1972), result in a decline of the aldosterone response to ACTH and may eventually reduce responses to other exogenous factors and also to sodium deficiency. Several workers have examined the possibility that the suppression of responsiveness is due to an ensuing positive sodium balance, suppression of renin release and plasma level of renin, resulting in inhibition of the biosynthetic process for aldosterone. Although treatment with high dosage of ACTH did suppress plasma renin activity in the dog (GANONG et al., 1971), but not in man [NEWTON and LARAGH, 1968 (1); MULLER, personal communication], concurrent sodium depletion to sustain a high blood level of renin did not prevent the adrenal inhibition. The inhibition may be related to the changes of sodium and potassium balance acting through direct ionic mechanisms, as described above. But aldosterone biosynthesis can also be inhibited by protracted administration of glucocorticoids in man [SPARK et al., 1968; NEWTON and LARAGH, 1968 (2)] and the rat (MULLER, 1970), and it seems possible that the effect may be due to a direct effect of high levels of glucocorticoids on the glomerulosa cells by a process requiring identification.

E. Time Course of Action on Aldosterone Biosynthesis

Stores of aldosterone in human adrenals appear to be insufficient to sustain secretion rate for more than a few minutes (NEHER, 1958). The aldosterone content of sodium replete sheep adrenal glands varies in the range 0.10 to 0.47 μg/gland (COGHLAN and BLAIR-WEST, 1967) so that at a basal secretion rate of 2 μg/h the store would maintain the secretion for 6 to 30 min but such a store would be emptied in about 2 min in very severe sodium depletion. Although storage may be greater in sodium deficiency (DUFAU and KLIMAN, 1968) it is clear that the aldosterone secretion rate of the normal animal is due to continuing aldosterone biosynthesis and that high steady state secretion rates must be due to increased production. It is evident also that the biosynthetic mechanism has a short response time. Infusions of Ang. II, KCl or ACTH into the adrenal arterial blood supply to the sheep or the dog adrenal increasd aldosterone secretion in a matter of minutes only (BLAIR-WEST et al., 1962; GANONG et al., 1962). The time-course of response to high levels of these stimuli in the sodium-replete sheep has been measured formally by collecting 3-min samples of adrenal venous blood beginning when the intra-adrenal infusion is started [BLAIR-WEST et al., 1970 (3)]. Increase of aldosterone secretion was usually seen in 3 to 6 min and the maximal responses (up to 0.2 μg/min) were achieved in 9 to 15 min. This rapid response, despite low storage of the hormone, indicates that even in the sodium-replete state the glomerulosa cells, and more particularly a necessary set of enzymic mechanisms, are present and capable of synthesizing large quantities of aldosterone from early precursors such as cholesterol, because a common site of action of the three stimuli is at the step cholesterol to pregnenolone.

States of continuous high secretion of aldosterone in response to exogenous stimulation may not persist indefinitely, but different explanations seem to apply depending on stimulus and species used. The human adrenal may remain responsive to continuous i.v. infusion of Ang. II for several days (AMES et al., 1965). The dog may also sustain a high aldosterone response, as measured by urinary excretion, for many days (URQUHART et al., 1963), but the increase was transient in hypophysectomized dogs on high-sodium diet (DAVIS et al., 1969). Prolonged systemic infusion of Ang. II in the sheep maintained a high aldosterone secretion for periods of up to 8 h only [BLAIR-WEST et al., 1963 (1)] and although the reversal may be ascribed to a fall of plasma potassium concentration in some instances, a similar transient rise of aldosterone was seen when Ang. II was infused into the adrenal arterial blood without change of plasma potassium. A persistent stimulation of aldosterone secretion has been reported in rat following very high dosage of renin or Ang. II (MASSON and TRAVIS, 1968; DUFAU and KLIMAN, 1968) but this animal tends to lose sodium under these circumstances. In each study with prolonged infusion of Ang. II, the pressor effect was sustained and sometimes enhanced. Prolonged treatment with high dosage of ACTH does not sustain an augmented level of aldosterone and this has been detailed above. The present limited knowledge of biosynthetic events does not permit definition of the cause of transient responses to prolonged treatment with effective stimuli.

F. Biosynthetic Model

Consideration of the single effects of the four humoral factors, sodium, potassium, ACTH and Ang. II, the interactions between them, and the effects of sodium deficiency, provide a basis for constructing a biosynthetic model of the type drawn by MULLER (1971) for the rat (Fig. 1) and BLAIR-WEST et al. (1972) for the sheep. From analysis of *in-vivo* and *in-vitro* data on aldosterone mechanisms it is clear that each stimulus, when presented in sufficient strength, is an adequate condition for increased biosynthesis, and also that ACTH, Ang. II, and potassium stimulate the step cholesterol to pregnenolone. On currently available data, ACTH and Ang. II do not act on later steps. Prolonged treatment with renin — see below — may stimulate a later step (AGUILERA and MARUSIC, 1972). There are no data on the biosynthetic step affected by change of plasma sodium concentration. Ang. II may stimulate an even earlier step, involving the incorporation of acetate (LOMMER and WOLFF, 1966). Increase of potassium concentration may also promote the 11-hydroxylation step producing corticosterone from deoxycorticosterone (BURWELL et al., 1969) and potassium deficiency may exert an effect on aldosterone control by suppressing this step although the primary effect appeared to be after corticosterone [BAUMANN and MULLER, 1972 (1)]. The later step has been shown to be stimulated by high potassium in the rat both *in vivo* (BOYD et al., 1971) and *in vitro* (HANING et al., 1970).

There are several unresolved questions in Fig. 1. This is generally true for all models of aldosterone regulation because the information is not complete. First, there is a question of specificity of corticosteroid response. Ang. II or potassium or sodium changes in blood affect aldosterone secretion with small effects only on glucocorticoid secretion. Sodium deficiency has similar specificity. ACTH does not have this specificity, even though it appears to share a common early site of action with Ang. II and potassium in steroidogenesis. It seems unlikely from *in-vitro* studies e.g. MULLER (1971) and from time course studies *in vivo* [BLAIR-WEST et al., 1970 (3)] that specificity for aldosterone is due to inhibitory feedback on ACTH release, and therefore a more likely possibility is that receptors of the zona glomerulosa cells have a higher affinity for Ang. II than for ACTH. Increased corticosterone secretion due to high levels of Ang. II or sodium depletion may be due partly to release of corticosterone simultaneously with aldosterone from

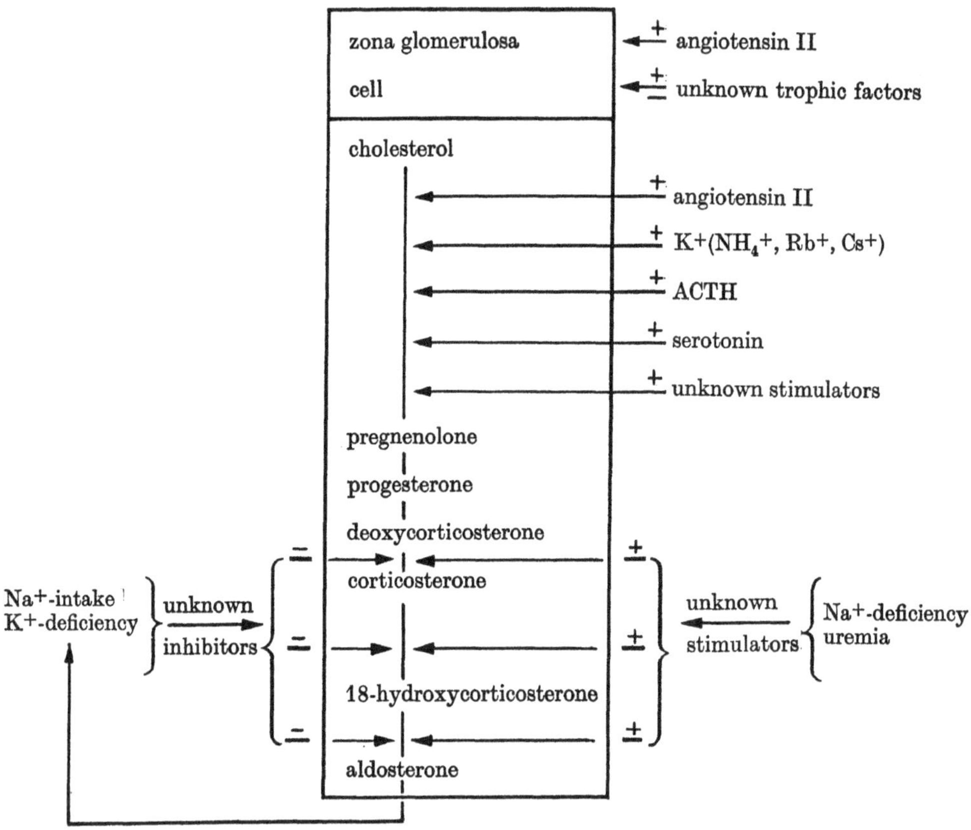

Fig. 1. Scheme of regulation of aldosterone biosynthesis in the rat (MULLER, 1971)

glomerulosa cells and partly to a small effect on steroidogenesis in the zona fasciculata, in view of findings in the hypophysectomized dog (GANONG et al., 1962; DAVIS, 1962) and in sodium-deficient dexamethazone-treated man (BLEDSOE et al., 1966).

Second, although a great deal of information has been accumulated concerning the biosynthetic reactions to many humoral factors and conditions that affect aldosterone secretion, there is little knowledge of how these external changes establish control over intracellular biosynthetic processes. There has been substantial confirmation of the proposition that ACTH action on the zona fasciculata is mediated by activation of adenyl cyclase promoting formation of cyclic AMP.

The adrenal cortical cell membrane appears to have an important role, in that particles such as ACTH seem unlikely to penetrate it, at least without difficulty, whilst their effects on aldosterone secretion *in vivo* can be detected in approximately 3 min [BLAIR-WEST et al. 1970 (3)]. Furthermore, Ang. II or high potassium failed to stimulate aldosterone production *in vitro* in calcium-free media (MULLER, 1971). Addition of ouabaine to incubation media may reduce aldosterone production (CUSHMAN, 1969) and corticosterone production (WELLEN and BENRAAD, 1969) or reduce aldosterone responses to added potassium or ACTH, without affecting corticosterone production (MULLER, 1971). In the sheep, intracarotid infusion of ouabaine for $4^1/_2$ h at 0.1 mg/h did not affect a high aldosterone secretion in response to sodium deficiency but a maximal response in glucocorticoid secretion was produced (DENTON et al., 1969). The effects observed with ouabaine could suggest direct biosynthetic consequences from alteration of intracellular concentrations of sodium and/or potassium but may indicate an alteration in the condition of receptors and excitatory processes located in the cell membrane. The *in-vivo* effect, inconsistent with *in-vitro* findings, suggests caution in attributing the final common pathway of all stimuli of aldosterone to changes of adrenal cell potassium content.

Studies of Ang. II action on smooth muscle cells have not provided a definition of the chemical nature of angiotensin receptors. RICHARDSON and BEAULNES (1971), studying distribution and action of Ang. II, free or bound to horse-radish peroxidase, argue in favour of an endothelial site of action, although there is doubt o the firmness of binding of the complex *in vivo*. The findings of KHAIRALLAH (1971) and BAUDOUIN and MEYER (1971) are consistent with the idea that Ang. II may enter cells and locate on receptors in mitochondrial or nuclear membranes. According to KHAIRALLAH, Ang. II bound on intracellular sites stimulated calcium-dependent protein synthesis, whilst BAUDOUIN and MEYER found that Ang. II caused calcium mobilization and increased calcium concentration in the myofilaments. These findings, whilst not necessarily applicable to Ang. II action on the adrenal glomerulosa raise the important possibilities for I. an intracellular action of Ang. II; II. the role of protein synthesis in the steroidogenic action of Ang. II and other factors, and III. the mechanism of zona glomerulosa hypertrophy in chronic sodium depletion.

Third, the mechanisms of sodium depletion and repletion and the effects of change of potassium balance have not yet been fully described, and nor have the more specific effects of change of adrenal arterial plasma potassium and sodium concentration. Concerning the direct action of the electrolytes, the high aldosterone secretion caused by increased plasma potassium concentration may be attributable to stimulation at early or late biosynthetic sites but there are no data on the site of action of reduced sodium concentration. Local and moderate increase of sodium concentration or reduction of potassium concentration rapidly reduced the high aldosterone secretion of sodium deficiency in the sheep [BLAIR-WEST et al., 1971 (2)] suggesting that the extracellular ionic levels or intracellular resultants can determine the throughput of aldosterone but it is not clear whether these ionic changes suppressed early site stimulation or inhibited later biosynthetic steps, e.g. DOC to corticosterone to aldosterone. Furthermore, it is not clear whether the ionic changes were suppressing conversions attributable to the ionic factors themselves or whether they were antagonizing stimulation by other factors, e.g. Ang. II, at earlier steps.

As detailed above, sodium loading reduces aldosterone responsiveness to exogenous stimulation and this effect may be directly due to inhibition by high local plasma sodium (BLAIR-WEST et al., 1965). Potassium deficiency also renders the *in-vitro* rat adrenal relatively incapable of producing aldosterone, but this is not likely to be due to local hypokalaemia alone, because increase of potassium does not restore aldosterone production (MULLER, 1971). However, it is likely that the effect is due to inhibition at a site later than production of DOC and that earlier conversions are not impaired. At the moment, the mechanisms by which local changes of ionic concentrations may oppose the increase of aldosterone caused by sodium depletion or by exogenous factors is not known. In addition, the biosynthetic mechanisms by which long-term procedures such as sodium deficiency or treatment with renin may affect the responsiveness of the adrenal glomerulosa are virtually unexamined. In this context, sodium deficiency is known to cause an increase in the width of the zona glomerulosa in rat and rabbit (DEANE et al., 1948; HARTROFT and EISENSTEIN, 1957; PALMORE and MULROW, 1967; MULLER and HUBER, 1969; SCOGGINS et al., 1970) and potassium depletion causes a narrowing (MULLER and HUBER, 1969). These changes may indicate a trophic action of circulating factors generated by sodium deficiency but there is evidence that the morphological changes are not necessarily correlated with functional changes, e.g. zona glomerulosa width was increased by sodium deficiency in hypophysectomized rats but the capacity for aldosterone production was less than in normal sodium-depleted rats (PALMORE and MULROW, 1967; LEE and DE WIED, 1968). The proposal that increased zona glomerulosa width may be due to increased blood levels of renin and angiotensin is weakened by the evidence of a narrowing in potassium-deficient rats, because potassium depletion could also stimulate renin release (BRUNNER et al., 1970).

G. Aldosterone Secretion in Response to Sodium Depletion

The data on aldosterone control in sodium deficiency are not complete. Briefly, the outstanding issues are the importance of ionic factors, the primacy of the renin/angiotensin system, the mechanism controlling the late step conversion of corticosterone to aldosterone, the problem of applying a model based mainly on short-term stimulation of aldosterone to the relatively chronic condition of sodium deficiency, and finally the evidence for hitherto unidentified factors in aldosterone regulation during sodium deficiency.

Aldosterone secretion rate and blood level are increased in man by salt restriction for a few days or by treatment with saliuretic agents. Primitive highland natives of New Guinea on chronic low sodium intake had blood aldosterone concentrations higher than native subjects on hospital diet in a coastal district or the levels established for Westernized man on a daily sodium intake of 100 mEq or more (SCOGGINS et al., 1970). A similar response to sodium deficiency has been measured in all Eutherian mammals tested, and there is evidence for a similar response in Metatheria (JOHNSTON et al., 1967; COGHLAN and SCOGGINS, 1967) and Amphibia (ULICK and FEINHOLTZ, 1968). Studies of lower mammals in natural habitats, low in sodium content, showed an aldosterone response consistent with experimental findings in the laboratory [BLAIR-WEST et al., 1968 (1)]. The increased width of zona glomerulosa described for sodium-deficient laboratory animals (see above) was also observed in lower mammalian species in natural low-sodium environments and this morphological reaction was associated with hypertrophy of the epithelial cells of the salivary ducts and proximal renal tubules (SCOGGINS et al., 1970).

GANONG (personal communicatioD) argues that the renin-angiotensin system acts as a trophic hormone for the zona glomerulosa and the idea may draw support from the observation of KHAIRALLAH (1971) that Ang. II infusion may stimulate DNA, RNA and protein synthesis in several tissues of the guinea pig. Against this proposal is the observation that the width of the zona glomerulosa is increased by a few days of sodium deficiency in the rat, but not by prolonged infusion of Ang. II (MARIEB and MULROW, 1965) except at very high doses (MARX and DEANE, 1963). Hypertrophy of the cells of the salivary ducts and proximal nephron in chronically sodium-depleted mammalian species appears similar to the hypertrophy seen in salivary glands of sheep depleted of sodium for only a few days in the laboratory [BLAIR-WEST et al., 1969 (2)] and these findings indicate a diversity of sites of increased protein synthesis during sodium deficiency. The hypertrophic changes in the salivary glands are associated with increased sensitivity of the secretory sites to the action of aldosterone [BLAIR-WEST et al., 1963 (2), 1968 (4)]. The sensitization of the parotid gland in sodium deficiency was not reproduced by Ang. II infusion and the nature of this mechanism has not been established. The possibility that the renin-angiotensin system may be the cause of the hypertrophy of the target organs of aldosterone in sodium deficiency has not yet been studied.

The logic of the biosynthetic model proposed by MULLER (1971) (Fig. 1), plus the evidence for low storage of aldosterone, requires that increased secretion of aldosterone in sodium deficiency is due to stimulation of the step cholesterol to pregnenolone, ensuring adequate provision of substrate, by one of the humoral factors, Ang. II or potassium (and perhaps sodium should be added for situations in which it is substantially reduced); stimulation of the late step, corticosterone to aldosterone, must also be involved. Alternatively, it has been suggested that corticosterone turnover is not substantially increased and that the major effect of sodium deficiency is a redistribution between products of corticosterone metabolism [BLAIR-WEST et al., 1970 (1), 1972].

It is not possible at present to define the intracellular ionic status of the adrenal glomerulosa of sodium-depleted animals. The importance and the possible role of intracellular ionic concentration has been an undecided question for a very long time (cf. DENTON et al., 1959; BLAIR-WEST et al., 1963), but the possibility that this mechanism determines aldosterone secretion independently of the chemical differences between humoral stimulants remains a matter of conjecture rather than knowledge. This is not to say that altered intracellular concentrations of sodium and potassium arising from extracellular changes may not help to determine aldosterone secretion in sodium depletion, but there are few data on this issue, and the nature of the intracellular events governing the biosynthetic mechanism is one of the most challenging questions in aldosterone control.

There is virtually no evidence that the rise of aldosterone secretion during sodium depletion is generated by increased plasma levels of ACTH or potassium in the studied species, other than rat. In rats, attention is presently being given to the importance of the small rise of plasma potassium observed during sodium depletion because the renin-angiotensin II system does not appear to be involved (BOYD and MULROW, 1972). It has not been established that the increment of potassium is necessary for the aldosterone response. In other species, potassium and ACTH plasma levels may influence the limit to which aldosterone rises during sodium depletion by influencing the biosynthetic throughput at early or late steps, but neither factor rises to initiate increased steroidogenesis under this stimulus.

If these two factors are excluded, the pathway for increased aldosterone in sodium deficiency should be stimulated by altered concentration of Ang. II and perhaps sodium in the milieu of the zona glomerulosa cells. The remaining possibility is that if the model does not satisfy all observations, it follows that there must be another factor involved in aldosterone biosynthesis in sodium deficiency.

There is already evidence for an as yet undefined mechanism promoting conversion of corticosterone to aldosterone (see below) and this is shown in Fig. 1.

Muller (1971) and Davis (1971) and earlier reviewers of aldosterone regulation have attributed a very minor role to changes of plasma sodium concentration. Data have been presented above showing the small but definite direct action of changes of plasma sodium and its interaction with other stimuli. The impact of increased adrenal arterial plasma sodium concentration, with or without concurrent reduction of potassium concentration, on aldosterone secretion in conscious sodium-deficient sheep is shown in Fig. 2. Sodium increase alone had only a slight effect

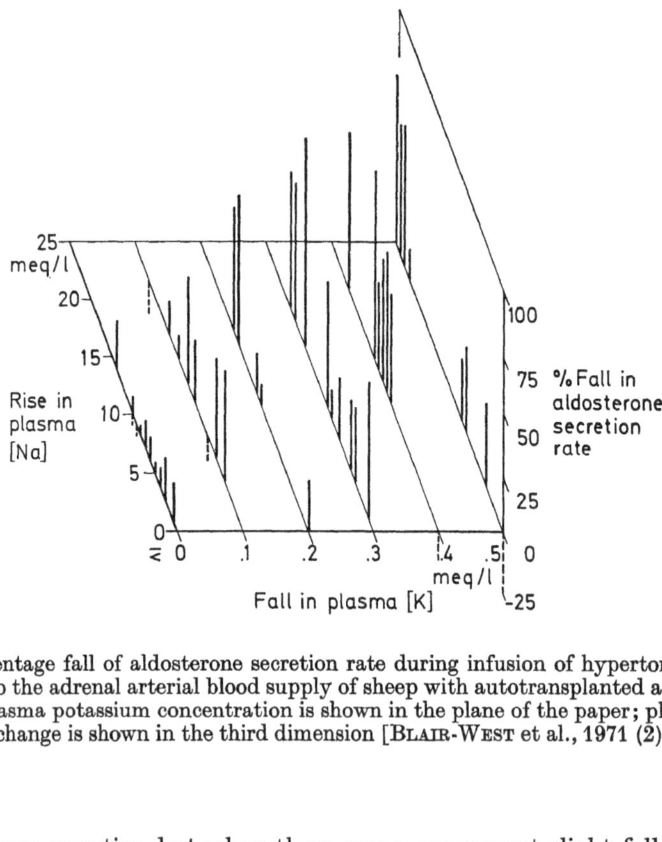

Fig. 2. Percentage fall of aldosterone secretion rate during infusion of hypertonic Na HCO_3 solutions into the adrenal arterial blood supply of sheep with autotransplanted adrenal gland. Change of plasma potassium concentration is shown in the plane of the paper; plasma sodium change is shown in the third dimension [Blair-West et al., 1971 (2)]

on aldosterone secretion but when there was a concurrent slight fall in the potassium concentration, aldosterone secretion rate was substantially reduced although it never reached the sodium-replete range. On simple quantitative grounds, it appears certain that the direct effect of plasma sodium concentration can be excluded as a major stimulant of aldosterone secretion in sodium deficiency. Indeed, it is not a necessary change during mild sodium depletion.

Therefore, confining attention to sodium deficiency and the model in Fig. 1, only Ang. II remains of the stimuli known to increase aldosterone secretion by direct action and of the factors known to stimulate the biosynthetic steps before corticosterone. If it should prove inadequate, like plasma sodium, there would be strong ground for assuming the existence of an additional humoral factor in aldosterone regulation.

H. The Renin-Angiotensin System

The many aspects of this system are given detailed attention throughout this volume and therefore only its contribution to the adrenal reaction during sodium depletion is of concern here. Sodium depletion is associated with a large number of systemic reactions, some of which may control the intake (Section J) or the output of sodium, resulting in restoration of the normal sodium status or maintenance of a position of minimal negative deviation. Although sodium deficiency causes reduction of intravascular and extracellular fluid volumes, there is some doubt as to whether these correlated changes are an essential part of the stimulation process for the high aldosterone secretion of a sodium-deficient animal (BLAIR-WEST et al., 1967; BULL et al., 1970). Arterial pressure may fall a little in severe sodium depletion but that stimulation of baroceptors in the renal afferent arteriole causes renin release is demonstrated by experimental studies in which renal arterial pressure was reduced sharply and by a large amount (SKINNER, PAGE and McCUBBIN, 1964; VANDER et al., 1967; BLAINE et al., 1970). BLAINE et al. (1970) and DAVIS et al. (1971) have recently provided strong evidence to establish the existence of a separate baroceptor facility in the control of renin secretion but it has not yet been shown that this mechanism has sufficient sensitivity to cause the increase of renin release during the earliest stages of sodium depletion.

The renin-angiotensin system satisfies a number of criteria for its acceptance as the major humoral mechanism stimulating aldosterone biosynthesis in sodium depletion. Some of these points have been treated in detail above. Excluding the situation in the rat, they are:

1. Infused Ang. II is a potent stimulus of aldosterone secretion in several species.

2. Ang. II stimulates aldosterone secretion by a direct action on the adrenal cortex; it stimulates predominately aldosterone and not glucocorticoid secretion, which is appropriate to the pattern of adrenal secretion seen in sodium depletion.

3. There are high correlations between plasma renin concentration or activity, blood Ang. II concentration, aldosterone secretion and sodium deficit in sodium-depletion experiments [NEWSOME and BARTTER, 1968; ROMERO et al., 1968; BLAIR-WEST et al., 1969 (1); GOCKE et al., 1969].

4. Bilateral nephrectomy of sodium-deficient hypophysectomized animals may reduce the high aldosterone sectretion down to the basal range. In the dog, the decline was complete in about 1 h [DAVIS et al., 1961 (1)]; in the sheep, the decline was delayed until the 6 to 12 h period after nephrectomy [BLAIR-WEST et al., 1964, 1968 (2)]. The difference may be due to a slower metabolism of renin in the sheep ($T^1/_2$ of the major component is 40 min), but there is data suggesting the disappearance rate in the dog is, in fact, slower (ASSAYKEEN et al., 1968). Different rates of decline of the adrenal enzymic systems which promote biosynthesis of aldosterone might cause aldosterone to fall at different rates after nephrectomy but rapid correction of sodium deficit in the sheep can suppress aldosterone secretion to basal in only 3 to 4 h [BLAIR-WEST et al., 1971 (4)].

The sodium-deficient rat does not show the same dependence on the presence of the kidneys (EILERS and PETERSON, 1964; MARIEB and MULROW, 1965). Recent studies in the Ang. II-immunized rabbit (LOWENSTEIN et al., 1971) suggest that the increase of aldosterone in response to sodium deficiency is not dependent on the renin-angiotensin system. The effective use of immunological techniques to abolish the action of circulating Ang. II completely requires considerable validation, and similar findings with renin antibodies in the dog [GANONG et al., 1965 (2)] were interpreted differently. The nephrectomy procedure, too, is not the simple unifactorial approach essential to examination of the role of Ang. II in sodium deficiency. BLAIR-WEST et al. [1968 (2)] and MULLER and HUBER (1969) have seen aldosterone responses to uraemic changes after nephrectomy. SLATER et al. (1965) have reported that aldosterone secretion did not fall to basal in sodium-deficient hypophysectomized dogs when the kidneys were removed from the circulation without major surgery. Studies with angiotensin antagonists or substances blocking renin or converting enzyme action may test with greater validity the role of Ang. II in the response to sodium deficiency. Experiments described later indicate the role is permissive (BLAIR-WEST et al., 1972).

Important results are coming from studies in anephric man. In an early report on one patient, BALIKIAN et al. (1968) found no increase in the plasma concentration or blood production rate of aldosterone after standing. BAYARD et al. (1970) also found no effect of postural change on aldosterone production but an increase was observed between dialyses that may have been due to accumulation of potassium. In a continuing collaborative study be members of the Peter Bent Brigham Hospital, Boston, and the Howard Florey Institute, Melbourne, it was found that isokalaemic hypovolaemia did not significantly increase plasma aldosterone concentration. ACTH infusion did not increase aldosterone levels either, suggesting that prolonged treatment with heparin in these patients may have caused a general suppression of aldosterone biosynthesis. There is strong evidence for this interpretation (FORD and BAILEY, 1966; CONN et al., 1966; ABBOTT et al., 1966).

Other groups have reported increases of plasma aldosterone concentration after standing or volume depletion in anephric patients. MCCAA et al. (1971) found plasma aldosterone was unaffected by erect posture but rose in response to volume depletion despite a fall in plasma potassium. MITRA et al. (1972) reported a significant increase of aldosterone after 2 h of quiet standing, which was not related to plasma renin, sodium or potassium, or to consistent change of plasma cortisol. WEIDMAN et al. (1972) found two groups amongst anephric patients, some with plasma aldosterone unresponsive to postural change, volume depletion or Ang. II infusion and some with consistent increase of plasma aldosterone following these procedures. MCCAA et al. (1971), MITRA et al. (1972) and WEIDMAN et al. (1972) found anephric patients who were sensitive to stimulation by potassium, Ang. II or ACTH showing that adrenal glomerulosa function can be maintained in these patients despite chronic use of heparin. The difference between these studies and the collaborative study at the Peter Bent Brigham Hospital may have been due to lower levels and frequency of heparin treatment and greater support of steroidogenesis by intermittent hyperkalaemia.

Contrary to the proposition of Ang. II as the major stimulus of aldosterone secretion in sodium deficiency are the following observations:

Group I: These findings test the proposition that rise of blood Ang. II concentration is a *sufficient* condition for aldosterone rise in sodium depletion.

I. Continuous intravenous or adrenal infusion of Ang. II did not sustain a high aldosterone secretion rate in the sodium-replete sheep [BLAIR-WEST et al., 1963 (1)]. On the other hand, sodium depletion caused a steady and sustained rise of aldosterone and therefore Ang. II may be only part of the stimulus.

II. Intravenous or adrenal arterial infusion of Ang. II did not cause significant increase of aldosterone secretion in mild sodium deficiency [BLAIR-WEST et al., 1970 (2)]. Further sodium loss or adrenal arterial infusion of KCl (FUNDER et al., 1969) or ACTH [BLAIR-WEST et al., 1963 (1)] increased aldosterone secretion in the same conditions. Therefore the rise of aldosterone during progressive sodium depletion may require a factor additional to any effect of the rise of blood Ang. II concentration.

III. Systemic infusion of Ang. II in sodium-replete man, reproducing the blood Ang. II concentrations measured in sodium deficiency, did not elevate plasma aldosterone concentration to the sodium deficient level (BOYD et al., 1969).

IV. Slight changes of posture, from recumbent to sitting, resulted in increased plasma aldosterone levels without change in aldosterone metabolic clearance rate or alteration of blood Ang. II concentration (BLAIR-WEST et al., 1972). MICHELAKIS and HORTON (1970) reported poor correlations between plasma renin activity and plasma aldosterone concentration for normal men on low sodium diet subjected to postural changes. More recently, BRUNNER et al. (1972) have compared peripheral blood levels of renin and urinary aldosterone in a very large number of patients with essential hypertension. The group with plasma renin levels suppressed below normal over a wide range of sodium status did not show an equivalent suppression of aldosterone.

V. Present knowledge of aldosterone biosynthesis seems incompatible with the proposal that the renin-angiotensin system is the major mechanism of aldosterone regulation in sodium depletion. It has been fairly consistently shown that there is a major discrepancy between the biosynthetic sites of action of Ang. II and sodium depletion. Ang. II stimulates at a site before corticosterone, probably cholesterol to pregnenolone; sodium deficiency in sheep, rat and probably dog acts mainly at a site after corticosterone.

The difference is shown in Fig. 3. Tritiated corticosterone was infused into the adrenal arterial supply of a) sodium depleted sheep or b) sheep given intravenous infusions of Ang. II to increase aldosterone secretion to the levels seen in sodium depletion. Ang. II reduced the percent conversion of corticosterone to aldosterone indicating an early site action, whereas moderate sodium deficiency caused increased conversion of corticosterone showing the primacy of a late site effect. In severe sodium deficiency the stimulus switched to act, like Ang. II, at a site before corticosterone or else stimulated a pathway that bypassed corticosterone. There was another important aspect. The specific activity of secreted aldosterone was nearly constant while the percent conversion rose. Assuming a constant rate of entry of tritiated corticosterone into the corticosterone pool, it appears likely that the rate of production of corticosterone was unchanged except in severe sodium depletion. This means that in repletion and mild depletion the precursor pool would have to be shed by secretion of some product other than corticosterone and also 18-OH corticosterone because its secretion is proportional to aldosterone in sodium depletion (ULICK et al., 1964). It has been argued that this compound may be 18-OH 11-dehydro-corticosterone (BLAIR-WEST et al., 1972). Stimuli acting before corticosterone e.g. Ang. II would then have a permissive role only, by providing an adequate supply of corticosterone.

Somewhat contrary to this analysis was the interpretation of findings during sodium depletion in the hypophysectomized dog (BINNION et al., 1965; DAVIS et al., 1966) and in man treated with dexamethazone (BLEDSOE et al., 1966) or children with hypopituitarism (RAITI et al., 1968). Increased corticosterone levels were interpreted as evidence that the primary site of action of sodium deficiency was before corticosterone. These results have been discussed [COGHLAN and BLAIR-WEST, 1967; BLAIR-WEST et al., 1970 (1)] and it remains uncertain whether the changes of corticosterone represent substantial and specific production from the aldosterone pathway. The mechanism in man will prove more difficult to define than in experimental animals. The evidence for an early site of stimulation by sodium depletion is consistent with observations that Ang. II stimulates aldosterone secretion by conversion of cholesterol and is taken as evidence for a major biosynthetic role for increased blood concentration of Ang. II.

The recent paper of AGUILERA and MARUSIC (1972) provides the first evidence for a late pathway site of action of the renin-angiotensin system. Using the isolated adrenal mitochondria preparation in the dog, they found that infusion of Ang. II or renin for up to 3 h did not stimulate corticosterone to aldosterone conversion, but treatment of dogs for 4 days with renin stimulated this conversion about two-fold relative to the rate in preparations from normal dogs. They argue that this means angiotensin has I. a site of stimulation before corticosterone shown by "acute" infusion experiments and II. a site after corticosterone during chronic

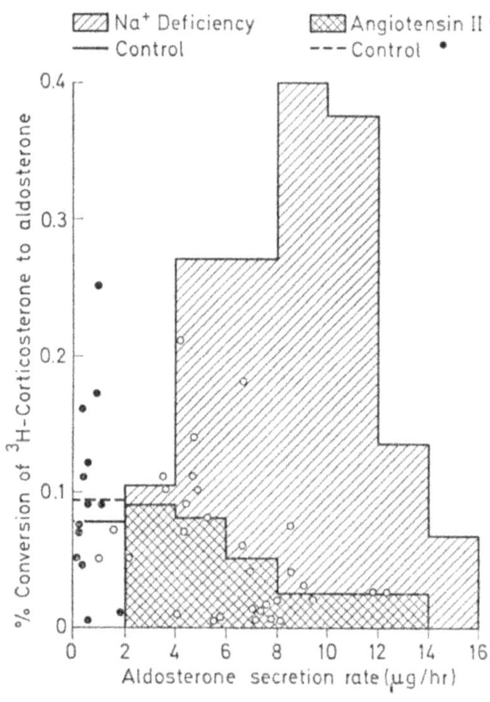

Fig. 3. Percentage conversion of ^{3}H-corticosterone to aldosterone by the autotransplanted sheep adrenal gland during stimulation of aldosterone secretion by adrenal infusion of Ang. II or by various degrees of sodium deficiency [BLAIR-WEST et al., 1969 (1)]

exposure to high blood levels of Ang. II, e.g. in sodium deficiency. Evidence was presented that the effect was not due to change of sodium balance or pituitary function. The result requires confirmation in species in which prolonged Ang. II infusion will sustain a high aldosterone secretion and because it is in these species that evidence has been gathered for the primacy of an early site of stimulation by sodium deficiency. It has already been established in the sheep that aldosterone secretion increases progressively throughout the first 24 h of sodium depletion by loss of parotid saliva but angiotensin infusion does not reproduce this effect [BLAIR-WEST et al., 1963 (1)]. That is, sodium depletion stimulates the biosynthetic step after corticosterone at a time when infused Ang. II has no effect at all on aldosterone biosynthesis.

Summarizing the results presented in Group I, it appears that an increase of blood Ang. II concentration during sodium deficiency may not be a *sufficient* stimulus for increased aldosterone secretion and therefore it may not be appropriate to treat it as the major stimulus. Other studies have been designed to test whether the usual *rise* of Ang. II concentration during sodium depletion is *necessary*.

Group II: Is there a *consistent* and *necessary* relation between blood Ang. II concentration and aldosterone secretion during change of sodium status? The following studies in the sheep suggest a negative answer.

I. When sodium-deficient sheep corrected their deficiency by drinking adequate $NaHCO_3$ solution, aldosterone fell to the replete level much more rapidly than renin and Ang. II [BLAIR-WEST et al., 1971 (4)]. This effect was attributed partly to ionic changes, particularly the important effect of small reduction of plasma potassium. However the same ionic changes alone, produced by adrenal arterial infusion of $NaHCO_3$ solution, did not produce the same degree of inhibition of aldosterone secretion [Fig. 2; BLAIR-WEST et al., 1971 (2)].

II. Characteristic rise and fall of aldosterone secretion with onset and correction of sodium deficiency were observed in experiments where blood Ang. II concentration was maintained relatively constant at a low, medium or high level in the sodium-deficient range (10 to 100 ng/ml) over a pariod of 4 days by continuous intravenous infusion of Ang. II or homologous sheep renin at constant rate [BLAIR-WEST et al , 1969 (1), 1970 (4)]. Ionic changes occurred although changes in aldosterone were consistently related to plasma sodium only. Plasma cortisol concentrations varied slightly and randomly. The data indicated that either ionic changes can have a spectacularly larger effect on aldosterone than has been attributed to them (Section C and F) in that they can reproduce the full rise and fall of aldosterone seen with sodium deficiency and its rapid correction or else an unidentified factor was operative. In further experiments, intravenous infusion of KCl was begun at the time the animals corrected sodium deficiency by rapidly drinking $NaHCO_3$ solution and the rate of Ang. II infusion was also increased slightly. Decrease of these two factors could then be prevented during correction of sodium deficiency. Aldosterone was sometimes observed to fall to basal when increase of plasma sodium was the only change observed. Such decrease cannot be produced by direct increase of adrenal arterial plasma sodium concentration alone [BLAIR-WEST et al., 1966 (1), 1971 (2)].

III. In these studies with continuous intravenous infusion of Ang. II, the usual rise of plasma renin concentration during the first 24 h of sodium depletion was blocked. The same result was achieved by infusion of Ang. II at 3 μg/h into the renal artery of uninephrectomized sheep but without effect on systemic blood Ang. II level, the angiotensin being metabolized in passage across the kidney [BLAIR-WEST et al., 1971 (5)]. Over 24 h sodium depletion during this infusion, aldosterone blood level rose normally. Fig. 4 (open circles) depicts the normal close relation between Ang. II and aldosterone concentrations in systemic blood during mild to moderate sodium deficiency. The determinations represented by closed circles represent observations on the same relation during renal arterial infusion of Ang. II when rise of plasma renin outside the normal sodium replete range was prevented. Aldosterone rose the usual extent with sodium deficiency though angiotensin did not increase outside the sodium-replete range. Plasma potassium in this experimental series was constant or decreased. The small fall of plasma sodium which occurred would not have accounted for this increase of blood aldosterone (Section C) and no significant change in cortisol secretion occurred. The data indicate that the increase of blood Ang. II to levels above the sodium-replete range is not necessary for the aldosterone response to sodium deficiency and strongly suggests that an additional factor is responsible biosynthetically.

The results of studies in Group II indicate that there is no necessary correlation between blood Ang. II and aldosterone secretion during change of sodium status in the sheep. Variations of ACTH or ionic factors were often inconsistent and small and therefore unlikely to account for the regular aldosterone responses. Additional factor(s) seem implicated but at the present there is no known substance with aldosterone stimulating property which has its blood level altered with consistent relation to sodium status. However there are experimental findings which show the possible importance of mechanisms involving the central nervous system.

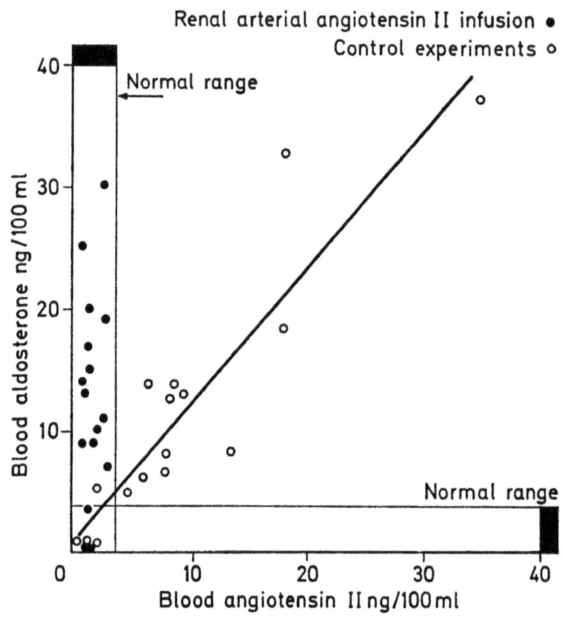

Fig. 4. Relation between blood aldosterone concentration and blood Ang. II concentration during sodium depletion in sheep: a) control experiments (open circles) and b) experiments with continuous infusion of Ang. II into the renal artery (closed circles). The normal ranges for sodium replete sheep are shown

J. Central Nervous Mechanisms Affecting Aldosterone Regulation

The sodium-deficient condition may provoke physiological reactions which are directed at increasing sodium intake, as well as the more evident processes which achieve sodium conservation. Evidence for sodium appetite in sodium deficiency is derived from studies of several mammalian species in the laboratory and in natural environments; the field has been reviewed by RICHTER (1956) and by DENTON (1965, 1967, 1969). DENTON has suggested that during the evolutionary process, the central nervous mechanisms governing sodium appetite are unlikely to have developed entirely separately in physiological integration from the hormonal processes controlling sodium conservation. Some interactions might be expected at the central nervous level. This idea has been strengthened by the increasing mass of evidence that central nervous mechanisms may affect renin release via neural or humoral paths (VANDER, 1967; MOGIL et al., 1969; MOUW and VANDER, 1970; PASSO et al., 1971), aldosterone secretion by processes not involving ACTH (BLAIR-WEST et al., 1960; BARTTER et al., 1964) and renal excretion of sodium perhaps by pathways not involving the renal nerves (ANDERSON et al., 1969; MOUW and VANDER, 1970). Of these, the subject of immediate concern here is the evidence indicating the existence of a central nervous process directly affecting aldosterone secretion.

The studies which directed attention away from the brain as the origin of possible mechanisms affecting aldosterone secretion were the work of DAVIS et al. r1961 (2)], who found that midbrain transection did not prevent the aldosterone [esponse to haemorrhage or thoracic inferior vena cava constriction, and BLAIR-WEST et al. (1960, 1964), who found that decerebrations down to the level of the rostral border of the pons did not suppress the high aldosterone secretion due to previous sodium depletion. However there were two unexplained findings in experiments of this type. In the experiments of BLAIR-WEST et al. (1960), pontine decerebration appeared to prevent the rapid decline of aldosterone secretion in response to rapid correction of sodium deficit by intravenous infusion of adequate NaCl solution. BARBOUR et al. (1965) reported that midcollicular decerebration caused an increase of aldosterone secretion in hypophysectomized, nephrectomized dogs. There are reports in man of diseases of the CNS which appear to cause reduced aldosterone secretion (KRIEGER and KRIEGER, 1964; BARBEAU et al., 1969). There is a substantial collection of data in the sheep indicating the existence of a central nervous process affecting aldosterone secretion.

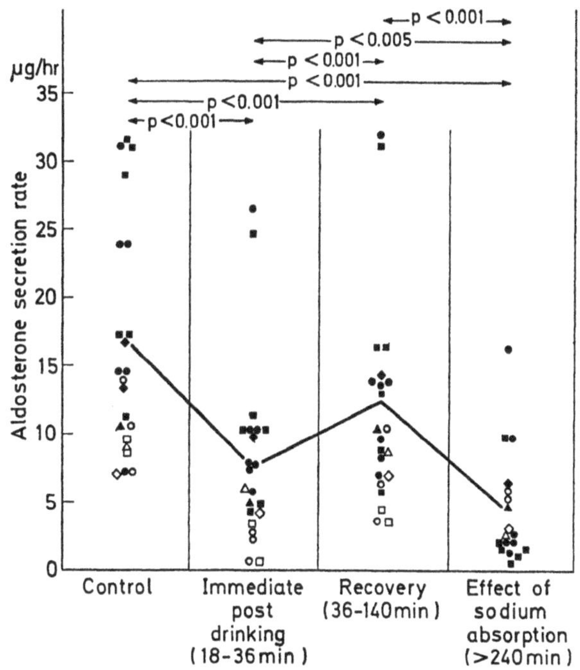

Fig. 5. Effect of voluntary satiation of sodium appetite by rapid drinking of 300 mEq/l $NaHCO_3$ solution on aldosterone secretion rate in sodium-deficient sheep with autotransplanted adrenal gland. Twenty-two experiments on eight animals are shown. Significance of changes of aldosterone secretion between intervals after drinking are shown (paired t-test). Mean values are shown by the continuous line

In sheep with adrenal transplant, the consummatory act of rapid satiation of salt appetite often causes a large, highly significant, evanescent decrease of aldosterone secretion over 18 to 36 min (Fig. 5) [BLAIR-WEST et al., 1966 (2)]. The effect reverses by 36 to 140 min after drinking. Subsequently aldosterone falls as a result of absorption of sodium from the gut. The rapid inhibition does not occur if the sodium is administered by tube into the rumen. Thus the central nervous events of satiation are the direct cause of the reaction. It is clear that a 40 to 50%

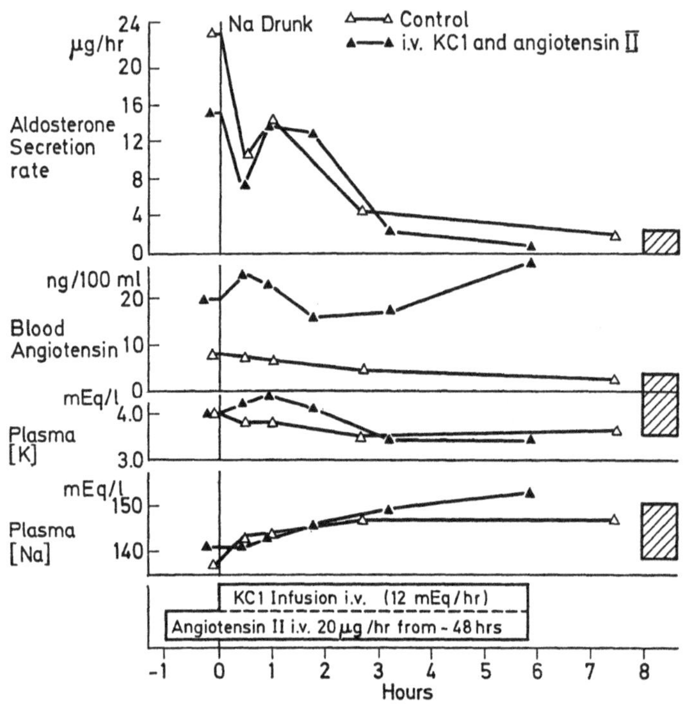

Fig. 6. Effect of voluntary satiation of sodium appetite by rapid drinking of 300 mEq/l $NaHCO_3$ solution on aldosterone secretion, blood Ang. II concentration and concentrations of potassium and sodium in plasma; a) control experiment (open triangles) and b) experiment with continuous i.v. infusions of Ang. II and KCl (closed triangles). Normal ranges for sodium-replete sheep are shown on the right

decrease of aldosterone secretion may occur without change of levels of Ang. II, cortisol, potassium or sodium. Furthermore, the effect occurred under conditions of long continuous infusion of Ang. II and intravenous KCl infusion to prevent reduction of blood Ang. II concentration or plasma potassium (Fig. 6). The effect is not seen in all animals.

Other experiments have been made in which the region of the adrenal transplant was infiltrated with procaine. Also, a slow adrenal arterial infusion of hypertonic NaCl has been begun before drinking to eliminate the possibility that the effect was due to exquisite sensitivity of the adrenal to the first influx of sodium into the circulation. In both cases the "psychic inhibition" occurred as under control conditions. This data clearly shows the existence of an unidentified humoral factor which can have a large effect on aldosterone secretion. It may involve sudden withdrawal of a stimulating factor or secretion of an inhibitory substance.

K. Summary of Aldosterone Regulation in Sodium Deficiency

The possibility that there is a single humoral stimulus with an associated unique biosynthetic reaction that controls aldosterone secretion in sodium deficiency seems to have been discounted by the present data in the mammalian species studied. Workers with different species have tended to interpret their results as representing different mechanisms rather than different parts of the same mechanism but this seems unwarranted when the mechanism of aldosterone regulation is known to be multifactoral. There has been only a little cross-checking of discrepant results between laboratories and species. It may be that the discrepancies are derived from differences of methodology and hypothesis under test so that several aspects of a complex mechanism have been revealed rather than intrinsically different mechanisms.

Ang. II may have a potent effect on aldosterone secretion; its blood level may increase with aldosterone during sodium depletion; its total withdrawal may be followed by a failure of aldosterone biosynthesis in sodium depletion. This evidence, accumulated over more than 10 years by classical *in-vivo* physiological techniques in several species has established a prima facie case for the importance of the renin-angiotensin system in the response to sodium deficiency. This case has been thoroughly described by DAVIS (1962, 1967, 1971) and GANONG et al. (1966). However, work in the sheep has built up an argument for the important role of a factor in addition to renin/angiotensin [BLAIR-WEST et al., 1963 (1), 1966; COGHLAN et al., 1971]. From the outset, findings in the rat have also indicated that some humoral stimulus other than Ang. II has the predominant governing role in sodium deficiency (EILERS and PETERSON, 1964; MARIEB and MULROW, 1965) and the major discrepancy is now firmly based (BOYD et al., 1971; MULLER, 1971). There is not sufficient compelling data in man, at the moment, to establish a particular case but work in anephric man is approaching definite conclusions.

The aldosterone stimulating properties of renin and Ang. II and the good correlations with aldosterone levels in sodium deficiency are not, by themselves, adequate grounds for the generalization of a dominant role for the renin-angiotensin system when it is taken into account that infusion of renin or Ang. II alone, to establish the blood Ang. II concentrations of sodium deficiency, is not sufficient to maintain the high aldosterone levels of sodium deficiency in man, sheep or rat. Therefore, and also in view of knowledge that the overall regulation of aldosterone is multifactorial, it seems possible that the blood level of Ang. II may be only one of a set of necessary conditions for the completely normal aldosterone response to sodium deficiency. Different results might then be expected after total withdrawal of the renin-angiotensin system and, in addition, some variability could derive from the degree of completeness of withdrawal of Ang. II by nephrectomy or by blockade of the complex renin-angiotensin system. Assuming the complete absence of Ang. II stimulation, a limited aldosterone response to sodium deficiency may indicate that the renin-Ang. II system is involved in but not necessary for the aldosterone response, which may be the situation in rats; almost total cessation of aldosterone secretion, as may be seen in nephrectomized sodium-depleted sheep or dogs, suggests a situation in which the renin-angiotensin system is essential for the biosynthetic response to this stimulus. It is important that in the arenal condition aldosterone biosynthesis can usually be stimulated by other mechanisms, e.g. trauma or hyperkalaemia, showing that the presence of Ang. II is not a prerequisite for a continuing capacity for high aldosterone secretion.

Experiments in sheep have indicated the existence of a process that seems to act conjointly with Ang. II to control aldosterone biosynthesis in sodium depletion

(Fig. 7). Sheep were sodium depleted by loss of parotid saliva and then nephrectomized. Dietary control of potassium intake prevented a rise of plasma potassium concentration so that aldosterone secretion was basal 24 h after nephrectomy. Dexamethazone was infused to suppress ACTH to basal and later Ang. II was infused in a series of increasing rates. Infusion of Ang. II at 1 to 2 μg/h increased the blood Ang. II concentration to 1 to 2 ng/100 ml which is in the range of the sodium-replete sheep. Infusion at 2 μg/h but not 1 μg/h restored peripheral blood aldosterone concentration to the high sodium deplete level before nephrectomy. This effect occurred without ionic change or alteration of blood cortisol level. Infusion of Ang. II at 20 μg/h did not further increase blood aldosterone level although blood Ang. II concentration rose to about 20 ng/100 ml which is the usual level for this degree of sodium deficiency.

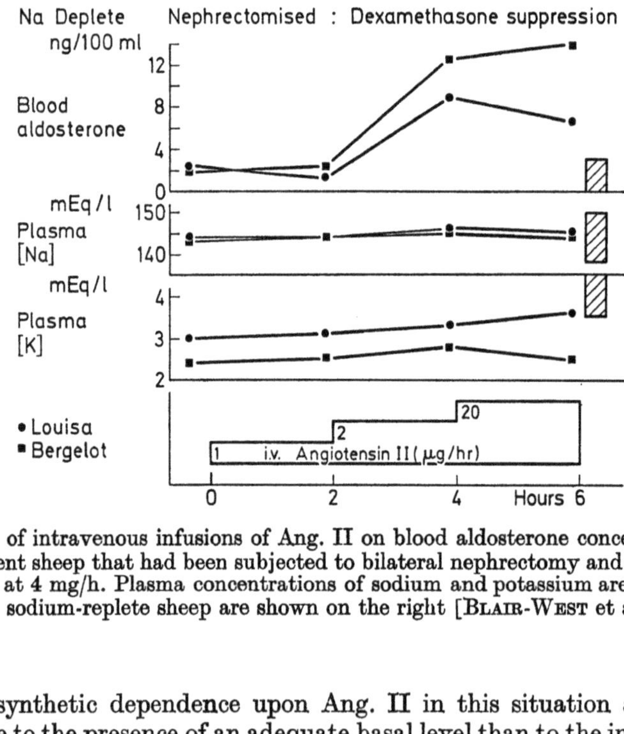

Fig. 7. Effect of intravenous infusions of Ang. II on blood aldosterone concentration in two sodium deficient sheep that had been subjected to bilateral nephrectomy and i.v. dexamethazone infusion at 4 mg/h. Plasma concentrations of sodium and potassium are shown. Normal ranges for sodium-replete sheep are shown on the right [Blair-West et al., 1970 (4)]

The biosynthetic dependence upon Ang. II in this situation appears to be related more to the presence of an adequate basal level than to the increase of level that may occur during the onset of sodium depletion. It can be argued, therefore, that where Ang. II appears to be essential for aldosterone biosynthesis its role may be mainly permissive [Blair-West et al., 1970 (4), 1972]. This is consistent with much of the biosynthetic data available. Ang. II may ensure an adequate supply of precursor by virtue of its established action at an early site in the biosynthetic pathway and an additional factor may regulate the conversions after corticosterone.

It has been suggested that the apparent difference of biosynthetic sites of action of Ang. II and sodium depletion may have resulted from differences in duration of exposure to Ang. II in biosynthetic experiments. One study that involved daily treatment of dogs with a renin preparation has shown a small induced effect on corticosterone to aldosterone conversion after 4 days (Aguilera and Marusic, 1972). However aldosterone secretion was not measured. It is mandatory to establish that such treatment is virtually specific for high aldosterone secretion and due to a direct action of Ang. II rather than secondary effects e.g. prolonged high blood pressure, ACTH release and change of sodium or potassium balance; any morphological change in the adrenal cortex would require careful evaluation. The time for the change from early to late site of stimulation in these experiments seems long in view of the observation that stimulation of conversion of corticosterone to aldosterone by sodium deficiency may be achieved in less than 24 h in the sheep [Blair-West et al., 1970 (1)].

A major point still at issue concerns the biosynthetic site predominately stimulated by sodium deficiency. Early studies in dogs and man were interpreted to favour control of an early site of conversion consistent with the apparent site of action of Ang. II. More recent studies in dogs (Davis et al., 1968; Aguilera and Marusic, 1972) suggest later sites, more consistent with the findings in sheep and rats. Alternatively and perhaps more consistent with the bulk of the biosynthetic data, it seems possible that more than one step can be regulated. The mode of stimulation by sodium deficiency may depend on the status of the whole set of effective humoral factors, Ang. II, ACTH and ionic concentrations and may vary with the extent of sodium deficiency and the potassium balance. Evidence for more than one site of stimulation with variation of sodium status may be seen in the results of Baniukewicz et al. (1968) in the rat, and Blair-West et al. [1970 (1)] in the sheep. As well as the possibility of multiple sites of stimulation, the lack of accord between results for different species and even for the same species using different experimental design, may arise from utilization of different pathways (Blair-West et al., 1972). Corticosterone conversion might be bypassed during very severe sodium depletion in the sheep [Blair-West et al., 1970 (1)] or during potassium depletion in the rat [Baumann and Muller, 1972 (2)]. Corticosterone to aldosterone conversion was substantially reduced in both of these studies but aldosterone secretion was very high in the former and production was only mildly reduced in the latter. A possible alternative pathway could involve the formation and utilization of 18-OH-progesterone. The total process may include inhibition of corticosterone conversion by end-product inhibition or by by-product inhibition through 18-OH-corticosterone production which has been shown by Raman et al. (1966).

In view of the predominance of arguments favouring late site control of aldosterone in sodium deficiency, recent biosynthetic experiments have sought to identify the stimulus with high specificity for this site. The authors have presented from their own studies the case for a factor additional to those known to affect aldosterone secretion. A similar conclusion was reached by Muller (1971). An important alternative possibility is that one or more of the known factors may have this property. Aguilera and Marusic (1972) have evidence that this may occur after long-term exposure to renin. If confirmed, this result would support existing evidence for the primacy of the renin-angiotensin mechanism without helping to explain the observations in sheep and rats that do not fit that proposition.

Recent studies in rats have raised the possibility that the factor may be plasma potassium concentration (Boyd et al., 1971; Boyd and Mulrow, 1972). They attributed the steady increase of aldosterone in sodium deficiency to the associated small nocturnal increase of plasma potassium concentration and found that a similar small potassium increase stimulated aldosterone production by adrenal cortex *in vitro*. Their contention of a late site effect of changed external potassium concentration is consistent with other *in-vitro* results [Haning et al., 1970; Baumann and Muller, 1972 (2)]. Earlier evidence of high sensitivity of the biosynthetic process to very small change of plasma potassium concentration in conscious sheep is also compatible [FUNDER et al., 1969; BLAIR-WEST et al., 1971 (2)]. Although it may be shown that the adrenal glomerulosa is highly sensitive to plasma potassium change in many species it needs to be established whether the proposed potassium stimulus in sodium-deficient rats depends on the transient rise of plasma potassium concentration or whether the aldosterone response would be observed independently of that change.

Much more work needs to be done on the biosynthetic site of action of the potassium stimulus and the ionic changes in the adrenal glomerulosa in sodium deficiency. Further attention should be paid to the mechanism of stimulation of biosynthesis by changes of levels of humoral factors. The recent biosynthetic findings with potassium and prolonged treatment with renin do not seem to provide a generally applicable explanation of aldosterone biosynthesis in sodium deficiency. The results may be revealing processes that are part of a more complex mechanism in which the specificity is in the aldosterone response and a number of biosynthesis sites or even pathways can be influenced by more than one intracellular event, arising from several possible external stimuli. It seems likely that there are humoral stimuli yet to be defined.

References

ABBOTT, E. C., GORNALL, A. G., SUTHERLAND, D. J. A., STIEFEL, M., LAIDLAW, J. C.: The influence of a heparin-like compound on hypertension, electrolytes and aldosterone in man. Canad. med. Ass. J. **94**, 1155 (1966).

AGUILERA, G., MARUSIC, E. T.: Role of the renin-angiotensin system in the biosynthesis of aldosterone. Endocrinology **89**, 1524 (1971).

AMES, R. P., BORKOWSKI, A. J., SICINSKI, A. M., LARAGH, J. H.: Prolonged infusions of angiotensin II and norepinephrine and blood pressure electrolyte balance, and aldosterone and cortisol secretion in normal man and in cirrhosis with ascites. J. clin. Invest. **44**, 1171 (1965).

ANDERSON, B., DALLMAN, M. F., OLSSON, K.: Evidence for a hypothalamic control of renal sodium excretion. Acta Physiol. scand. **75**, 496 (1969).

ASSAYKEEN, T. A., OTSUKA, K., GANONG, W. F.: Rate of disappearance of exogenous dog renin from the plasma of nephrectomized dogs. Proc. Soc. exp. Biol. (N. Y.) **127**, 306 (1968).

BALIKIAN, H. M., BRODIE, A. H., DALE, S. L., MELBY, J. C., TAIT, J. F.: Effect of posture on the metabolic clearance rate, plasma concentration and blood production rate of aldosterone in man. J. clin. Endocr. **28**, 1630 (1968).

BANIUKIEWICZ, S., BRODIE, A., FLOOD, C., MOTTA, M., OKAMOTO, M., TAIT, J. F., TAIT, S. A. S., BLAIR-WEST, J. R., COGHLAN, J. P., DENTON, D. A., GODING, J. R., SCOGGINS, B. A., WINTOUR, E. M., WRIGHT, R. D.: Adrenal biosynthesis of steroids in vitro and in vivo using continuous superfusion and infusion procedures. In: Functions of the Adrenal Cortex, Vol. 1, p. 153 (MCKERNS, K. W., Ed.). Amsterdam: North Holland 1968.

BARBEAU, A., GILLO-JOFFROY, L., BOUCHER, R., NOWACZYNSKI, W., GENEST, J.: Renin-aldosterone system in Parkinson's Disease. Science **165**, 291 (1969).

BARBOUR, B. H., SLATER, J. D. H., CASPER, A. G. T., BARTTER, F. C.: On the role of the central nervous system in control of aldosterone secretion. Life Sci. **4**, 1161 (1965).

BARTTER, F. C., BARBOUR, B. H., CARR, A. A., DELEA, C. S.: On the role of potassium and of the central nervous system in the regulation of aldosterone secretion. In: Aldosterone, p. 221 (BAULIEU, E. E., ROBEL, P., Eds.). Oxford: Blackwell 1964.

BAUDOUIN, M., MEYER, P.: Subcellular individualization of angiotensin receptors in smooth muscle cells. In: Hypertension '72, p. 495 (GENEST, J., KOIW, E., Eds). Berlin - Heidelberg - New York: Springer 1972.

BAUMANN, K., MULLER, J.: (1) Influence of potassium intake upon the final steps of aldosterone biosynthesis in the rat. II. 11 beta-hydroxylation. Acta endocr. (Kbh.) **69**, 718 (1972).

BAUMANN, K., MULLER, J.: (2) Influence of potassium intake upon the final steps of aldosterone biosynthesis in the rat. I. 18-hydroxylation and 18-hydroxydehydrogenation. Acta endocr. (Kbh.) **69**, 701 (1972).

BAUMBER, J. S., DAVIS, J. O., JOHNSON, J. A., WITTY, R. T.: Increased adrenocortical potassium in association with increased biosynthesis of aldosterone. Amer J. Physiol. **220**, 1094 (1971).

BAYARD, F., COOKE, C. R., BERTINS, I. Z., TILLER, D. J., KOWARSKI, A., WALKER, W. G., MIGEON, C. J.: Plasma aldosterone levels and plasma renin activity in normal subjects and anephritic patients: effect of posture and sodium. Proc. IIIrd. Int. Congress Hormonal Steroids Excerpta Medica Int. Congr. Series **210**, 39 (1970).

BIGLIERI, E. G., SCHAMBELAN, M., SLATON, P. E., Jr.: Effect of adrenocorticotropin on desoxycorticosterone, corticosterone and aldosterone excretion. J. clin. Endocr. **29**, 1090 (1969).

BIGLIERI, E. G., SLATON, P. E., KRONFIELD, S. J., DECK, J. B.: Primary aldosteronism with unusual secretory pattern. J. clin. Endocr. **27**, 715 (1967).

BINNION, P. F., DAVIS, J. O., BROWN, T. C., OLICHNEY, M. J.: Mechanisms regulating aldosterone secretion during sodium depletion. Amer. J. Physiol. **208**, 655 (1965).

BLAINE, E. H., DAVIS, J. O., WITTY, R. T.: Renin release after haemorrhage and after suprarenal aortic constriction in dogs without sodium delivery to the macula densa. Circulat. Res. **27**, 1081 (1970).

BLAIR-WEST, J. R., BOYD, G. W., COGHLAN, J. P., DENTON, D. A., GODING, J. R., WINTOUR, M., WRIGHT, R. D.: (2) Aldosterone secretion in relation to homeostasis of body fluids, p. 207. Int. Congr. Series 87, Proc. 23rd, Int. Congr. Physiol. Sci. Excerpta med. (Amst.) 1966.

BLAIR-WEST, J. R., BOYD, G. W., COGHLAN, J. P., DENTON, D. A., WINTOUR, M., WRIGHT, R. D.: The role of circulating fluid volume and related physiological parameters in the control of aldosterone secretion. Aust. J. exp. Biol. med. Sci. **45**, 1 (1967).

BLAIR-WEST, J. R., BRODIE, A., COGHLAN, J. P., DENTON, D. A., FLOOD, C., GODING, J. R., SCOGGINS, B. A., TAIT, J. F., TAIT, S. A. S., WINTOUR, E. M., WRIGHT, R. D.: (1) Studies on the biosynthesis of aldosterone using sheep adrenal transplant: Effect of sodium depletion on the conversion of corticosterone to aldosterone. J. Endocr. **46**, 453 (1970).

BLAIR-WEST, J. R., CAIN, M. D., CATT, K. J., COGHLAN, J. P., DENTON, D. A., FUNDER, J. W., SCOGGINS, B. A., STOCKIGT, J. R., WRIGHT, R. D.: Further facets of aldosterone regulation, p. 572. Int. Congr. Series **219**. Excerpta med. (Amst.) 1972.

BLAIR-WEST, J. R., CAIN, M., CATT, K. J., COGHLAN, J. P., DENTON, D. A., FUNDER, J. W., SCOGGINS, B. A., WINTOUR, E. M., WRIGHT, R. D.: (4) The mode of control of aldosterone secretion, p 33 Proc. 4th Int. Congr. Nephrol Basel, New York: Karger 1970.

BLAIR-WEST, J. R., CAIN, M., CATT, K., COGHLAN, J. P., DENTON, D. A., FUNDER, J. W., SCOGGINS, B. A., WRIGHT, R. D.: (1) Aldosterone regulation and biosynthesis, p. 276. Int. Congr. Series 184, Proc. 3rd. Int. Congr. Endocrin. Excerpta med. (Amst.) 1969.

BLAIR-WEST, J. R., CAIN, M. D., CATT, K. J., COGHLAN, J. P., DENTON, D. A., FUNDER, J. W., SCOGGINS, B. A., WRIGHT, R. D.: (4) The dissociation of aldosterone secretion and systemic renin and angiotensin II levels during the correction of sodium deficiency. Acta endocr. (Kbh.) **66**, 229 (1971).

BLAIR-WEST, J. R., COGHLAN, J. P., DENTON, D. A., FUNDER, J. W., SCOGGINS, B. A., WRIGHT, R. D.: (1) The effect of the heptapeptide (2-8) and the hexapeptide (3-8) fragments of angiotensin II on aldosterone secretion. J. clin. Endocr. **32**, 575 (1971).

BLAIR-WEST, J. R., COGHLAN, J. P., DENTON, D. A., FUNDER, J. W., SCOGGINS, B. A., WRIGHT, R. D.: (2) The effect of adrenal arterial infusion of hypertonic $NaHCO_3$ solution on aldosterone secretion in sodium deficient sheep. Acta endocr. (Kbh.) **66**, 448 (1971).

BLAIR-WEST, J. R., COGHLAN, J. P., DENTON, D. A., FUNDER, J. W., SCOGGINS, B. A., WRIGHT, R. D.: (3) Effects of prostaglandin E_1 upon the steroid secretion of the adrenal of the sodium deficient sheep. Endocrinology 88, 367 (1971).

BLAIR-WEST, J. R., COGHLAN, J. P., DENTON, D. A., FUNDER, J. W., SCOGGINS, B. A., WRIGHT, R. D.: (5) Inhibition of renin secretion by systemic and intrarenal angiotensin infusion during onset of Na depletion. Amer. J. Physiol. **220**, 1309 (1971).

BLAIR-WEST, J. R., COGHLAN, J. P., DENTON, D. A., GODING, J. R., MUNRO, J., WRIGHT, R. D.: The effect of neuroaxial ablations upon the secretion of electrolyte-active steroid. Proc. physiol. Soc. July 9, 1960, J. Physiol. (Lond.) **153**, 52 (1960).

BLAIR-WEST, J. R., COGHLAN, J. P., DENTON, D. A., GODING, J. R., MUNRO, J. A., PETERSON, R. E., WINTOUR, M.: Humoral stimulation of adrenocortical secretion. J. clin. Invest. **41**, 1606 (1962).

BLAIR-WEST, J. R., COGHLAN, J. P., DENTON, D. A., GODING, J. R., WINTOUR, M., WRIGHT, R. D.: (1) The control of aldosterone secretion. Recent. Prog. Hormone Res. **19**, 311 (1963).

BLAIR-WEST, J. R., COGHLAN, J. P., DENTON, D. A., GODING, J. R., WINTOUR, M., WRIGHT, R. D.: Effect of variations of plasma sodium concentration on the adrenal response to angiotensin II. Circulat. Res. **17**, 386 (1965).

BLAIR-WEST, J. R., COGHLAN, J. P., DENTON, D. A., GODING, J. R., WINTOUR, M., WRIGHT, R. D.: (1) The direct effects of increased sodium concentration in adrenal arterial blood on corticosteroid secretion in sodium deficient sheep. Aust. J. exp. Biol. med. Sci. **44**, 455 (1966).

Blair-West, J. R., Coghlan, J. P., Denton, D. A., Munro, J. A., Wintour, M., Wright,. R. D.: The effect of bilateral nephrectomy and midcollicular decerebration with pinealectomy and hypophysectomy on the corticosteroid secretion of sodium deficient sheep. J. clin. Invest. 43, 1576 (1964).

Blair-West, J. R., Coghlan, J. P., Denton, D. A., Goding, J. R., Wintour, M., Wright, R. D.: (2) The effect of nephrectomy on aldosterone secretion in the conscious sodium-depleted hypophysectomized sheep. Aust. J. exp. Biol. med. Sci. 46, 295 (1968).

Blair-West, J. R., Coghlan, J. P., Denton, D. A., Goding, J. R., Wintour, M., Wright, R. D.: (3) The local action of ammonium, calcium and magnesium on adrenocortical secretion. Aust. J. exp. Biol. med. Sci. 46, 361 (1968).

Blair-West, J. R., Coghlan, J. P., Denton, D. A., Goding, J. R., Wright, R. D.: (2) The effect of aldosterone, cortisol and corticosterone upon the sodium and potassium content of sheep's parotid saliva. J. clin. Invest. 42, 484 (1963).

Blair-West, J. R., Coghlan, J. P., Denton, D. A., Nelson, J. F., Orchard, E., Scoggins, B. A., Wright, R. D., Myers, K., Junqueira, C. L.: (1) Physiological, morphological and behavioural adaption to a sodium deficient environment by wild native Australian and introduced species of animals. Nature (Lond.) 217, 922 (1968).

Blair-West, J. R., Coghlan, J. P., Denton, D. A., Nelson, J., Wright, R. D., Yamauchi, A.: (2) Ionic, histological and vascular factors in the reaction of the sheeps' parotid to high and low mineralocorticoid status. J. Physiol. (Lond.) 205, 563 (1969).

Blair-West, J. R., Coghlan, J. P., Denton, D. A., Scoggins, B. A., Wintour, E. M., Wright, R. D.: (2) Effect of change of sodium balance on the corticosteroid response to angiotensin II. Aust. J. exp. Biol. med. Sci. 48, 253 (1970).

Blair-West, J. R., Coghlan, J. P., Denton, D. A., Scoggins, B. A., Wintour, E. M., Wright, R. D.: (3) The onset of effects of ACTH, angiotensin II and raised plasma potassium concentration on the adrenal cortex. Steroids 15, 433 (1970).

Blair-West, J. R., Coghlan, J. P., Denton, D. A., Scott, D., Wright, R. D.: (4) The role of aldosterone in renal sodium conservation during sodium depletion. Aust. J. exp. Biol. med. Sci. 46, 525 (1968).

Bledsoe, T., Island, D. P., Liddle, G. W.: Studies on the mechanism through which sodium depletion increases aldosterone biosynthesis in man. J. clin. Invest. 45, 524 (1966).

Bojesen, E.: Concentrations of aldosterone and corticosterone in peripheral plasma of rats. The effects of salt depletion, potassium loading and intravenous injections of renin and angiotensin II. Europ. J. Steroids 1, 145 (1966).

Boyd, G. W., Adamson, A. R., James, V. H. T., Peart, W. S.: The role of the renin-angiotensin system in the control of aldosterone in man. Proc. roy. Soc. Med. 62, 1253 (1969).

Boyd, J., Marusic, E., Mulrow, P.: Effect of potassium on aldosterone biosynthesis by rat adrenal mitochondria. Clin. Res. (abstract) 16, 262 (1968).

Boyd, J. E., Mulrow, P. J.: Further studies of the influence of potassium upon aldosterone production in the rat. Endocrinology 90, 299 (1972).

Boyd, J. E., Palmore, W. P., Mulrow, P. J.: Role of potassium in the control of aldosterone secretion in the rat. Endocrinology 88, 556 (1971).

Brunner, H. R., Baer, L., Sealey, J. E., Ledingham, J. G., Laragh, J. H.: The influence of potassium administration and of potassium deprivation on plasma renin in normal and hypertensive subjects. J. clin. Invest. 49, 2128 (1970).

Brunner, H. R., Laragh, J. H., Baer, L., Newton, M. A., Goodwin, F. T., Krakoff, L. R., Bard, R. H., Buhler, F. R.: Essential hypertension: Renin and aldosterone, heart attack and stroke. New Engl. J. Med. 286, 441 (1972).

Bull, M. B., Hillman, R. S., Cannon, P. J., Laragh, J. H.: Renin and aldosterone secretion in man as influenced by changes in electrolyte balance and blood volume. Circulat. Res. 27, 953 (1970).

Burwell, L. R., Davis, W. W., Bartter, F. C.: Studies on the loci of action of stimuli to the biogenesis of aldosterone. Proc. roy. Soc. Med. 62, 1254 (1969).

Cannon, P. J., Ames, R. P., Laragh, J. H.: Relation between potassium balance and aldosterone secretion in normal subjects and in patients with hypertensive or renal tubular disease. J. clin. Invest. 45, 865 (1966).

Carpenter, C. C. J., Davis, J. O., Ayers, C. R.: Relation of renin, angiotensin II and experimental renal hypertension to aldosterone secretion. J. clin. Invest. 40, 2026 (1961).

Coghlan, J. P., Blair-West, J. R.: Aldosterone. In: Hormones in Blood, Vol. 2, 2nd ed., p. 391 (Gray, C. H., Bacharach, A. L., Eds.). New York: Academic Press 1967.

Coghlan, J. P., Blair-West, J. R., Denton, D. A., Scoggins, B. A., Wright, R. D.: Perspectives in aldosterone and renin control. Aust. N. Z. J. Med. 2, 178 (1971).

Coghlan, J. P., Scoggins, B. A.: The measurement of aldosterone, cortisol and corticosterone in the blood of the wombat (Vombatus hirsutus Perry) and the kangaroo (Macropus giganteus). J. Endocr. 39, 445 (1967).

CONN, J. W., ROVNER, D. R., COHEN, E. L., ANDERSON, J. E., Jr.: Inhibition by heparinoid of aldosterone biosynthesis in man. J. clin. Endocr. **26**, 527 (1966).
CUSHMAN, P., Jr.: Inhibition of aldosterone secretion by ouabain in dog adrenal tissue. Endocrinology **84**, 808 (1969).
DAVIS, J. O.: The control of aldosterone secretion. Physiologist **5**, 65 (1962).
DAVIS, J. O.: The regulation of aldosterone secretion. In: The Adrenal Cortex, p. 203 (EISENSTEIN, A. B., Ed.). Boston: Little, Brown and Comp. 1967.
DAVIS, J. O.: The renin-angiotensin system in the control of aldosterone secretion. In: Kidney Hormones, p. 173 (FISHER, J. W., Ed.). London, New York: Academic Press 1971.
DAVIS, J. O., ANDERSON, E., CARPENTER, C. C. J., AYERS, C. R., HAYMAKER, W., SPENCE, W. T.: (2) Aldosterone and corticosterone secretion following midbrain transection. Amer. J. Physiol. **200**, 437 (1961).
DAVIS, J. O., AYERS, C. R., CARPENTER, C. J.: (1) Renal origin of an aldosterone-stimulating hormone in dogs with thoracic caval constriction and in sodium-depleted dogs. J. clin. Invest. **40**, 1466 (1961).
DAVIS, J. O., BLAINE, E. H., JOHNSON, J. A., WITTY, R. T.: New observations on renin release by the non-filtering kidney. In: Hypertension '72, p. 56 (GENEST, J., KOIW, E., Eds.) Berlin - Heidelberg - New York: Springer 1972.
DAVIS, J. O., URQUHART, J., HIGGINS, J. T., Jr.: The effects of alterations of plasma sodium and potassium concentrations on aldosterone secretion. J. clin. Invest. **42**, 597 (1963).
DAVIS, W. W., BURWELL, L. R., BARTTER, F. C.: Inhibition of the effects of angiotensin II on adrenal steroid production by dietary sodium. Proc. nat. Acad. Sci. (Wash.) **63**, 718 (1969).
DAVIS, W. W., BURWELL, L. R., CASPER, A. G. T., BARTTER, F. C.: Sites of action of sodium depletion on aldosterone biosynthesis in the dog. J. clin. Invest. **47**, 1425 (1968).
DAVIS, W. W., BURWELL, L. R., KELLEY, G., CASPER, A. G. T., BARTTER, F. C.: Studies of the loci of stimulation of aldosterone biosynthesis during sodium depletion. Biochem. biophys. Res. Commun. **22**, 218 (1966).
DEANE, H. W., SHAW, J. H., GREEP, R. O.: The effect of altered sodium or potassium intake on the width and cytochemistry on the zona glomerulosa of the rat's adrenal cortex. Endocrinology **43**, 133 (1948).
DENTON, D. A.: Evolutionary aspects of the emergence of aldosterone secretion and salt appetite. Physiol. Rev. **45**, 80 (1965).
DENTON, D. A.: Salt appetite. Handbook of Physiology, Alimentary Canal, p. 433. I. Washington: Amer. Physiol. Soc. 1967.
DENTON, D. A.: Salt appetite. Nutr. Abstr. Rev. **39**, 1043 (1969).
DENTON, D. A., GODING, J. R., WRIGHT, R. D.: Control of adrenal secretion of electrolyte-active steroids. Brit. med. J. **1959 II**, 447 and 522.
DUFAU, M. L., KLIMAN, B.: Pharmacologic effects of angiotensin-II-amide on aldosterone and corticosterone secretion by the intact anaesthetized rat. Endocrinology **82**, 29 (1968).
EILERS, E. A., PETERSON, R. E.: Aldosterone secretion in the rat. In: Aldosterone, p. 251 (BAULIEU, E. E., ROBEL, P., Eds.). Oxford: Blackwell 1964.
FICHMAN, M. P., LITTENBERG, G. D., BROOKER, G., HORTON, R.: Effect of prostaglandin (PGA_1) on blood pressure, renal and adrenal function in man. Proc. Council for High Blood Pressure Research, Cleveland October 1971. Circulat. Res. **31**, 19 (1972).
FORD, H. C., BAILEY, R. E.: The effect of heparin on aldosterone secretion and metabolism in primary aldosteronism. Steroids **7**, 30 (1966).
FUNDER, J. W., BLAIR-WEST, J. R., COGHLAN, J. P., DENTON, D. A., SCOGGINS, B. A., WRIGHT, R. D.: Effect of Plasma (K^+) on the secretion of aldosterone. Endocrinology **85**, 381 (1969).
GANN, D. S., DELEA, C. S., GILL, J. R., Jr., THOMAS, J. P., BARTTER, F. C.: Control of aldosterone secretion by change of body potassium in normal man. Amer. J. Physiol. **207**, 104 (1964).
GANONG, W. F.: Effects of sympathetic activity and ACTH on renin and aldosterone secretion. In: Hypertension, p. 4 (GENEST, J., KOIW, E., Eds.) Berlin - Heidelberg - New York: Springer 1972.
GANONG, W. F., BIGLIERI, E. G., MULROW, P. J.: Mechanisms regulating adrenocortical secretion of aldosterone and glucocorticoids. Recent Progr. Hormone Res. **22**, 381 (1966).
GANONG, W. F., BORYCZKA, A. T., SHACKLEFORD, R.: (2) Effect of renin on adrenocortical sensitivity to ACTH and angiotensin II in dogs. Endocrinology **80**, 703 (1967).
GANONG, W. F., BORYCZKA, A. T., SHACKLEFORD, R., CLARK, R. M., CONVERSE, R. P.: (1) Effect of dietary sodium restriction on adrenal cortical response to ACTH. Proc. Soc. exp. Biol. (N. Y.) **118**, 792 (1965).
GANONG, W. F., LEE, T. C., VAN BRUNT, E. E., BIGLIERI, E. G.: (2) Aldosterone secretion in dogs immunized with hog renin. Endocrinology **76**, 1141 (1965).

Ganong, W. F., Mulrow, P. J., Boryczka, A., Cera, G.: Evidence for a direct effect of angiotensin-II on adrenal cortex of the dog. Proc. soc. Exp. Biol. (N. Y.) **109**, 381 (1962).
Ganong, W. F., Pemberton, D. L., Van Brunt, E. E.: (1) Adrenocortical responsiveness to ACTH and angiotensin II in hypophysectomized dogs and dogs treated with large doses of glucocorticoids. Endocrinology **81**, 1147 (1967).
Genest, J., Nowaczynski, W., Koiw, E., Sandor, T.: Adrenocortical function in essential hypertension. In: Essential Hypertension, p. 126 (Bock, K. D., Cottier, P. T., Eds.). Berlin-Göttingen-Heidelberg: Springer 1960.
Gocke, D. J., Gerten, J., Sherwood, L. M., Laragh, J. H.: Physiological and pathological variations of plasma angiotensin II in man. Circulat. Res. **24**, **25** (Suppl. I), I—131 (1969).
Gross, F., Brunner, H., Ziegler, M.: Renin-angiotensin system, aldosterone, and sodium balance. Recent Progr. Hormone Res. **21**, 119 (1965).
Haning, R., Tait, S. A. S., Tait, J. F.: In vitro effects of ACTH, angiotensin, serotonin and potassium on steroid output and conversion of corticosterone to aldosterone by isolated adrenal cells. Endocrinology **87**, 1147 (1970).
Hartroft, P. M., Eisenstein, A. B.: Alterations in the adrenal cortex of the rat induced by sodium deficiency; correlation of histological changes with steroid hormone secretion. Endocrinology **60**, 641 (1957).
Hilton, J. C., Scian, L. F., Westermann, C. D., Nakano, J., Kruesi, O. R.: Vasopressin stimulation of the isolated adrenal glands: nature and mechanism of hydrocortisone secretion. Endocrinology **67**, 298 (1960).
Johnston, C. I., Davis, J. O., Hartfort, P. M.: Renin-angiotensin system, adrenal steroids and sodium depletion in a primitive mammal, the American opossum. Endocrinology **81**, 633 (1967).
Kaplan, N. M.: The biosynthesis of adrenal steroids: effects of angiotensin II, adrenocorticotropin, and potassium. J. clin. Invest. **44**, 2029 (1965).
Kaplan, N. M., Bartter, F. C.: The effect of ACTH, renin, angiotensin II, and various precursors on biosynthesis of aldosterone by adrenal slices. J. clin. Invest. **41**, 715 (1962).
Khairallah, P. A., Robertson, A. L., Davila, D.: In: Hypertension '72, p. 212 (Genest, J., Koiw, E., Eds.) Berlin - Heidelberg - New York: Springer 1972.
Kinson, G. A., Singer, B.: Sensitivity to angiotensin and adrenocorticotrophic hormone in the sodium deficient rat. Endocrinology **83**, 1108 (1968).
Krieger, D. T., Krieger, H. P.: Aldosterone excretion in pretectal disease. J. clin. Endocr. **24**, 1055 (1964).
Laragh, J. H., Angers, M., Kelly, W. G., Lieberman, S.: Hypotensive agents and pressor substances. The effect of epinephrine, norepinephrine, angiotensin II and others on the secretory rate of aldosterone in man. J. Amer. med. Ass. **174**, 234 (1960).
Lee, T. C., De Wied, D.: Somatotropin as the non-ACTH factor of anterior pituitary origin for the maintenance of enhanced aldosterone secretory responsiveness of dietary sodium restriction in chronically hypophysectomized rats. Life Sci. **7**, 35 (1968).
Lommer, D., Wolff, H. P.: Stimulation of the in vitro biosynthesis of corticosteroids by angiotensin II. Experientia (Basel) **22**, 699 (1966).
Lowenstein, J., Boyd, G. W., Rippon, A., James, V. H. T., Peart, W. S.: Increased aldosterone in response to sodium deficiency in the angiotensin II-immunized rabbit. In: Hypertension, p. 481 (Genest, J., Koiw, E., Eds.) Berlin - Heidelberg - New York: Springer 1972.
Marieb, N. J., Mulrow, P. J.: Role of the renin-angiotensin system in the regulation of aldosterone secretion in the rat. Endocrinology **76**, 657 (1965).
Marusic, E. T., Mulrow, P. J.: Stimulation of aldosterone biosynthesis in adrenal mitochondria by sodium depletion. J. clin. Invest. **46**, 2101 (1967).
Marx, A., Deane, H. W.: Histophysiologic changes in the kidney and adrenal cortex in rats on a low-sodium diet. Endocrinology **73**, 317 (1963).
Masson, G. M. C., Travis, R. H.: Effects of renin on aldosterone secretion in the rat. Canad. J. Physiol. Pharmacol. **46**, 11 (1968).
McCaa, R. E., Read, V. H., Bower, J. D., McCaa, C. S., Guyton, A. C.: Adrenal cortical responses to haemodialysis, ACTH and angiotensin II in anephric man. Circulation **44** (Suppl. II), II—67 (1971).
McDonald, I. R., Goding, J. R., Wright, R. D.: Transplantation of the adrenal gland of the sheep to provide access to its blood supply. Aust. J. exp. Biol. med. Sci. **36**, 83 (1958).
Michelakis, A. M., Horton, R.: The relationship between plasma renin and aldosterone in normal man. Circulat. Res. **26** and **27** (Suppl. I), I—185 (1970).
Mitra, S., Genuth, S. M., Berman, L. B., Vertes, V.: Aldosterone secretion in anephric patients. New Engl. J. Med. **286**, 61 (1972).
Mogil, R. A., Itskovitz, H. D., Russell, J. H., Murphy, J. J.: Renal innervation and renin activity in salt metabolism and hypertension. Amer. J. Physiol. **216**, 693 (1969).

MOUW, D. R., VANDER, A. J.: Evidence for brain Na receptors controlling renal Na excretion and plasma renin activity. Amer. J. Physiol. **219**, 822 (1970).

MULLER, J.: (1) Aldosterone stimulation in vitro. I. Evaluation of assay procedure and determination of aldosterone-stimulating activity in a human urine extract. Acta endocr. (Kbh.) **48**, 283 (1965).

MULLER, J.: (2) Aldosterone stimulation in vitro. II. Stimulation of aldosterone production by monovalent cations. Acta endocr. (Kbh.) **50**, 301 (1965).

MULLER, J.: Aldosterone-stimulating in vitro. III. Site of action of different aldosterone-stimulating substances on steroid biosynthesis. Acta endocr. (Kbh.) **52**, 515 (1966).

MULLER, J.: Decreased aldosterone production by rat adrenal tissue in vitro due to treatment with 9-fluorocortisol, dexamethasone and adrenocorticotrophin in vivo. Acta endocr. (Kbh.) **63**, 1 (1970).

MULLER, J.: Regulation of aldosterone biosynthesis. Monographs of Endocrinology. Berlin-Heidelberg-New York: Springer 1971.

MULLER, J., HUBER, R.: Effects of sodium deficiency, potassium deficiency, and uremia upon the steroidogenic response of rat adrenal tissue to serotonin, potassium ions, and adrenocorticotropin. Endocrinology **85**, 43 (1969).

MULLER, A. F., RIONDEL, A. M., MANNING, E. L.: Effect of corticotrophin on secretion of aldosterone. Lancet **1956 II**, 1021.

MULLER, J., ZIEGLER, W. H.: Stimulation of aldosterone biosynthesis in vitro by serotonin. Acta endocr. (Kbh.) **59**, 23 (1968).

MULROW, P. J., GANONG, W. F., CERA, G., KULJIAN, A.: The nature of the aldosterone stimulating factor in dog kidneys. J. clin. Invest. **41**, 505 (1962).

NEHER, R.: Aldosterone and other adrenocortical hormones in human adrenals and adrenal tumours. In: An International Symposium on Aldosterone, p. 11 (MULLER, A. F., O'CONNOR, C. M., Eds.). Boston: Little, Brown and Comp. 1958.

NEWSOME, H. H., BARTTER, F. C.: Plasma renin activity in relation to serum sodium concentration and body fluid balance. J. clin. Endocr. **28**, 1704 (1968).

NEWTON, M. A., LARAGH, J. H.: (1) Effect of corticotropin on aldosterone excretion and plasma renin in normal subjects, in essential hypertension and in primary aldosteronism. J. clin. Endocr. **28**, 1006 (1968).

NEWTON, M. A., LARAGH, J. H.: (2) Effects of glucocorticoid administration on aldosterone excretion and plasma renin in normal subjects, in essential hypertension and in primary aldosteronism. J. clin. Endocr. **28**, 1014 (1968).

PALMORE, W. P., ANDERSON, R., MULROW, P. J.: Role of the pituitary in controlling aldosterone production in sodium-depleted rats. Endocrinology **86**, 728 (1970).

PALMORE, W. P., MARIEB, N. J., MULROW, P. J.: Stimulation of aldosterone secretion by sodium depletion in nephrectomized rats. Endocrinology **84**, 1342 (1969).

PALMORE, W. P., MULROW, P. J.: Control of aldosterone secretion by the pituitary gland. Science **158**, 1482 (1967).

PASSO, S. S., ASSAYKEEN, T. A., OTSUKA, K., WISE, B. L., GOLDFIEN, A., GANONG, W. F.: Effect of stimulation of the medulla oblongata on renin secretion in dogs. Neuroendocrinology **7**, 1 (1971).

PEART, W. S.: The renin-angiotensin system. Pharmacol. Rev. **17**, 143 (1965).

RAITI, S., KOWARSKI, A., WELDON, V. V., MIGEON, C. J.: Secretion of cortisol, corticosterone and aldosterone in children with hypopituitarism. John Hopkins Med. J. **122**, 229 (1968).

RAMAN, P. B., SHARMA, D. C., DORFMAN, R. I.: Studies on aldosterone biosynthesis in vitro. Biochemistry **5**, 1795 (1966).

RAYYIS, S. S., HORTON, R.: Effect of angiotensin II on adrenal and pituitary function in man. J. clin. Endocr. **32**, 539 (1971).

REID, I. A., McDONALD, I. R.: The renin-angiotensin system in a marsupial (*Trichosurus vulpecula*). J. Endocr. **44**, 231 (1969).

RICHARDSON, J. B., BEAULNES, A.: The cellular site of action of angiotensin. J. Cell. Biol. **51**, 419 (1971).

RICHTER, C. P.: Salt appetite of mammals: its dependence on instinct and metabolism. In: L'Instinct dans le Comportement des Animaux et de l'Homme, p. 577. Paris: Masson et Cie. 1956.

ROMERO, J. C., STANELONI, R. J., DUFAU MARIA, L., DOHMEN, R., BINIA, A., KLIMAN, B., FASCIOLO, J. C.: Changes in fluid compartments, renal hemodynamics, plasma renin and aldosterone secretion induced by low sodium intake. Metabolism **17**, 10 (1968).

SCOGGINS, B. A., BLAIR-WEST, J. R., COGHLAN, J. P., DENTON, D. A., MYERS, K., NELSON, J. F., ORCHARD, ELSPETH, WRIGHT, R. D.: The physiological and morphological response of mammals to changes in their sodium status. In: Hormones and the Environment, Memoirs of the Society for Endocrinology (U. K.), p. 577. Cambridge: Cambridge University Press 1970.

SCOGGINS, B. A., COGHLAN, J. P., CRAN, E., DENTON, D. A., FAN, J., MCDOUGALL, J., ODDIE, C., SHULKES, A.: Experimental studies on the metabolism of ACTH induced hypertension. Proc. Int. Soc. Hypertension, Milan, 1972. Clin. Sci. (in press).

SEALEY, J. E., CLARK, I., BULL, M. B., LARAGH, J. H.: Potassium balance and the control of renin secretion. J. clin. Invest. **49**, 2119 (1970).

SKINNER, S. L., MCCUBBIN, J. W., PAGE, I. H.: Control of renin secretion. Circulat. Res. **15**, 64 (1964).

SLATER, J. D. H., BARBOUR, B. H., HENDERSON, H. H., CASPER, A. G. T., BARTTER, F. C.: Physiological influence of the kidney on the secretion of aldosterone, corticosterone and cortisol by the adrenal cortex. Clin. Sci. **28**, 219 (1965).

SLATON, P. E., SCHAMBELAN, M., BIGLIERI, E. G.: Stimulation and suppression of aldosterone secretion in patients with an aldosterone-producing adenoma. J. clin. Endocr. **29**, 239 (1969).

SPARK, R. F., GORDON, S. J., DALE, S. L., MELBY, J. C.: Aldosterone production after suppression of corticotropic secretory activity. Arch. intern. Med. **122**, 394 (1968).

SPAT, A., SOLYO, J., STURCZ, J., MESZAROS, I., LUDWIG, E.: Effect of angiotensin superfusion on the rate of aldosterone production by incubated rat adrenals. Acta physiol. Acad. Sci. hung. **35**, 149 (1969).

TAIT, S. A. S., SCHULSTER, D., OKAMOTO, M., FLOOD, C., TAIT, J. F.: Production of steroids by in vitro superfusion of endocrine tissue. II. Steroid output from bisected whole, capsular and decapsulated adrenals of normal intact, hypophysectomized and hypophysectomized-nephrectomized rats as a function of time of superfusion. Endocrinology **86**, 360 (1970).

ULICK, S., FEINHOLTZ, E.: Metabolism and rate of secretion of aldosterone in the bullfrog. J. clin. Invest. **47**, 2523 (1968).

ULICK, S., NICOLIS, G. L., VETTER, K. K.: Relationship of 18-hydroxycorticosterone to aldosterone. In: Aldosterone, p. 3 (BAULIEU, E. E., ROBEL, P., Eds.). Oxford: Blackwell 1964.

URQUHART, J., DAVIS, J. O., HIGGINS, J. T., Jr.: Effects of prolonged infusion of angiotensin II in normal dogs. Amer. J. Physiol. **205**, 1241 (1963).

VANDER, A. J.: Control of renin release. Physiol. Rev. **47**, 359 (1967).

VANDER, A. J.: Direct effects of potassium on renin secretion and renal function. Amer. J. Physiol. **219**, 455 (1970).

VENNING, E. H., DYRENFURTH, I., DOSSETOR, J. B., BECK, J. C.: Influence of alterations in sodium intake on urinary aldosterone response to corticotropin in normal individuals and patients with essential hypertension. Metabolism **II**, 254 (1962).

VEYRAT, R., BRUNNER, H. R., MANNING, E. L., MULLER, A. F.: Inhibition de l'activite de la renine plasmatique par le potassium. J. Urol. Nephrol. **73**, 271 (1967).

WEIDMANN, P., HORTON, R., FRANKLIN, S., FICHMAN, M., GRAL, T., LUPU, A., MAXWELL, M.: Dynamic studies of aldosterone in anephric man. Clin. Res. **22**, 201 (1972).

WELLEN, J. J., BENRAAD, T. J.: Effect of ouabain on corticosterone biosynthesis and on potassium and sodium concentration in calf adrenal tissue in vitro. Biochim. biophys. Acta (Amst.) **183**, 110 (1969).

WILLIAMS, G. H., ROSE, L. I., DLUHY, R. G., DINGMAN, J. F., LAULER, D. P.: Aldosterone response to sodium restriction and ACTH stimulation in panhypopituitarism. J. clin. Endocr. **32**, 27 (1971).

YANKOPOULOS, N. A., DAVIS, J. O., COTLOVE, E., TRAPASSO, M.: Mechanisms of myocardial edema in dogs with congestive cardiac failure. Amer. J. Physiol. **199**, 603 (1960).

Effects of Aldosterone on Blood Pressure, Water, and Electrolytes

F. Gross

Today it may be considered an anachronism to discuss aldosterone in a volume on angiotensin, since, during recent years, an increasing number of observations have been reported that cast doubts on the significance of angiotensin for the regulation of aldosterone secretion (Blair-West et al., 1968, 1971; Palmore et al., 1969; Müller, 1971, 1972; Boyd et al., 1972). However, the fact that the secretion of aldosterone is under multifactorial control should not divert from the results that prove a close relationship between the renin-angiotensin system and the aldosterone-producing cells of the adrenal cortex. It has been stressed repeatedly that angiotensin should not be characterized as the aldosterone-stimulating hormone or factor, because this might create the impression that no other factor but angiotensin has such an action (Gross, 1967). However, it would also be incorrect to disregard all the findings that clearly demonstrate a close humoral connection between the kidney and the zona glomerulosa of the adrenal cortex [Brown et al., 1972 (2)].

Besides angiotensin, ACTH, potassium supply, and sodium deficiency stimulate the release of aldosterone, but there is increasing evidence that additional humoral factors, so far not identified, may participate in the control of aldosterone secretion, especially in the state of sodium deficiency (Blair-West et al., 1971; Coghlan et al., 1971; Palkovits et al., 1971; Boyd et al., 1972; Müller, 1972). The regulation of aldosterone secretion is a complex mechanism involving various humoral factors and also affected by feedback mechanisms and the state of sodium balance. Apparently contradictory findings may be explained by different experimental conditions with respect to sodium and potassium balance and the duration of the study. In the rat, an aldosterone-stimulating effect of angiotensin could be demonstrated in sodium deficiency (Kinson and Singer, 1968), a state that also sensitizes the adrenal glomerular zone to ACTH (Ganong and van Brunt, 1968). Hence, measurements of plasma renin activity and the secretion rate of aldosterone in physiological and pathological conditions, especially in hypertension, should be related to sodium intake and excretion (Laragh et al., 1966; Brunner et al., 1972; Gross, 1972; Möhring et al., 1972; Wisenbaugh et al., 1972).

Aldosterone is characterized as the sodium-conserving hormone of the adrenal cortex, although, quantitatively, it contributes to the total reabsorption of sodium within the kidney only to a minor degree (Roemmelt et al., 1949; Pitts, 1951). However, its action on sodium transport is not limited to the kidney, but is extended to most epithelial cells where sodium is reabsorbed. Besides preserving sodium, aldosterone facilitates potassium excretion to a major degree by favoring an exchange of the two cations. Among other essential electrolytes, magnesium is similarly affected (Hanna and MacIntyre, 1960; Horton and Biglieri, 1962), whereas equivocal effects have been reported for calcium. The actions of either endogenous or exogenous aldosterone on electrolyte balance depend not only on the amounts secreted or administered, but also on the time during which they act. Consequently, one has to distinguish between acute effects of aldosterone, seen after a short-lasting stimulation of the endogenous production or after the giving of a single dose of the hormone, and effects obtained after repeated administration over a period of several days or weeks or at a continuously increased secretion rate due to adrenal hyperplasia or tumor formation of the glomerular zone.

Aldosterone is called a mineralocorticoid, a simplified term coined several years prior to the isolation and identification of the hormone and originally applied to deoxycorticosterone and deoxycortisol (Reichstein's substance S). Shortly after its isolation, but at a time when the chemical structure was still unknown, aldosterone was called electrocortin, which indicated its effect on sodium and potassium balance (SIMPSON et al., 1953, 1954). It is evident that a hormone whose prime function is the maintenance of sodium balance should be characterized otherwise than as mineralocorticoid, but the term has been generally accepted. The sodium-conserving effect is not specific for aldosterone, but is also observed with other steroids, such as deoxycorticosterone and 9α-fluorocortisol (9α-FF), and to a certain degree also with 11-deoxycortisol (substance S) and 18-hydroxydeoxycorticosterone (KAGAWA and PAPPO, 1962; PORTER and KIMSEY, 1971). For pharmacokinetic reasons some of these compounds are more suitable than aldosterone for the study of the actions of mineralocorticoids on sodium transport in the intact animal. Glucocorticoids, such as corticosterone, cortisol, and cortisone, also exert a mild sodium-retaining effect, but only in doses between 10 and 100 times higher than those of aldosterone. On the other hand, aldosterone has a mild glucocorticoid-like effect, which, however, is demonstrable only in a dosage range far beyond that affecting sodium transport (SCHULER et al., 1954).

Pharmacokinetics of Aldosterone

When aldosterone is administered either for substitution or for studies of its effects in the intact animal, its pharmacokinetics have to be considered. The biological half-life of aldosterone is shorter than that of deoxycorticosterone or of other corticosteroids and varies, according to the species, between 20 and 40 min (TAIT et al., 1961). This means that, for a satisfactory substitution, aldosterone should be injected either subcutaneously or intramuscularly every 3 to 4 h, but two to three injections at 12- or 8-h intervals may be satisfactory, especially if the hormone is given in oily solution. The most efficient form of administration is the subcutaneous implantation of pellets, which, however, has the disadvantage that, in the early phase after implantation, relatively large amounts of the hormone are absorbed from the depot, which may substantially exceed normal secretion rates [GROSS and SCHMIDT, 1958 (2)]. Various esters have been prepared, such as the 21-acetate or the 21-trimethylacetate, the actions of which are prolonged if compared with that of free aldosterone. However, the half-lives of deoxycorticosterone-21-acetate and especially deoxycorticosterone-21-trimethylacetate are longer, and these compounds are therefore more suitable for long-range substitution therapy than aldosterone or its esters. The former opinion that aldosterone and deoxycorticosterone-acetate differ not only quantitatively but also qualitatively from each other must probably be ascribed to the distinct pharmacokinetics of the two corticoids [GROSS and LICHTLEN, 1958 (2)].

In addition to the biological half-life, the metabolic clearance rate of aldosterone has been determined. In man it was found to be 0.86 to 1.64 ml/min (CHEVILLE et al., 1966) or 0.85 to 1.50 ml/min (LOMMER et al., 1968; VECSEI et al.,

1969); when calculated for 24 h, values of 1,200 to 2,400 l were obtained (TAIT et al., 1961; BALIKIAN et al., 1968). In patients with essential hypertension a decrease in metabolic clearance rate was found, being in the order of 867 l/day versus 1,480 l/day in normotensive control subjects; simultaneously, the secretion rate of aldosterone was slightly reduced (NOWACZYNSKI et al., 1971). Despite this reduction, plasma concentration of aldosterone had a tendency to rise.

Not only are 90 to 100% of the free aldosterone extracted in the liver, but also about 90% of the metabolites are formed there. The rate of extraction is directly proportional to the hepatic blood flow. About 60% of the metabolites have been identified so far, the main ones being 3α, 5β-tetrahydro-aldosterone-3-mono-glucuronide (THA-glucuronide) and aldosterone-18-glucuronide, formerly also described as acid-labile or acid-hydrolyzable conjugate. The original assumption that the latter was a 3-oxo-conjugate (AYRES et al., 1957) was not confirmed in later studies (BOUGAS et al., 1964). Whereas the THA-glucuronide is almost exclusively formed within the liver, the conjugation of aldosterone with glucuronic acid in position 18 takes place to a major part within the kidney, which is responsible for the production of about 10 to 15% of the total metabolites of aldosterone and extratcs about 20% (14 to 27%) of free aldosterone.

Aldosterone and Blood-Pressure Regulation

Complete removal of the adrenals is followed by a slow reduction in blood pressure, negative sodium and positive potassium balance, a decrease in intravascular and extracellular fluid volume, and an increase in non-protein nitrogen. Muscular weakness, apathy, and fatigue occur, and without adequate hormonal substitution or at least administration of sodium the animals die within 5 to 8 days. Among the various adrenocortical hormones — the glucocorticoids cortisol or corticosterone and the mineralocorticoid aldosterone — it is the latter that is of vital significance and the absence of which is responsible for the fatal outcome of bilateral adrenalectomy. The inability to maintain sodium balance subsequent to diminished sodium reabsorption in the kidney and the resulting impairment of homeostasis is the cause of death in the absence of aldosterone. However, in experimental animals, such as rats, rabbits, or dogs, it is not necessary to substitute aldosterone to maintain life after adrenalectomy, but deoxycorticosterone can completely replace aldosterone, and adrenalectomized dogs can be kept in good condition for years solely by the administration of deoxycorticosterone (GROSS, 1948; GROSS and MEIER, 1951; GROSS and DETTBARN, 1956). Aldosterone restores diminished blood pressure in adrenalectomized rats within 60 min (FRIEDMAN et al., 1958) as well as in adrenalectomized dogs [GROSS and LICHTLEN, 1958 (2)].

There is little evidence that aldosterone affects blood pressure directly in acute experiments. In intact or nephrectomized rats a slight increase in blood pressure was described after subcutaneous or intravenous injection of d,l-aldosterone in doses of 20 to 40 µg (FRIEDMAN et al., 1958). In recent studies in decerebrate rabbits a mild rise in blood pressure was obtained when aldosterone was infused at a rate of 6 µg/kg for 5 h. This effect was more pronounced when the animals had had 1% saline as drinking fluid prior to the experiment than when they had been kept on a low-sodium diet (BURSTYN et al., 1971). After topical application of aldosterone to the carotid sinus region in rabbits, blood pressure rose rapidly (BURSTYN and HORROBIN, 1970), but it is doubtful that this acute effect is related to the increase in blood pressure that develops subsequent to prolonged overdosage or high secretion rates of aldosterone.

It may be assumed that aldosterone acts on blood pressure by means of its influence on sodium balance. The fall in blood pressure after adrenalectomy is mainly the consequence of a reduced intravascular volume and the disturbed sodium balance and, to a certain degree, potassium balance. The response to pressor substances is diminished and can be restored by aldosterone (Friedman et al., 1958). A comparable decrease in pressor response can be obtained in dogs by repeated administration of saluretics, such as hydrochlorothiazide, which indicates that it is the loss of sodium that is responsible for the reduced pressor effects of epinephrine or angiotensin (Bock and Gross, 1960).

From these observations it may be concluded that aldosterone and similarly acting corticosteroids, when given for substitution in the adrenalectomized state, exert their action by restoring negative sodium and positive potassium balances. Consequently, in normotensive animals and in the presence of a normally functioning adrenal cortex, aldosterone has no direct blood-pressure elevating effect, and, similarly, other mineralocorticoids are also devoid of such an action (Friedman et al., 1958). However, in certain experimental conditions, such as after administration of bacterial endotoxins in cats, aldosterone was able to restore vascular response to epinephrine within a short period (Bein and Jaques, 1960; Bein, 1962). Unfortunately, this antitoxic effect could not be demonstrated unequivocally in the treatment of toxin-induced shock in experimental animals and in man (Spink and Vick, 1961, 1962).

Blood-Pressure Raising Effect of Aldosterone and Other Mineralocorticoids

Administration of aldosterone over a period of at least 10 days, but preferably of 3 to 4 weeks, induces an increase in the systemic blood pressure of rats, provided that sufficient sodium is administered, either in the diet or in the drinking fluid. The dose of aldosterone necessary to cause an elevation of blood pressure depends on the form of application. If the free alcohol is given in oily solution, 0.25 mg d-aldosterone daily, preferably administered in divided doses at 12-h intervals, may suffice, but only if the animals have saline to drink. If d-aldosterone-acetate or -trimethylacetate is administered in oily solution, a single daily dose of 0.25 mg will produce hypertension, but results will be more consistent if half the dose is given twice daily at 12-h intervals. The most reliable results are obtained when aldosterone is administered in the form of pellets, implanted subcutaneously in a dose of 25 to 50 mg. The continuous absorption of the hormone from the depot is the most efficient way of achieving a long-lasting overdosage comparable in effect to that of an aldosterone-producing tumor.

Various authors have reported different threshold doses of aldosterone for the production of hypertension in rats (Gross et al., 1955, 1956, 1957; Gaunt et al., 1957; Kumar et al., 1957; Gornall et al., 1960; Hall and Hall, 1965, 1967), and it may be assumed that the strains of rats used in individual laboratories vary in their sensitivity to the hormone and to salt. In recent years the significance of hereditary factors for the response to salt-induced hypertension has been emphasized (Dahl et al., 1962, 1964) and has received much wider attention than at the time when the first studies on the blood-pressure raising effect of aldosterone were undertaken (Gross et al., 1955, 1957). Variations in the biosynthetic pathways of cortical hormones, e. g. the ratio of 18-OH-deoxycorticosterone to corticosterone, may be at least partly responsible for high sensitivity or resistance to salt (Rapp and Dahl, 1971), but more work is necessary.

Deoxycorticosterone-acetate or -trimethylacetate, either given by injection of oily solution (2.5 mg daily) or of microcrystalline suspension (50 mg/kg once a week) or implanted as pellets (2 to 4 pellets of 25 mg each), produced, in our hands, more reliable increases in blood pressure than aldosterone. However, other investigators have not confirmed this observation and have found aldosterone-acetate the more potent corticoid, providing it is injected twice daily in oily solution (HALL and HALL, 1967). When a mixture of 1% saline and 5% sucrose solution was given as drinking fluid, salt intake was increased, since fluid consumption was twice or three times that with saline alone. Whereas, without aldosterone, mild hypertension developed when saline and sucrose were offered together, in the presence of high doses of the hormone (0.25 mg daily in divided doses) the degree of hypertension was similar whether 1% saline or a mixture of saline and sucrose was given (HALL and HALL, 1965).

Besides dietary factors, unilateral nephrectomy also leads to the development of hypertension. The removal of half the nephron population obviously diminishes the ability of the animal to adjust itself to the sodium-retaining effect of mineralocorticoids, and the increase in intravascular and extracellular fluid volume, which accompanies prolonged administration of aldosterone or other mineralocorticoids, is more pronounced when renal mass is reduced. The animals should preferably weigh between 60 and 90 g at the beginning of the experiment and should not exceed 120 g; otherwise the hypertensive response is irregular and less marked, particularly if the hormones are injected in oily solution.

Hypertension due to aldosterone or deoxycorticosterone is a sodium-induced form of hypertension and does not develop if a sodium-deficient diet is offered (GROSS et al., 1956; GOODWIN et al., 1969). It is not known whether the negative potassium balance, which accompanies sodium retention, affects blood pressure; however, it may have a mitigating rather than an intensifying influence on the development of hypertension. Bilateral adrenalectomy does not facilitate the development of mineralocorticoid hypertension (GROSS, 1957; HALL and AYACHI, 1971).

Of the laboratory animals, only rats respond to overdosage of mineralocorticoids with hypertension; neither the rabbit nor the dog shows a comparable reaction, regardless of the dosage and the duration of treatment. A rise in blood pressure was described in hamsters (STROIA et al., 1954) and chicken (STAMLER et al., 1951), but no further studies were undertaken. In rabbits, high doses of aldosterone, administered repeatedly over 10 days, induce pleural and peritoneal effusions, severe hypokalemia, and paralysis of skeletal and smooth muscles, leading to head-drop phenomenon, ataxia, and excessive filling of the bowel and bladder, which have a reduced muscular tone [GROSS and SCHMIDT, 1958 (2)]. In the dog, results are controversial. In our own studies, even high doses of either aldosterone or deoxycorticosterone — also in association with saline as drinking fluid — did not provoke marked hypertension, and similar observations have been reported earlier (SUMMERS, 1948). In unilaterally nephrectomized dogs an increase in blood pressure was obtained (RODBARD and FREED, 1942), and, more recently, sustained hypertension was induced by long-term overdosage of DOCA, but, after withdrawal of the steroid, blood pressure returned to normal values (WISENBAUGH et al., 1965). The reason why no hypertension develops in dogs and rabbits is not known.

Since other signs of mineralocorticoid overdosage, such as sodium and water retention and potassium loss, are similar to those seen in rats, differences in electrolyte metabolism cannot be responsible for the failure to develop hypertension. In man, both aldosterone and deoxycorticosterone may produce hypertension comparable in various ways to that seen in the rat. The first observations were made in patients suffering from Addison's disease, who were treated with deoxycorticosterone-acetate and who had high blood pressure besides retaining sodium and water, which resulted in edema formation (FERREBEE et al., 1939; SOFFER et al., 1940; THORN, 1941). The best example of the blood-pressure elevating effect of mineralocorticoids is the syndrome of primary aldosteronism caused by tumor formation of the zona glomerulosa of the adrenal cortex (CONN, 1955). The symptoms are directly comparable to those seen after overdosage of mineralocorticoids in the rat or in man: sodium retention, potassium loss, increased intravascular and extracellular fluid volume, increased fluid turnover, hypertension, but generally no edema formation such as occurs after overdosage of DOCA in Addisonian patients. Elevated plasma levels of DOC may be the consequence of 11β-hydroxylase or 17-hydroxylase deficiency; they were observed in a few patients with endocrine disorders and hypertension (BIGLIERI et al., 1966, 1968; BROWN and STROTT, 1971). Increased secretion of deoxycorticosterone (DOC) without tumor formation and with normal aldosterone secretion has recently been described in some patients with hypertension [BROWN et al., 1972 (1)]. The activity of the renin-angiotensin system was suppressed in most of them, and intermittent hypokalemia was observed. It is impossible to determine whether hypertension was the consequence of the increased formation of DOC in these cases, but if it were, it would be another example of the various possible ways in which the adrenal cortex may be involved in the pathogenesis of hypertension.

A characteristic finding in either overdosage of mineralocorticoids or endogenous overproduction of aldosterone is the disappearance of renin from the kidneys (GROSS and SULSER, 1956; GROSS, 1958). Renin activity is suppressed independently of the development of hypertension in rats and rabbits [GROSS and SCHMIDT, 1958 (1, 2)], provided that sodium is administered in adequate amounts (GROSS et al., 1956; SOKABE et al., 1963; GOODWIN et al., 1969). An inverse relationship between sodium balance and production or release of renin from the kidney is demonstrable under various experimental conditions and occurs in experimental mineralocorticoid hypertension in rats as well as in primary aldosteronism due to tumor formation of the zona glomerulosa or to hyperplasia of the adrenal cortex (CONN, 1964; GROSS et al., 1965; BROWN et al., 1968). In normal subjects and in patients with essential hypertension a similar inverse relationship between plasma renin activity or aldosterone excretion and sodium intake or excretion was found (LARAGH et al., 1966; BRUNNER et al., 1972).

Mineralocorticoid hypertension is accompanied by cardiac hypertrophy, and at a later stage severe vascular lesions are seen, which are reminiscent of periarteritis nodosa. Perivascular proliferative inflammation with granuloma formation may occur, and hyaline or fibrinoid necrosis of the arterial media is found as well as intima proliferation, which may partly occlude the lumen of the vessels and has been characterized as proliferative panarteritis (SELYE et al., 1943; SALGADO and SELYE, 1952; HALL and HALL, 1967). The kidneys are larger than in control rats, and compensatory hypertrophy after removal of one kidney is more pronounced than in rats without overdosage of mineralocorticoids. Microangiographic studies revealed an early dilatation of the efferent arterioles, which was related to some failure of the afferent arteriole. The afferent arteriole may lose the ability to contract adequately, with the consequence that the glomerulus and postglomerular vessels are perfused at an elevated pressure. Subsequently, lesions occur in the vasculature under the influence of high pressure (HEPTINSTALL and HILL, 1967; HILL and HEPTINSTALL, 1968). The renal glomeruli are severely damaged, the capillary loops may be hyalinized, the capillary membranes are thickened, and the space between the glomerular tuft and the Bowman capsule is either obliterated or full of hyaline material and cellular debris. The tubular epithelia are flat, the cell structure is irregular, and hyaline casts may fill the tubular lumen.

The lesions observed are not specific for the mineralocorticoids, but are the consequence of hypertension together with excessive sodium retention. Although this type of renal damage is comparable to nephrosclerotic lesions, which, after stenosis of one renal artery, occur in the contralateral kidney, hypertension due to mineralocorticoid overdosage cannot be considered a special type of renal hypertension. Whereas in renal hypertension the renin-angiotensin system may contribute to the increase in blood pressure, this is not the case in mineralocorticoid hypertension, in which the renal pressor system is suppressed. It may be assumed that the elevated pressure is responsible for the damage seen in various vascular beds, mainly in the kidneys and the areas supplied by the mesenteric arteries. How far the sodium retention contributes to the vascular lesions and to the proliferative inflammation found especially in the perivascular space is not known, but the fact that in sensitive rats similar changes are observed when large amounts of salt are administered without simultaneous administration of mineralocorticoids demonstrates that sodium alone is of pathogenic significance.

Eclampsia-Like Syndrome

During mineralocorticoid hypertension the pressor response to exogenous renin and angiotensin is increased [Gross and Lichtlen, 1958 (1)]. When high doses of either renin or angiotensin are given to rats with hypertension subsequent to overdosage of DOCA or aldosterone and salt, a characteristic syndrome develops, which has been called the eclampsia-like syndrome, because, besides severe hypertension and vascular damage, convulsions may occur (Masson et al., 1952, 1953, 1962). Whereas, in mineralocorticoid hypertension, the renin-angiotensin system is supressed, the high levels of exogenous renin or angiotensin aggravate vascular damage under these conditions. Such a situation is comparable to secondary aldosteronism in malignant hypertension (Laragh et al., 1960; Brown et al., 1971; Möhring et al., 1972).

Metacorticoid Hypertension

Hypertension produced by overdosage of mineralocorticoids may become self-sustaining after some time, so that no further administration of mineralocorticoids or salt is necessary. Metacorticoid hypertension has been observed after overdosage of deoxycorticosterone and salt (Green, 1953; Sturtevant, 1958); that it has not been described with aldosterone is probably because this hormone is more expensive and has not been made so freely available as DOCA. Metacorticoid hypertension is characterized by increased cardiovascular reactivity, vascular lesions, disturbances in salt and water metabolism, and reduced life expectancy (Sturtevant, 1958). It is probably caused by irreversible vascular lesions induced by high blood pressure and sodium retention. This form of hypertension is not easily reproducible, and certain strains of rats may be more sensitive to it than others, but no systematic studies have been performed in this direction. Metacorticoid hypertension has been compared with essential hypertension in man (Green, 1953), but it is certainly not justified to relate two types of hypertension that differ fundamentally in their etiology and pathogenesis. On the other hand, recent findings on the effectiveness of aldosterone antagonists in patients with essential hypertension and suppressed renin response indicate that, at least in some cases of essential hypertension, mineralocorticoids may be involved in the pathogenesis [Spark and Melby, 1971; Brown et al., 1972 (1); Liddle, in press].

Adrenal Regeneration Hypertension

This type of hypertension, which develops in rats after unilateral adrenalectomy and nephrectomy and enucleation of the second adrenal, was originally regarded as a type of mineralocorticoid hypertension depending on a high sodium intake mostly in the form of 1% saline (Skelton, 1959). However, it was not possible to demonstrate an increased secretion of aldosterone at any time after removal of the adrenals; on the contrary, the hormone was secreted only in minute amounts when blood pressure increased (Brogi and Pellegrino, 1959; Gaunt, 1969). Nor is high salt intake essential, since, in sensitive rats, hypertension was also obtained when water was given as drinking fluid [Rapp, 1964 (2); Hall et al., 1966]. The regenerating adrenal tissue, which completely substitutes the function of the intact adrenals, did not produce increased amounts of cortical hormones, which fact explains the development of hypertension (Masson et al., 1958; Gaunt et al., 1959; Skelton, 1959).

When the pattern of adrenocortical hormone secretion necessary for the maintenance of adrenal regeneration hypertension was investigated, it was found that, after removal of the adrenal regenerate, hypertension was sustained either by 0.1 mg aldosterone daily or by a combination of 0.1 mg aldosterone and 1 mg corticosterone. Corticosterone alone, in doses of 2.5 mg and 1.0 mg, was also sufficient to maintain hypertension, but, with the higher dose, thymus involution was observed, indicating that the amount of hormone exceeded that produced by the adrenal regenerate. It was concluded that the regenerated adrenal tissue secretes a mixture of aldosterone and corticosterone (Hall et al., 1967).

Subsequent studies revealed that mineralocorticoids other than aldosterone might be responsible for the development of adrenal regeneration hypertension, namely 18-hydroxy-deoxycorticosterone (18-OH-DOC) or deoxycorticosterone. 18-OH-DOC (Cortes et al., 1963), which is secreted by the rat adrenal in amounts similar to those of corticosterone [Melby et al., 1972 (1, 2); Gaunt et al., in press], has a weak mineralocorticoid activity (Kagawa and Pappo, 1962; Birmingham et al., 1968). In the rat, it had about 6% of the action of DOCA (Kagawa and Pappo, 1962), and in the isolated toad bladder, effectiveness was between 16 and 50% of that of DOCA, according to its action on sodium transport within 6 h (Porter and Kimsey, 1971). Adrenal regenerates incubated *in vitro* produced increased amounts of 18-OH-DOC (Birmingham et al., 1968; de Nicola et al., 1969), and *in-vivo* studies revealed an increased secretion rate of this corticoid 6 weeks after adrenal enucleation. At that time, when the rats had developed severe hypertension, only 18-OH-DOC was secreted in amounts that exceeded those in control rats, whereas corticosterone, DOC, and aldosterone secretion reached normal values. In studies on secretory rates of corticoids, DOC was not found to be increased, but plasma levels of this mineralocorticoid were elevated after 2 weeks, reached a maximum after 3 weeks, and subsequently fell slowly to control values (Brown et al., 1972; Gaunt et al., in press). The plasma levels measured 3 weeks after adrenal enucleation exceeded even those determined after implantation of 50 mg of DOCA as pellets, a dose that induced a degree of hypertension similar to that caused by adrenal enucleation (Brown et al., 1972). Other investigators observed an increased secretion rate of DOC in adrenal regeneration hypertension 4 weeks after the operation (Rapp, 1969).

On the basis of these and other findings it was suggested that the regenerating adrenal cortex may have a changing secretory pattern of hormones. During the first few days after enucleation, the adrenal produces an unidentified sodium-retaining factor, the action of which disappears before hypertension develops. Subsequently, high plasma concentrations of DOC are demonstrable, which are sufficient to cause hypertension. Progression and maintenance at a time when DOC secretion has fallen to control levels may be due to increased secretion of 18-OH-DOC, and finally a self-sustaining type of metacorticoid hypertension may occur (GAUNT et al., in press).

The fact that adrenal regeneration hypertension is the consequence of an increased production of mineralocorticoids is evident from the preventive action of spironolactone and from the reduced activity of the renin-angiotensin system (DUNIHUE et al., 1963; RAPP, 1964).

Effects of Hypertension on the Production and Secretion of Aldosterone

The mineralocorticoids, especially aldosterone, should be regarded not only as agents capable of producing hypertension by itself but also as substances with an intermediary function in other forms of hypertension, mainly those of renal origin. Since the close interrelationship between the renin-angiotensin system and the secretion of aldosterone was first described, numerous data have been reported, clearly showing that either the eliciting mechanisms of renal hypertension or the effects of chronically elevated blood pressure on kidney function may act on the production and secretion of aldosterone. Aldosterone secretion may be primarily affected by activation of the renin-angiotensin system such as follows stenosis of one renal artery in the presence of a normal kidney. The sequence of events under these conditions is: reduced renal blood flow, increased release of renin and subsequently increased formation of angiotensin, stimulation of aldosterone secretion, retention of sodium, increased intravascular and extracellular fluid volume. The release of both renin and aldosterone was increased under these conditions (SINGER et al., 1963), and an initial phase of positive sodium balance has also been shown recently (MÖHRING et al., 1971, 1972; GROSS et al., 1972). In this type of hypertension the ischemic kidney continues to produce and release renin in disproportionately large amounts, which continuously stimulate aldosterone secretion despite a positive sodium balance. Under these circumstances, aldosterone contributes to the development and maintenance of hypertension by its sodium-retaining effect, and consequently removal of the adrenals is followed by a fall in blood pressure, which can only partly be restored to hypertensive levels by administration of aldosterone (GROSS, 1960).

If blood pressure exceeds a critical value of about 180 mmHg systolic, sodium balance may become negative owing to a pressure-induced natriuresis in the contralateral kidney (MÖHRING et al., 1972; DAUDA et al., 1973). The consequence is a further stimulation of the renin-angiotensin system in the ischemic kidney and an increase in aldosterone secretion, with the result of secondary aldosteronism. Secondary aldosteronism in malignant hypertension was first described in man (LARAGH et al., 1960) at a time when it was not possible to determine either renin or angiotensin concentrations in plasma, but these observations have been confirmed by various authors [BROWN et al., 1971, 1972 (2)]. One consequence of high renin release may be a further increase in blood pressure, to which the elevated secretion of aldosterone may contribute, although it has to be considered mainly an attempt to reestablish sodium balance. In patients with malignant hypertension, excessive stimulation of aldosterone-producing cells by either angiotensin or another so far unknown factor may induce persistent hypersecretion of aldosterone, resulting in a disturbed feedback control (MCALLISTER et al., 1971).

The increased production of aldosterone in experimental renal hypertension is also evident from studies on the biosynthesis of aldosterone in vitro and in vivo. In adrenals taken from rats with renal hypertension due to unilateral clamping of the renal artery in the presence of an untouched kidney, aldosterone production was increased (MÜLLER and GROSS, 1969). When the conversion of radioactive-labeled precursors of aldosterone was investigated in rats, an increased conversion of tritiated progesterone and deoxycorticosterone into aldosterone was found, indicating an elevated production of the hormone (VECSEI et al., 1971; VECSEI and MÜNTER, in press).

The situation is different in renal hypertension due to stenosis of the remaining renal artery in the unilaterally nephrectomized rat. In such cases the activity of the renin-angiotensin system is comparable to that of control rats but relatively elevated if compared with unilaterally nephrectomized rats, in which the activity of the renin-angiotensin system is reduced and plasma renin concentration diminished. The reduction in renal mass together with the decrease in blood flow to the remaining kidney results in a positive sodium balance and increased intravascular volume without evidence of an elevated secretion of aldosterone. The sequence of events in this case is: removal of one kidney, clamping of the remaining renal artery, relative increase in activity of the renin-angiotensin system, positive sodium balance, increased intravascular volume, and later on increase in total peripheral resistance (LEDINGHAM and COHEN, 1964; GUYTON and COLEMAN, 1969; GUYTON et al., 1970).

Adrenals of rats with this type of hypertension showed no elevated production of aldosterone *in vitro* (MÜLLER and GROSS, 1969), and also the *in-vivo* conversion of labeled precursors to aldosterone was not increased (VECSEI and MÜNTER, in press). The significance of a positive sodium balance for this type of hypertension could be demonstrated by removal of the clip from the renal artery. This procedure was followed not only by a fall in blood pressure, but also by a marked excretion of sodium in the rat (LIARD and PETERS, 1970), whereas in sheep the reduction in blood pressure was not accompanied by urinary sodium loss (BLAIR-WEST et al., 1970). Although it has not been demonstrated so far, it may be assumed that aldosterone is of significance for the development and maintenance of renal hypertension in the unilaterally nephrectomized rat.

The fact that neither the secretion of aldosterone nor the activity of the renin-angiotensin system exceeds values measured in normotensive control rats does not exclude the possibility that in view of the positive sodium balance and the increased intravascular and extracellular fluid volume both angiotensin and aldosterone are produced and released in inadequately high amounts. It has been stressed previously that the normal secretory rate of a hormone-producing gland may not correspond to the actual conditions. When sodium balance is positive, a normal secretory rate of aldosterone is relatively too high, and, conversely, it would be too low in case of a negative sodium balance. The same is true of the activity of the renin-angiotensin system, which, although not beyond normal, is relatively stimulated in the unilaterally nephrectomized rat in which hypertension is produced by ischemia of the remaining kidney. Under this condition the remaining kidney is partly protected from the elevated systemic blood pressure, since the clip, at least in the early phase, prevents the pressure increase necessary to cause natriuresis. For this reason the remaining, clamped kidney will only rarely become a sodium-losing kidney comparable to the contralateral companion of an ischemic kidney, and consequently secondary aldosteronism is less frequent than in the presence of a contralateral unclamped kidney exposed to very high blood pressure.

Effects of Aldosterone on Electrolytes

Studies on the regulation of sodium and potassium balance by aldosterone have to distinguish between acute effects of a single dose of the hormone and effects of repeated doses given at intervals that provide a continuous action of the hormone. Furthermore, the presence or absence of endogenous aldosterone and other cortical hormones may influence the action of administered hormones. The sodium-retaining and kaliuretic effects of a single dose of aldosterone are best demonstrable in adrenalectomized animals, such as rat, dog, or sheep [GROSS and LICHTLEN, 1958 (2)].

The influence of aldosterone on sodium-potassium linked transport is not limited to the kidney but extends to other secretory glands and various epithelial structures, such as the salivary glands (SIMPSON and TAIT, 1952), the sweat glands (McCONAHAY et al., 1964; DOBSON and SLEGERS, 1971), or the colon (EDMONDS and MARRIOTT, 1969; CHARRON et al., 1969; THOMPSON and EDMONDS, 1971). Studies on sodium and potassium balances have been undertaken with aldosterone and deoxycorticosterone-acetate in intact rats (MÖHRING et al., 1970), dogs, and man (AUGUST et al., 1958; STRAUSS and EARLEY, 1959; MILLS, 1962; WRIGHT et al., 1969).

The acute action of aldosterone on sodium-potassium linked transport is similar in all vertebrate species investigated, but recently a certain refractoriness to the renal effects of aldosterone was reported in the golden hamster (GAUNT et al., 1971). Over a wide dosage range aldosterone did not produce sodium retention in adrenalectomized hamsters, but increased potassium excretion. Large doses elicited diuresis and natriuresis, which were attributed to the mild glucocorticoid activity of aldosterone, demonstrable with high doses administered to adrenalectomized animals (DESAULLES, 1958).

The site of action of aldosterone in the nephron has been studied by micropuncture methods in adrenalectomized rats. In the state of severe adrenal insufficiency, transit time was prolonged in the proximal tubules and transtubular sodium reabsorption diminished; fractional sodium reabsorption was not reduced, but even slightly increased as a consequence of the prolonged transit time (HIERHOLZER et al., 1965, 1966; HIERHOLZER, 1968; CORTNEY, 1969). However, impaired proximal sodium transport was found when the proximal tubules were perfused at a constant flow rate. In doses corresponding to daily secretion rates, aldosterone, within about 1 h, restored proximal sodium and fluid transport (HIERHOLZER et al., 1966; HIERHOLZER, 1968). This action was not specific for aldosterone, but was also obtained with cortisone, yet not with dexamethasone, which is devoid of any sodium-retaining effect. The action of aldosterone on the impaired sodium transport in the proximal tubules was prevented by actinomycin D (WIEDERHOLT, 1966; HIERHOLZER, 1968), which had originally been found to inhibit the effect of aldosterone on sodium transport in the toad bladder (EDELMAN et al., 1963; CRABBÉ and DE WEER, 1964; SHARP and LEAF, 1966). Besides affecting sodium transport, aldosterone also modified net potassium reabsorption in the proximal tubule and induced a decrease in $TF/P[K^+]$ in free-flow experiments during osmotic diuresis (WIEDERHOLT et al., 1972).

In intact rats, direct effects of aldosterone on proximal sodium transport are difficult to demonstrate. When the endogenous secretion of aldosterone was suppressed by the provision of 1% saline as drinking fluid for 4 weeks, fractional sodium reabsorption in the proximal tubules was diminished and sodium excretion increased (Stumpe and Ochwadt, 1968). Under such conditions, aldosterone normalized the proximal reabsorptive capacity (Stumpe and Ochwadt, 1968). In young rats, which did not yet have a well-developed regulation of aldosterone secretion, aldosterone enhanced proximal sodium reabsorption much as it did in adult rats (Čapek et al., 1968).

Aldosterone increased sodium transport not only in the proximal and distal tubules, but also in the collecting ducts, where it reduced leak permeability for sodium (Uhlich et al., 1969). As a consequence of the diminished sodium permeability a decreased efflux of radioactive sodium from the collecting ducts was obtained, and the transcellular concentration gradient for sodium increased in the collecting ducts (Uhlich et al., 1970). Although it has not yet been measured directly, it may be assumed that potassium secretion in the collecting ducts is also facilitated by aldosterone.

It has been suggested that aldosterone may contribute to the phenomenon of "potassium adaptation", which is observed after administration of a high-potassium diet and consists of the reduced toxicity of an acute potassium load (Alexander and Levinsky, 1968; Wright et al., 1971). Rats adapted to potassium excreted a potassium load more rapidly than nonadapted rats, in which plasma potassium concentration rose to higher levels than in controls. After adrenalectomy, potassium adaptation was no longer demonstrable but could be maintained by supplements of DOCA (Alexander and Levinsky, 1968). Potassium adaptation was also observed in rats on a low-sodium diet, which had an increased secretion of potassium in the distal tubules and the collecting ducts.

Chronic Effects of Aldosterone on Electrolytes

Repeated administration of mineralocorticoids has different effects on electrolytes and on blood pressure, depending on the dosage and the treatment schedule. After an initial retention of sodium, the kidney "escapes" this action of mineralocorticoids, whereas the negative potassium balance and the effect on blood pressure remain, the latter becoming more pronounced as administration of the mineralocorticoid continues.

Among the mineralocorticoids, DOCA has been more extensively studied than aldosterone with respect to chronic effects on electrolyte balances, but the two hormones differ mainly quantitatively from each other, owing to their different pharmacokinetics. The transient nature of the effect of DOCA on sodium balance was observed in dog (Ragan et al., 1940) and man (McGavack et al., 1946), shortly after the corticoid had been made available in sufficient amounts. The term "escape phenomenon", however, was not applied until 1958 (August et al., 1958; Relman et al., 1958), since when it has been in general use. All mammalian species studied, dog (Ragan et al., 1940), cat (Winter and Ingram, 1943), rabbit (Dawborn and Ross, 1967), rat (Suki et al., 1968; Thompson and Edmonds, 1971), and man (McGavack et al., 1946; August et al., 1958; Relman et al., 1958), escape from the sodium-retaining effect of mineralocorticoids.

Variations in the onset of the escape depend on the doses and pharmacokinetics of the corticoids, the sodium intake, and the amount of total body sodium. The kidney escapes from the sodium-retaining effect not only of exogenous mineralocorticoids but also of endogenous aldosterone, as is the case in various forms of aldosteronism, especially primary aldosteronism due to adenoma formation or adrenal hyperplasia (CONN et al., 1964). The contralateral kidney in renal hypertension induced by clamping one renal artery can also be considered a sodium-escaped kidney (GROSS et al., 1965).

Electrolyte Balance Studies

Renal escape of the sodium-retaining effect of mineralocorticoids does not occur unless a certain amount of sodium and water has been retained and consequently intravascular volume and extracellular fluid volume have been increased. The higher the sodium intake at the beginning of the administration of the mineralocorticoid is, the more rapidly will the critical expansion of the intravascular volume, which precedes the actual escape, be reached. As a consequence of the renal escape from the sodium-retaining effect, sodium balance is reestablished, but the initially retained sodium is not eliminated (LUFT and SJÖGREN, 1951; DAVIS and HOWELL, 1953; AUGUST et al., 1958; CONN et al., 1964; BIGLIERI et al., 1969; ELLINGHAUS, 1971), and the increase in total body sodium is maintained as long as the mineralocorticoid is given. After discontinuation of the mineralocorticoid, sodium balance becomes negative for several days, until the retained amount of sodium is excreted.

Simultaneously with the excretion of sodium, potassium is retained [DAVIS and HOWELL, 1953; ELLINGHAUS, 1971; MÖHRING and MÖHRING, 1972 (1)]. The new equilibrium in sodium balance achieved by the renal escape from the sodium-retaining effect of mineralocorticoids corresponds to a resetting of the regulation of total body sodium in response to the increased extracellular fluid volume.

In contrast to the escape from the sodium-retaining effect is the continued negative potassium balance, which induces hypokalemia and a decrease in total exchangeable potassium. The consequences of a persisting potassium loss may be more severe than those of the initial sodium retention, as can be demonstrated in animal species that are especially sensitive to potassium deprivation, such as the rabbit. Weakness and paralysis of skeletal muscles and of some smooth muscles may develop, the severity increasing as the sodium intake rises [GROSS and SCHMIDT, 1958 (1, 2)]. On the other hand, studies with aldosterone in dog and man have revealed that potassium loss may be prevented by a sodium-restricted diet (HOWELL and DAVIS, 1954; MULLER et al., 1955; DAWBORN, 1969). The negative potassium balance and the resultant hypokalemia, which occur under normal or elevated sodium intake, are the consequence of renal potassium excretion.

No evidence was obtained for extrarenal, e.g. fecal, potassium loss during continuous administration of aldosterone for several days, nor was there any indication that potassium was redistributed between the intracellular and extracellular fluid spaces (DAWBORN, 1969). In man, loss of potassium in the feces may occasionally contribute to the hypokalemia of primary aldosteronism (ROSS and HURST, 1965). However, fecal potassium loss under the influence of either endogenous aldosterone production or administration of mineralocorticoids did not reach values comparable to those seen in hyperaldosteronism induced by abuse of laxatives (WOLFF et al., 1968). In rabbits, prolonged administration of aldosterone did also elicit fecal loss of potassium, but urinary excretion of potassium was reduced at first, leading to a positive balance. Despite this fact, hypokalemia developed, probably as a consequence of potassium moving into the intracellular fluid space (DAWBORN and ROSS, 1967; DAWBORN and WATSON, 1968). After several days, renal excretion of potassium rose and, together with the still elevated fecal excretion, led to a further lowering of plasma potassium. The initial retention of potassium was accompanied by sodium retention, from which the animals rapidly escaped (DAWBORN and ROSS, 1967). Hypokalemia was accompanied by a fall in plasma magnesium concentration, which was attributed to a shift of magnesium from the extracellular to the intracellular fluid space, similar to that suggested for potassium (DAWBORN and WATSON, 1968) (see also below).

In recent balance studies on rats during DOCA administration, evidence was obtained for a biphasic course of the escape phenomenon [MÖHRING et al., 1970; MÖHRING and MÖHRING, 1972 (1)]. After an initial phase of sodium retention and potassium loss lasting approximately 24 h, both sodium and potassium excretion returned to control levels. This early normalization was followed by a second phase, during which sodium balance remained in equilibrium, whereas potassium balance became negative again. The escape phenomenon was only demonstrable during the night, the period of the main activity of the rat, when it consumes most of its food. During the first phase of the escape, sodium reabsorption and potassium secretion in the distal parts of the nephron were diminished, and consequently the balances of the two electrolytes were restored. In the second phase, proximal sodium reabsorption was reduced and distal sodium load increased, which led to an increase in sodium-potassium exchange, with the result of a normal sodium and an elevated potassium excretion [MÖHRING et al., 1970; MÖHRING and MÖHRING, 1972 (1)]. When aldosterone was continuously infused into rats, escape from the sodium-retaining effect occurred only within 4 days (THOMPSON and EDMONDS, 1971). Under these conditions, diurnal variations in sodium excretion persisted when high doses of aldosterone were given and when sodium intake was controlled by constant infusion of 0.9% saline.

In contrast to aldosterone and DOCA, another mineralocorticoid, 9α-FF, did not induce the typical escape phenomenon in intact rats (HAACK et al., 1972), whereas in dog or man a typical sodium-retaining effect was demonstrable, from which the kidney escaped (STRAUSS and EARLEY, 1959; MILLS, 1962; WRIGHT et al., 1969). No positive sodium balance was obtained in rats when 9α-FF was given in doses ranging from 0.1 to 1.0 mg daily. Potassium excretion, however, rose more than with corresponding doses of DOCA. In the doses used, 9α-FF had a marked glucocorticoid-like effect, including symptoms such as increased urinary volume and weight loss. In some contrast to these data are observations that 9α-FF induced an initial sodium retention and subsequent escape in rats when it was given in association with a low-calcium diet (SUKI et al., 1968). Simultaneously with sodium retention, urinary calcium excretion rose, whereas potassium excretion remained unaltered. Further studies with 9 α-FF, especially regarding its pharmacokinetics, are necessary before final conclusions can be drawn as to how this steroid compares with other mineralocorticoids with respect to influences on electrolyte balances.

In dogs, DOCA caused an initial retention of sodium, which was related to sodium intake, but the excess of excreted potassium did not correspond quantitatively to the amount of sodium retained (ELLINGHAUS, 1971). During a high sodium intake, a rapid onset of escape was seen, but weight gain during this period did not correspond to the expected increase in extracellular fluid volume. This discrepancy was explained by a shifting of water from the intra- to the extracellular space during the phase of sodium retention (ELLINGHAUS, 1971) or by the fact that retained sodium chloride had been sequestered without concomitant fluid retention in compartments other than extracellular space, such as bone (DAWBORN, 1969).

When DOCA was given to pregnant dogs, sodium was retained and escape occurred after some days, but potassium excretion never exceeded control values

(ROBB et al., 1970). Since kaliuresis induced by DOCA could be abolished in nonpregnant dogs by the administration of estrogens (JOHNSON et al., 1970), the absence of kaliuresis in pregnant dogs during DOCA treatment was attributed to the increased production of estrogens. On the other hand, the sodium-retaining effects of DOCA and of estrogens are additive when the two hormones are given together, suggesting that they act at different sites of the nephron. Although no comparable balance studies have been carried out in human pregnancy, it may be assumed that sodium retention and increase in extracellular fluid volume, which are not accompanied by hypokalemia and negative potassium balance, are consequences of the simultaneous increase in aldosterone and estrogen secretion. With respect to potassium balance, the "physiological" secondary aldosteronism during pregnancy differs from the pathological states of secondary aldosteronism, such as liver cirrhosis or some forms of renal artery stenosis, in which hypokalemia is often observed.

Apart from the kidney, no other target organs of aldosterone escape in a similar way from its sodium-retaining effect. The failure to escape has been demonstrated in the gut of rabbit (DAWBORN and ROSS, 1967), rat (THOMPSON and EDMONDS, 1971), and man (AUGUST et al., 1958; CHARRON et al., 1969; EDMONDS, 1972), and in the sweat and salivary glands of man (GIBÍNSKI et al., 1970; HEIDLAND et al., 1972). This difference between the kidney and other tissues where aldosterone acts on sodium reabsorption makes it probable that the mechanism underlying renal sodium escape is related either to specific effects of aldosterone on various parts of the nephron or to factors that interfere with the action of aldosterone within the kidney but not in other organs (see below).

Mechanism of Renal Sodium Escape

Despite numerous attempts to elucidate the mechanism by which the kidney escapes the sodium-retaining effect of mineralocorticoids, the data available do not give a clear answer. Since sodium intake determines the onset of the escape phenomenon, it was obvious to relate the escape mechanism with changes brought about by sodium retention, in particular the initial increase in extracellular fluid volume. It may be assumed that once extracellular fluid volume has surpassed a critical value, the renal tubules become resistant to the action of aldosterone [KRAMER et al., 1969; MÖHRING and MÖHRING, 1972 (2)]. However, nothing is known about how and where the kidney receives information on variations in extracellular fluid volume. Volume receptors have been localized in the left atrium, and in acute experiments increased filling of the left atrium by negative pressure-breathing or by inflating a balloon was followed by an increase in urinary volume (GAUER and HENRY, 1963; BRENNAN et al., 1971), but no effect on sodium excretion was observed under these experimental conditions. Acute changes obtained by such maneuvers cannot be compared with the slow increase in intravascular volume following the retention of sodium and water after administration of mineralocorticoids and may, therefore, not be of significance for the escape mechanism.

Besides physical factors, humoral factors have also been studied with respect to their influence on the renal sodium escape mechanism. However, the so-called natriuretic factors, which have been discussed most often in this context, have not been clearly defined so far and cannot be considered intrarenal antagonists to the sodium-retaining action of mineralocorticoids. The search for the renal sodium escape mechanism is handicapped by the fact that most information on the site of action of aldosterone under various conditions has been obtained by micropuncture studies, which have undoubtedly made a substantial contribution to the knowledge of renal physiology, but which have their technical limitations and may interfere with regulatory functions.

The simple explanation that the escape phenomenon is nothing but the response of the kidney to an increase in extracellular fluid volume is complicated by the fact that changes in intravascular and extravascular compartments of the total extracellular fluid space may be of different significance for the regulation of sodium reabsorption. Humoral and physical factors and their effects on sodium reabsorption have recently been extensively studied (WINDHAGER, 1969; ORLOFF and BURG, 1971; SCHRIER and DE WARDENER, 1971), but it is still not known what role they play in renal sodium escape.

Depending on the experimental conditions chosen, expansion of intravascular or extracellular fluid volume either diminishes, or has no effect on, proximal fractional sodium reabsorption (DAVIS et al., 1969; SONNENBERG and SOLOMON, 1969; DAUGHARTY et al., 1972), and the decrease in proximal sodium reabsorption may or may not be accompanied by increased sodium excretion (BRENNER and BERLINER, 1969; DAVIS et al., 1969). These observations have been made by means of micropuncture studies in dogs and rats. Sodium excretion may increase when the sodium load delivered to the distal tubules exceeds its transport capacity (BRENNER and BERLINER, 1969), but, in rats, reduced distal sodium reabsorption with no effect on proximal tubular reabsorption was found after infusion of hypertonic saline (GIEBISCH et al., 1964; LASSITER et al., 1964; CORTNEY et al., 1965). Furthermore, it has to be considered that, besides proximal and distal tubules, the collecting ducts also participate in sodium reabsorption, and physical or humoral factors may affect sodium transport in collecting-duct cells (HELLER, 1971). In rats, sodium excretion was enhanced after injection of small amounts of isotonic saline, which had no influence on glomerular filtration rate or fractional sodium reabsorption in the proximal or distal tubules (HELLER, 1971).

The role of expanded intravascular and extracellular fluid volumes has also been studied in DOCA-escaped dogs. At the onset of escape, fractional sodium reabsorption in the proximal tubules was unchanged [KNOX et al., 1970; SCHNEIDER et al., 1971 (1, 2)], which indicated diminished sodium reabsorption in the distal nephron. The close functional connection between intravascular volume and renal sodium reabsorption during the escape state was also obvious from the finding that, after infusion of albumin, DOCA-escaped dogs excreted more sodium than nonescaped control dogs, although reduction in proximal sodium reabsorption did not differ (KNOX et al., 1970). In dogs (WRIGHT et al., 1969) and rats (SONNENBERG, 1971; MÁLYUSZ et al., 1972), diminished proximal reabsorption of sodium has also been made responsible for the escape phenomenon, but all other data support the interpretation that the reduced distal transport is essential for the increase in urinary sodium excretion.

In DOCA-escaped dogs, mild dehydration was followed by normalization of intravascular volume, but increased sodium excretion was not affected. On the other hand, since hydration of sodium-depleted dogs and the subsequent increase in intravascular volume did not prevent the diminished elimination of a sodium load, it was suggested that the interstitial fluid volume might be more significant than the intravascular volume for the control of sodium excretion (HIGGINS, 1971). However, the lack of methods for direct determination of interstitial fluid volume and the impossibility of strict separation of the two extracellular fluid compartments make conclusions difficult.

The Renin-Angiotensin System and Sodium Escape

The close correlation between sodium balance and the activity of the renin-angotensin system suggests that humoral factors are involved in the escape mechanism. In the kidney that has escaped the sodium-retaining effect of mineralocorticoids, renin activity is reduced, and after several weeks of either DOCA or aldosterone administration the amount of renin extractable from the kidney is negligible. Extractable renin disappears from the escaped kidney long after the onset of escape, but suppressed production of renin may be preceded by its diminished release, which results in reduced plasma renin activity. Although data are lacking as to the early action of mineralocorticoids on the renin-angiotensin system, it may be assumed that renin release decreases in response to an increase in intravascular volume, and that at the time of renal escape very little or no renin is released (GROSS et al., 1965).

Attempts to demonstrate the significance of the renin-angiotensin system for the escape phenomenon have given divergent results. When the aorta was constricted above the origin of the renal arteries in both DOCA-escaped and control dogs, proximal sodium reabsorption rose markedly in the control animals only [SCHNEIDER et al., 1971 (1)]. In the DOCA-escaped dogs the suppressed renin activity was made responsible for the abolished increase in proximal tubular reabsorption. Additional constriction of the aorta enhanced plasma renin activity both in control and in DOCA-escaped dogs, but the absolute increase was much smaller in the DOCA-treated than in the control dogs [SCHNEIDER et al., 1971 (1)]. In dogs with cardiac failure, DOCA reduced the renin activity in the kidneys to a similar extent as in intact dogs, but, despite the low renin activity, dogs in severe cardiac failure did not escape the sodium-retaining effect of DOCA (JOHNSTON et al., 1968). The fact that in a special pathological situation a regulatory mechanism may not function in the same way as under normal conditions is not contradictory to its physiological significance. It may be claimed that escape from the sodium-retaining effect of mineralocorticoids does not occur when the activity of the renin-angiotensin system is high, but the possibility that escape may be prevented when the renin activity is low cannot be excluded.

Suppressed renin release from the kidney during mineralocorticoid administration and disappearance of extractable renin have no influence on the concentration of plasma renin substrate, which remains unchanged. This observation demonstrates that the relationship between renin and its substrate does not simply depend on the plasma concentration of the enzyme (CARRETERO and GROSS, 1967). During the state of mineralocorticoid escape the activity of the renin system is only transiently suppressed, but not at all eliminated as after bilateral nephrectomy. A remarkable stability of plasma renin substrate concentration has also been observed when sodium intake was varied. With low sodium intake and subsequent increase in renin activity, plasma substrate concentration did not differ from that obtained when sodium intake was high and renin activity low (GROSS et al., 1972).

If one assumes that renin, by means of angiotensin, acts on the efferent arterioles in the kidney [SCHMID, 1968; KRAHÉ et al., 1970, 1971; REGOLI and GAUTHIER, 1971 (1, 2)], the suppressed formation of angiotensin would result in a reduced tone of the efferent arteriole and a diminished intravascular resistance. Independent of the increase in blood pressure, which is only observed in rats and man after prolonged administration of mineralocorticoids and which occurs much later than the escape from their sodium-retaining effect, the escape phenomenon might be considered a consequence of a change in intrarenal hemodynamics.

Isolated perfused kidneys from DOCA-treated rabbits respond differently from kidneys of untreated animals (KRAHÉ et al., 1970). When the kidneys were perfused with a red-cell suspension in Tyrode's solution free of renin substrate, the control kidneys reacted with an increase in glomerular filtration rate, in filtration fraction, and in intravascular resistance when plasma substrate was added to the perfusate. The kidneys from DOCA-treated rabbits, which had escaped from the sodium-retaining effect of DOCA, showed no such response when renin substrate was added, which indicates that not only the stores, but also the endogenous release of renin and of angiotensin were diminished. So far it is not clear how significant these findings are for what happens in the intact animal during the phase of resistance to mineralocorticoids, especially with regard to the incomplete sodium reabsorption found in the isolated organ, but with an improved technique (HOFBAUER et al., 1973) the isolated kidney may become a suitable means to obtain further insight into the escape mechanism.

It has already been mentioned that dogs with experimental congestive heart failure subsequent to an aorta-to-vena cava (A-V) fistula failed to escape from the sodium-retaining effect of DOCA despite renin-depleted kidneys (JOHNSTON et al., 1968). It was assumed that reduction of glomerular filtration rate and subsequently diminished delivery of sodium to the distal parts of the nephron were responsible for the inability of the kidney to escape sodium retention. When saline was infused, fractional proximal sodium reabsorption fell in both DOCA-escaped and non-escaped dogs with heart failure, but in the latter, sodium excretion rose by only one fourth as much as in escaped dogs. It was concluded that enhanced sodium reabsorption in the distal tubules may have contributed to the inability to escape. If the escape phenomenon were mainly the consequence of a change in intrarenal hemodynamics, it would not be surprising that in the state of congestive heart failure the kidney responded differently to influences that would otherwise induce changes in intrarenal vascular resistance. In dogs that did not escape the sodium-retaining effect of DOCA, urinary potassium excretion did not rise, and no hypokalemia occurred (JOHNSTON et al., 1968).

In conclusion, although the significance of the renin-angiotensin system for the escape mechanism has not been definitely proved, and despite the fact that some experimental observations have been brought up against a prevailing role of renin depletion in the resistance of the nephron to the sodium-retaining effect of mineralocorticoids, it is difficult not to regard the renin-angiotensin system as being closely involved in the renal response to mineralocorticoids. Such a participation of angiotensin in the response to mineralocorticoids is probably limited to an intrarenal hemodynamic action, which explains the unique position of the kidney if compared with other target organs of mineralocorticoids that are unable to escape the sodium-retaining effect. The inability of extrarenal organs to escape despite the suppression of plasma renin concentration indicates that angiotensin may affect sodium transport only within the kidney and may in this respect be of no significance to other tissues. Isorenins of extrarenal origin, such as the one found in the submandibulary gland of male mice, do not respond to variations in sodium intake or prolonged administration of mineralocorticoids and are probably not involved in the regulation of sodium balance.

Effect of Aldosterone on Calcium and Magnesium Balances

In contrast to the regulation of sodium and potassium, that of the two bivalent cations is apparently not primarily affected by mineralocorticoids. Injection of single doses of aldosterone reduced calcium excretion in normal man (LAMBERG et al., 1964), and infusion of aldosterone diminished excretion of calcium and magnesium in adrenalectomized man, but moderately increased phosphate output (LEVIN and CADE, 1965). On the other hand, in patients with Addison's disease, the reduced excretion of magnesium was restored towards normal when aldosterone was administered (HORTON and BIGLIERI, 1962). Acute effects of aldosterone on renal handling of calcium and magnesium gave no indication that the hormone might influence tubular reabsorption of the two cations (LEMANN et al., 1970).

Repeated administration of aldosterone or DOCA was followed by a negative magnesium balance (HANNA and MACINTYRE, 1960). An increase in daily urinary excretion of magnesium was observed in rats (MAHY and MUNDAY, 1963) and sheep (SCOTT and DOBSON, 1965), as well as in dogs that had escaped the sodium-retaining effect of DOCA (MASSRY et al., 1968). Another mineralocorticoid, 9α-FF, increased calcium excretion in rats (SUKI et al., 1967). As a result of the negative balance, hypomagnesemia may develop (MAHY and MUNDAY, 1963). In primary aldosteronism, negative magnesium balance and low plasma concentration of magnesium may also occur (HORTON and BIGLIERI, 1962), resulting eventually in reduced urinary excretion of magnesium (HORTON and BIGLIERI, 1962; KAPITOLA and KÜCHEL, 1964). Hypomagnesemia is also currently found in patients with Bartter's syndrome. Since no direct effect on the renal tubular transport of magnesium or calcium could be observed, it was suggested that the mineralocorticoids act upon magnesium excretion indirectly by the expansion of ECFV (MASSRY et al., 1969).

A special observation was reported in rabbits, in which prolonged infusion of aldosterone reduced plasma concentration of both potassium and magnesium without changing the external balance. It was supposed that the hormone had promoted a transfer of the two ions from extracellular fluid spaces into the cells (DAWBORN and WATSON, 1968). Parallel changes in potassium and magnesium excretion or transport have been seen in various experimental and pathological conditions.

In magnesium-depleted rats, aldosterone secretion was elevated, leading to an increased muscle sodium concentration and a diminished concentration of potassium (GINN et al., 1967), but secretion of corticosterone was reduced. On the other hand, no consistent effect of magnesium depletion on aldosterone secretion was found in man (COPE and PEARSON, 1963), which indicates that the hormone is not of primary significance for the regulation of magnesium balance.

Mechanism of Aldosterone Action on Electrolyte Transport

It is not within the scope of this contribution to refer in detail to studies on the molecular basis underlying the action of aldosterone on sodium and potassium transport in the renal tubules or other epithelial structures, but rather to give a summary of some of the most significant findings. In these investigations wide use has been made of the isolated toad bladder *(Bufo marinus)* and the skin of the frog *(Rana temporaria)*, which served as models for sodium transport in the distal renal tubules. Since aldosterone exerts its effect on renal sodium transport only after a latent period of between 60 and 90 min, it was supposed that it might act by the formation or activation of an intermediate (CRABBÉ, 1963). Subsequently, evidence was presented that aldosterone induced the de-novo synthesis of proteins by stimulating RNA synthesis (EDELMAN et al., 1963; WILLIAMSON, 1963). In toad-bladder cells, tritiated aldosterone is concentrated in the nuclear region, as was shown by autoradiographic methods, and may be displaced from nuclear binding sites by other mineralocorticoids, such as 9α-FF (Porter and Edelman, 1964; Porter et al., 1964). Besides the nuclear fraction, a cytoplasmatic fraction of mineralocorticoid-binding proteins has been characterized (Ausiello and Sharp, 1968; Edelman, 1972).

In kidney cells, aldosterone also induces the formation of various aldosterone-binding proteins, which are localized in the nuclear, cytosol, mitochondrial, and microsomal fractions [Fanestil and Edelman, 1966 (1); Herman et al., 1968]. In the nuclear fraction, binding of aldosterone could be inhibited by 9α-FF, but not by 6α-methylprednisolone or 17α-isoaldosterone, which are devoid of mineralocorticoid activity (Herman et al., 1968). Aldosterone antagonists of the spirolactone type (SC 14266) prevented the uptake of tritiated aldosterone by the cytosol and nuclear fractions of specific binding proteins (Fanestil, 1968). The binding activity for aldosterone of the newly formed proteins obviously depends on intact SH groups of cystine or methionine (Edelman, 1968; Herman et al., 1968).

The fact that aldosterone is responsible for the *de-novo* synthesis of specific proteins has been demonstrated by the inhibiting effect of actinomycin D, which blocks m-RNA synthesis, and by the addition of puromycin or cycloheximide, which interfere with protein synthesis at the ribosomal level and prevent the action of aldosterone in the toad bladder [Fanestil and Edelman, 1966 (2); Edelman, 1968].

When aldosterone acts on the kidney, first the cytosol fraction is synthesized and forms a complex with aldosterone; this gives rise to the synthesis of the nuclear protein fraction, which subsequently generates the chromatin complex (Edelman, 1972; Funder et al., 1972). Hence the cytosol fraction may be considered the precursor of the nuclear fractions. *De-novo* synthesis of RNA in toad-bladder cells was not accelerated by aldosterone (Vančura et al., 1971), and similar observations were made with nuclear fractions from heart and kidney of adrenalectomized rats (Liu et al., 1972).

The aldosterone-induced proteins activate mitochondrial enzymes, providing sufficient substrates of oxidative metabolism are available (Edelman, 1968; Fanestil et al., 1968). The specific proteins may stimulate NADH-linked oxidative phosphorylation (Edelman, 1968, 1969), but an increase in other mitochondrial enzymes was also found in toad-bladder cells exposed to aldosterone (Kirsten et al., 1968, 1970). It was concluded that aldosterone, by means of aldosterone-binding proteins, may regulate sodium transport by supplying energy for the extrusion of sodium from the cells (Edelman, 1968; Lipton and Edelman, 1971). However, opinions are divided about whether aldosterone facilitates the entrance of sodium from the luminal site into the cells (Sharp and Leaf, 1963; Crabbé, 1969) or, at the cell basis, the extrusion into the peritubular space (Lipton and Edelman, 1971). As was shown in isolated epithelial cells of the toad bladder, aldosterone may accelerate a rate-limiting step for the entry of sodium into the cells at the mucosal site (Handler et al., 1972; Leaf and Macknight, 1972) and for the active sodium transport across the basal membrane (Lipton and Edelman, 1971; Crabbé, 1972). Although there is good evidence that aldosterone favors the apical entrance of sodium into the cells, and that in this way more sodium is made available to the transport system, it has not been excluded that the hormone may provide energy to the sodium pump mechanism responsible for the removal of sodium from the cell into the peritubular space.

Effect of Aldosterone on ATPase Activity

After adrenalectomy in rats, the activity of the sodium- and potassium-dependent ATPase falls slowly to low levels (CHIGNELL and TITUS, 1966; LANDON et al., 1966), which are restored by substitution with corticosterone, but not by aldosterone (JØRGENSEN, 1969). Recently it has been shown that the duration of exposure to the hormone action is of significance for the result obtained. In adrenalectomized rats, aldosterone increased the activity of the sodium- and potassium-dependent ATPase between 14 and 24 h after removal of the adrenal, whereas corticosterone was ineffective. After 24 to 48 h, however, aldosterone had only a partial effect, while glucocorticoids restored the ATPase activity to normal levels (JØRGENSEN, 1969; HENDLER et al., 1972). The increase in activity of the ATPase was most pronounced in the outer renal medulla, but was insignificant in the outer cortex. It was supposed that aldosterone may induce *de-novo* synthesis of the enzyme, but only as a consequence of a sustained action of the hormone on sodium reabsorption (JØRGENSEN, 1972).

Summary

Within the 15 years that have elapsed since the stimulating effect of angiotensin on the secretion of aldosterone was first reported, this observation has been repeatedly confirmed, but it has also become evident that the regulation of aldosterone secretion is much more complex than it seemed originally. Plasma concentrations of potassium and of sodium, ACTH—at least when sodium supply is reduced—and possibly additional so far unidentified factors participate in the adjustment of aldosterone secretion to changes in sodium balance. The role of aldosterone in the regulation of blood pressure and its contribution to the pathophysiological mechanisms of some types of hypertension are also far from clear. Despite some contradictory findings it may be stated that aldosterone has no acute blood-pressure raising effect. The increase in blood pressure that develops after repeated administration of high doses together with salt has all the features of mineralocorticoid hypertension such as is seen after high doses of deoxycorticosterone acetate. Because of its short duration of action, aldosterone has to be given as the free alcohol at least twice daily and as the acetate or a similar ester once daily. The characteristic reduction in renal renin content and plasma renin concentration is seen with both aldosterone and deoxycorticosterone. This process is reversible, and normal renin levels are restored after withdrawal of the steroids. The mechanisms responsible for the increase in blood pressure are unknown, but mineralocorticoid hypertension cannot be explained simply by the increase in plasma or blood volume.

Experimental mineralocorticoid hypertension has a clinical correlate in primary aldosteronism and in the rare cases of increased production of deoxycorticosterone. In adrenal regeneration hypertension an initial increase in deoxycorticosterone secretion has been observed, which is subsequently replaced by an elevated secretion of 18-OH-deoxycorticosterone. The latter steroid is a weak mineralocorticoid, which, when given together with salt, produces hypertension comparable to that caused by deoxycorticosterone. For obvious reasons, there is no clinical correlate to adrenal regeneration hypertension, but essential hypertension with suppressed response to stimuli of renin release has been ascribed to an elevated secretion of a mineralocorticoid other than aldosterone or deoxycorticosterone. However, attempts to demonstrate an increased secretion rate of any known mineralocorticoid that might cause hypertension and a suppressed response of the renin system to hemodynamic stimuli or drugs have so far not been successful. Since not only spironolactone, but also other diuretics reduce blood pressure and restore the renin response to usual stimuli in essential hypertension, it can be assumed that the reduced sensitivity of the renin-releasing mechanism is the consequence of an increase in plasma or extracellular volume. It remains to be shown what causes the expansion of extracellular space in this condition or why such a response is found only in some patients with essential hypertension.

High blood pressure can also have an indirect effect on aldosterone secretion, as it has in renal artery stenosis; the contralateral, non-stenosed kidney loses sodium when blood pressure exceeds a critical value, so that the renin-angiotensin system and aldosterone secretion are stimulated. The result is secondary aldosteronism, with high aldosterone secretion and elevated renin release, but without edema formation. Such a vicious circle—hypertension, sodium loss, increased renin release, and formation of angiotensin, which stimulates aldosterone secretion but may also increase blood pressure further—is present in the acute phase of malignant hypertension. Sodium supply may relieve symptoms under such conditions, whereas administration of diuretics will have an aggravating effect.

Aldosterone increases fractional sodium reabsorption at all sites of the nephron and favors potassium excretion in the distal tubules. These acute effects on sodium and potassium excretion are easily demonstrable in adrenalectomized animals, but are difficult to show in intact ones. When aldosterone is given repeatedly, the kidney escapes the sodium-retaining effect, as it does after repeated administration of other mineralocorticoids, probably by reducing distal sodium reabsorption. Diminished sodium reabsorption may be due partly to extracellular fluid expansion after repeated administration of aldosterone, but it is not known how changes in extracellular fluid space are perceived and transmitted to the tubular epithelium. The decreased renin release and the reduced intrarenal formation of angiotensin may be of significance in the escape of the kidney from the sodium-retaining effect of aldosterone and other mineralocorticoids. Hence, it may be that angiotensin and aldosterone have complementary actions within the kidney, the main target organ of aldosterone. The more aldosterone is available, the less angiotensin will be produced within the kidney, and vice versa. In this sense, the kidney's escape from the sodium-retaining action of aldosterone is the converse of its efforts to conserve sodium by stimulating the renin-angiotensin system in sodium deficiency. It must be admitted, however, that, although the overall effects appear relatively straightforward, the way aldosterone, renin, angiotensin, and other factors are interrelated will not be disentangled until our understanding of the renin-angiotensin system is more complete than now.

References

ALEXANDER, E. A., LEVINSKY, N. G.: An extrarenal mechanism of potassium adaptation. J. clin. Invest. **47** 740—748 (1968).

AUGUST, J. T., NELSON, D. H., THORN, G. W.: Response of normal subjects to large amounts of aldosterone. J. clin. Invest. **37**, 1549—1555 (1958).

AUSIELLO, D. A., SHARP, G. W. G.: Localization of physiological receptor sites for aldosterone in the bladder of the toad, *Bufo marinus*. Endocrinology **82**, 1163—1169 (1968).

AYRES, P. J., GARROD, O., TAIT, S. A. S., TAIT, J. F., WALKER, G., PEARLMAN, W. H.: The use of (16-^{3}H) aldosterone in studies on human peripheral blood. In: Ciba Foundation Colloquia on Endocrinology, Vol. 11: "Hormones in Blood", p. 309—326 (WOLSTENHOLME, G. E. W., MILLAR, E. C. P., Eds.). London: Churchill 1957.

BALIKIAN, H. M., BRODIE, A. H., DALE, S. L., MELBY, J. C., TAIT, J. F.: Effect of posture on the metabolic clearance rate, plasma concentration and blood production rate of aldosterone in man. J. clin. Endocr. **28**, 1630—1640 (1968).

BEIN, H. J.: Aldosterone and alterations in circulatory reactivity following endotoxins. In: Shock, Pathogenesis and Therapy. An International Symposium, p. 162—168 (BOCK, K. D., Ed.). Berlin-Göttingen-Heidelberg: Springer 1962.

BEIN, H. J., JAQUES, R.: The antitoxic effect of aldosterone. Experientia (Basel) **16**, 24—26 (1960).

BIGLIERI, E. G., HERRON, M. A., BRUST, N.: 17-Hydroxylation deficiency in man. J. clin. Invest. **45**, 1946—1954 (1966).

BIEGLIERI, E. G., SLATON, P. E., Jr., SCHAMBELAN, M., KRONFIELD, S. J.: Hypermineralocorticoidism. Amer. J. Med. **45**, 170—175 (1968).

BIGLIERI, E. G., SCHAMBELAN, M., SLATON, P. E., Jr.: Effect of adrenocorticotropin on desoxycorticosterone, corticosterone and aldosterone excretion. J. clin. Endocr. **29**, 1090—1101 (1969).

BIRMINGHAM, M. K., MACDONALD, M. L., ROCHEFORT, J. G.: Adrenal function in normal rats and in rats bearing regenerated adrenal glands. In: Functions of the Adrenal Cortex, Vol. 2, p. 647—689 (MCKERNS, K. W., Ed.). New York: Appleton Century Crofts 1968.

BLAIR-WEST, J. R., COGHLAN, J. P., DENTON, D. A., GODING, J. R., WINTOUR, M., WRIGHT, R. D.: The effect of nephrectomy on aldosterone secretion in the conscious sodium-depleted hypophysectomized sheep. Aust. J. exp. Biol. med. Sci. **46**, 295—318 (1968).

BLAIR-WEST, J. R., CAIN, M. C., CATT, K. J., COGHLAN, J. P., DENTON, D. A., FUNDER, J. W., NELSON, J. F., SCOGGINS, B. A., WRIGHT, R. D.: Role of the kidney in experimental renovascular hypertension. Circulat. Res. **26** (Suppl. 2), 149—158 (1970).

BLAIR-WEST, J. R., CAIN, M. D., CATT, K. J., COGHLAN, J. P., DENTON, D. A., FUNDER, J. W., SCOGGINS, B. A., WRIGHT, R. D.: The dissociation of aldosterone secretion and systemic renin and angiotensin II levels during the correction of sodium deficiency. Acta endocr. (Kbh.) **66**, 229—247 (1971).

BOCK, K. D., GROSS, F.: Abschwächung pressorischer Wirkungen durch Sali-Diuretica. Naunyn-Schmiedebergs Arch. exp. Path. Pharmak. **238**, 339—347 (1960).

BOUGAS, J., FLOOD, C., LITTLE, B., TAIT, J. F., TAIT, S. A. S., UNDERWOOD, R.: Dynamic aspects of aldosterone metabolism. In: Aldosterone, A Symposium, p. 25—50 (BAULIEU, E. E., ROBEL, P., Eds.). Oxford: Blackwell Scientific Publications 1964.

BOYD, G. W., ADAMSON, A. R., ARNOLD, M., JAMES, V. H. T., PEART, W. S.: The role of angiotensin II in the control of aldosterone in man. Clin. Sci. **42**, 91—104 (1972).

BRENNAN, L. A., Jr., MALVIN, R. L., JOCHIM, K. E., ROBERTS, D. E.: Influence of right and left atrial receptors on plasma concentrations of ADH and renin. Amer. J. Physiol. **221**, 273—278 (1971).

BRENNER, B. M., BERLINER, R. W.: Relationship between extracellular volume and fluid reabsorption by the rat nephron. Amer. J. Physiol. **217**, 6—12 (1969).

BROGI, M. P., PELLEGRINO, C.: The secretion of corticosterone and aldosterone by the rat adrenal cortex regenerating after enucleation. J. Physiol. (Lond.) **146**, 165—179 (1959).

BROWN, J. J., CHINN, R. H., DAVIES, D. L., DÜSTERDIECK, G., FRASER, R., LEVER, A. F., ROBERTSON, J. I. S., TREE, M., WISEMAN, A.: Plasma electrolytes, renin, and aldosterone in the diagnosis of primary hyperaldosteronism. Lancet **1968 II**, 55—59.

BROWN, J. J., DÜSTERDIECK, G., FRASER, R., LEVER, A. F., ROBERTSON, J. I. S., TREE, M., WEIR, R. J.: Hypertension and chronic renal failure. Brit. med. Bull. **27**, 128—135 (1971).

BROWN, J. J., FERRISS, J. B., FRASER, R., LEVER, A. F., LOVE, D. R., ROBERTSON, J. I. S., WILSON, A.: (1) Apparently isolated excess deoxycorticosterone in hypertension. A variant of the mineralocorticoid-excess syndrome. Lancet **1972 II**, 243—247.

BROWN, J. J., FRASER, R., LEVER, A. F., ROBERTSON, J. I. S.: (2) Aldosterone: Physiological and pathophysiological variations in man. Clinics in Endocrinology and Metabolism **1**, 397—449 (1972).

BROWN, R. D., STROTT, C. A.: Plasma deoxycorticosterone in man. J. clin. Endocr. **32**, 744—750 (1971).

BROWN, R. D., GAUNT, R., GISOLDI, E., SMITH, N.: The role of deoxycorticosterone in adrenal regeneration hypertension. Endocrinology **91**, 921—924 (1972).

BRUNNER, H. R., LARAGH, J. H., BAER, L., NEWTON, M. A., GOODWIN, F. T., KRAKOFF, L. R., BARD, R. H., BÜHLER, F. R.: Essential hypertension: Renin and aldosterone, heart attack and stroke. New Engl. J. Med. **286**, 441—449 (1972).

BURSTYN, P. G., HORROBIN, D. F.: Possible mechanism of action for aldosterone-induced hypertension. Lancet **1970 I**, 973—976.

BURSTYN, P. G., HORROBIN, D. F., LLOYD, I. J.: The effect of intravenous aldosterone on arterial pressure in the rabbit and its modification by variations in diet. J. Endocr. **50**, 653—657 (1971).

ČAPEK, K., FERNANDEZ, J., DLOUHÁ, H.: Natriumresorption im proximalen Konvolut der jungen Rattenniere. Pflügers Arch. ges. Physiol. **300**, R 24—R 25 (1968).

Carretero, O., Gross, F.: Renin substrate in plasma under various experimental conditions in the rat. Amer. J. Physiol. **213**, 695—700 (1967).

Charron, R. C., Leme, C. E., Wilson, D. R., Ing, T. S., Wrong, O. M.: The effect of adrenal steroids on stool composition, as revealed by *in vivo* dialysis of faeces. Clin. Sci. **37**, 151—167 (1969).

Cheville, R. A., Luetscher, J. A., Hancock, E. W., Dowdy, A. J., Nokes, G. W.: Distribution, conjugation, and excretion of labelled aldosterone in congestive heart failure and in controls with normal circulation: Development and testing of a model with an analog computer. J. clin. Invest. **45**, 1302—1316 (1966).

Chignell, C. F., Titus, E.: Effect of adrenal steroids on a Na^+- and K^+-requiring adenosine triphosphatase from rat kidney. J. biol. Chem. **241**, 5083—5089 (1966).

Coghlan, J. P., Blair-West, J. R., Denton, D. A., Scoggins, B. A., Wright, R. D.: Perspectives in aldosterone and renin control. Aust. N. Z. J. Med. **2**, 178—197 (1971).

Conn, J. W.: Primary aldosteronism: A new clinical syndrome. J. Lab. clin. Med. **45**, 661—664 (1955).

Conn, J. W.: Plasma renin activity in primary aldosteronism. Importance in differential diagnosis and in research of essential hypertension. J. Amer. med. Ass. **190**, 222—225 (1964).

Conn, J. W., Knopf, R. F., Nesbit, R. M.: Primary aldosteronism: present evaluation of its clinical characteristics and of the results of surgery. In: Aldosterone. A Symposium, p. 327—352 (Baulieu, E. E., Robel, P., Eds.). Oxford: Blackwell Scientific Publications 1964.

Cope, C. L., Pearson, J.: Aldosterone secretion in magnesium deficiency. Brit. med. J. **1963 II**, 1385—1386.

Cortés, J. M., Péron, F. G., Dorfman, R. I.: Secretion of 18-hydroxydeoxycorticosterone by the rat adrenal gland. Endocrinology **73**, 713—720 (1963).

Cortney, M. A.: Renal tubular transfer of water and electrolytes in adrenalectomized rats. Amer. J. Physiol. **216**, 589—598 (1969).

Cortney, M. A., Mylle, M., Lassiter, W. E., Gottschalk, C. W.: Renal tubular transport of water, solute, and PAH in rats loaded with isotonic saline. Amer. J. Physiol. **209**, 1199—1205 (1965).

Crabbé, J.: Site of action of aldosterone on the bladder of the toad. Nature (Lond.) **200**, 787—788 (1963).

Crabbé, J.: The mechanism of action of aldosterone. In: Progress in Endocrinology, p. 41—46 (Gual, C., Ed.). Amsterdam: Excerpta Medica Foundation 1969.

Crabbé, J.: Hormonal influences on transepithelial sodium transport: Aldosterone vs insulin. J. Steroid Biochem. **3**, 229—235 (1972).

Crabbé, J., de Weer, P.: Action of aldosterone on the bladder and skin of the toad. Nature (Lond.) **202**, 298—299 (1964).

Dahl, L. K., Heine, M., Tassinari, L.: Effects of chronic excess salt ingestion. Evidence that genetic factors play an important role in susceptibility to experimental hypertension. J. exp. Med. **115**, 1173—1190 (1962).

Dahl, L. K., Heine, M., Tassinari, L.: Effects of chronic excess salt ingestion. Vascular reactivity in two strains of rats with opposite genetic susceptibility to experimental hypertension. Circulation **30** (Suppl. 2), 11—22 (1964).

Dauda, G., Möhring, J., Hofbauer, K. G., Homsy, E., Miksche, U., Orth, H., Gross, F.: The vicious circle in acute malignant hypertension of rats. Clin. Sci. **45** (Suppl. 1), 251—255 (1973).

Daugharty, T. M., Ueki, I. F., Nicholas, D. P., Brenner, B. M.: Comparative renal effects of isoncotic and colloid-free volume expansion in the rat. Amer. J. Physiol. **222**, 225—235 (1972).

Davis, B. B., Walter, M. J., Murdaugh, H. V.: Renal response to graded saline challenge. Amer. J. Physiol. **217**, 1604—1607 (1969).

Davis, J. O., Howell, D. S.: Comparative effect of ACTH, cortisone and DCA on renal function, electrolyte excretion and water exchange in normal dogs. Endocrinology **52**, 245—255 (1953).

Dawborn, J. K.: The effect of prolonged intravenous infusion of aldosterone in a normal human subject. Med. J. Aust. **1969 I**, 1079—1082.

Dawborn, J. K., Ross, E. J.: The effect of prolonged administration of aldosterone on sodium and potassium turnover in the rabbit. Clin. Sci. **32**, 559—570 (1967).

Dawborn, J. K., Watson, L.: Effect of prolonged administration of aldosterone on potassium and magnesium metabolism in the rabbit. Med. J. Aust. **1968 II**, 304—307.

Desaulles, P.: Comparison of the effects of aldosterone, cortexone and cortisol on adrenalectomized rats under various salt loads. In: Aldosterone. An International Symposium, p. 29—38 (Muller, A. F., O'Connor, C. M., Eds.). London: Churchill 1958.

Dobson, R. L., Slegers, J. F. G.: The effect of aldosterone on sweating in the cat. J. invest. Derm. **56**, 337—339 (1971).

DUNIHUE, F. W., VAN B. ROBERTSON, W., MACHANIC, B.: Effect of adrenal enucleation and of the spironolactone SC-8109 on granularity of rat juxtaglomerular cells. Endocrinology **72**, 859—864 (1963).

EDELMAN, I. S.: Intracellular action of aldosterone on sodium transport. In: Renal Transport and Diuretics, p. 139—151 (THURAU, K., JAHRMÄRKER, H., Eds.). Berlin-Heidelberg-New York: Springer 1968.

EDELMAN, I. S.: Intracellular action of aldosterone on sodium transport. In: Progress in Endocrinology, p. 24—25 (GUAL, C., Ed.). Amsterdam: Excerpta Medica Foundation 1969.

EDELMAN, I. S.: The initiation mechanism in the action of aldosterone on sodium transport. J. Steroid Biochem. **3**, 167—172 (1972).

EDELMAN, I. S., BOGOROCH, R., PORTER, G. A.: On the mechanism of action of aldosterone on sodium transport: The role of protein synthesis. Proc. nat. Acad. Sci. (Wash.) **50**, 1169—1177 (1963).

EDMONDS, C. J.: Effect of aldosterone on mammalian intestine. J. Steroid Biochem. **3**, 143—149 (1972).

EDMONDS, C. J., MARRIOTT, J. C.: The effect of aldosterone on the electrical activity of the rat colon. J. Endocr. **44**, 363—377 (1969).

ELLINGHAUS, K.: Sodium and potassium balance during the administration of desoxycorticosterone in dogs with differing dietary sodium intakes. Pflügers Arch. ges. Physiol. **322**, 347—354 (1971).

FANESTIL, D. D.: Mode of spirolactone action: Competitive inhibition of aldosterone binding to kidney mineralocorticoid receptors. Biochem. Pharmacol. **17**, 2240—2242 (1968).

FANESTIL, D. D., EDELMAN, I. S.: (1) Characteristics of the renal nuclear receptors for aldosterone. Proc. nat. Acad. Sci. (Wash.) **56**, 872—879 (1966).

FANESTIL, D. D., EDELMAN, I. S.: (2) On the mechanism of action of aldosterone on sodium transport: Effects of inhibitors of RNA and of protein synthesis. Fed. Proc. **25**, 912—916 (1966).

FANESTIL, D. D., HERMAN, T. S., FIMOGNARI, G. M., EDELMAN, I. S.: In: Regulatory Functions of Biological Membranes. Biochim. Biophys. Acta Library Series Vol. II, p. 177ff. (JARNEFELT, J., Ed.). Amsterdam: Elsevier 1968.

FERREBEE, J. W., RAGAN, C., ATCHLEY, D. W., LOEB, R. F.: Desoxycorticosterone esters; certain effects in treatment of Addison's disease. J. Amer. med. Ass. **113**, 1725—1731 (1939).

FRIEDMAN, S. M., FRIEDMAN, C. L., NAKASHIMA, M.: Effects of aldosterone on blood pressure and electrolyte distribution in the rat. Amer. J. Physiol. **195**, 621—627 (1958).

FUNDER, J. W., FELDMAN, D., EDELMAN, I. S.: Specific aldosterone binding in rat kidney and parotid. J. Steroid Biochem. **3**, 209—218 (1972).

GANONG, W. F., VAN BRUNT, E. E.: Control of aldosterone secretion. In: The Adrenocortical Hormones. Handbook of Experimental Pharmacology, Vol. 14, Part 3, p. 4—116 (WENDLER DEANE, H., RUBIN, B. L., Eds.). Berlin-Heidelberg-New York: Springer 1968.

GAUER, O. H., HENRY, J. P.: Circulatory basis of fluid volume control. Physiol. Rev. **43**, 423—481 (1963).

GAUNT, R.: The functions of the enucleate adrenal. Trans. N. Y. Acad. Sci. **31**, 256—260 (1969).

GAUNT, R., ULSAMER, G. J., CHART, J. J.: Aldosterone and hypertension. Arch. int. Pharmacodyn. **110**, 114—118 (1957).

GAUNT, R., GROSS, F., RENZI, A. A., CHART, J. J.: The adrenal cortex in hypertension (with particular reference to adrenal regeneration hypertension). In: Hypertension. The First Hahnemann Symposium on Hypertensive Disease, p. 219—232 (MOYER, J., Ed.). Philadelphia: Saunders 1959.

GAUNT, R., GISOLDI, E., SMITH, N.: Refractoriness to renal effects of aldosterone in the golden hamster. Endocrinology **89**, 63—69 (1971).

GAUNT, R., MELBY, J. C., DALE, S. L., GREKIN, R. J., BROWN, R. D.: Adrenal regeneration hypertension. In: Proceedings of the Fourth International Congress of Endocrinology. Amsterdam: Excerpta Medica (in press).

GIBÍNSKI, K., GIEC, L., NOWAK, S., KOKOT, F.: Mineralocorticoids and sweat gland function. Acta biol. med. germ. **25** 201—205 (1970).

GIEBISCH, G., KLOSE, R. M., WINDHAGER, E. E.: Micropuncture study of hypertonic sodium chloride loading in the rat. Amer. J. Physiol. **206**, 687—693 (1964).

GINN, H. E., CADE, R., MCCALLUM, T., FREGLEY, M.: Aldosterone secretion in magnesium-deficient rats. Endocrinology **80**, 969—971 (1967).

GOODWIN, F. J., KNOWLTON, A. I., LARAGH, J. H.: Absence of renin suppression by deoxycorticosterone acetate in rats. Amer J. Physiol. **216**, 1476—1480 (1969).

GORNALL, A. G., GRUNDY, H. M., KOLADICH, C. J.: Studies on aldosterone. III. Chronic effect on the blood pressure of rats. Canad. J. Biochem. **38**, 43—50 (1960).

GREEN, D. M.: Experimental hypertension. Ann. intern. Med. **39**, 333—344 (1953).

Gross, F.: Kombinierte Wasser- und Kochsalzbelastungen an normalen und nebennierenlosen Hunden. II. Mitteilung. Helv. physiol. pharmacol. Acta 6, 426—454 (1948).
Gross, F.: Experimentelle Methoden zur Beurteilung blutdrucksenkender Pharmaka. Naunyn-Schmiedebergs Arch. exp. Path. Pharmak. 232, 161—197 (1957).
Gross, F.: Renin und Hypertensin, physiologische oder pathologische Wirkstoffe? Klin. Wschr. 36, 693—706 (1958).
Gross, F.: Adrenocortical function and renal pressor mechanisms in experimental hypertension. In: Essential Hypertension. An International Symposium, p. 92—111 (Bock, K. D., Cottier, P. T., Eds.). Berlin-Göttingen-Heidelberg: Springer 1960.
Gross, F.: The regulation of aldosterone secretion by the renin-angiotensin system under various conditions. Acta endocr. (Kbh.) 56 (Suppl. 124), 41—64 (1967).
Gross, F.: Niere und Hochdruck. Klin. Wschr. 50, 621—635 (1972).
Gross, F., Dettbarn, W. D.: Water and salt loading in adrenalectomized dogs treated with cortexone, aldosterone and 9α-fluorocortisol. Acta endocr. (Kbh.) 22, 335—370 (1956).
Gross, F., Lichtlen, P.: (1) Verstärkung der pressorischen Wirkung von Renin, drucksteigernden Peptiden und adrenergischen Wirkstoffen nach Nephrektomie und bei Überdosierung von Cortexon und Kochsalz an der Ratte. Naunyn-Schmiedebergs Arch. exp. Path. Pharmak. 233, 323—337 (1958).
Gross, F., Lichtlen, P.: (2) Further evidence for a qualitative difference between aldosterone and cortexone. In: Aldosterone. An International Symposium, p. 39—50 (Muller, A. F., O'Connor, C. M., Eds.). London: Churchill 1958.
Gross, F., Meier, R.: Versuch zur Differenzierung der Wirkungen verschiedener Nebennierenrinden-Steroide auf den Wasser- und Elektrolytstoffwechsel. Schweiz. med. Wschr. 81, 1013—1018 (1951).
Gross, F., Schmidt, H.: (1) Überdosierung von Cortexon (DOC) und Kochsalz beim Kaninchen. Naunyn-Schmiedebergs Arch. exp. Path. Pharmak. 232, 408—418 (1958).
Gross, F., Schmidt, H.: (2) Aldosterone overdosage in the rabbit. Acta endocr. (Kbh.) 28, 467—478 (1958).
Gross, F., Sulser, F.: Pressorische Substanzen in den Nieren experimentell hypertonischer Ratten. Naunyn-Schmiedebergs Arch. exp. Path. Pharmak. 229, 374—380 (1956).
Gross, F., Loustalot, P., Meier, R.: Vergleichende Untersuchungen über die hypertensive Wirkung von Aldosteron und Desoxycorticosteron. Experientia (Basel) 11, 67—68 (1955).
Gross, F., Loustalot, P., Sulser, F.: Die Bedeutung von Kochsalz für den Cortexon-Hochdruck der Ratte und den Gehalt der Nieren an pressorischen Substanzen. Naunyn-Schmiedebergs Arch. exp. Path. Pharmak. 229, 381—388 (1956).
Gross, F., Loustalot, P., Meier, R.: Production of experimental hypertension by aldosterone. Acta endocr. (Kbh.) 26, 417—423 (1957).
Gross, F., Brunner, H., Ziegler, M.: Renin-angiotensin system, aldosterone, and sodium balance. Recent Progr. Hormone Res. 21, 119—167 (1965).
Gross, F., Dauda, G., Kazda, S., Kynčl, J., Möhring, J., Orth, H.: Increased fluid turnover and the activity of the renin-angiotensin system under various experimental conditions. Circulat. Res. 31 (Suppl. 2), 173—181 (1972).
Guyton, A. C., Coleman, T. G.: Quantitative analysis of the pathophysiology of hypertension. Circulat. Res. 24 (Suppl. 1), 1—14 (1969).
Guyton, A. C., Coleman, T. G., Bower, J. D., Granger, H. J.: Circulatory control in hypertension. Circulat. Res. 27 (Suppl. 2), 135—147 (1970).
Haack, D., Homsy, E., Möhring, B., Möhring, J.: Effects of 9α-fluorhydrocortisone, DOCA, and cortisone acetate on 24-hour and 12-hour urinary sodium, potassium, and water excretions in rats. Naunyn-Schmiedebergs Arch. Pharmakol. 274 (Suppl.), R 46 (1972).
Hall, C. E., Ayachi, S.: Dose-effect relationship in desoxycorticosterone hypertension: Reduced sensitivity in adrenalectomized rats and its possible significance to the etiology of adrenal regeneration hypertension. Can. J. Physiol. Pharmac. 49, 139—146 (1971).
Hall, C. E., Hall, O.: Hypertension and hypersalimentation. I. Aldosterone hypertension. Lab. Invest. 14, 285—294 (1965).
Hall, C. E., Hall, O.: The comparative hypertensive activities of the acetates of d-aldosterone and deoxycorticosterone. Acta endocr. (Kbh.) 54, 399—410 (1967).
Hall, C. E., Holland, O. B., Hall, O.: The sodium chloride requirement in adrenal-regeneration hypertension. Arch. Path. 81, 247—256 (1966).
Hall, C. E., Holland, O. B., Hall, O.: Comparative abilities of aldosterone and corticosterone singly and together to sustain adrenal-regeneration hypertension following adrenalectomy. Circulation 36 (Suppl. 2), 130 (1967).
Handler, J. S., Preston, A. S., Orloff, J.: Effect of ADH, aldosterone, ouabain, and amiloride on toad bladder epithelial cells. Amer. J. Physiol. 222, 1071—1074 (1972).
Hanna, S., MacIntyre, J.: The influence of aldosterone on magnesium metabolism. Lancet 1960 II, 348—350.

HEIDLAND, A., KREUSSER, B., HENNEMANN, H., KNAUF, H., WIEGAND, M.: Excretion of the mono- and bivalent ions in the relation to flow rate in Bartter's and Pseudo-Bartter's syndrome in parotid salivary. Comparative studies to the syndrome of Conn. Klin. Wschr. **20**, 959—966 (1972).

HELLER, J.: Micropuncture study of the mechanism of natriuresis after a short infusion of isotonic saline in rats. Physiol. bohemoslov. **20**, 139—145 (1971).

HENDLER, E. D., TORRETTI, J., KUPOR, L., EPSTEIN, F. H.: Effects of adrenalectomy and hormone replacement on Na-K ATPase in renal tissue. Amer. J. Physiol. **222**, 754—760 (1972).

HEPTINSTALL, R. H., HILL, G. S.: Steroid-induced hypertension in the rat. A study of the effects of renal artery constriction on hypertension caused by desoxycorticosterone. Lab. Invest. **16**, 751—767 (1967).

HERMAN, T. S., FIMOGNARI, G. M., EDELMAN, I. S.: Studies on renal aldosterone-binding proteins. J. biol. Chem. **243**, 3849—3856 (1968).

HIERHOLZER, K.: Intrarenal action of steroid hormones on sodium transport. In: Renal Transport and Diuretics, p. 153—171 (THURAU, K., JAHRMÄRKER, H., Eds.). Berlin-Heidelberg-New York: Springer 1968.

HIERHOLZER, K., WIEDERHOLT, M., HOLZGREVE, H., GIEBISCH, G., KLOSE, R. M., WINDHAGER, E. E.: Micropuncture study of renal transtubular concentration gradients of sodium and potassium in adrenalectomized rats. Pflügers Arch. ges. Physiol. **285**, 193—210 (1965).

HIERHOLZER, K., WIEDERHOLT, M., STOLTE, H.: Hemmung der Natriumresorption im proximalen und distalen Konvolut adrenalektomierter Ratten. Pflügers Arch. ges. Physiol. **291**, 43—62 (1966).

HIGGINS, J. T.: Role of extracellular volume in diuretic response to saline loading, and Role of plasma volume in control of proximal tubular sodium reabsorption. Amer. J. Physiol. **220**, 1367—1372 and 1373—1378 (1971).

HILL, G. S., HEPTINSTALL, R. H.: Steroid-induced hypertension in the rat. Amer. J. Path. **52**, 1—20 (1968).

HOFBAUER, K. G., ZSCHIEDRICH, H., RAUH, W., ORTH, H., GROSS, F.: Reaction of endogenous renin with exogenous renin substrate within the isolated perfused rat kidney. Proc. Soc. exp. Biol. (N. Y.) **142**, 796—799 (1973).

HORTON, R., BIGLIERI, E. G.: Effect of aldosterone on the metabolism of magnesium. J. clin. Endocr. **22**, 1187—1192 (1962).

HOWELL, D. S., DAVIS, J. O.: Relationship of sodium retention to potassium excretion by the kidney during administration of desoxycorticosterone acetate to dogs. Amer. J. Physiol. **179**, 359—363 (1954).

JOHNSON, J. A., DAVIS, J. O., BAUMBER, J. S., SCHNEIDER, E. G.: Effects of estrogens and progesterone on electrolyte balances in normal dogs. Amer. J. Physiol. **219**, 1691—1697 (1970).

JOHNSTON, C. I., DAVIS, J. O., ROBB, C. A., MACKENZIE, J. W.: Plasma renin in chronic experimental heart failure and during renal sodium "escape" from mineralocorticoids. Circulat. Res. **22**, 113—125 (1968).

JØRGENSEN, P. L.: Regulation of the ($Na^+ + K^+$) activated ATP hydrolyzing enzyme system in rat kidney. Biochim. biophys. Acta (Amst.) **192**, 326—334 (1969).

JØRGENSEN, P. L.: The role of aldosterone in the regulation of ($Na^+ + K^+$)-ATPase in rat kidney. J. Steroid Biochem. **3**, 181—191 (1972).

KAGAWA, C. M., PAPPO, R.: Na retention with 18-OH-DOC. Renal electrolyte effects of synthetic 18-hydroxylated steroids in adrenalectomized rats. Proc. Soc. exp. Biol. (N. Y.) **109**, 982—985 (1962).

KAPITOLA, J., KÜCHEL, O.: Nebennierenrinde und Magnesiumstoffwechsel. Klin. Wschr. **42**, 954—958 (1964).

KINSON, G. A., SINGER, B.: Sensitivity to angiotensin and adrenocorticotrophic hormone in the sodium deficient rat. Endocrinology **83**, 1108—1116 (1968).

KIRSTEN, E., KIRSTEN, R., LEAF, A., SHARP, G. W. G.: Increased activity of enzymes of the tricarboxylic acid cycle in response to aldosterone in the toad bladder. Pflügers Arch. ges. Physiol. **300**, 213—225 (1968).

KIRSTEN, E., KIRSTEN, R., SHARP, G. W. G.: Effects of sodium transport stimulating substances on enzyme activities in the toad bladder. Pflügers Arch. ges. Physiol. **316**, 26—33 (1970).

KNOX, F. G., SCHNEIDER, E. G., DRESSER, T. P., LYNCH, R. E.: Natriuretic effect of increased proximal delivery in dogs with salt retention. Amer. J. Physiol. **219**, 904—910 (1970).

KRAHÉ, P., HOFBAUER, K. G., GROSS, F.: Effects of endogenous renin on the function of the isolated kidney. Life Sci. **9** (Part I), 1317—1320 (1970).

Krahé, P., Hofbauer, K. G., Gross, F.: Effects of angiotensin infusion on the isolated rabbit kidney. Proc. Soc. exp. Biol. (N. Y.) **137**, 1324—1327 (1971).

Kramer, K., Boylan, J. W., Keck, W.: Regulation of total body sodium in the mammalian organism. Nephron **6**, 379—387 (1969).

Kumar, D., Hall, A. E. D., Nakashima, R., Gornall, A. G.: Studies on aldosterone. II. Hypertension as a cumulative effect of aldosterone administration. Canad. J. Biochem. **35**, 113—118 (1957).

Lamberg, B. A., Paloheimo, J., Torsti, P.: Changes in the urinary excretion of calcium after intravenous injection of aldosterone. Acta med. scand. **179** (Suppl. 412), 205—213 (1964).

Landon, E. J., Jazab, N., Forte, L.: Aldosterone and sodium-potassium-dependent ATPase activity of rat kidney membranes. Amer. J. Physiol. **211**, 1050—1056 (1966).

Laragh, J. H., Ulick, S., Januszewicz, V., Deming, Q. B., Kelly, W. G., Lieberman, S.: Aldosterone secretion and primary and malignant hypertension. J. clin. Invest. **39**, 1091—1106 (1960).

Laragh, J. H., Sealey, J. E., Sommers, S. C.: Patterns of adrenal secretion and urinary excretion of aldosterone and plasma renin activity in normal and hypertensive subjects. Circulat. Res. **18** (Suppl. 1), 158—174 (1966).

Lassiter, W. E., Mylle, M., Gottschalk, C. W.: Net transport movement of water and urea in saline diuresis. Amer. J. Physiol. **260**, 669—673 (1964).

Leaf, A., Macknight, A. D. C.: The site of the aldosterone induced stimulation of sodium transport. J. Steroid Biochem. **3**, 237—245 (1972).

Ledingham, J. M., Cohen, R. D.: Changes in the extracellular fluid volume and cardiac output during the development of experimental renal hypertension. Canad. med. Ass. J. **90**, 292—294 (1964).

Lemann, J., Jr., Piering, W. F., Lennon, E. J.: Studies of the acute effects of aldosterone and cortisol on the interrelationship between renal sodium, calcium and magnesium excretion in normal man. Nephron **7**, 117—130 (1970).

Levin, D. M., Cade, R.: Intravenous d-aldosterone in man. Circulation **32** (Suppl. 2), 135—136 (1965).

Liard, J. F., Peters, G.: Mechanism of the fall in blood pressure after "unclamping" in rats with Goldblatt-type hypertension. Experientia (Basel) **26**, 743—745 (1970).

Liddle, G. W.: Evidence that the adrenal cortex plays a role in the pathogenesis of essential hypertension with suppressed renin response. In: Proceedings of the Fourth International Congress of Endocrinology. Amsterdam: Excerpta Medica (in press).

Lipton, P., Edelman, I. S.: Effects of aldosterone and vasopressin on electrolytes of toad bladder epithelial cells. Amer. J. Physiol. **221**, 733—741 (1971).

Liu, D. K., Liew, C. C., Gornall, A. G.: Aldosterone effects on nuclear and mitochondrial RNA synthesis in heart and kidney. Fed. Proc. **31**, 283 (1972).

Lommer, D., Düsterdieck, G., Jahnecke, J., Vecsei, P., Wolff, H. P.: Sekretion, Plasmakonzentration, Verteilung, Stoffwechsel und Ausscheidung von Aldosteron bei Gesunden und Kranken. Klin. Wschr. **46**, 741—751 (1968).

Luft, R., Sjögren, B.: A comparative study of the metabolic effect of adrenocorticotrophic hormone (ACTH), cortisone, and desoxycorticosterone acetate (DCA). Stanf. med. Bull. **9**, 218—230 (1951).

Mahy, B. W. J., Munday, K. A.: Hypomagnesaemia following aldosterone administration in rats. J. Physiol. (Lond.) **168**, 22 P—23 P (1963).

Málytusz, M., Mendoza-Osorio, V., Ochwadt, B.: Kidney function in rats with experimental DOCA-induced hypertension. Pflügers Arch. ges. Physiol. **332**, 28—39 (1972).

Masson, G. M. C., Corcoran, A. C., Page, I. H.: Renal and vascular lesions elicited by renin in rats with desoxycorticosterone hypertension. Arch. Path. **53**, 217—225 (1952).

Masson, G. M. C., Corcoran, A. C., Page, I. H., del Greco, F.: Angiotonin induction of vascular lesions in desoxycorticosterone-treated rats. Proc. Soc. exp. Biol. (N. Y.) **84**, 284—287 (1953).

Masson, G. M. C., Koritz, S. B., Peron, F. G.: Corticosteroid formation in regenerating rat adrenals. Endocrinology **62**, 229—233 (1958).

Masson, G. M. C., Mikasa, A., Yasuda, H.: Experimental vascular disease elicited by aldosterone and renin. Endocrinology **71**, 505—512 (1962).

Massry, S. G., Coburn, J. W., Chapman, L. W., Kleeman, C. R.: The effect of long-term desoxycorticosterone acetate administration on the renal excretion of calcium and magnesium. J. Lab. clin. Med. **71**, 212—219 (1968).

Massry, S. G., Coburn, J. W., Kleeman, C. R.: Renal handling of magnesium in the dog. Amer. J. Physiol. **216**, 1460—1467 (1969).

McAllister, R. G., van Way, C. W., III., Dayani, K., Anderson, W. J., Temple, E., Michelakis, A. M., Coppage, W. S., Jr., Oates, J.: Malignant hypertension: Effect of therapy on renin and aldosterone. Circulat. Res. **28** (Suppl. 2), 160—173 (1971).

McConahay, T. P., Robinson, S., Newton, J. L.: D-aldosterone and sweat electrolytes. J. appl. Physiol. **19**, 575—579 (1964).

McGavack, T. H., Saccone, A., Vogel, M., Harris, R.: Craniopharyngioma with panhypopituitarism: Case report with clinical and pathological study. J. clin. Endocr. **6**, 776—796 (1946).

Melby, J. C., Dale, S. L., Grekin, R. J., Gaunt, R., Wilson, T. E.: (1) 18-Hydroxy-11-deoxycorticosterone (18-OH-DOC) secretion in experimental and human hypertension. In: Hypertension — 1972, p. 350—360 (Genest, J., Koiw, E., Eds.). Berlin-Heidelberg-New York: Springer 1972.

Melby, J. C., Dale, S. L., Grekin, R. J., Gaunt, R., Wilson, T. E.: (2) 18-Hydroxy-11-deoxycorticosterone (18-OH-DOC) secretion in experimental and human hypertension. Recent Prog. Hormone Res. **28**, 287—339 (1972).

Mills, I. H.: Sodium-retaining steroids in non-oedematous patients. Production of oedema and heart-failure. Lancet **1962 I**, 1264—1267.

Möhring, J., Möhring, B.: (1) Reevaluation of the DOCA escape phenomenon. Amer. J. Physiol. **223**, 1237—1245 (1972).

Möhring, J., Möhring, B.: (2) Evaluation of sodium and potassium balance in rats. J. appl. Physiol. **33**, 688—692 (1972).

Möhring, J., Möhring, B., Just, S.: Beschreibung des DOCA-escape Phänomens bei Ratten. Naunyn-Schmiedebergs Arch. Pharmakol. **266**, 406—407 (1970).

Möhring, J., Näumann, H. J., Möhring, B., Philippi, A., Gross, F.: Sodium balance and plasma renin activity in renal hypertensive rats. Europ. J. clin. Invest. **1**, 384 (1971).

Möhring, J., Dauda, G., Haack, D., Hofbauer, K. G., Homsy, E., Näumann, H. J., Orth, H., Gross, F.: Malignant phase of renal hypertension in rats. Europ. J. clin. Invest. **2**, 297 (1972).

Müller, J.: Regulation of Aldosterone Biosynthesis. Monographs on Endocrinology, Vol. 5. Berlin-Heidelberg-New York: Springer 1971.

Müller, J.: Gibt es ein Renin-Angiotensin-Aldosteron-System? Schweiz. med. Wschr. **102**, 1105—1112 (1972).

Müller, J., Gross, F.: Effects of experimental renal hypertension on aldosterone biosynthesis by rat adrenal tissue. Acta endocr. (Kbh.) **60**, 669—680 (1969).

Muller, A. F., Mach, E., Naegeli, H.: Comparison of the effect of aldosterone and cortexone (desoxycorticosterone) on electrolyte excretion in man. Acta endocr. (Kbh.) **20**, 113—130 (1955).

de Nicola, A. F., Oliver, J. T., Birmingham, M. K.: Corticosteroid synthesis in adrenal enucleated rats before the onset of hypertension. Endocrinology **85**, 1205—1208 (1969).

Nowaczynski, W., Kuchel, O., Genest, J.: A decreased metabolic clearance rate of aldosterone in benign essential hypertension. J. clin. Invest. **50**, 2184—2190 (1971).

Orloff, J., Burg, M.: Kidney. Ann. Rev. Physiol. **33**, 83—130 (1971).

Palkovits, M., de Jong, W., van der Wal, B., de Wied, D.: The aldosterone secretory response to sodium restriction in chronically hypophysectomized corticotrophin-maintained rats as a function of duration and amount of growth hormone treatment. J. Endocr. **50**, 407—411 (1971).

Palmore, W. P., Marieb, N. J., Mulrow, P. J.: Stimulation of aldosterone secretion by sodium depletion in nephrectomized rats. Endocrinology **84**, 1342—1351 (1969).

Pitts, R. F.: Effects of adrenal cortical hormones on renal function. In: Adrenal Cortex. Transactions of the Third Conference. Josiah Macy, Jr., Foundation Conference Program, p. 11—53 (Ralli, E. P., Ed.). New York 1951.

Porter, G. A., Edelman, I. S.: The action of aldosterone and related corticosteroids on sodium transport across the toad bladder. J. clin. Invest. **43**, 611—620 (1964).

Porter, G. A., Kimsey, J.: Verification that 18-hydroxydesoxycorticosterone (18-OH-DOC) has mineralocorticoid activity. Clin. Res. **19**, 196 (1971).

Porter, G. A., Bogoroch, R., Edelman, I. S.: On the mechanism of action of aldosterone on sodium transport: The role of RNA synthesis. Proc. nat. Acad. Sci. (N. Y.) **52**, 1326—1333 (1964).

Ragan, C., Ferrebee, J. W., Phyfe, P., Atchley, D. W., Loeb, R. F.: A syndrome of polydipsia and polyuria induced in normal animals by desoxycorticosterone acetate. Amer. J. Physiol. **131**, 73—78 (1940).

Rapp, J. P.: (1) Effect of an aldosterone antagonist on electrolytes and juxtaglomerular granularity in adrenal regeneration hypertension. Endocrinology **75**, 326—332 (1964).

Rapp, J. P.: (2) Electrolyte and juxtaglomerular changes in adrenal regeneration hypertension. Amer. J. Physiol. **206**, 93—104 (1964).

Rapp, J. P.: Deoxycorticosterone production in adrenal regeneration hypertension: *in vitro vs. in vivo* comparison. Endocrinology **84**, 1409—1420 (1969).

Rapp, J. P., Dahl, L. K.: 18-Hydroxy-deoxycorticosterone secretion in experimental hypertension in rats. Circulat. Res. 28 (Suppl. 2), 153—159 (1971).

Regoli, D., Gauthier, R.: (1) Etude sur le rôle intrarénal de la rénine: effets des vasoconstricteurs sur le rein isolé de lapin. Un. méd. Can. 100, 733—739 (1971).

Regoli, D., Gauthier, R.: (2) Site of action of angiotensin and other vasoconstrictors on the kidney. Canad. J. Physiol. Pharmac. 49, 608—612 (1971).

Relman, A. S., Stewart, W. K., Schwartz, W. B.: A study of the adjustments to sodium- and water-retaining hormones in normal subjects. J. clin. Invest. 37, 924—925 (1958).

Robb, C. A., Davis, J. O., Johnson, J. A., Blaine, E. H., Schneider, E. G., Baumber, J. S.: Mechanisms regulating the renal excretion of sodium during pregnancy. J. clin. Invest. 49, 871—880 (1970).

Rodbard, S., Freed, S. C.: The effect of desoxycorticosterone acetate on the blood pressure of the dog. Endocrinology 30, 365—368 (1942).

Roemmelt, J. C., Sartorius, O. W., Pitts, R. F.: Excretion and reabsorption of sodium and water in the adrenalectomized dog. Amer. J. Physiol. 159, 124—136 (1949).

Ross, E, J., Hurst, P. E.: Effect of prolonged administration of aldosterone and corticosterone on plasma and urinary electrolytes on man. Clin. Sci. 28, 91—98 (1965).

Salgado, E., Selye, H.: Protection by hypophysectomy against some of the toxic effects of corticoid hormone overdosage. J. clin. Endocr. 12, 974 (1952).

Schmid, H. E., Jr.: Action of angiotensin in normal, adrenalectomized, and renal hypertensive trained dogs. Nephron 5, 265—281 (1968).

Schneider, E. G., Dresser, T. P., Lynch, R. E., Knox, F. G.: (1) Sodium reabsorption by proximal tubule of dogs with experimental heart failure. Amer. J. Physiol. 220, 952—957 (1971).

Schneider, E. G., Dresser, T. P., Lynch, R. E., Knox, F. G.: (2) Glomerulotubular balance in dogs with chronic salt retention. Nephron 8, 46—56 (1971).

Schrier, R. W., de Wardener, H. E.: Tubular reabsorption of sodium ion: Influence of factors other than aldosterone and glomerular filtration rate (I and II). New Engl. J. Med. 285, 1231—1243 and 1292—1303 (1971).

Schuler, W., Desaulles, P., Meier, R.: Electrocortin-Wirkung im Glykogentest. Experientia (Basel) 10, 142 (1954).

Scott, D., Dobson, A.: Aldosterone and the metabolism of magnesium and other minerals in the sheep. Quart. J. exp. Physiol. 50, 42—56 (1965).

Selye, H., Hall, C. E., Rowley, E. M.: Malignant hypertension produced by treatment with desoxycorticosterone acetate and sodium chloride. Canad. med. Ass. J. 49, 88—92 (1943).

Sharp, G. W. G., Leaf, A.: Studies on the biological action of aldosterone *in vitro*. J. clin. Invest. 42, 978 (1963).

Sharp, G. W. G., Leaf, A.: Studies on the mode of action of aldosterone. Recent Progr. Hormone Res. 22. 431—466 (1966).

Simpson, S. A., Tait, J. F.: Quantitative method for the bioassay of the effect of adrenal cortical steroids on mineral metabolism. Endocrinology 50, 150—161 (1952).

Simpson, S. A., Tait, J. F., Wettstein, A., Neher, R., von Euw, J., Reichstein, T.: Isolierung eines neuen kristallisierten Hormons aus Nebennieren mit besonders hoher Wirksamkeit auf den Mineralstoffwechsel. Experientia (Basel) 9, 333—335 (1953).

Simpson, S. A., Tait, J. F., Wettstein, A., Neher, R., von Euw, J., Schindler, O., Reichstein, T.: Konstitution des Aldosterons, des neuen Mineralocorticoids. Experientia (Basel) 10, 132—133 (1954).

Singer, B., Losito, C., Salmon, S.: Aldosterone and corticosterone secretion rates in rats with experimental renal hypertension. Acta endocr. (Kbh.) 44, 505—518 (1963).

Skelton, F. R.: Adrenal regeneration and adrenal regeneration hypertension. Physiol. Rev. 39, 162—182 (1959).

Soffer, L. J., Engel, F. L., Oppenheimer, B. S.: Treatment of Addison's disease with desoxycorticosterone acetate by intramuscular injections and subcutaneous implantation of pellets. J. Amer. med. Ass. 115, 1860—1866 (1940).

Sokabe, H., Mikasa, A., Yasuda, H., Masson, G. M. C.: Adrenal cortex and renal pressor function. Circulat. Res. 12, 94—100 (1963).

Sonnenberg, H.: The renal response to blood volume expansion in the rat: Proximal tubular function and urinary excretion. Canad. J. Physiol. Pharmac. 49, 525—535 (1971).

Sonnenberg, H., Solomon, S.: Mechanism of natriuresis following intravascular and extracellular volume expansion. Canad. J. Physiol. Pharmac. 47, 153—159 (1969).

Spark, R. F., Melby, J. C.: Hypertension and low plasma renin activity: Presumptive evidence for mineralocorticoid excess. Ann. intern. Med. 75, 831—836 (1971).

Spink, W. W., Vick, J. A.: Reversal of experimental endotoxin shock with a combination of aldosterone and metaraminol. Proc. Soc. exp. Biol. (N. Y.) 107, 777—779 (1961).

SPINK, W. W., VICK, J. A.: Canine endotoxin shock: Reversal with aldosterone and angiotensin II (Hypertensin). Proc. Soc exp. Biol. (N. Y.) **109**, 521—522 (1962).

STAMLER, J., PICK, R., KATZ, L. N.: Effects of desoxycorticosterone acetate on cholesterolemia, blood pressure and atherogenesis in chicks. Circulation **4**, 262—269 (1951).

STRAUSS, M. B., EARLEY, L. E.: An inquiry into the role of "sodium-retaining" steroids in the homeostasis of body sodium in man. Trans. Ass. Amer. Phycns **72**, 200—206 (1959).

STROIA, L. N., BOHR, D. F., VOCKE, L.: Experimental hypertension in the hamster. Amer. J. Physiol. **139**, 154—158 (1954).

STUMPE, K. O., OCHWADT, B.: Wirkung von Aldosteron auf die Natrium- und Wasserresorption im proximalen Tubulus bei chronischer Kochsalzbelastung. Pflügers Arch. ges. Physiol. **300**, 148—160 (1968).

STURTEVANT, F. M.: The biology of metacorticoid hypertension. Ann. intern. Med. **49**, 1281—1293 (1958).

SUKI, W. N., SCHWETTMANN, R. S., RECTOR, F. C., Jr., SELDIN, D. W.: The effect of chronic mineralocorticoid administration on calcium excretion. Clin. Res. **15**, 372 (1967).

SUKI, W. N., SCHWETTMANN, R. S., RECTOR, F. C., Jr., SELDIN, D. W.: Effect of chronic mineralocorticoid administration on calcium excretion in the rat. Amer. J. Physiol. **215**, 71—74 (1968).

SUMMERS, J. E.: Desoxycorticosterone acetate and blood pressure of dogs on a high sodium chloride intake. Amer. J. Physiol. **154**, 119—121 (1948).

TAIT, J. F., TAIT, S. A. S., LITTLE, B., LAUMAS, K. R.: The disappearance of 7-^{3}H-d-aldosterone in the plasma of normal subjects. J. clin. Invest. **40**, 72—80 (1961).

THOMPSON, B. D., EDMONDS, C. J.: Comparison of effects of prolonged aldosterone administration on rat colon and renal electrolyte excretion. J. Endocr. **50**, 163—169 (1971).

THORN, G. W.: Treatment of Addison's disease. J. clin. Endocr. **1**, 76—86 (1941).

UHLICH, E., BALDAMUS, C. A., ULLRICH, K. J.: Einfluß von Aldosteron auf den Natriumtransport in den Sammelrohren der Säugetierniere. Pflügers Arch. ges. Physiol. **308**, 111—126 (1969).

UHLICH, E., HALBACH, R., ULLRICH, K. J.: Einfluß von Aldosteron auf den Ausstrom markierten Natriums aus den Sammelrohren der Ratte. Pflügers Arch. ges. Physiol. **320**, 261—264 (1970).

VANČURA, P., SHARP, G. W. G., MALT, R. A.: Kinetics of RNA synthesis in toad bladder epithelium: Action of aldosterone during the latent period. J. clin. Invest. **50**, 543—551 (1971).

VECSEI, P., MÜNTER, R.: Conversion of precursors to aldosterone in vivo. In: Proceedings of the Fourth International Congress of Endocrinology. Amsterdam: Excerpta Medica (in press).

VECSEI, P., DÜSTERDIECK, G., JAHNECKE, J., LOMMER, D., WOLFF, H. P.: Secretion and turnover of aldosterone in various pathological states. Clin. Sci. **36**, 241—256 (1969).

VECSEI, P., MÜNTER, R., KAZDA, S., NÄUMANN, H. J.: Erhöhte „in vivo"-Konversion von Desoxycorticosteron in Aldosteron bei renal hypertonischen Ratten. Acta endocr. (Kbh.) **66** (Suppl. 152), 60 (1971).

WIEDERHOLT, M.: Mikropunktionsuntersuchungen am proximalen und distalen Konvolut der Rattenniere über den Einfluß von Actinomycin D auf den mineralocorticoidabhängigen Na-Transport. Pflügers Arch. ges. Physiol. **292**, 334—342 (1966).

WIEDERHOLT, M., BEHN, C., SCHOORMANS, W., HANSEN, L.: Effect of aldosterone on sodium and potassium transport in the kidney. J. Steroid Biochem. **3**, 151—159 (1972).

WILLIAMSON, H. E.: Mechanism of antinatriuretic action of aldosterone. Biochem. Pharmacol. **1?**, 1449—1450 (1963).

WINDHAGER, E. E.: Kidney, water, and electrolytes. Ann. Rev. Physiol. **31**, 117—172 (1969).

WINTER, C. A., INGRAM, W. R.: Observations on the polyuria produced by desoxycorticosterone acetate. Amer. J. Physiol. **139**, 710—718 (1943).

WISENBAUGH, P. E., BOGATY, G. V., HILL, R. W.: Deoxycorticosterone acetate hypertension in dogs. Lab. Invest. **14**, 2140—2149 (1965).

WISENBAUGH, P. E., GARST, J. B., HULL, C., FREEDMAN, R. J., MATTHEWS, D. N., HADADY, M.: Renin, aldosterone, sodium and hypertension. Amer. J. Med. **52**, 175—185 (1972).

WOLFF, H. P., VECSEI, P., KRUCK, F., ROSCHER, S., BROWN, J. J., DÜSTERDIECK, G. O., LEVER, A. F., ROBERTSON, J. I. S.: Psychiatric disturbance leading to potassium depletion, sodium depletion, raised plasma-renin concentration, and secondary hyperaldosteronism. Lancet **1968 I**, 257—261.

WRIGHT, F. S., KNOX, F. G., HOWARDS, S. S., BERLINER, R. W.: Reduced sodium reabsorption by the proximal tubule of DOCA-escaped dogs. Amer. J. Physiol. **216**, 869—875 (1969).

WRIGHT, F. S., STRIEDER, N., FOWLER, N. B., GIEBISCH, G.: Potassium secretion by distal tubule after potassium adaptation. Amer. J. Physiol. **221**, 437—448 (1971).

Adrenal Medulla

M. J. PEACH

Release of adrenal catecholamines by angiotensin was first demonstrated by BRAUN-MENENDEZ et al. (1940), using a crude peptide preparation. Further studies concerning angiotensin-adrenal medullary interactions did not occur until almost 20 years later when RENSON et al. (1959) reported that after cocaine administration angiotensin II caused contraction of the nictitating membrane and the α-adrenergic blocking agent, phenoxybenzamine, blocked this effect. At about the same time, HAAS and GOLDBLATT (1959) showed that infusions of a ganglionic stimulant, dimethylphenylpiperazinium iodide (DMPP), potentiated cardiovascular responses to Ang. II. This DMPP-induced facilitation of responses to Ang. II was abolished by bilateral adrenalectomy or administration of phentolamine (KANEKO et al., 1961). Adrenalectomy in rats was reported to decrease the vasopressor action of Ang. II, and direct perfusion of rat adrenals with Ang. II caused an increase in catecholamine output (CESSION and CESSION-FOSSION, 1963). FELDBERG and LEWIS (1964) demonstrated that injections of Ang. II into the central stump of the celiac artery in the eviscerated cat induced marked adrenal catecholamine release. The threshold dose of Ang. II administered via the celiac artery was 1 to 2 ng, while the intravenous threshold dose was 100 ng. In a subsequent study the intravenous administration of renin was reported to induce the secretion of adrenal catecholamines (FELDBERG and LEWIS, 1965). Stimulation of isolated canine adrenals perfused via the superior mesenteric artery required large doses (8 µg) of Ang. II (VOGT, 1965), but ROBINSON (1967) reported that the isolated, retrogradely perfused adrenal of the dog was very sensitive to Ang. II, with a threshold dose of less than 1 ng. *In-vivo* studies in the dog estimating plasma catecholamines indicated that Ang. II (i.-v. infusion 0.05 µg/kg/min or i.-v. injections of 0.5 µg/kg) evoked adrenal catecholamine release (PEACH et al., 1966); the other *in-vivo* (STASZEWSKA-BARCZAK and VANE, 1967; STASZEWSKA-BARCZAK and KONOPKA-ROGATKO, 1967), *in-situ* (POISNER and DOUGLAS, 1966) and *in-vitro* (PEACH et al., 1971) studies in the cat on adrenal chromaffin stimulation by Ang. II yielded results compatible with the findings of FELDBERG and LEWIS (1964). Ang. II is a potent secretogogue in the isolated, retrogradely perfused rabbit adrenal (PEACH et al., 1970) and also stimulates the isolated human adrenal to release catecholamines (PEACH, unpublished observation). Stimulation of the human adrenal is dose-dependent with a threshold dose of about 5 ng. In the bovine adrenal medulla, Ang. II is reported to have only a marginal stimulatory effect (COMLINE et al., 1968).

Ang. II-induced adrenal medulla stimulation is not inhibited by bilateral splanchnicotomy, spinal block with a local anesthetic or the administration of hexamethonium, pentolinium, morphine, 5-hydroxytryptamine, histamine, bradykinin, kalliden and eledoisin (FELDBERG and LEWIS, 1965; LEWIS and REIT, 1966; STAZEWSKA-BARCZAK and VANE, 1967). In addition, when the adrenal medulla is made tachyphylactic to Ang. II, responses to other secretogogues (e.g., acetylcholine, bradykinin, nicotine) are not affected (FELDBERG and LEWIS, 1965; STASZEWSKA-BARCZAK and VANE, 1967; PEACH et al., 1971). In isolated adrenal medullary cells of the gerbil, Ang. II has been shown to depolarize the chromaffin cell membrane (DOUGLAS et al., 1967). This depolarizing effect was not altered by the administration of hexamethonium and atropine in doses that completely inhibited acetylcholine-, nicotine- and pilocarpine-induced membrane depolarization. All these studies indicate that angiotensin has a direct stimulatory effect on adrenal chromaffin tissue.

Immediately after the administration of blocking doses of nicotine (during depolarization-phase blockade), angiotensin-induced adrenal catecholamine secretion is blocked (LEE and TRENDELENBURG, 1967; PEACH et al., 1971). In contrast, Ang. II responses are markedly potentiated during late phase (postdepolarization) nicotine blockade (LEE and TRENDELENBURG, 1967; KOVACIC and ROBINSON, 1970). The administration of non-depolarizing nicotinic receptor-blocking agents (e.g. hexamethonium; pentolinium; 4,4'-biphenylene bis-[(2-oxoethylene)-bis-(2,2-diethoxyethyl) dimethylammonium Br] referred to as DMAE) also results in potentiation of angiotensin-induced adrenal catecholamine release (STASZEWSKA-BARCZAK and VANE, 1967; STASZEWSKA-BARCZAK and KONOPKA-ROGATKO, 1967; PEACH, 1971; PEACH and WESTFALL, 1972). These studies support the findings of DOUGLAS et al. (1967) by demonstrating that angiotensin-evoked catecholamine release is prevented by (nicotine-induced) chromaffin-membrane depolarization and secondly that the direct secretory effect of Ang. II is independent of any cholinergic mechanism.

In a report on the *in-situ* perfused adrenal of the cat, POISNER and DOUGLAS (1966) reported that Ca^{2+} was required for release of catecholamines by Ang. II. This requirement for extracellular Ca^{2+} was confirmed in the isolated dog (ROBINSON, 1967) and cat adrenal (PEACH et al., 1971). It would appear that angiotensin depolarizes the chromaffin-cell membrane, which then results in a net transfer of extracellular Ca^{2+} into the cell. It is not known if angiotensin has the ability to effect the translocation of intracellular Ca^{2+} and induce secretion-coupling without depolarizing the cell membrane; however, this would seem unlikely.

Analogs of angiotensin have been studied in the adrenal medulla and their activities relative to angiotensin have been determined (FELDBERG and LEWIS, 1965; STASZEWSKA-BARCZAK and KONOPKA-ROGATKO, 1967; PEACH, 1971; PEACH et al., 1971). Angiotensin structure-activity relationship studies in the adrenal medulla are summarized in Table 1. Structural requirements established for stimulation of medullary catecholamine secretion are as follows: 1) there must be at least six amino acids in the peptide chain (residues 3 to 8 of Ang. II); 2) a tyrosine residue is required as the fourth residue of the Ang. II molecule; 3) the imidazole ring of histidine must be in position no. 6; and 4) proline must be adjacent to the eigth amino-acid residue. From these structural studies it was also determined that the C-terminal residue did not have to be an aromatic amino acid for activity in adrenal chromaffin tissue. For myotropic activity, however, the C-terminal aromatic amino acid is required.

Another observation of interest generated by the peptide structural studies in the adrenal was the marked activity (95% relative to Ang. II) of Ang. I. In the isolated, retrogradely perfused adrenal, Ang. I-induced catecholamine release is not affected by the administration of Ang. II-antibody or an inhibitor of converting enzyme, *Bothrops jararaca*-venom pentapeptide (PEACH et al., 1971; PEACH, 1972). These studies suggest that Ang. I acts directly on the adrenal medulla to release catecholamines. Various studies suggest that Ang. I and Ang. II interact with the same adrenal chromaffin receptor (PEACH, 1971; PEACH and WESTFALL, 1972).

Table 1. *Angiotensin structure activity in adrenal medulla*

Peptide No.	Amino-acid residues								Relative activity (%)	
	Asp 1	Arg 2	Val 3	Tyr 4	Ile 5	His 6	Pro 7	Phe 8	Pressor/ Oxytocic	Adrenal catecholamine release
1	α-L-Asp	Arg	Val	Tyr	Val	His	Pro	Phe	100/100	100
2	α-L-Asp	Arg	Val	Tyr	Ile	His	Pro	Phe	100/100	100
3	α-L-Asp (NH_2)	Arg	Val	Tyr	Val	His	Pro	Phe	100/100	100
4	β-L-Asp	Arg	Val	Tyr	Val	His	Pro	Phe	200/200	200
5	α-D-Asp	Arg	Val	Tyr	Val	His	Pro	Phe	200/200	200
6	Suc	Arg	Val	Tyr	Val	His	Pro	Phe	50/51	40
7	Ile	Arg	Val	Tyr	Ile	His	Pro	Phe	25/20	35
8	Arg	Arg	Vai	Tyr	Ile	His	Pro	Phe	35/75	15
9		α-L-Asp (NH_2)	Val	Tyr	Ile	His	Pro	Phe	20/?	12
10		Arg	Val	Tyr	Ile	His	Pro	Phe	22/18	17
11			Val	Tyr	Val	His	Pro	Phe	0.1/?	0.2
12			Vai	Tyr	Ile	His	Pro	Phe	2/6	6
13	α-L-Asp (NH_2)	D-Arg	Val	Tyr	Val	His	Pro	Phe	2.5/?	2.5
14	α-L-Asp	Arg	Ala	Tyr	Ile	His	Pro	Phe	40/42	35
15	α-L-Asp	Arg	Val	D-Tyr	Val	His	Pro	Phe	0/?	0.2
16	α-L-Asp (NH_2)	Arg	Val	D-Tyr	Val	His	Pro	Phe	0/?	0.1
17	α-L-Asp	Arg	Val	Phe	Val	His	Pro	Phe	10/?	5
18	α-L-Asp (NH_2)	Arg	Val	Phe	Val	His	Pro	Phe	6/?	5
19	α-L-Asp	Arg	Val	p-OMe-Tyr	Ile	His	Pro	Phe	1/3	3
20	α-L-Asp	Arg	Val		Val	His	Pro	Phe	15/?	13
21	α-L-Asp	Arg	Val	Tyr	Aia	His	Pro	Phe	10/12	10
22	α-L-Asp (NH_2)	Arg	Val	Tyr	Val	D-His	Pro	Phe	0.07/?	0.05
23	α-L-Asp	Arg	Val	Tyr	Ile	Ala	Pro	Phe	0.1/0.1	2
24	α-L-Asp	Arg	Val	Tyr	Ile	His	Ala	Phe	0.1/0.1	2
25	α-L-Asp	Arg	Val	Tyr	Ile	His	Pro	Ala	0.1/0.1	25
26	α-L-Asp	Arg	Val	Tyr	Ile	His	Pro	Tyr	83/100	70
27	α-L-Asp	Arg	Val	Tyr	Iie	His	Pro	p-OMe-Tyr	33/35	75
28	α-L-Asp	Arg	Val	Tyr	Ile	His	Pro	Amino phenyl butyric acid	10/8	45

29	α-L-Asp	Arg	Val	Tyr	Ile	His	Pro	Amino phenyl isobutyric acid	0.1/0.1	7
30	α-L-Asp	Arg	Val	Tyr	Iie	His	Pro	Phe-His	15/20	38
31	α-L-Asp	Arg	Val	Tyr	Tyr	Val	His	Pro-Phe	1/?	0.1
32	α-L-Asp (NH_2)	Arg	Val	Tyr	Tyr	Vai	His	Pro-Phe	1/?	0.1
33	α-L-Asp	Arg	Val	Tyr	Ile	His	Pro	Phe-His-Leu	?/2	95
34	α-L-Asp (NH_2)	Arg	Vai	Tyr	Val	His	Pro	Phe-Pro-Phe	0.2/?	0.2
35	α-L-Asp	Arg	Val	Tyr	Ile	His	Pro	Phe-His-Leu Leu-Val-Tyr-Ser	5/5	7

Feldberg and Lewis (1965): 1, 3, 4, 5, 6, 9, 11, 15, 16, 17, 18, 31, 32, 34.
Staszewska-Barczak and Konopka-Rogatko (1967): 1, 3, 13, 16, 18, 20, 22.
Peach, Bumpus and Khairallah (1971): 2, 3, 10, 12, 25, 33, 35.
Peach (1971): 2, 25, 26, 27, 28, 29, 33, 35.
Peach (unpublished observations): 7, 8, 14, 19, 21, 23, 24, 30.

It remains to be determined if catecholamines contribute to the cardiovascular responses produced by Ang. I or renin administration.

Both the injection of renin (1 to 2 Goldblatt units) and the infusion of large doses of Ang. II *in vivo* have been reported to induce adrenal medullary tachyphylaxis. FELDBERG and LEWIS (1965), using a crude renin preparation, reported that renin abolished medullary responses to Ang. II and bradykinin but not to acetylcholine. Later studies in the adrenal with continuous administration of Ang. II showed no cross-tachyphylaxis between angiotensin and bradykinin (STASZEWSKA-BARCZAK and VANE, 1967; PEACH et al., 1971). There was cross-tachyphylaxis in chromaffin tissue, however, between Ang. II, Ang. I, heptapeptide (amino-acid residues 2 to 8 of Ang. II) and several 8-substituted analogs of Ang. II (PEACH et al., 1971; and PEACH, 1971). Tachyphylaxis develops very rapidly when μg doses are administered, but stimulation of catecholamine secretion can be sustained when low doses of angiotensin are used. Catecholamine release *in vivo* was sustained during 10-min i.-v. infusions of Ang. II in doses of 0.05 or 0.1 μg/kg/min (PEACH et al., 1966; PEACH and FORD, 1968). WERNING et al. (1969) reported that 30-min i.-a. infusion of Ang. II also resulted in elevated plasma catecholamines. In isolated, retrogradely perfused adrenals, 30-min perfusions of Ang. I or Ang. II in amounts of up to 50 ng/ml induced catecholamine secretion that was maintained at constant levels for the duration of peptide administration (PEACH et al., 1971).

In addition to the direct stimulatory effect of Ang. II on adrenal chromaffin tissue, it appears that angiotensin may also initiate indirect centrally mediated stimulation of the adrenal medulla (SEVERS et al., 1966). The pressor response following an intraventricular injection of Ang. II in the cat is attenuated by the parenteral administration of P-286 (N,N-di-isopropyl-N′-isoamyl-N′-diethylaminoethylurea). GARDIER et al. (1960) reported that P-286 caused a relatively specific block of adrenal medullary catecholamine secretion. In the isolated, retrogradely perfused adrenal of the cat, continuous perfusion of P-286 (10 or 100 μg/ml) abolishes catecholamine secretion induced by KCl, nicotine or Ang. II (PEACH, unpublished observations). The direct as well as the centrally mediated effects of angiotensin on the adrenal medulla are blocked by P-286.

On the basis of all the studies reviewed above, it is very easy to establish that angiotensin stimulates the release of catecholamines from the adrenal medulla. It is difficult, however, to determine 1) whether the catecholamines released play any significant role in cardiovascular responses to angiotensin and 2) whether adrenal catecholamines contribute to the production or maintenance of renal hypertension. Several studies with angiotensin have been carried out in adrenalectomized animals. SALMOIRAGHI and MCCUBBIN (1954) reported that adrenalectomy in dogs had no effect on pressor responses to Ang. II. Later studies in the cat, dog and rabbit showed that vasopressor responses to i.-v. injections or infusions of Ang. II were not altered following acute, bilateral adrenalectomy (FELDBEG and LEWIS, 1964; PEACH and FORD, 1968; PEACH et al., 1970). There may be some species differences, however, since angiotensin-induced increases in arterial pressure are attenuated in adrenalectomized rats (GROSS and SULSER, 1957; CESSION and CESSION-FOSSION, 1963). In the cat, the effects of adrenalectomy on pressor responses to Ang. II also depend on the route of peptide administration. When angiotensin is administered intra-arterially, the resultant pressor responses are decreased by bilateral adrenalectomy (FELDBERG and LEWIS, 1964). LEE and TRENDELENBURG (1967) showed that depolarization-phase nicotine blockade or adrenalectomy resulted in identical decreases in arterial blood pressure responses induced by i.-a. injections of Ang. II. These studies with intra-arterial injections of octapeptide are of particular interest since the primary site of endogenous Ang. II formation may be the lung (NG and VANE, 1968). If Ang. II is generated predominantly in the lung, then the highest systemic circulating titer would be arterial and the peptide should be administered i.-a. for evaluation.

Some studies have demonstrated that the catecholamines released by Ang. II also play a role in modulating blood flow. After i.-v. administration, Ang. II produced vasodilation in skeletal muscle of limbs and this vasodilatation was inhibited by β-adrenergic blockade and adrenal ligation (WHITE and ROSS, 1966). In a subsequent paper these authors reported that adrenal catecholamines modulated cardiac, pressor and flow responses to angiotensin (ROSS and WHITE, 1966). Ang. II-induced elevation of plasma catecholamines was reported to result in an increase in plasma free fatty acids and glycerol (TRINER et al., 1967). These metabolic changes were blocked by acidosis or reserpine treatment and were associated with increases in circulating catecholamines. All these studies strongly implicate a catecholamine contribution to hemodynamic and metabolic changes associated with the administration of Ang. II. It remains to be determined where Ang. I fits into this peptide-adrenal medullary interrelationship.

Numerous evaluations of the role of adrenal catecholamines in the development or maintenance of renal hypertension have been attempted. GOLDBLATT et al. (1934) showed that unilateral adrenalectomy and demedullation of the other adrenal did not alter experimental renal hypertension in dogs. Several other investigators have reported that the absence of adrenal medullary tissue does not affect the development or maintenance of renal hypertension (FASCIOLO, 1938; PAGE, 1938; FREGLY, 1957, 1960; FINCH and LEACH, 1970). All of these other studies involved bilateral adrenalectomy or surgical bilateral medullectomy to eliminate adrenal chromaffin tissue. In contrast, chemical adrenal medullosclerosis in dogs (achieved by intramedullary injections of 40% sterile Na-salicylate) has been reported to prevent the development of arterial hypertension induced by clamping the renal arteries (TURAI et al., 1961). The balance of information certainly favors the opinion that the adrenal medulla does not affect the acute or sustained phases of renal hypertension. This conclusion, however, is based on the measurement of a single parameter — arterial blood pressure. In view of the catecholamine-induced changes in hemodynamics, blood flow and metabolism associated with exogenously administered Ang. II, it would seem logical to consider this role for catecholamines in renal hypertension. In a Goldblatt hypertensive model, catecholamines affected flow, and caused hemodynamic and metabolic changes without altering total peripheral resistance as estimated by arterial blood pressure recordings. Certainly, however, at *present* there is little evidence in favor of a significant role played by the adrenal medulla in renal hypertension.

References

BRAUN-MENENDEZ, E., FASCIOLO, J. C., LELOIR, L. F., MUNOZ, J. M.: Farmacologia de la hipertensina. Rev. Soc. argent. Biol. **16**, 398 (1940).

CESSION, G., CESSION-FOSSION, A.: Action excito-surrenalienne de l'angiotensine chez le rat. C. R. Soc. Biol. (Paris) **157**, 1830 (1963).

COMLINE, R. S., SILVER, M., SINCLAIR, D. G.: The effects of bradykinin, angiotensin and acetylcholine on the bovine adrenal medulla. J. Physiol. (Lond.) **196**, 339 (1968).

DOUGLAS, W. W., KANNO, T., SAMPSON, S. R.: Effects of acetylcholine and other medullary secretogogues and antagonists on the membrane potential of adrenal chromaffin cells: an analysis employing techniques of tissue culture. J. Physiol. (Lond.) 188, 107 (1967).

FASCIOLO, J. C.: Papel de las grandulas adrenales en la genesis de la hipertension arterial por isquemia renal. Rev. Soc. argent. Biol. **14**, 25 (1938).

FELDBERG, W., LEWIS, G. P.: The action of polypeptides on the adrenal medulla: Release of adrenaline by bradykinin and angiotensin. J. Physiol. (Lond.) **171**, 98 (1964).
FELDBERG, W., LEWIS, G. P.: Further studies on the effects of peptides on the suprarenal medulla of cats. J. Physiol. (Lond.) **178**, 239 (1965).
FINCH, L., LEACH, G. F. H.: Does the adrenal medulla contribute to the maintenance of experimental hypertension? Europ. J. Pharmacol. **11**, 388 (1970).
FREGLY, M. J.: Adrenal glands in the development of renal hypertension in rats. Amer. J. Physiol. **191**, 542 (1957).
FREGLY, M. J.: Production of hypertension in adrenalectomized rats given hypertonic salt solution to drink. Endocrinology **66**, 240 (1960).
GARDIER, R. W., ABRELU, B. E., RICHARDS, A. B., HERRLICH, H. C.: Specific blockade of the adrenal medulla. J. Pharmacol. exp. Ther. **130**, 340 (1960).
GOLDBLATT, H., LYNCH, J., HANZAL, R. F., SUMMERVILLE, W. W.: Studies on experimental hypertension. I. The production of persistent elevation of systolic blood pressure by means of renal ischemia. J. exp. Med. **59**, 347 (1934).
GROSS, F., SULSER, F.: Der Einfluß der Nebennieren auf die blutdrucksteigernde Wirkung von Renin und auf pressorische Substanzen in den Nieren. Naunyn-Schmiedebergs Arch. Pharmakol. exp. Path. **230**, 274 (1957).
HAAS, E., GOLDBLATT, H.: Effects of an antihypertensive drug, pentolinium. Amer. J. Physiol. **196**, 763 (1959).
KANEKO, Y., MCCUBBIN, J. W., PAGE, I. H.: Ability of vasoconstrictor drugs to cause adrenal medullary discharge after "lsensitization" by ganglion stimulation agents. Circulat. Res. **9**, 1247 (1961).
KOVACIC, B., ROBINSON, R. L.: Drug-induced secretion of catecholamines by the perfused adrenal gland of the dog during nicotine blockade. J. Pharmacol. exp. Ther. **175**, 178 (1970).
LEE, F. L., TRENDELENBURG, U.: Muscarinic transmission of preganglionic impulses to the adrenal medulla of the cat. J. Pharmacol. exp. Ther. **158**, 73 (1967).
LEWIS, G. P., REIT, E.: Further studies on the actions of peptides on the superior cervical ganglion and suprarenal medulla. Brit. J. Pharmacol. **26**, 444 (1966).
NG, K. K. F., VANE, J. R.: Fate of angiotensin I in the circulation. Nature (Lond.) **218**, 144 (1968).
PAGE, I. H.: The effect of bilateral adrenalectomy on arterial blood pressure of dogs with experimental hypertension. Amer. J. Physiol. **122**, 352 (1938).
PEACH, M. J.: Adrenal medullary stimulation induced by angiotensin I, angiotensin II and analogues. Circulat. Res., Suppl. II to **28**, **29**, 11—107 (1971).
PEACH, M. J.: Effects of converting enzyme inhibition on peptide induced adrenal medullary stimulation. Fed. Proc. (1972) (inpress).
PEACH, M. J., BUMPUS, F. M., KHAIRALLAH, P. A.: Release of adrenal catecholamines by angiotensin I. J. Pharmacol. exp. Ther. **176**, 366 (1971).
PEACH, M. J., CLINE, W. H., DAVILA, D., KHAIRALLAH, P. A.: Angiotensin-catecholamine interactions in the rabbit. Europ. J. Pharmacol. **11**, 286 (1970).
PEACH, M. J., CLINE, W. H., WATTS, D. T.: Release of adrenal catecholamines by angiotensin II. Circulat. Res. **19**, 571 (1966).
PEACH, M. J., FORD, G. D.: The actions of angiotensin II on canine myocardial and plasma catecholamines. J. Pharmacol. exp. Ther. **162**, 92 (1968).
PEACH, M. J., WESTFALL, T. C.: Potentiation of adrenal medullary responses to angiotensin by DMAE *in vitro*. J. Pharmacol. exp. Ther. (1972) (in press).
POISNER, A. M., DOUGLAS, W. W.: The need for calcium in adrenomedullary secretion evoked by biogenic amines, polypeptides and muscarinic agents. Proc. Soc. exp. Biol. (N. Y.) **123**, 62 (1966).
RENSON, J., BARAC, G., BACQ, Z. M.: Effects de deux angiotensin sympathetiques sur la pression arterieile et la membrane nictitante du chat. C. R. Soc. Biol. (Paris) **153**, 1621 (1959).
ROBINSON, R. L.: Stimulation of the catecholamine output of the isolated perfused adrenal gland of the dog by angiotensin and bradykinin. J. Pharmacol. exp. Ther. **156**, 252 (1967).
ROSS, G., WHITE, F. N.: Role of catecholamine release in cardiovascular responses to angiotensin. Amer. J. Physiol. **211**, 1419 (1966).
SALMOIRAGHI, G., MCCUBBIN, J. W.: Effect of adrenalectomy on pressor responsiveness to angiotensin and renin. Circulat. Res. **2**, 280 (1954).
SEVERS, W. B., DANIELS, A. E., SMOOKLER, H. H., KINNARD, W. J., BUCKLEY, J. P.: Interrelationship between angiotensin II and the sympathetic nervous system. J. Pharmacol. exp. Ther. **153**, 530 (1966).
STASZEWSKA-BARCZAK, J., KONOPKA-ROGATKO, K.: Pressor activity and release of catecholamines by angiotensin and some of its analogues. Bull. Acad. Pol. sci. Cl. 2. **25**, 503 (1967).

STASZEWSKA-BARCZAK, J., VANE, J. R.: The release of catecholamines from the adrenal medulla by peptides. Brit. J. Pharmacol. **30**, 655 (1967).
TRINER, L., HEULLY, M. C., NAHAS, G. G.: Metabolic effects of angiotensin. Amer. J. Physiol. **213**, 1545 (1967).
TURAI, I., PAPAHAGI, E., MANDACHE, F., HOVER, G.: The part played by the adrenal medulla and cortex in the pathogenesis of arterial hypertension. J. cardiovasc. Surg. (Toronto) **2**, 381 (1961).
VOGT, M.: Release of medullary amines from the isolated perfused adrenal gland of the dog. Brit. J. Pharmacol. **24**, 561 (1965).
WERNING, C., SCHONBECK, M., ZIEGLER, W. H., BAUMANN, K., GYSLING, E., WEIDMANN, P., SIEGENTHALER, W.: Die Adrenalin- und Noradrenalinausscheidung während Angiotensin II-Infusionen in die Arteria carotis beim narkotisierten Hund. Klin. Wschr. **47**, 640 (1969).
WHITE, F. N., ROSS, G.: Adrenal dependent circulatory responses to angiotensin in the cat. Amer. J. Physiol. **210**, 1118 (1966).

Central Neurogenic Effects of Angiotensin

C. John Dickinson and Carlos M. Ferrario

With 4 Figures

"Our experiments indicate that renin probably acts through the autonomic nervous system, but a direct vasoconstrictor action is not excluded". Thus said Scarff and Martin, in 1941, after they had observed the remarkable reduction in the pressor effect of renin which occurred when general anesthesia was given to animals. Their conclusion, though remarkably prophetic was not entirely accurate, as they failed to recognize that the pressor effects were mediated by angiotensin rather than by renin itself. In later years however, very little further was heard about any neurogenic effects of renin or angiotensin, though it is interesting to find that Braun-Menendez et al. (1940) recognized that angiotensin could provoke the release of catecholamines from the adrenal medulla, a phenomenon rediscovered nearly 23 years later by Feldberg and Lewis (1963). Other effects of angiotensin have now been recognized in the periphery, and the second section of this chapter is concerned with such effects, principally the facilitation of transmission in sympathetic ganglia and sensitization of the neurovascular effector in the postganglionic nerve terminals in such a way that the effects of locally released norepinephrine are augmented (McCubbin and Page, 1963). The latter effect may depend in part upon the prevention of re-uptake of released norepinephrine (Peach et al., 1969).

In early experiments with purified angiotensin (reviewed by Page and Bumpus, 1961) the materials had been injected into various vascular beds and because its pressor effect following injection into the internal carotid artery was no greater than its pressor effect following intravenous injection, the possible effect of angiotensin upon the central nervous system had been generally discounted. However, Bickerton and Buckley (1961) had noticed that if a dog's head was perfused from a donor animal, the trunk of the recipient, connected to its head only by the spinal cord, showed a rise in blood pressure if large quantities of angiotensin were injected into the brain circulation. The amounts of angiotensin used were very high (in the order of 1.0 to 2.0 μg/kg). Since it was possible to abolish the pressor response by a sympatholytic agent, the authors concluded that angiotensin could stimulate the sympathetic nervous system.

At approximately the same time, Dickinson and McCubbin (1961) attempted to test the hypothesis that cerebrovascular resistance might have an influence on systemic arterial pressure by infusing angiotensin into the vertebral arteries of dogs. However, they observed no greater pressor effect when angiotensin was delivered to the vertebral arteries than when it was given into a vein. In retrospect, their failure to observe a specific effect on the brain stem was simply due to the use of too high an infusion rate, possibly combined with the slight but appreciable depressant effects of barbiturate anesthesia. Since many observers had reported that barbiturate anesthesia depressed the pressor response to renin or angiotensin (Bingel and Claus, 1910; Dock et al., 1942; Pickering and Printzmetal, 1938;

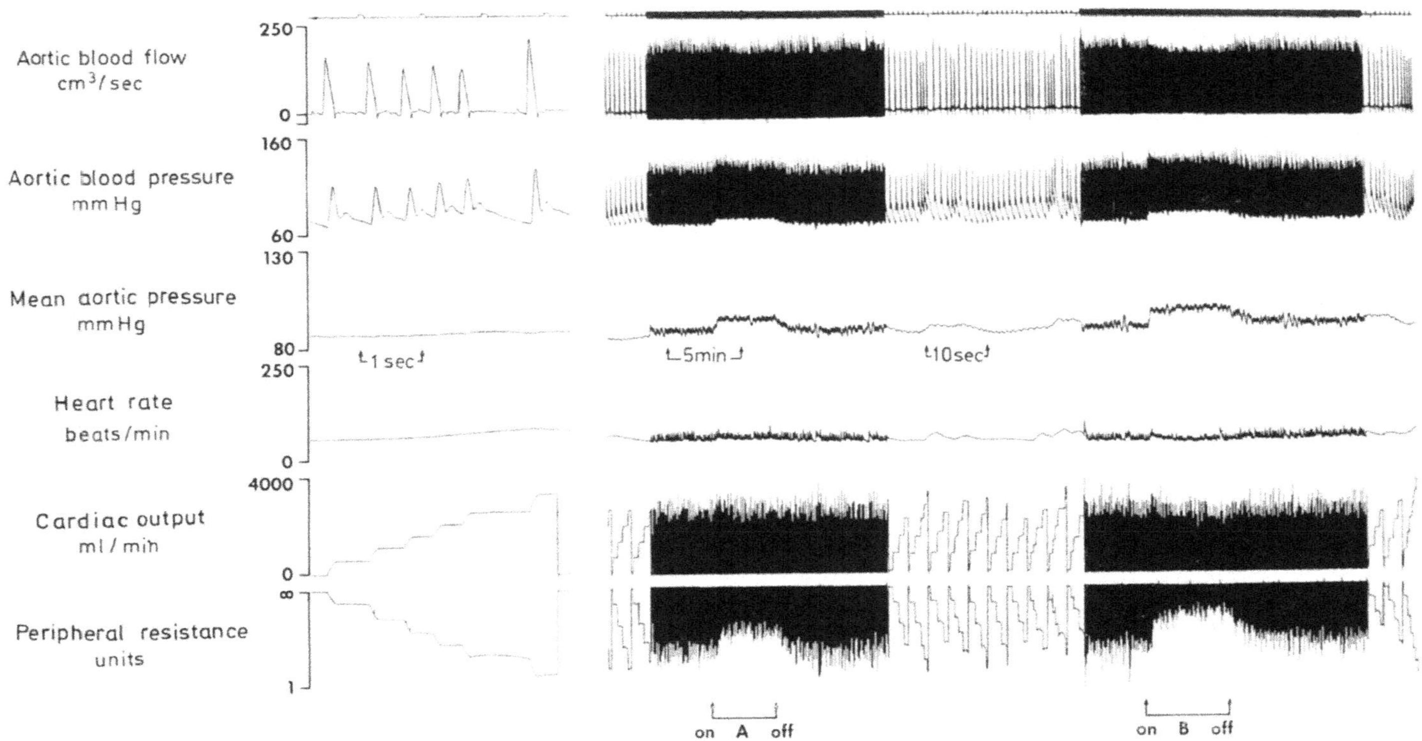

Fig. 1. Pressor effect of angiotensin infused into the vertebral arteries. From above down: aortic blood flow; pulsatile aortic blood pressure; mean aortic blood pressure; heart rate; cardiac output; peripheral resistance (Aortic pressure divided by cardiac output). To obtain cardiac output the heart stroke volume was displayed as vertical steps added and re-cycled every 4 sec (see expanded times traces); to obtain peripheral resistance mean aortic pressure was electronically and continuously computed at 4-sec intervals. Signal mark A: infusion of 1.0 $ng/kg^{-1}/min^{-1}$ angiotensin into the vertebral arteries; B: same, at 3.5 $ng/kg^{-1}/min^{-1}$. Both infusion rates were without effect when angiotensin was delivered into a vein (FERRARIO et al., 1970, by kind permission)

Page and Helmer, 1940), Dickinson (1965) and Yu and Dickinson (1965, 1971) infused angiotensin into the vertebral arteries of unanesthetized rabbits, delivering the drug into a catheter inserted by way of the subclavian artery with its tip lying at the vertebral artery origin. They reported a 10- to 15-fold increase in sensitivity when angiotensin was given by this means into the hind brain circulation, compared to the rise in blood pressure when it was given into a vein. In one case convulsions and enormous rises in blood pressure occurred each time angiotensin was given, and Dickinson (1965) interpreted this as evidence that angiotensin constricted cerebral arteries, as he had suggested in his hypothesis of long-term blood pressure

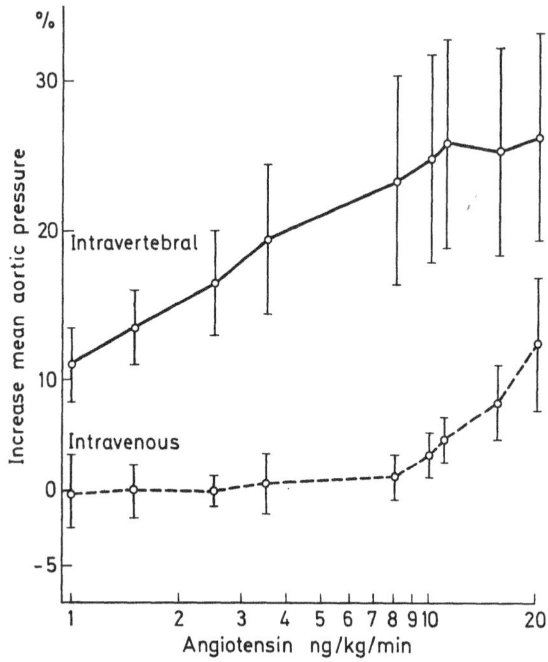

Fig. 2. Dose response curve obtained for infusions of angiotensin at various rates either into the vertebral arteries or intravenously. Values are means of blood pressure elevations in mmHg (± SD) obtained from at least ten measurements in nine dogs (Ferrario et al., 1970, by kind permission)

regulation. He also suggested that the progressive pressor effect of small doses of angiotensin (Dickinson and Lawrence, 1963; Dickinson and Yu, 1967) might have been due to stimulation of the central vasomotor apparatus by angiotensin, because these authors observed that the progressive rise in blood pressure resulting from low infusion rates could be blocked by adrenergic neurone-blocking agents.

Scroop and Lowe (1968) were the first to show that the phenomenon (i.e. increased rise of blood pressure resulting from infusion of angiotensin into a vertebral artery) could be obtained in a consistent manner in greyhounds anesthetized with morphine and chloralose, and these results were confirmed in mongrel dogs by Ferrario et al. (1970) (Figs. 1 and 2). The opportunity of observing the phenomenon during anesthesia made it possible to note the onset and characteristics of the response more exactly than had been possible in consicous animals, and both groups of investigators confirmed the rapid onset of the pressor response and its extremely low threshold. Since a response could be produced with infusion rates as low as 0.1 ng/kg^{-1}/min^{-1} (LOWE and SCROOP, 1969) this phenomenon provides the most sensitive bio-assay of angiotensin known. However, the rapidity of the response made it extremely unlikely that it was exerted through brain-stem ischemia, predominantly at least, because such responses take approximately 2 min to develop (DICKINSON and MCCUBBIN, 1963).

Site of Action of Angiotensin in the Brain Stem

The previous experiments provided the bases for elucidation of the site at which angiotensin exerts pressor effects at such low concentrations. The hypothalamus and midbrain were excluded from consideration as a site of activity when GILDENBERG (1969) reported that section of the dog's brain stem at the level of the mesencephalon failed to abolish the response to angiotensin administered into

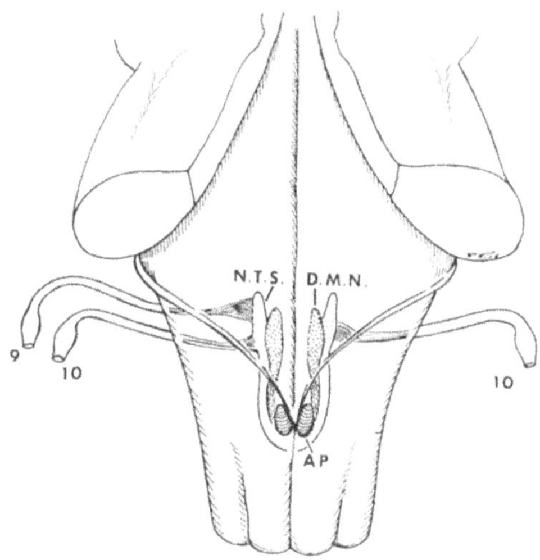

Fig. 3. Dorsal aspect of pons and medulla of the dog. The area postrema (A. P.) communicates with the nucleus of the solitary tract (N. T. S.), the terminus for sensory fibers from the sinus nerve which enter the brain stem through the glossopharyngeal nerve (9); the N. T. S. lies in juxtaposition to the dorsal motor nucleus (D. M. N.) of the vagus nerve (10) (FERRARIO et al., 1972, by kind permission)

vertebral arteries. GILDENBERG, FERRARIO and MCCUBBIN (unpublished observations) then proceeded to conduct a series of experiments in which the distribution of the circulation of the vertebral arteries was altered by ligation of the basilar artery exposed through the roof of the dog's mouth. When a silver clip was applied at the lowermost part of the basilar artery, just below the cervicocranial anastomosis, the pressor response disappeared. Thus, it was concluded that the area responsible for the central effects of angiotensin lay in the lower medulla (for review see FERRARIO, GILDENBERG and MCCUBBIN, 1972). These results were independently confirmed by JOY and LOWE [1970 (1)] who injected Indian ink into the vertebral arteries at the same speed at which they had injected angiotensin and correlated the distribution of the marker with the action. Fig. 3 shows diagrammatically the main structures of the brain stern of the dog.

Of the neurological structures within this area of the lower medulla, the area postrema and the tractus solitarius were possible sites of angiotensin activity. Since angiotensin would not be expected to penetrate the blood-brain barrier, it was considered probable that it would act in a place where the blood-brain barrier was absent. The area postrema appeared the most likely site since it can be stained by intravascular injection of trypan blue (WISLOCKI and PUTNAM, 1924), which is evidence for the existence of a gap in the blood-brain barrier. Microinjections of angiotensin directly into the area postrema were reported by UEDA (1968) to cause systemic pressor responses; similar injections into adjacent areas did not.

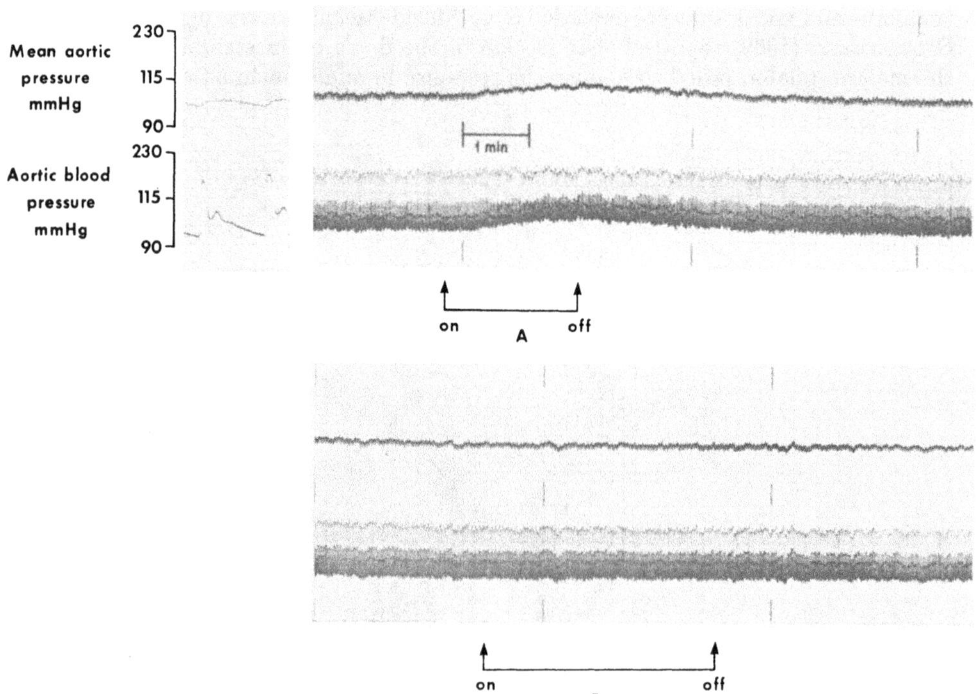

Fig. 4. Blood pressure response to the infusion of 4.5 ng/kg/min of angiotensin into the vertebral arteries before A) and its disappearance after B) bilateral coagulation of the area postrema (FERRARIO, GILDENBERG and McCUBBIN, unpublished)

The credit for determining that bilateral ablation of the area postrema abolished the specific pressor response to injection of angiotensin into the vertebral arteries is due to JOY and LOWE [1970 (2)]. GILDENBERG et al. (1971) were able to block the response reversibly by cooling the area postrema locally. JOY (1971) has established that both area postrema need to be ablated to prevent the response altogether. Fig. 4 illustrates the effect of bilateral thermocoagulation of the area postrema on the pressor response to infusion of angiotensin in the vertebral arteries.

The histological appearance of the area postrema suggests that it may have a chemoreceptor function. In view of its intimate connections to the baroreceptor reflex paths MOREST (1967) and FERRARIO et al. (1972) envisage the possibility that angiotensin may modify inhibitory activity reaching medullary vasomotor effector neurons. They point out the observation of BARRETT et al. (1971) and SWEET and BRODY (1970) that the injection of angiotensin into the vertebral arteries inhibited the reflex vasodilatation in the dog's hind limb which normally occurred in response to a pressor stimulus as evidence of some such inter-relationship.

It is possible that angiotensin may in some way modulate outflow of the autonomic nervous system since connections have been shown to exist between the area postrema and the nucleus of the solitary tract (MOREST, 1967); the latter receives fibers from the glossopharyngeal and carotid sinus nerves, constituting a major relay station for baroreceptor afferent integration (GABRIEL and SELLER, 1970). In this connection, it is interesting that renin has recently been demonstrated by GANTEN et al. (1971) to occur in brain tissue of nephrectomized dogs, despite the fact that it does not cross the blood-brain barrier. That the central autonomic effects of angiotensin may play a significant role in overall reflex cardiovascular adjustments has been shown recently by KATIC et al. (1971). They observed a fall rather than an increase in blood pressure after dogs with ablated area postremas were bled at a rate of 34 ml/min for 10 to 15 min. They concluded that the central cardivascular effects of angiotensin play a significant role in the response to hemorrhage of moderate severity.

Additional Sites of Action of Angiotensin in the Brain

SEVERS et al. (1966) observed that angiotensin could cause a pressor response after intraventricular injection, presumably by stimulating suprapontine structures. They also review previous observations along similar lines (DEUBEN and BUCKLEY, 1970; VOLICER and LOEW, 1971). In addition, the recently observed stimulatory action of angiotensin on the release of vasopressin (MOUW et al., 1971) and thirst (FITZIMONS et al., 1963; EPSTEIN et al., 1970; ANDERSSON and WESTBYE, 1970; FITZSIMONS, 1971; DANIELS-SEVERS et al., 1971) provides further evidence for an important action of angiotensin on brain structures above the tentorium. However, the pressor effects are only observable in relatively large doses, and, as mentioned before, angiotensin has rather unspectacular immediate effects on blood pressure when infused into the carotid artery. However, the long-term effects on fluid balance mediated by thirst and vasopressin stimulation could be of great importance in the change of long-term blood pressure regulation through alteration of the renal threshold of fluid excretion in relation to blood pressure (GUYTON, 1961) and it could also explain the well-known tendency for patients with high levels of circulating renin and angiotensin to have low plasma-sodium concentrations (BROWN et al., 1967).

Hemodynamic Features of the Pressor Response to Administration of Angiotensin via the Vertebral Arteries

LOWE and his colleagues (LOWE and SCROOP, 1969; SCROOP and LOWE, 1969) were inclined to attribute most of the pressor effects of angiotensin to inhibition of vagal inhibitory activity. These authors observed cardiac acceleration and increased cardiac output, with little change in total peripheral resistance. On the other hand, FERRARIO et al. (1970), using chronically implanted flowmeters, usually found a consistent increase in peripheral resistance (Fig. 1), with only occasional increases in cardiac output as a notable feature. They recorded both cardiac rate and cardiac output as substantially unchanged. GILDENBERG (unpublished observations) observed that bretylium tosylate abolished the pressor response. Fukiyama, Ferrario and McCubbin (unpublished) measured the efferent activity in various parts of the sympathetic nervous system. In the majority of cases, infusion of angiotensin into an intravertebral artery did not change cardiac nerve activity, bur frequently increased pre-ganglionic splanchnic vasomotor discharge. Renal nerve activity usually diminished, presumably as a result of the rise of blood pressure. In rabbits, Rosendorf et al. (1970) and Yu and Dickinson (1971), found evidence of a central effect of angiotensin on the sympathetic nervous system, and Ueda et al. (1969) found that in man, too the response involved the sympathetic nervous system. The recent work of Joy (1971) suggests that even in the greyhound there is a residual pressor response mediated through the sympathetic nervous system and accounting for 50 to 70% of the pressor response obtainable when vagi are intact.

Mode of Action of Angiotensin on the Brain Stem

Fukiyama et al. (1971) were able to sustain a rise in blood pressure for 7 days while angiotensin was infused into the vertebral artery of an unanesthetized dog, and Sweet et al. (1971) have confirmed this. It may be relevant that there is a close correlation between the concentration of angiotensin and that of norepinephrine in different parts of the brain (Fischer-Ferraro et al., 1971). The observation of Daniels and Buckley (1968), that the pressor effect of angiotensin elicited from the forebrain can be prevented by the removal of calcium ions, again raises the possibility of a central adrenergic pressor mechanism stimulated by the peptide. Further work will be necessary to determine the precise mode of action of angiotensin in the brain stem. Dickinson and Yu (1967) observed small but significant differences in the response to norepinephrine, which had a greater effect when given into the vertebral arteries of a conscious rabbit than when administered by intravenous infusion. Dickinson (unpublished) has been unable to confirm this effect in anesthetized dogs. However, the phenomenon would repay further investigation, and it might also be interesting to investigate the possible synergism of restriction of blood flow and administration of angiotensin into the brain stem circulation.

Summary

In rabbits, dogs and man angiotensin effects a greater rise of blood pressure, both acutely and in the long term, when infused into the vertebral arteries than when given intravenously. The phenomenon is mainly, and probably wholly, due to a specific stimulatory effect of angiotensin on the area postrema in the distal medulla, where the blood-brain barrier is deficient. The hemodynamic response usually involves wide-spread constriction of arterioles mediated through the sympathetic nervous system, but a rise in cardiac output, mediated by decreased vagal parasympathetic activity, may play some part in the response; in the greyhound this type of response seems to be particularly important.

References

Andersson, B., Westbye, O.: Synergistic action of sodium and angiotensin on brain mechanisms controlling water and salt balance. Nature (Lond.) **228**, 75 (1970).

Barrett, J. P., Ingenito, A. J., Procita, L.: Influence of the carotid sinus on centrally mediated peripheral cardiovascular effects of angiotensin II. J. Pharmacol. exp. Ther. **176**, 692 (1971).

Bickerton, R. K., Buckley, J. P.: Evidence for a central mechanism in angiotensin induced hypertension. Proc. Soc. exp. Biol. (N. Y.) **106**, 834 (1961).

BINGEL, A., CLAUS, R.: Weitere Untersuchungen über die blutdrucksteigernde Substanz der Niere. Dtsch. Arch. klin. Med. **100**, 412 (1910).

BRAUN-MENENDEZ, E., FASCIOLO, J. C., LELOIR, L. F., MUNOZ, J. M.: Farmacologia de la hipertensina. Rev. Soc. argent. Biol. **16**, 398 (1940).

BROWN, J. J., LEVER, A. F., ROBERTSON, J. I. S.: Plasma renin concentration in human hypertension. Amer. Heart J. **74**, 413 (1967).

DANIELS, A. E., BUCKLEY, J. P.: Relation of the centrally evoked pressor effect of angiotensin II to calcium ion. Europ. J. Pharmac. **4**, 152 (1968).

DANIELS-SEVERS, A., OGDEN, E., VERNIKOS-DANELLIS, J.: Centrally mediated effects of angiotensin II in the unanesthetized rat. Physiol. Behav. **7**, 785 (1971).

DEUBEN, R. R., BUCKLEY, J. P.: Identification of a central site of action of angiotensin II. J. Pharmac. exp. Ther. **175**, 139 (1970).

DICKINSON, C. J.: Neurogenic hypertension. Oxford and Edinburgh: Blackwell Scientific Publications 1965.

DICKINSON, C. J., LAWRENCE, J. R.: A slowly developing pressor response to small concentrations of angiotensin; its bearing on the pathogenesis of chronic renal hypertension Lancet **1963 I**, 1354.

DICKINSON, C. J., MCCUBBIN, J. W.: Pressor effects of increased cerebrospinal fluid pressure and vertebral artery occlusion with and without anesthesia. Circulat. Res. **12**, 190 (1963).

DICKINSON, C. J., MCCUBBIN, J. W.: Evidence cited by DICKINSON, C. J. (1965) Loc. Cit. p. 158 and plate 16.

DICKINSON, C. J., YU, R.: Mechanisms involved in the progressive pressor response to very small amounts of angiotensin in conscious rabbits. Circulat. Res. **20** and **21** (Suppl. II), II—157 (1967).

DOCK, W., SHIDLER, F., MOY, B.: The vasomotor center essential in maintaining renal hypertension. Amer. Heart J. **23**, 513 (1942).

EPSTEIN, A. N., FITZSIMONS, J. T., BARBARA, J.: Drinking induced by injection of angiotensin into the brain of the rat. J. Physiol. (Lond.) **210**, **457** (1970).

FELDBERG, W., LEWIS, G. P.: The action of peptides on the adrenal medulla. Release of adrenaline by bradykinin and angiotensin. J. Physiol. (Lond.) **171**, 98 (1964).

FERRARIO, C. M., DICKINSON, C. J., MCCUBBIN, J. W.: Central vasomotor stimulation by angiotensin. Clin. Sci. **39**, 239 (1970).

FERRARIO, C. M., GILDENBERG, P. L., MCCUBBIN, J. W.: Cardiovascular effects of angiotensin mediated by the central nervous system. Circulat. Res. **30**, 257 (1972).

FISCHER-FERRARO, C., NAHMOD, V. E., GOLDSTEIN, D. J., FINKIELMAN, S.: Angiotensin and renin in rat and dog brain. J. exp. Med. **133**, 353 (1971).

FITZSIMONS, J. T.: The effect on drinking of peptide precursors of angiotensin II injected into the rat's diencephalon. J. Physiol. (Lond.) **214**, 295 (1971).

FITZSIMONS, J. T., SIMONS, B. J.: The effect on drinking in the rat of intravenous infusion of angiotensin given alone or in combination with other stimuli of thirst. J. Physiol. (Lond.) **203**, 45 (1969).

FUKIYAMA, K., MCCUBBIN, J. W., PAGE, I. H.: Chronic hypertension elicited by infusion of angiotensin into the vertebral arteries of unanesthetized dogs. Clin. Sci. **40**, 283 (1971).

GABRIEL, M., SELLER, M.: Interaction of baroreceptor afferents from carotid sinus and aorta at the nucleus tractus solitarii. Pflügers Arch. ges. Physiol. **318**, 7 (1970).

GANTEN, D., MINNICH, J. L., GRANGER, P., HAYDUK, K., BRECHT, H. M., BARBEAU, A., BOUCHER, R., GENEST, J.: Angiotensin forming enzyme in brain tissue. Science **173**, 64 (1971).

GILDENBERG, P. L.: Localization of a site of angiotensin vasopressor activity in the brain. Physiologist **12**, 235 (abstract) (1969).

GILDENBERG, P. L., FERRARIO, C. M., ALFIDI, J. W., MCCUBBIN, J. W.: Localization of central nervous system vasopressor activity of angiotensin. Proc. XXVth International Congress of Physiological Sciences, 1971.

GUYTON, A. C.: Physiologic regulation of arterial pressure. Amer. J. Cardiol. **8**, 401 (1961).

JOY, M. D.: The intramedullary connections of the area postrema involved in the central cardiovascular response to angiotensin II. Clin. Sci. **41**, 89 (1971).

JOY, M. D., LOWE, R. D.: (1) The site of cardiovascular action of angiotensin II in the brain. Clin. Sci. **39**, 327 (1970.

JOY, M. D., LOWE, R. D.: (2) Evidence that the area postrema mediates the central cardiovascular response to angiotensin II. Nature (Lond.) **228**, 1303 (1970).

KATIC, F., JOY, M. D., LAVERY, H., LOWE, R. D., SCROOP, G. C.: Role of central effects of angiotensin in response to hemorrhage in the dog. Lancet **1971 II**, 1354.

LOWE, R. D., SCROOP, G. C.: The cardiovascular response to vertebral artery infusions of angiotensin in the dog. Clin. Sci. **37**, 593 (1969).

McCUBBIN, J. W., PAGE, I. H.: Neurogenic component of chronic renal hypertension. Science **139**, 210 (1963).

MOREST, K.: Experimental study of the projections of the nucleus of the tractus solitarius and the area postrema in the cat. J. Comp. Neurol. **130**, 277 (1967).

MOUW, D., BONJOUR, J. P., MALVIN, R. L., VANDER, A.: Central action of angiotensin in stimulating ADH release. Amer. J. Physiol. **220**, 239 (1971).

PAGE, I. H., BUMPUS, F. M.: Angiotensin. Physiol. Rev. **41**, 331 (1961).

PAGE, I. H., HELMER, O. M.: A crystalline pressor substance (angiotonin) resulting from the reaction between renin and renin-activator. J. exp. Med. **71**, 29 (1940).

PEACH, M. J., BUMPUS, F. M., KHAIRALLAH, P. A.: Inhibition of norepinephrine uptake in hearts by angiotensin II and analogs. J. Pharmacol. exp. Ther. **167**, 291 (1969).

PICKERING, G. W., PRINZMETAL, M.: Some observations on renin, a pressor substance contained in normal kidney, together with a method for its biological assay. Clin. Sci. **3**, 211 (1938).

ROSENDORF, C., LOWE, R. D., LAVERY, H., CRANSTON, W. I.: Cardiovascular effects of angiotensin mediated by the central nervous system of the rabbit. Cardiovasc. Res. **4**, 36 (1970).

SCARFF, R. W., MARTIN, N. H.: Experiments with renin. Brit. J. exp. Path. **22**, 309 (1941).

SCROOP, G. C., LOWE, R. D.: Central pressor effect of angiotensin mediated by the parasympathetic nervous system. Nature (Lond.) **220**, 1331 (1968).

SCROOP, G. C., LOWE, R. D.: Efferent pathways of the cardiovascular response to vertebral artery infusions of angiotensin in the dog. Clin. Sci. **37**, 605 (1969).

SEVERS, W. B., DANIELS, A. E., SMOOKLER, H. H., KINNARD, W. S., BUCKLEY, J. P.: Interrelationship between angiotensin II and the sympathetic nervous system. J. Pharmacol. exp. Ther. **153**, 530 (1966).

SWEET, C. S., BRODY, M. J.: Central inhibition of reflex vasodilitation by angiotensin and reduced renal pressure. Amer. J. Physiol. **219**, 1751 (1970).

SWEET, C. S., KADOWITZ, P., BRODY, M. J.: Arterial hypertension elicited by prolonged intravertebral infusion of angiotensin II in the conscious dog. Amer. J. Physiol. **221**, 1640 (1971).

UEDA, H.: Renine-angiotensine system and central nervous system. Proc. 5th Europ. Congr. Cardiol. 249 (1968).

UEDA, H., UCHIDA, Y., UEDA, K., GONDARIA, T., KATAYAMA, S.: Centrally mediated vasopressor effect of angiotensin II in man. Jap. Heart J. **10**, 243 (1969).

VOLICER, L., LOEW, C.: Penetration of angiotensin II into the brain. Neuropharmacol. **10**, 631 (1971).

WISLOCKI, G. B., PUTNAM, T. J.: Further observations on the anatomy and physiology of the areae postremae. Anat. Rec. **27**, 151 (1924).

YU, R., DICKINSON, C. J.: Neurogenic effects of angiotensin. Lancet **1965 II**, 1276.

YU, R., DICKINSON, C. J.: The progressive pressor response to angiotensin in the rabbit. The role of the sympathetic nervous system. Arch. int. Pharmacodyn. **191**, 24 (1971).

Peripheral Effects of Angiotensin on the Autonomic Nervous System

J. W. McCubbin

With 1 Figure

An important link between neurogenic and renal factors in the genesis of renal hypertension is probably to be found in the multiple actions of angiotensin on the peripheral autonomic nervous system. It is remarkable that discovery of these actions commenced only after 20 years of study of the well-known direct vasoconstrictor action of angiotensin. There was one exception, and this was the first clear demonstration that angiotensin has a direct action on the peripheral autonomic nervous system. In 1940, Braun-Menéndez et al. provided convincing evidence in cross-transfusion experiments that angiotensin can cause adrenal medullary discharge. Release of adrenal catecholamines by angiotensin receives thorough treatment in Chapter 20. The subject was then to lie dormant until recent years when the action of angiotensin on the autonomic nervous system attracted the interest of many investigators and new information is now accruing rapidly. Unfortunately, it is still too early to assess whether or not these newly discovered actions of angiotensin play an important physiologic role in cardiovascular regulation.

Parasympathetic Nervous System and Sympathetic Ganglia

Robertson and Rubin (1958, 1962) functionally denervated the guinea-pig ileum using botulinium toxin and showed that this procedure greatly reduced response to angiotensin, though response to acetylcholine was unchanged; response to nicotine was abolished. Shortly thereafter, Khairallah and Page (1961) demonstrated that response of the isolated guinea-pig ileum to angiotensin was reduced 60 to 70% when it was treated with atropine; the inhibition was reversed by addition of neostigmine. Morphine, known to prevent release of acetylcholine from nerve endings in this preparation, also inhibited response to angiotensin. These groups of experiments thus demonstrated that angiotensin could stimulate parasympathetic nerve tissue and elicit a contractile response mediated by acetylcholine. Feldberg and Lewis (1964) then demonstrated that angiotensin presumably had a direct ganglionic-stimulant action. When given by close intra-arterial injection into the superior cervical ganglion, it caused contraction of the ipsilateral nictitating membrane. The response was abolished by removal of the ganglion or section of the postganglionic, but not the preganglionic, nerve trunk. Angiotensin falls into the class of non-nicotinic ganglion stimulants since the response was not blocked by ganglion-blocking agents (Lewis and Reit, 1965; Trendelenburg, 1966).

Somewhat similar experiments by Haefely et al. (1965) and Panisset (1967) demonstrated that angiotensin is also able to modulate transmission through sympathetic ganglia. Small doses inhibited contraction of the nictitating membrane and release of acetylcholine in response to electrical stimulation of the preganglionic sympathetic nerve trunk. Large doses, on the other hand, were found to facilitate transmission. Machová and Boška (1967), using electrophysiological methods, confirmed the observation that angiotensin injected intra-arterially to the cat's superior cervical ganglion enhances ganglionic transmission, but their results differ from those of Haefely et al. and Panisset, in that injection of very large doses continued to cause enhanced transmission rather than inhibition.

In contrast to the effect of angiotensin on response of the nictitating membrane to electrical stimulation of its nerve supply, response to intra-arterially injected norepinephrine is reduced by prior administration of angiotensin by the same route (Cervoni and Reit, 1971). Inhibition of response was considered to be the consequence of ischemia due to the local vasoconstrictor action of angiotensin.

Cardiac Innervation

Angiotensin is apparently able to stimulate the myocardium through its sympathetic nerve supply. Farr and Grupp (1967) showed that 0.1 to 1.0 mcg/kg of angiotensin given intravenously to dogs increased the cardiac rate and force of contraction and that these effects were abolished when the caudal cervical sympathetic ganglia were crushed (crushing the stellate ganglia had no effect on response, leading the authors to conclude that there is an important species difference as regards the major cardiac sympathetic ganglia in dogs). Farr and Grupp (1971) later showed that cardiac effects similar to those produced by intravenous injection could be obtained by giving angiotensin locally into the blood supply of the caudal cervical ganglion, but not when given into the coronary circulation. They concluded that these effects of angiotensin are due to ganglion stimulation. Again (see above), angiotensin behaved as a non-nicotinic ganglion-stimulating agent since the cardiac effects were not prevented by administration of hexamethonium. Krasney et al. (1967) injected angiotensin directly into the right coronary artery and obtained an immediate increase in heart rate, causing them to conclude that angiotensin also acts on the sympathetic nervous system within the myocardium. The effects were prevented by adrenergic- but not by ganglion-blocking agents.

Thompson (1970) found the accelerator response to sympathetic nerve stimulation in perfused rabbit hearts to be increased during infusion of angiotensin but that the infusion of angiotensin had no effect on response to injection of norepinephrine; this is analogous to the different effects of infusion of angiotensin on systemic pressor responses to release of endogenous norepinephrine compared with responses to injected norepinephrine (see below).

It is questionable whether the cardiac effects of angiotensin demonstrated in these experiments ever play any physiologic role since, as emphasized by Finch and Leach (1969), the doses required to produce stimulation are large.

Innervation of Peripheral Vasculature

There is a clear interaction between the vasoconstrictor effects of angiotensin and those produced by sympathetic nerve activity. Zimmerman (1962) and Page and McCubbin (1963) demonstrated that the vasoconstrictor action of angiotensin in the dog's perfused hind limb is reduced by sympathectomy. Zimmerman (1962) showed additionally that responsiveness is restored when sympathetic activity is made to return by electrical stimulation of the cut distal end of the sympathetic nerve trunk. He also demonstrated that responsiveness to angiotensin in the hind limb is reduced when sympathetic activity is eliminated by section of the spinal cord or by pharmacological ganglion blockade.

The reverse interaction, modification by angiotensin of response to release of norepinephrine at sympathetic nerve endings, was reported by McCubbin and Page (1963). They demonstrated that responses to ephedrine and tyramine, which release endogenous norepinephrine, are enhanced by infusion of small amounts of angiotensin, and that the enhanced responses persisted even when tachyphylaxis to the direct vasoconstrictor action of angiotensin was produced. These changes in responsiveness induced by angiotensin appear clearly not to involve ganglion stimulation or modification of ganglionic transmission since tyramine has no known action on sympathetic ganglia; rather, the effect must result from some action at or near sympathetic nerve endings. Reflex vasoconstrictor responses in the perfused splanchnic bed associated with occlusion of the common carotid arteries were also enhanced by infusion of angiotensin (McCubbin and Page, 1963). In contrast to the effect on responses to ephedrine and tyramine, infusion of angiotensin had little or no effect on pressor responsiveness to injected norepinephrine. This action of angiotensin has also been demonstrated in man. Kaneko et al. (1966) infused subpressor amounts of angiotensin and observed increases in response to ephedrine and tyramine but not to norepinephrine. They obtained similar results in patients with essential hypertension. In contrast, control responses to ephedrine and tyramine were already increased in patients with renovascular hypertension and infusion of angiotensin caused no further increase.

Further evidence for an interaction between the two pressor systems was supplied by Zimmerman and Gomez (1965) who demonstrated that infusion of angiotensin into the dog's perfused paw caused increased vasoconstrictor responses to electrical stimulation of the postganglionic sympathetic chain, which is consistent with Zimmerman's (1962) earlier experiment in which he showed that sympathectomy reduced response to angiotensin. McGregor (1965) also found that contractile responses to angiotensin in the rat's isolated, perfused mesenteric bed are increased by administration of norepinephrine or electrical stimulation of the sympathetic nerves. Thoenen et al. (1965) demonstrated increased responsiveness of the isolated, perfused cat's spleen to electrical stimulation of the postganglionic sympathetic nerves when angiotensin was infused. Additionally, Sakurai and Hashimoto (1965) reported that infusion of angiotensin into isolated perfused rabbit ears caused enhancement of vasoconstrictor responses to norepinephrine and tyramine.

Other experiments also point to the inter-relationship between the two systems. Laverty (1963), using the perfused rat's hind limb, McGiff and Fasy (1965), using the dog's renal circulation, and Scroop and Whelan (1966), employing the circulation of the hand in man, all demonstrated that vascular responses to angiotensin were reduced or abolished when the respective sympathetic nerve supplies were cut or blocked pharmacologically. The response of the guinea-pig vas deferens to electrical stimulation was enhanced by angiotensin (Benelli et al., 1964) as were the responses of spirally cut aortic strips to tyramine (Khairallah et al., 1966) and responses of isolated rabbit atria to tyramine (Illanes et al., 1967). Day and Owen (1968) reported that the perfused rabbit's ear artery responded feebly to angiotensin but that the response was markedly increased during electrical stimulation of the sympathetic nerves; they also report, in contrast to the majority of other observations, that angiotensin depressed response to tyramine and norepinephrine. Sato and Masuyama (1971) observed that infusion of angiotensin into a rat's hind limb perfused with Tyrode's solution caused enhancement of response to injected norepinephrine. Tachyphylaxis to angiotensin occurred readily but responsiveness could be restored promptly by infusion of norepinephrine. Day and Owen (1969) studied the effects of infusion of angiotensin on responses to tyramine, norepinephrine and electrical stimulation of the spinal cord in pithed rats. Pressor amounts of angiotensin increased responses to tyramine and electrical stimulation but had little effect on response to norepinephrine.

The nature of the action of angiotensin on the sympathetic nervous system that results in enhanced cardiovascular responsiveness is not yet established. It might involve facilitation of release of endogenous stores of norepinephrine or prevention of uptake of released norepinephrine at the nerve ending, or both. Each possibility has its proponents. The effects of angiotensin on uptake and release of norepinephrine have been given thorough consideration in a recent Symposium [Fed. Proc. **31**, 1331 [1972)].

Production of Hypertension Through an Action on the Sympathetic Nervous System

Following the observation of Dickinson and Lawrence (1963) that chronic infusion of angiotensin into rabbits in dosages that initially had no effect on arterial pressure eventually caused sustained hypertension, McCubbin et al. (1965) repeated the experiment in dogs using somewhat different techniques. Angiotensin was infused intravenously at the rate of 10 mcg/kg/day or less. Initially there was no effect on arterial pressure but after from 1 to 3 days it began to rise and increased progressively until sustained hypertension was established. Rise in pressure was due entirely to increased total peripheral resistance. The remarkable feature of the hypertension was its lability; minor environmental stimuli that before the infusion had no discernable effect on pressure would cause mean arterial pressure to leap as much as over 100 mmHg during the infusion. An example of this changed responsiveness is shown in Fig. 1. In parallel with the progressive rise in pressure and appearance of hyper-responsiveness, there was accompanying increase in response to intravenous injections of tyramine. Both the hypertension and exaggerated responses to environmental stimuli were abolished by treatment with guanethidine.

Yu and Dickinson (1965) estimated sympathetic-nerve activity in rabbits chronically infused with initially subpressor amounts of angiotensin by serial injections of a short-acting ganglion blocking agent. They report that neural activity increased steadily during the first few days after start of the infusion.

Kezdi and Nomura (1968) infused subpressor amounts of angiotensin into dogs for 3 weeks and produced small sustained rises in pressure. The carotid sinus nerves were than cut, the purpose being to cause an increase in sympathetic discharge, and there was a further rise in pressure that was due to increase in peripheral resistance. Recordings of pre- and postganglionic sympathetic nerve activity before and during the infusions suggested that angiotensin was exerting its effect at the periphery rather than upon central vasomotor centers.

Monkeys have also received infusions of subpressor amounts of angiotensin for periods of 26 to 30 days (Forsyth et al., 1971). As in dogs, there was a delayed onset of rise in pressure; the hypertension plateaued after about 5 days and rise in pressure at the end of the infusion period was due entirely to increased peripheral resistance. Also as in dogs, environmental stresses produced much more marked pressor episodes in the infused than in the non-infused animals. These authors also

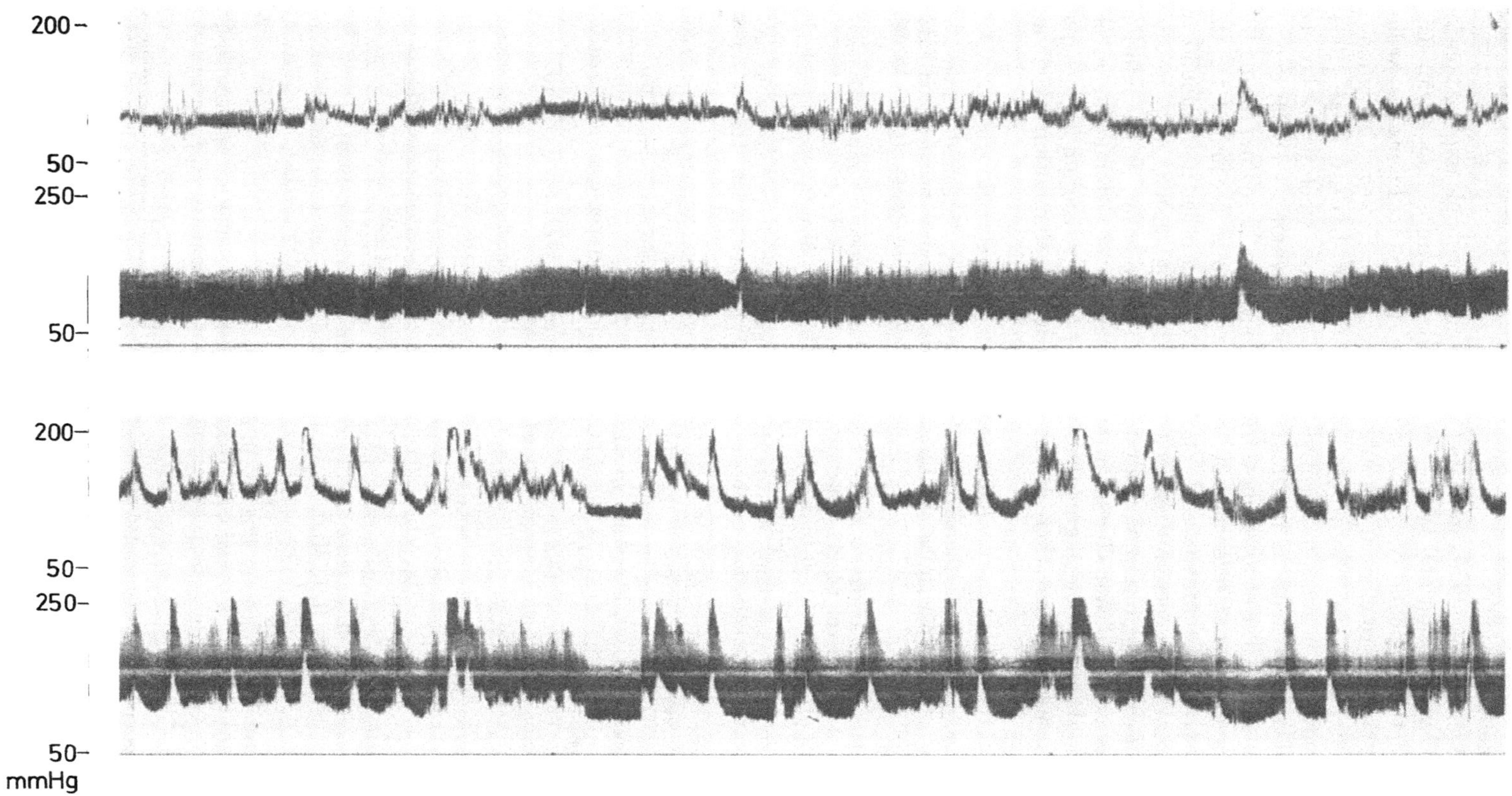

Fig. 1. Mean and pulsatile pressure of unanesthetized dog during control period (above) and then after 2 weeks of infusion of 10 mcg/kg/day of angiotensin (below). Laboratory equally quiet during both periods and dog rested comfortably during both recordings. Note highly exaggerated responses to subdued laboratory activity following infusion of angiotensin

concluded that small amounts of angiotensin can potentiate sympathetically mediated vasomotor activity.

All the foregoing experiments indicate that the most probable explanation for appearance of hypertension and lability of arterial pressure is that angiotensin has an action on the peripheral sympathetic nervous system that intensifies cardiovascular responsiveness to efferent sympathetic dischange. However, retention of sodium and water may also play a role, at least in man. Laragh et al. (1964) observed a progressive increase in sensitivity to angiotensin when it was infused over several days in patients, as in Dickinson and Lawrence's (1963) experiments in rabbits. Laragh et al. demonstrated a net gain in sodium during the period and suggested that retention of sodium and water accounted for the increasing sensitivity. Dickinson and Yu (1967), on the other hand, found in rabbits that total adrenalectomy reduced but did not abolish the progressive pressor effect of chronic infusion of small dosages of angiotensin. At low infusion rates there was no significant change in renal excretion of sodium and water. At higher rates (above 0.05 mcg/kg/min) there was a negative sodium balance due entirely to urinary sodium loss; there was no change in fecal elimination of sodium.

References

Ames, R. P., Borkowski, A. J., Sicinski, A. M., Laragh, J. H.: Prolonged infusions of angiotensin II and norepinephrine and blood pressure, electrolyte balance, and aldosterone and cortisol secretion in normal man and in cirrhosis with ascites. J. clin. Invest. **44**, 1171 (1965).

Benelli, G., Della Bella, D., Gandini, A.: Angiotensin and peripheral sympathetic nerve activity. Brit. J. Pharmacol. **22**, 211 (1964).

Braun-Menéndez, E., Fasciolo, J. C., Leloir, L. F., Muñoz, J. M.: Farmacologia de la hipertensina. Rev. Soc. argent. Biol. **16**, 398 (1940).

Cervoni, P., Reit, E.: Interactions between angiotensin and bloodborne exogenous norepinephrine on the cat nictitating membrane *in vivo*. J. Pharmacol. exp. Ther. **177**, 633 (1971).

Day, M. D., Owen, D. A. A.: The interaction between angiotensin and sympathetic vasoconstriction in the isolated artery of the rabbit ear. Brit. J. Pharmacol. **34**, **499** (1968).

Day, M. D., Owen, D. A. A.: Potentiation of responses to endogenously released noradrenaline in the pithed rat. Arch. int. Pharmacodyn. **179**, 469 (1969).

Dickinson, C. J., Lawrence, J. R.: A slowly developing pressor response to small concentrations of angiotensin. Lancet **1963 I**, 1354.

Dickinson, C. J., Yu, R.: Mechanism involved in the progressive pressor response to small concentrations of angiotensin. Circulat. Res. **21**, 157 (1967).

Farr, W. C., Grupp, G.: Sympathetically mediated effects of angiotensin on dog heart in situ. J. Pharmacol. exp. Ther. **156**, 528 (1967).

Farr, W. C., Grupp, G.: Ganglionic stimulation: mechanism of the positive inotropic and chronotropic effects of angiotensin. J. Pharmacol. exp. Ther. **177**, 48 (1971).

Feldberg, W., Lewis, G. P.: The action of peptides on the adrenal medulla. Release of adrenaline by bradykinin and angiotensin. J. Physiol. (Lond.) **171**, 98 (1964).

Finch, L., Leach, G. D. H.: The role of the sympathetic nervous system in the cardiovascular responses to angiotensin in the pithed rat. Brit. J. Pharmacol. **36**, 481 (1969).

Forsyth, R. P., Hoffbrand, B. I., Melmon, K. L.: Hemodynamic effects of angiotensin in normal and environmentally stressed monkeys. Circulation **54**, 119 (1971).

Haefely, W. A., Hurlimann, A., Thoenen, H.: Effect of bradykinin and angiotensin on ganglionic transmission. Biochem. Pharmacol. **14**, 1393 (1965).

Illanes, A., Perez-Olea, J., Quevedo, M., Ortiz, A., Lazo, M.: Influence of angiotensin on the effects of tyramine upon the contractile force of isolated rabbit atria. J. Pharmacol. exp. Ther. **158**, 487 (1967).

Kaneko, Y., Takeda, T., Nakajima, K., Ueda, H.: Effects of angiotensin on the pressor response to tyramine in normotensive subjects and hypertensive patients. Circulat. Res. **19**, 673 (1966).

Kezdi, P., Nomura, G.: Potentiation of sympathetic output by chronic angiotensin infusion and the effect of altered carotid sinus mechanism. Hypertension **16**, 39 (1968).

Khairallah, P. A., Page, I. H.: Mechanism of action of angiotensin and bradykinin on smooth muscle in situ. Amer. J. Physiol. **200**, 51 (1961).

KHAIRALLAH, P. A., PAGE, I. H., TURKER, R. K.: Potentiation of vascular myotropic responses by metanephrine and other noncatecholamines. Circulat. Res. **19**, 538 (1966).
KRASNEY, J. A., THOMPSON, J. L., LOWE, R. F.: Cardiac effects of angiotensin injections into perfused right coronary artery. Amer. J. Physiol. **213**, 134 (1967).
LAVERTY, R.: A nervously mediated action of angiotensin in anaesthetised rats. J. Pharm. Pharmacol. **15**, 63 (1963).
LEWIS, G. P., REIT, E.: The action of angiotensin and bradykinin on the superior cervical ganglion of the cat. J. Physiol. (Lond.) **179**, 538 (1965).
MACHOVÀ, J., BOŠKA, D.: A study of the action of angiotensin on the superior cervical ganglion in comparison with other ganglion stimulating agents. Europ. J. Pharmacol. **1**, 233 (1967).
MCCUBBIN, J. W., DEMOURA, R. S., PAGE, I. H., OLMSTED, F.: Arterial hypertension elicited by subpressor amounts of angiotensin. Science **149**, 1394 (1965).
MCCUBBIN, J. W., PAGE, I. H.: Neurogenic component of chronic renal hypertension. Science **139**, 210 (1963).
MCCUBBIN, J. W., PAGE, I. H.: Renal pressor system and neurogenic control of arterial pressure. Circulat. Res. **12**, 553 (1963).
MCGIFF, J. C., FASY, T. M.: The relationship of the renal vascular activity of angiotensin II to the autonomic nervous system. J. clin. Invest. **44**, 1911 (1965).
MCGREGOR, D. D.: The effect of sympathetic nerve stimulation on vasoconstrictor responses in perfused mesenteric blood vessels of the rat. J. Physiol. (Lond.) **177**, 21 (1965).
PAGE, I. H., MCCUBBIN, J. W.: Mechanisms by which ganglioplegics and atropine enhance cardiovascular responsiveness. Amer. J. Physiol. **205**, 1 (1963).
PANISSET, J. C.: Effect of angiotensin on release of acetylcholine from preganglionic and post-ganglionic nerve endings. Canad. J. Physiol. and Pharmacol. **45**, 313 (1967).
ROBERTSON, P. A., RUBIN, D.: An indirect action of angiotensin I on smooth muscle. Nature (Lond.) **182**, 867 (1958).
ROBERTSON, P. A., RUBIN, D.: Stimulation of intestinal nervous elements by angiotensin. Brit. J. Pharmacol. **19**, 5 (1962).
SAKURAI, T., HASHIMOTO, Y.: The vasoconstrictor action of angiotensin in relation to catecholamine. Jap. J. Pharmacol. **15**, 223 (1965).
SATO, R., MASUYAMA, Y.: Interaction of angiotensin and noradrenaline in rat's hindlimb preparation. Jap. Circulat. J. **35**, 505 (1971).
SCROOP, G. C., WHELAN, R. F.: A central vasomotor action of angiotensin in man. Clin. Sci. **30**, 79 (1966).
THOENEN, H., HURLIMAN, A., HAEFELY, W.: The effect of angiotensin on the response to postganglionic sympathetic stimulation of the cat spleen; lack of facilitation of norepinephrine liberation. Med. et pharmacol. exp. **13**, 379 (1965).
THOMPSON, J. L.: Effect of angiotensin on the cardioaccelerator response to sympathetic nerve stimulation in isolated rabbit hearts. Proc. Soc. exp. Biol. (N. Y.) **135**, 825 (1970).
TRENDELENBURG, U.: Observations on the ganglion stimulating action of angiotensin and bradykinin. J. Pharmacol. exp. Ther. **154**, 418 (1966).
YU, R., DICKINSON, C. J.: Neurogenic effects of angiotensin. Lancet **1965 II**, 1276.
ZIMMERMAN, B. G.: Effect of acute sympathectomy on responses to angiotensin and norepinephrine. Circulat. Res. **11**, 780 (1962).
ZIMMERMAN, B. G., GOMEZ, J.: Increased response to sympathetic stimulation in the cutaneous vasculature in presence of angiotensin. Int. J. Neuropharmacol. **4**, 185 (1965).

Angiotensin on Vascular Smooth Muscle

DAVID F. BOHR

Angiotensin is a potent agonist that causes contraction of vascular smooth muscle. The resultant vasoconstriction in the intact organism has important physiological and pathophysiological implications which are reflected in a number of recent reviews (PEART, 1965; GROSS et al., 1968; SOMLYO and SOMLYO, 1970). These extensive and excellent surveys have lightened my burden. In these reviews and in the recent literature I have covered, credit is given to the pioneer investigations in this already mature field; historical survey is omitted in the current review. Although I have restricted coverage to the past few years, I have found that in this period research has been adequately active to justify an attempt to describe the current state of the art. Contributions dealing with the effect of angiotensin on vascular smooth muscle have been primarily descriptive, yet enough of these bits of information have accumulated and are falling into place so that some mechanistic interpretations now seem appropriate.

Direct and Indirect Action

Before considering in detail the effects that angiotensin has on vascular smooth muscle, it should be helpful to review the evidence as to whether these effects are the results of direct or of indirect actions of this polypeptide on the vascular smooth muscle. On the one hand, angiotensin is known to act directly on the vascular smooth muscle cell to initiate a sequence of events that leads to its contraction; alternatively, angiotensin may alter the contractile state of vascular smooth muscle indirectly by its influence on the nervous system control of this muscle. It is often difficult to differentiate between the direct action of angiotensin and the contractile effect that it may induce by altering the properties of autonomic nerve endings in the vascular wall. Two types of indirect action must be considered: 1) Angiotensin may inhibit the uptake of norepinephrine by the nerve endings, and thereby potentiate its action and that of the sympathetic nervous system by permitting a higher concentration of the catecholamine to have access to the alpha receptors of the vascular smooth muscle cell. 2) Angiotensin may actually cause the release of norepinephrine or other neurohumoral agents from nerve terminals in the vessel wall.

The following generalizations bearing on the relative importance of direct and indirect effects of angiotensin on vascular smooth muscle appear to be borne out by the literature reviewed below: 1) There is better evidence supporting angiotensin inhibition of norepinephrine uptake by nerve endings than there is supporting its action via the release of norepinephrine from nerve endings. 2) The more simple the biological system studied, the more difficult it is to demonstrate an indirect action of angiotensin; there is very little evidence for this indirect effect from studies on isolated vascular smooth muscle whereas studies of the pressor response in the intact animal suggest that the indirect action of angiotensin may be important. 3) There may be some individuality among vascular smooth muscles from various sites in the body with respect to the relative contribution of the direct and indirect action of angiotensin, but uniformly in vascular smooth muscle the direct action seems to be more important than it is in other smooth muscle, such as that of the colon and ileum.

The following studies bearing on the issue of whether angiotensin inhibits norepinephrine uptake have generated results which support the proposition. KHAIRALLAH et al. (1971) observed that during the infusion of angiotensin there was a decrease in norepinephrine uptake in the kidney and uterus. PANISSET and BOURDOIS (1968) found that angiotensin decreased the uptake of labelled norepinephrine in the perfused vascular bed of the cat. In contrast, PALS et al. (1968) found no decrease in norepinephrine-H^3 in the rat heart and spleen during angiotensin infusion whereas the uptake in these tissues was diminished in the presence of cocaine or desipramine.

Other evidence bearing on the influence of angiotensin on norepinephrine uptake arises from studies of the influence of angiotensin on the response to norepinephrine or to sympathetic nerve stimulation. If angiotensin inhibits sequestration of norepinephrine by the nerve terminals, the response of the smooth muscle to this catecholamine should be potentiated in the presence of angiotensin. KHAIRALLAH et al. (1971) confirmed earlier findings that the constrictor response of the rabbit ear artery to norepinephrine is potentiated in the presence of angiotensin. PALAIC and LEMORVAN (1971) found that the response of guinea-pig aortic strip to norepinephrine was potentiated during angiotensin tachyphylaxis, suggesting that under this condition angiotensin might be blocking the uptake of norepinephrine by adrenergic nerve endings. PANISSET and BOURDOIS (1968) noted that the constrictor response of the mesenteric vessels of the cat to norepinephrine or nerve stimulation was potentiated by the presence of angiotensin. This potentiation of a norepinephrine response by angiotensin is not confined to arterial vessels; KADOWITZ et al. (1971) observed it in isolated saphenous vein. PALS et al. (1968) described at least minimal angiotensin potentiation of the pressor response to norepinephrine in the pithed cat. This potentiation, however, was not as great as that produced by cocaine or by desipramine.

If angiotensin is capable of potentiating the response to norepinephrine by blocking its sequestration, then perhaps antibodies to angiotensin, which should prevent its action on the nerve terminals, should depress the response to norepinephrine. KHAIRALLAH et al. (1971) found that angiotensin antibodies depressed the response to norepinephrine in the rabbit ear, and WORCEL et al. (1970) found that angiotensin antibodies diminished the pressor response to exogenous norepinephrine in the anesthetized rat.

From this review of the current findings it seems appropriate to conclude that angiotensin does inhibit the uptake of norepinephrine by nerve terminals in the vessel wall and that this inhibition can cause potentiation of the response of the vascular smooth muscle to norepinephrine. There is, however, a major concern that must be entertained regarding the validity of this functional evidence that angiotensin blocks the uptake of norepinephrine by nerve terminals. PANISSET and BOURDOIS (1968) have observed that in the chronically denervated cat angiotensin still potentiates the response of mesenteric vessels to norepinephrine, and the potentiation is even greater than in the normally innervated vessel. It is possible that angiotensin, by some direct action on the smooth muscle, produces this norepinephrine-potentiating effect.

The other postulated indirect action of angiotensin would result from its release of effective concentrations of norepinephrine from the nerve endings.

Although LIEBAU et al. (1965) presented evidence that this happens in isolated vessels from various species, including man, more recent studies argue that this is not an important phenomenon. KIRAN and KHAIRALLAH (1969) found that a concentration of angiotensin of 10^{-5} g/ml was required to displace norepinephrine from storage granules in the nerve endings of the rabbit aorta. This concentration is approximately 1000 times that required to reduce the uptake of norepinephrine in this system.

One functional corollary of the possibility that angiotensin may cause a release of norepinephrine from the nerve endings is in the tachyphylaxis that characterizes the response of isolated vascular smooth muscle to angiotensin. LIEBAU et al. (1965) have hypothesized that the failure of response of this tissue to repeated stimulation by angiotensin is the result of a depletion of the catecholamine stores in the nerve endings. They observed that with isolated blood vessels tachyphylaxis to angiotensin was reversed by exposure to norepinephrine 10^{-6} g/ml for 10 min. They also reported that cocaine prevented this reversal by norepinephrine, and that tachyphylaxis occurred more readily in vessels from animals that had been pretreated with reserpine. WALTER and BASSENGE (1969) and PALAIC and LEMORVAN (1971), however, were unable to demonstrate any reversal of tachyphylaxis by incubation with norepinephrine.

Since the vasoconstrictor response to tyramine is dependent on the release of norepinephrine from sites where it is sequestered, it should be possible to get insight regarding the effect of angiotensin on these pools by studying the effect of one of these agents on the response produced by the other. PALS et al. (1968) observed no effect of angiotensin on the pressor response of the pithed cat to tyramine. This response was, however, depressed by desipramine or cocaine. On the other hand, PALAIC and LEMORVAN (1971), using guinea pig aortic strip, found that once the muscle was made tachyphylactic to angiotensin, it failed to respond to tyramine. They interpreted this as indicating that angiotensin blocked access of tyramine to the site in the nerve terminal from which it causes norepinephrine release. They also observed that during complete tachyphylaxis to tyramine, the vascular smooth muscle was still capable of a maximal response to angiotensin. This suggests that the maximal response does not depend on the ability of angiotensin to release norepinephrine from tyramine-sensitive catecholamine stores.

This functional evidence that norepinephrine release is not an important factor in the response of vascular smooth muscle to angiotensin is supported by extensive observations indicating that alpha adrenergic receptor blocking agents, and other blocking agents, have little or no effect on the vascular response to angiotensin. If angiotensin produces its effect on vascular smooth muscle indirectly through the release of catecholamines, then this response should be eliminated by agents that block the action of this biogenic amine. The bulk of the current evidence supports the conclusion that blockade of alpha adrenergic receptors by either phentolamine or phenoxybenzamine does not alter the response of isolated blood vessels, or of an isolated perfused organ, to angiotensin (MAZURKIEWICZ-KWILECKI, 1968; THIND and PETERSON, 1968; WALTER and BASSENGE, 1969; AYERS et al., 1970; MCNEILL et al., 1970; PALAIC and LEMORVAN, 1971; VOTH et al., 1971). On the other hand, WARD and GAUTIERI (1969) reported that phenoxybenzamine caused a decrease in the constrictor response of the human placenta to angiotensin. Evidence bearing on the effect of alpha adrenergic blockade on the pressor response of the intact animal is divided. DAY and OWEN (1970) reported that alpha adrenergic blockade did not reduce the pressor response to angiotensin in the conscious cat. On the other hand, CHRYSSANTHOU et al. (1971) observed that phentolamine caused a shift to the right of the dose-response curve to angiotensin when a pressor response to this agent was studied in anesthetized pentolinium-blocked rats. It must be recognized, however, that in the intact animal an observed decrease in the response to angiotensin produced by alpha adrenergic blockade could be the result of a loss of the effectiveness of the elevated concentration of catecholamines resulting from a blockade by angiotensin of the uptake of endogenous norepinephrine by the nerve endings.

The use of reserpine to study the neurogenic component of an angiotensin response has also furnished ambivalent results. DiSalvo and Fell (1970) found no difference between renal vasoconstrictor responses in normal and reserpinized dogs. On the other hand, Drimal (1968) found a reduction in the coronary constrictor action of angiotensin following reserpine treatment. Day and Owen (1970) and Chryssanthou et al. (1971) described a decrease in the pressor response to angiotensin after reserpine pretreatment, in the cat and rat, respectively. In interpreting these reserpine studies it must be remembered that, in addition to eliminating the neurogenic effect, this agent is capable of a direct action on the calcium metabolism of the vascular smooth muscle cell (Carrier and Shibata, 1967).

Beta receptor blockade has no effect on the response to angiotensin of the rat portal vein (Voth et al., 1971) or on the pressor response to angiotensin in the intact cat (Day and Owen, 1970). Reports of the effect of propranolol on the response of the rabbit aorta to angiotensin indicate either that it has no effect (Thind and Peterson, 1968) or that it potentiates the response (Mazurkiewicz-Kwilecki, 1968).

Ganglionic blockade has no effect on the response to angiotensin of the rabbit aorta (Thind and Peterson, 1968) or the pressor response of the conscious cat (Day and Owen, 1970). Brunner et al. (1972) observed that treatment of the intact rat with a ganglionic blocker increased the amount of antibody required to prevent the pressor response to a standard dose of angiotensin. This observation they interpret as indicating that the autonomic nervous system "exerts some moderating influence on receptor affinity to angiotensin II". In this case it must decrease the "affinity" since the "affinity" increases with autonomic blockade.

The response to angiotensin is not altered when cholinergic receptors are blocked with atropine in the rat portal vein (Voth et al., 1971), the rabbit aorta (Thind and Peterson, 1968), or the rabbit ear (Blair-West et al., 1968). This absence of effect of atropine on the response of isolated vascular smooth muscle to angiotensin is in marked contrast to its inhibiting effect on the response of gut smooth muscle to angiotensin (Khairallah and Page, 1961). Blair-West et al. (1968) have demonstrated that blockade of serotonin receptors with methysergide or of histamine receptors with mepyramine fails to alter the response of the resistance vessels of the rabbit ear to angiotensin.

Further support for the preponderance of the direct effect of angiotensin on the vascular smooth muscle cell is seen in the failure of denervation to alter the renal vascular response to angiotensin (Geller and Kendrick, 1968; DiSalvo and Fell, 1970). It should also be pointed out that angiotensin is a potent activator of the smooth muscle of the sheep umbilical artery, which presumably is not innervated (Dyer, 1970). It has been noted, too, that the response to angiotensin of the isolated perfused kidney is greater than the response *in situ* (Korner et al., 1967; Geller and Kendrick, 1968). Additional evidence in support of the greater importance of the direct action of angiotensin on vascular smooth muscle is found in the observations of Drimal (1968) and Walter and Bassenge (1969), that angiotensin causes only constriction of the coronary vascular smooth muscle. If norepinephrine were released from nerve endings by angiotensin it would be expected to cause relaxation rather than contraction of the coronary vessels

(BOHR, 1967). A final bit of evidence that may be mustered in support of the absence of an indirect effect of angiotensin on vascular smooth muscle is the finding by BLAIR-WEST et al. (1968) that the response of the rabbit ear artery to angiotensin is highly dependent on the sodium concentration of the physiological salt solution perfusate whereas the response of this resistance system to norepinephrine is not.

In summary, there is little evidence to suggest that the contraction of vascular smooth muscle produced by angiotensin is dependent to any significant degree on the ability of this polypeptide to release norepinephrine from adrenergic nerve terminals in the vessel wall. However, angiotensin may augment the effects of norepinephrine and the sympathetic nervous system by blocking the uptake of norepinephrine in the nerve terminals. More evidence is needed before this neurogenic action of angiotensin can be quantified.

Tachyphylaxis and Autopotentiation

Repeated stimulation of vascular smooth muscle with angiotensin results in responses which may sequentially decrease, increase, or remain unchanged. Which of these trends will prevail depends upon the following variables: 1) the frequency of stimulation; 2) the concentration of angiotensin; 3) the anatomical site of origin of the muscle; 4) the species of origin of the muscle; and 5) the environment of the muscle. Recent studies of these phenomena have not only generated descriptive observations regarding tachyphylaxis and autopotentiation, but have also formed a basis for interesting speculation about the mechanism of action of angiotensin related to its receptor system.

Within the past several years studies have been made comparing the degree of tachyphylaxis evidenced by isolated vascular smooth muscle from different sources. KHAIRALLAH et al. (1966) noted greater tachyphylaxis in vascular smooth muscle from the cat than in that from the rabbit; BOHR and UCHIDA (1967) described differences in the degree of tachyphylaxis among different vessels from the dog, with no response of the small renal artery to angiotensin; and WALTER and BASSENGE (1969) observed tachyphylaxis in isolated vascular smooth muscle from coronary, renal, and carotid arteries. Tachyphylaxis in smooth muscle from the guinea-pig aorta has been extensively studied by GODFRAIND (1970) and by PALAIC and LEMORVAN (1971). It has been observed in isolated uterine artery from human beings (GOUGH and DYER 1971) and in perfused mesenteric (SHEHADEH et al. 1969) and coronary (DRIMAL, 1968) arteries.

On the other hand, the rabbit aorta, which is by all odds the isolated vascular smooth muscle most studied for its response to angiotensin, does not display tachyphylaxis. Its failure to show tachyphylaxis has been convincingly demonstrated by ALTURA and ALTURA [1970 (1)] who found that repeated stimulation over a 10-h study period failed to induce a change in the maximum response. However, the rabbit aorta showed some decrease in response to submaximal concentrations of angiotensin, causing the ED-50 to shift from 2.5×10^{-8} M at the outset to 10^{-7} at the end of the 10-h incubation period. BOHR and UCHIDA (1967) have shown that this diminution in angiotensin response was not due to tachyphylaxis since it occurred with the passage of time in the bath of physiological salt solution whether or not the aortic smooth muscle was stimulated repeatedly with angiotensin. Also in the category of vessels that show very little tachyphylaxis to angiotensin is the arterial system of the perfused rabbit ear (BLAIR-WEST et al., 1968). *In vivo* there is much less tendency than in the isolated system for tachyphylaxis to angiotensin to develop. LUMBERS and WHALEN (1970) observed no tachyphylaxis in the vasoconstrictor response of the human forearm to angiotensin, and the reproducibility of the pressor responses to angiotensin has been documented in all of the laboratories where this device is used for assay of renin activity.

The most satisfactory concept for handling the mechanism of tachyphylaxis of vascular smooth muscle to the angiotensin response is that of receptor occupancy. The angiotensin molecule occupies the receptor site and thereby prevents its activation by other angiotensin molecules to which the tissue is subsequently exposed. This possible mechanism is supported by the observation made by several investigators (KHAIRALLAH et al., 1966; BOHR and UCHIDA, 1967; WALTER and BASSENGE, 1969) that when tissue made tachyphylactic by exposure to angiotensin is treated with a solution containing angiotensinase activity, or with Dowex-50 which absorbs angiotensin, the tachyphylaxis diminishes. These procedures which remove the angiotensin occupying the receptor site, presumably make this site available again for activation by angiotensin. KHAIRALLAH et al. (1966) presented additional evidence along these lines in their finding that the angiotensinase activity of blood vessel wall is inversely related to the tendency of that particular vessel to develop tachyphylaxis. GOODFRIEND and LIN (1970) observed that I_2-labelled angiotensin became bound to tissues that it activated and was removed only very slowly by rinsing the tissue. In this study using rabbit aorta, the bound angiotensin which could not be removed by rinsing could be removed by treatment of the tissue with unlabelled angiotensin. The fact that angiotensin tachyphylaxis is not as conspicuous as it is in isolated tissues may be due to the fact that there are large amounts of angiotensinase in the circulating plasma.

WALTER and BASSENGE (1969) suggest that tachyphylaxis is not due to depletion of norepinephrine stores; they were unable to reverse tachyphylaxis by incubating the tissue in norepinephrine, to reload the stores.

Several lines of evidence have been developed which might be interpreted as indicating that the process of angiotensin tachyphylaxis may be dependent at least somewhat on mechanisms other than receptor occupancy. One non-specific effect of angiotensin that might alter subsequent vascular responses is described by GODFRAIND (1970) in his studies on the electrolyte composition of helical strips of guinea-pig aorta. He observed that treatment with acetylcholine caused the tissue to lose potassium and to gain an equal amount of sodium. He noted that the presence of angiotensin reduced to less than half, the magnitude of the sodium-potassium exchange, and speculates that angiotensin might activate a coupling between an inward movement of calcium and an outward movement of sodium. Activation of such an exchange system would explain the tendency of angiotensin to reduce the sodium depletion produced by acetylcholine. It might also account for the increase in tissue responsiveness after treatment with angiotensin that has been observed in various experiments. Possibly also related to a non-specific electrolyte effect of angiotensin is the observation by GODFRAIND (1968) that in some tissues made tachyphylactic to angiotensin there is also a loss of sensitivity in response to bradykinin and to histamine. Although such observations argue that one must be alert to a general non-specific effect of angiotensin, current evidence suggests that the primary process responsible for tachyphylaxis is a specific receptor occupancy.

Quite opposite to the tachyphylactic effect are the potentiated responses that are occasionally observed following repeated angiotensin stimulations. In one study, GODFRAIND (1968) observed that exposure of the tissue to high concentrations of angiotensin (2×10^{-6} M) caused potentiation of subsequent responses to low doses of angiotensin at a time when responses to high doses of angiotensin were depressed. GODFRAIND (1970) has also observed that subjecting a helical strip of guinea pig aorta to repeated, increasing angiotensin concentrations (10^{-10} to 10^{-6} M) may increase the maximum response by as much as 150%. In this case the ED-50 was not changed. He postulates that this change in responsiveness may be related to the effect, described above, of angiotensin on a sodium-calcium exchange system. PALAIC and LEMORVAN (1971) found that more ^{14}C-angiotensin was taken up by guinea-pig aorta made tachyphylactic to angiotensin than was taken up by this tissue under control conditions. They postulate that under the stimulation of angiotensin the cell may develop an increased number of receptor sites. Under proper conditions this phenomenon might account for the observed autopotentiation of the angiotensin response.

Angiotensin Receptors

Substantial evidence from experiments with radioactive angiotensin indicates that this agonist is bound to a specific physiologically active receptor site in vascular smooth muscle (GOODFRIEND and LIN, 1970; BAUDOUIN et al., 1971). In the rabbit aorta this binding site is completely loaded when the concentration of angiotensin is 10^{-7} M. This is the concentration that produces maximum contractile response. Furthermore, the rate of loading and unloading of the radioactive tag on this binding site parallels the rate of tension development and relaxation following stimulation of the aorta. BAUDOUIN et al. (1971) estimated that the concentration of the receptor substance in the aortic wall is 8×10^{-12} moles/gram. GOODFRIEND and LIN (1970) calculated it to be 10^{-12} moles/gram in the tissues that they studied, and further estimated that if the molecular weight of the receptor site protein was 100,000 it would constitute one millionth of the target cell protein.

There is conflicting evidence in the literature regarding the uniformity of angiotensin receptor sites. Using five structural analogues of Ang. II, MEYER et al. (1970) studied the ratio of their functional activity on isolated colon and uterus from the rat and on rabbit aorta strips. They reasoned that if the receptors in the three organs were the same, similar ratios of activity of the analogues would be expected. Since the ratios were not the same, they concluded that there were either two or three different types of receptors in these tissues. These observations refute those of ARAKAWA et al. (1962) who found similar ratios of various analogues in their ability to produce a pressor response in the rat and to cause contraction of rat uterus. AIKEN and VANE (1970) also using activity ratios, concluded that Ang. I and Ang. II act on the same receptor site.

Two recent studies suggest that the angiotensin receptor may be a labile structure. Using an indirect technique of antibody requirements for neutralization of an angiotensin pressor response in the rat, BRUNNER et al. (1972) concluded that the avidity of the receptor for the angiotensin molecule could be altered by changes in salt intake, by nephrectomy or by ganglionic blockade. PALAIC and LEMORVAN (1971), in a more direct study, observed that when the guinea-pig aortic strip was made tachyphylactic to angiotensin, using non-radioactive angiotensin, this tissue was capable of binding an increased amount of radioactive angiotensin. This observation suggested to them that administration of angiotensin caused the induction of new binding sites.

An observation by BAUDOUIN et al. (1972) gives some insight into the mechanism by which a combination of angiotensin with its receptor site might initiate the contractile response of vascular smooth muscle. They observed the rate of efflux of ^{45}Ca from a preparation of vesicular cell fragments of rabbit aorta. When angiotensin was added to this preparation, the calcium efflux rate was accelerated. This suggests that the combination of angiotensin with its receptor may be directly responsible for the release of activator calcium in the smooth muscle cell.

Heterogeneity of Vascular Smooth Muscle in Its Responsiveness to Angiotensin

Angiotensin, through its direct constrictor action on vascular smooth muscle, has gained the reputation of being the most potent physiologically-occurring pressor agent. However, its ability to cause contraction is not at all uniform for vascular smooth muscle from different sites in the body, and the extent of the contraction it produces is generally less than that produced by alpha adrenergic receptor activation. The disparity in its ability to produce contraction of vascular smooth muscle from different sites is evident in Table 1, in which the maximum tension that can be developed by angiotensin is expressed as percent of the maxi-

Table 1. *Angiotensin response expressed as % of maximum response to epinephrine or norepinephrine*

Vessel	% of maximum response	Adapted from
Rabbit aorta	55	ALTURA and ALTURA (1971)
Rabbit aorta	65	SOMLYO and SOMLYO (1971)
Rabbit pulmonary artery	21	SOMLYO and SOMLYO (1971)
Dog large renal artery	6	SOMLYO and SOMLYO (1971)
Dog small renal artery	0	BOHR and UCHIDA (1967)
Human uterine artery	45	GOUGH and DYER (1971)
Sheep umbilical artery	328	DYER (1970)

mum contraction that can be produced by epinephrine or norepinephrine. The basis for this individuality is usually thought to be due to differences in receptor population in the various vascular smooth muscles. The selection of alpha adrenergic agonists for comparison is based on the fact that the maximum response to these agonists tends to be as great as that to any agonist. This is not true in the case of the sheep umbilical artery where serotonin produces the greatest response and the maximum response to angiotensin is 87% of the response to serotonin. Although the threshold and ED-50 expressed on a molar basis for angiotensin are, in general, considerably lower than those for epinephrine or for norepinephrine, it is evident that for most vascular smooth muscle the maximum response to angiotensin is less than that to the catecholamine. Interestingly, vascular smooth muscle from the renal artery is particularly deficient in its ability to contract in response to angiotensin.

Not only does the effectiveness of angiotensin as a constrictor vary from one vascular bed to another, but its effectiveness differs greatly in the sequential segments of a given vascular bed. JÄRHULT (1971) has described a study of these individualities in a skeletal muscle bed of the cat. Again, the effectiveness of angiotensin on each of the vascular segments was compared with that of norepinephrine. Both angiotensin and norepinephrine were effective constrictors of the precapillary resistance vessels. Angiotensin is a more effective constrictor of the precapillary sphincter than is norepinephrine, as judged by its effect on the capillary filtration coefficient. The author points out that the precapillary sphincter normally is primarily under the control of local regulatory phenomena so that any agent which decreases flow through a vascular bed by constricting precapillary resistance vessels tends to cause relaxation of the precapillary sphincter. Angiotensin is unusual in that it is capable of overriding this local dilator influence; norepinephrine does not, and its administration results in an increase in capillary filtration coefficient. In the next segment of the vascular tree, angiotensin was found to be a more potent constrictor of the postcapillary resistance vessels than was norepinephrine. There was a net fluid accumulation in the tissues under the influence of angiotensin, indicating that there was an increase in postcapillary resistance. Control of the small resistance venules apparently differs from that of the larger capacity vessels since the latter are more effectively constricted by norepinephrine than they are by angiotensin.

There is much evidence to suggest that all veins do not respond uniformly to angiotensin. HEDWALL et al. (1970), measuring small vein pressures in constant rate perfusion systems, conclude that angiotensin produces greater venoconstriction in the dog gracilis than in the hind paw. HYMAN (1969) saw no constrictor effect of angiotensin on the pulmonary vein in a preparation in which this vein was constricted by norepinephrine. KADOWITZ et al. (1971) observed that low concentrations of angiotensin enhanced the constrictor response of the saphenous vein of the dog to sympathetic nerve stimulation but failed to enhance its response to injected norepinephrine. This led them to the conclusion that angiotensin enhances transmitter release in this vein.

Angiotensin has a potent renal vasoconstrictor action which, earlier studies to the contrary, does not depend on renal innervation (GELLER and KENDRICK, 1968; DISALVO and FELL, 1970). Studies designed to examine the effect of angiotensin on the intrarenal components of the vascular bed have given varying results. CARRIÈRE and BIRON (1970) observed that intraarterial infusion of angiotensin produced a decrease in renal blood flow without decreasing glomerular filtration. The resultant increase in filtration fraction could have been due to a predominant constriction of the efferent arterioles. CARRIÈRE and FRIBORG (1969), using the krypton washout technique, developed evidence which indicated that the subcapsular region of the cortex was more readily constricted than was the inner cortex. Medullary flow also decreased under the influence of angiotensin. Recently NISSEN and GALSKOV (1972) have studied flow distribution in the cat kidney, taking advantage of the fact that in this animal the outer cortex is drained by subcapsulary veins whereas the inner cortex is drained by arcuate veins. It is possible to measure flow from these two drainage systems separately. Angiotensin produced equal flow reduction in the two venous systems whereas catecholamines produced greater constriction in the inner cortex. The pronounced constrictor action of angiotensin in the intact kidney stands in contrast to its relatively weak contracting action in the isolated renal artery (BOHR and UCHIDA, 1967; SOMLYO and SOMLYO, 1971). Recent observations by UCHIDA and OHTSU, personal communication, indicate that angiotensin causes relaxation of the renal vein. It is noteworthy that this unusual effect of angiotensin occurs in the vascular segment which is exposed to the highest concentration of renin and angiotensin in the blood.

Smooth muscle from isolated pulmonary artery contracts in response to angiotensin (AIKEN and VANE, 1970), but angiotensin is not as potent as eledoisin (POPOVIC et al., 1968) or norepinephrine (SOMLYO and SOMLYO, 1971) in producing contraction. Studies on the *in situ* perfused lobe of the lung demonstrate that angiotensin produces constriction of the pulmonary artery but does not produce constriction of the pulmonary vein (HYMAN, 1969).

Angiotensin has been found to be a potent constrictor of the coronary vascular bed, both when studied in the *in situ* perfused coronary system (DRIMAL, 1968) and when helical strips from these vessels were studied in the isolated bath (WALTER and BASSENGE, 1969). In either case there is a striking tendency for the coronary smooth muscle to show tachyphylaxis to the angiotensin response.

The constrictor action of angiotensin on the mesenteric vascular bed has been studied extensively. The constriction here may be the result of both a direct effect of angiotensin on the vascular smooth muscle and its augmentation of the adrenergic response (PANISSET and BOURDOIS, 1968). The constrictor response to angiotensin shows rapid tachyphylaxis (SHEHADEH et al., 1969) and is diminished in the presence of a high level of constrictor tone initiated by norepinephrine (ŠTOLC, 1969). MCNEILL et al. (1970) have presented evidence that the major basis for mesenteric vasoconstriction during hemorrhage in the cat is an increase in circulating angiotensin and vasopressin, and is not related to an increase in adrenergic activity. Angiotensin produces an increase in splenic vascular resistance, but unlike norepinephrine, fails to produce contraction of the splenic capsule (AYERS et al., 1970; GREENWAY and STARK, 1970).

Arterial perfusion of the rabbit ear is still a popular system for studying the constrictor response to angiotensin (BLAIR-WEST et al., 1968; KHAIRALLAH et al., 1971). Recent studies have demonstrated that angiotensin also has a constrictor action on the umbilical artery (DYER, 1970), the uterine artery (GOUGH and DYER, 1971), and the placenta (WARD and GAUTIERI, 1969).

Interventions that Alter the Angiotensin Response

Many of the studies of the past few years that deal with the action of angiotensin on vascular smooth muscle have explored the effects of various interventions on the magnitude of this response. The logic of this procedure rests largely on the premise that, if the mechanism of action of the intervention is known, then the result of the experiment will give some insight as to the mechanism of action of angiotensin. Of course, there may also be the hope that having defined the action of a given intervention *in vitro*, it may be used to manipulate the angiotensin response in the intact organism. Conversely, the intervention may be used to define the action of angiotensin in the intact organism, but this is justified only when the intervention has the specificity of action of an antibody.

In Table 2, comparisons are made between the effects of specific interventions on the angiotensin response and the response to epinephrine or norepinephrine. A difference in the effects of a given intervention may be caused by one or both of the following: 1) The intervention may differentially influence the agonist-receptor interaction. Since both the agonist and its receptor site are different, the individuality of the influence of an intervention may reflect the fact that it alters one agonist or its receptor and not the other. 2) There may be subtle differences in the individual events of the overall contractile process which affect the response to the two agonists. These differences may be in the nature of membrane excitation, the excitation-contraction coupling, the metabolic processes supporting contraction and relaxation, or in the actual chemo-mechanical transducing by the contractile protein. An example of this type of individuality is a difference in the extent to which the response to a given agonist depends on activator calcium from extracellular and from intracellular sources. A generalization which may be emerging is that whereas the contractile response to catecholamines utilizes calcium from either intracellular or extracellular sources, the response to angiotensin depends more exclusively on activator calcium from intracellular sources. This is in contrast to the contractile response to depolarizing concentrations of KCl, which depends almost exclusively on calcium from extracellular sources.

VAN BREEMEN et al. (1972) have demonstrated that the trivalent cation lanthanum has properties which make it a particularly valuable tool with which to produce an intervention in the response of vascular smooth muscle. Lanthanum displaces calcium from all extracellular binding sites, and acting on the vascular smooth muscle membrane hinders influx and efflux of calcium ions. These authors took advantage of these properties to develop a "lanthanum technique" for measuring intracellular calcium content of vascular smooth muscle. By placing a seg-

Table 2. *Various interventions; relative influence on response of vascular smooth muscle to angiotensin and to catecholamines*

Intervention	Vessel	Influence of intervention on response to: Angiotensin		Epi or norepi	References
La 0.5 mM	rabbit aorta	depressed	=	depressed	VAN BREEMEN et al. (1972)
Mn 0.5 mM	rabbit aorta	depressed	>	depressed	SULLIVAN and BRIGGS (1968)
Cd 0.1 mM	rabbit aorta	no change		depressed	PERRY et al. (1967)
Cd 50 μg/ml	rabbit aorta	depressed	<	depressed	THIND et al. (1970)
SKF-525 A 10 μg/ml	rabbit aorta	depressed	<	depressed	KALSNER et al. (1970)
Mg-free	rabbit aorta	augmented		depressed	ALTURA and ALTURA (1971)
Glucose-free	rabbit aorta	depressed	<	depressed	ALTURA and ALTURA (1970)
Decreased [Na] 40 mM	rabbit ear artery	depressed		no change	BLAIR-WEST et al. (1968)
Increased [Na] 40 mM	rabbit ear artery	depressed		no change	BLAIR-WEST et al. (1968)
KCl depolarization	rabbit aorta	no change		depressed	SULLIVAN and BRIGGS (1968)
Iproveratrile	rat portal vein	depressed	=	depressed	VOTH et al. (1971)
Alpha methyl dopa	constriction denervated hind limb, dog	augmented		no change	PRIVITERA and MOHAMMED (1970)

ment of rabbit aorta in a calcium-free physiological salt solution containing lanthanum [2 mM], the efflux of intracellular calcium was blocked and extracellular bound calcium was displaced. The content of calcium remaining in the vascular segment is probably all intracellular. Utilizing this technique for measuring intracellular calcium content, these authors demonstrated that exposure of the vascular segment to a depolarizing concentration of KCl caused an increase in the rate of calcium influx whereas exposure of the segment to a concentration of norepinephrine capable of producing maximum contraction did not alter calcium influx. They also calculated that the increase in rate of calcium influx induced by KCl was appropriate to account for the rate of tension development produced by this agent. Further corroboration of the flux data was presented in their observation that lanthanum prevented the contractile response produced by depolarizing concentrations of KCl (which produced its effect by increasing membrane permeability to extracellular calcium), but did not prevent contraction produced by norepinephrine. They concluded that norepinephrine produced a contractile response by the release of intracellularly-bound calcium. Once the segment had been made to contract in response to norepinephrine, it would not contract again. Angiotensin was also capable of producing a single response in the lanthanum-treated preparation. Regardless of which of these agonists was used first, neither produced a second response. This observation was used as evidence that norepinephrine and angiotensin utilize a similar pool of intracellularly sequestered calcium for activation of the contractile protein. However, other observations which I will cite suggest that there may be a difference in the calcium pools used by angiotensin and by norepinephrine. The disparity in these interpretations may be accounted for by the possibility that lanthanum displaces calcium from some pools, in the plasma membrane for instance, which may be differentially influenced by norepinephrine and angiotensin.

Manganese is another cation which has been shown to alter membrane permeability to calcium (KEENE et al., 1972). SULLIVAN and BRIGGS (1968) have observed that manganese depresses the response to angiotensin more than it does that to catecholamines.

The use of cadmium as an intervention to alter vascular response to angiotensin has been of some interest since this cation, administered to the intact animal, produces hypertension (THIND et al., 1969). Aortic strips from rabbits made hypertensive by this technique were significantly less responsive to angiotensin than were strips from normotensive control rabbits. Similarly paradoxical is the observation of THIND et al. (1970) that cadmium added to the physiological salt solution bathing a segment of normal rabbit aorta depresses the contractile response to both angiotensin and norepinephrine. Tracings shown in their publication suggest that cadmium has a greater depressant effect on the norepinephrine response than on the response to angiotensin. PERRY et al. (1967) found that cadmium, 0.1 mM, almost completely inhibited an epinephrine response whereas it produced no effect, or slightly potentiated, a response to angiotensin. These differences, although clear-cut, do not lend themselves to evident mechanistic interpretations. They do, however, parallel the observation (KALSNER et al., 1970) that the agent SKF-525A, which seems to block membrane permeability to extracellular calcium, depresses the response to norepinephrine more than it does that to angiotensin. These observations could be interpreted as indicating that the angiotensin response is less dependent on external calcium than is the response to norepinephrine.

The ALTURAS, using exacting dose-response studies, have defined several differences between the responses of rabbit aorta to angiotensin and to norepinephrine through the use of the intervention technique. They found (ALTURA and ALTURA, 1971) that after a 1-h exposure to a magnesium-free physiological salt solution, the response to angiotensin was augmented whereas that to epinephrine was depressed. After exposure to a glucose-free physiological salt solution both responses were depressed but the effect on the norepinephrine response was greater [ALTURA and ALTURA, 1970 (1)]. These authors also compared the rate of development of mechanical responses to various agonists as the rabbit aorta accumulated calcium during a 3-h incubation period in physiological salt solution. The development of responsiveness to epinephrine closely paralleled the accumulation of calcium in the artery segment whereas the development of responsiveness to angiotensin was slower [ALTURA and ALTURA, 1970 (2)]. This suggests that these two agonists use different calcium pools, the one used by angiotensin accumulating more slowly.

Because of the interest in sodium as a cation important in the development of arterial hypertension, studies have been carried out in various systems to evaluate the effect of varying concentrations of this cation on the vascular response to angiotensin. BLAIR-WEST et al. (1968) reported that 40 mM increases or decreases in sodium concentration depressed the constrictor response of the rabbit ear artery to angiotensin, but had little effect on its response to norepinephrine. However, similar studies on the rabbit aorta indicate that this degree of change in sodium concentration produces a pronounced effect on the response to epinephrine (SITRIN and BOHR, 1971). BRUNNER et al. (1972) observed that rats on a high sodium intake require a greater amount of angiotensin antibody to neutralize the pressor response to a standard dose of angiotensin. They interpret this as indicating that an increase in sodium intake causes an increase in "avidity" of the Ang. II receptor. Other interpretations of this observation would appear to be in order. BERGMANN et al. (1971) have made the puzzling observation that angiotensin made up in saline elicits a significantly greater pressor response in various animals than it does when made up in distilled water. They propose that sodium complexes with the polypeptide to produce a conformational change which makes it more active.

Electrolytes and the Mechanism of the Contractile Response to Angiotensin

Most vascular smooth muscle mounted in physiological salt solution remains completely relaxed unless the contractile process is activated by some humoral agonist. Our understanding of the contractile process of vascular smooth muscle is that this contractile process is initiated by the delivery of free calcium ions to the environment of the contractile protein (SPARROW et al., 1970). A solution to the problem of how angiotensin produces contraction of vascular smooth muscle must then answer the question as to how it produces an increase in activator calcium concentration. The concentration in the cell at any moment is the net result of processes that tend to deliver free calcium to this environment, on the one hand, and, on the other, those that tend to remove calcium from this environment. Angiotensin might increase the rate of delivery of calcium to the environment of the contractile protein by increasing membrane permeability to calcium, permitting more rapid diffusion of calcium from its high concentration outside of the cell, or by releasing calcium from bound intracellular sites. Additionally, it might accelerate an active pump that exchanges intracellular sodium for extracellular calcium. Alternatively angiotensin might bring about an increase in the net concentration of calcium in this environment by slowing down the rate of removal of calcium. It might do this either by impairing sequestration of calcium in cellular binding sites or by slowing a calcium efflux pump.

SOMLYO and SOMLYO (1971), measuring membrane potentials in various types of vascular smooth muscle, observed that the fall in membrane potential produced by angiotensin was about one-half as great as that produced by norepinephrine. This was roughly parallel to the magnitude of contraction produced by these two agonists. They speculate that the fall in membrane potential reflects an increase in membrane permeability produced by the agonist and that this change in membrane permeability might permit an increase in Ca influx. GODFRAIND (1970). on the basis of observations of the effect of angiotensin on the sodium and calcium concentrations in helical strips of guinea-pig aorta, speculates that angiotensin may activate a pump that couples the inward movement of calcium and the outward movement of sodium. VILLAMIL et al. (1970) report that chronic infusion of angiotensin results in an increase in both calcium and sodium content in the blood vessel wall. Their flux studies indicate that membrane permeability to sodium is greatly increased with an increase in intracellular sodium concentration. Studies bearing on the influence of angiotensin on sodium fluxes are difficult to interpret since it is not clear how an alteration in these fluxes might influence the concentration of activator calcium. Furthermore, the evidence with regard to the sodium flux problem is controversial. FRIEDMAN and FRIEDMAN (1965) report that angiotensin causes a net influx of sodium in vascular smooth muscle; this is in contrast to the evidence presented by TÜRKER et al. (1967) that angiotensin produces a marked increase in sodium efflux in vascular smooth muscle.

Probably the most direct evidence bearing on the action of angiotensin in controlling calcium concentration is that presented recently by BAUDOUIN et al. (1972). In studies of the calcium binding properties of membrane fragments from rabbit aorta, he noted that angiotensin in concentrations that are physiologically active caused an increase in the efflux rate of ^{45}Ca bound to the cell fragments.

Summary

The contraction of vascular smooth muscle in response to angiotensin is due primarily to direct action of the polypeptide on the vascular smooth muscle cell; the indirect neurogenic effects of angiotensin, at least in acute studies, are relatively minor. This direct contractile effect displays the phenomenon of tachyphylaxis. It appears probable in the light of current evidence that this phenomenon is due to receptor occupation by angiotensin. Receptor occupation has proven to be a valuable tool in identifying and quantifying angiotensin receptor distribution. Studies of these receptors constitute a most promising area for advance of our insight into this aspect of the problem which up to this point has been dealt with speculatively rather than with objective information.

Striking individualities in the direct constrictor action of angiotensin have been demonstrated in the various vascular beds. Similar heterogeneity is evidenced in its constrictor potency in the sequential segments of a given vascular bed.

Recently, a major approach to the understanding of the mechanism of the contractile response to angiotensin has employed studies of the effect of various interventions on the response. It is hoped that knowing the mechanism of action of the intervention, its effect on the angiotensin response will give insight into the mechanism of action of this polypeptide. Current best evidence suggests that angiotensin produces its contractile effect by causing the release of "activator calcium" from sequestered sites within the cell.

References

AIKEN, J. W., VANE, J. R.: The renin-angiotensin system: Inhibition of converting enzyme in isolated tissues. Nature (Lond.) **228**, 30 (1970).

ALTURA, B. M., ALTURA, B. T.: (1) Differential effects of substrate depletion on drug-induced contractions of rabbit aorta. Amer. J. Physiol. **219**, 1698 (1970).

ALTURA, B. M., ALTURA, B. T.: (2) Calcium content and force of drug-induced contractions of arterial muscle during recovery in vitro. Proc. Soc. exp. Biol. (N. Y.) **135**, 739 (1970).

ALTURA, B. M., ALTURA, B. T.: Influence of magnesium on drug-induced contractions and ion content in rabbit aorta. Amer. J. Physiol. **220**, 938 (1971).

ARAKAWA, K., SMEBY, B. R., BUMPUS, F. M.: Synthesis of succinyl^1-isoleucyl^5-angiotensin II and N(poly-O-acetyl-seryl)-isoleucyl^5-angiotensin II. J. Amer. chem. Soc. **84**, 1424 (1962).

AYERS, A. B., DAVIES, B. N., WITHRINGTON, P. G.: The responses of the isolated perfused spleen of man to sympathetic nerve stimulation, catecholamines, and polypeptides. Brit. J. Pharmacol. **40**, 575 P (1970).

BAUDOUIN, M., MEYER, P., WORCEL, M.: Specific binding of ^{3}H-angiotensin II in rabbit aorta. Biochem. biophys. Res. Commun. **42**, 434 (1971).
BAUDOUIN, M., MEYER, P., FERMANJIAN, S., MORGAT, J.: Calcium release induced by interaction of angiotensin with its receptors in smooth muscle cell microsomes. Nature **235**, 336 (1972).
BERGMANN, J., OEHME, P., JELÍNEK, J., CORT, J. H.: Potentiation of angiotensin and eledoisin activities by sodium chloride. Life Sci. **10**, 969 (1971).
BLAIR-WEST, J. R., HARDING, R., MCKENZIE, J. S.: Effect of sodium concentration on the vasoconstrictor action of angiotensin in the rabbit ear. Europ. J. Pharmacol. **4**, 77 (1968).
BOHR, D. F.: Adrenergic receptors in coronary arteries. In: New adrenergic blocking drugs: Their pharmacological, biochemical and clinical actions. Ann. Acad. Sci. (N. Y.) **139**, 799 (1967).
BOHR, D. F., UCHIDA, E.: Individualities of vascular smooth muscles in response to angiotensin. Circulat. Res. **20** and **21** (Suppl. II), II—135 (1967).
BRUNNER, H. R., CHANG, P., WALLACH, R., SEALEY, J. E., LARAGH, J. H.: Angiotensin II vascular receptors: Their avidity in relationship to sodium balance, the autonomic nervous system, and hypertension. J. clin. Invest. **51**, 58 (1972).
CARRIER, O., Jr., SHIBATA, S.: A possible role for tissue calcium in reserpine supersensitivity. J. Pharmacol. exp. Ther. **155**, 42 (1967).
CARRIÈRE, S., BIRON, P.: Effect of angiotensin I on intrarenal blood flow distribution. Amer. J. Physiol. **219**, 1642 (1970).
CARRIÈRE, S., FRIBORG, J.: Intrarenal blood flow and PAH extraction during angiotensin infusion. Amer. J. Physiol. **217**, 1708 (1969).
CHRYSSANTHOU, C., NELSON, E., TEICHNER, F., ANTOPOL, W.: The vasopressor effect of angiotensin in the rat and its inhibition by neotetrazolium. Fed. Proc. **30** (abstract), 450 (1971).
DAY, M. D., OWEN, D. A. A.: The effect of reserpine on the pressor responses to angiotensin in the conscious cat. Brit. J. Pharmacol. **39**, 414 (1970).
DISALVO, J., FELL, C.: Effects of angiotensin on canine renal blood flow. Proc. Soc. exp. Biol. (N. Y.) **133**, 1432 (1970).
DRIMAL, J.: Effects of angiotensin II on coronary smooth muscle. Europ. J. Pharmacol. **5**, 56 (1968).
DYER, D. C.: The pharmacology of isolated sheep umbilical cord blood vessels. J. Pharmacol. exp. Ther. **175**, 565 (1970).
FRIEDMAN, S. M., FRIEDMAN, C. L.: The emerging role of sodium and potassium in the regulation of vascular smooth muscle tension. In: Electrolytes and cardiovascular diseases, ed by E. BAJUSZ, pp 323—341. Basel: S. Karger 1965.
GELLER, R. G., KENDRICK, J. E.: Flow responses to angiotensin in innervated and denervated kidneys. Proc. Soc. exp. Biol. Med. **129**, 727 (1968).
GODFRAIND, T.: Réponse contractile de muscles lisses isolés à des stimulations répétées par l'angiotensine. Arch. int. Pharmacodyn. **176**, 464 (1968).
GODFRAIND, T.: Angiotensin auto-potentiation. Brit. J. Pharmacol. **40**, 542 (1970).
GOODFRIEND, T. L., LIN, S. Y.: Receptors for angiotensin I and II. Circulat. Res. **26** and **27** (Suppl. I), I—163 (1970).
GOUGH, E. D., DYER, D. C.: Responses of isolated human uterine arteries to vasoactive drugs. Amer. J. Obstet. Gynec. **110**, 625 (1971).
GREENWAY, C. V., STARK, R. D.: The vascular responses of the spleen to intravenous infusions of catecholamines, angiotensin and vasopressin in the anesthetized cat. Brit. J. Pharmacol. **38**, 583 (1970).
GROSS, F., KHAIRALLAH, P. A., MCGIFF, J. C.: Pharmacology of angiotensin. ed. by R. D. BUNAG. In: Renal hypertension, ed. by I. H. PAGE and J, W. MCCUBBIN, pp 134—159. Chicago: Year Book Medical Publishers, Inc. 1968.
HEDWALL, P. R., ABDEL-SAYED, W. A., SCHMIDT, P. G., ABBOUD, F. M.: Inhibition of venoconstrictor responses by prostaglandin E_1. Proc. Soc. exp. Biol. (N. Y.) **135**, 757 (1970).
HYMAN, A.: The direct effect of norepinephrine and of angiotensin on the pulmonary veins of intact dogs. J. Pharmacol. exp. Ther. **165**, 87 (1969).
JÄRHULT, J.: Comparative effects of angiotensin and noradrenaline on resistance, capacitance, and precapillary sphincter vessels in cat skeletal muscle. Acta physiol. scand. **81**, 315 (1971).
KADOWITZ, P. J., SWEET, C. S., BRODY, M. J.: Potentiation of adrenergic venomotor responses by angiotensin, prostaglandin $F_2\alpha$ and cocaine. J. Pharmacol. exp. Ther. **176**, 167 (1971).
KALSNER, S., NICKERSON, M., BOYD, G. N.: Selective blockade of potassium-induced contractions of aortic strips by β-diethyl-aminoethyl-diphenylpropylacetate (SKF 525A). J. Pharmacol. exp. Ther. **174**, 500 (1970).
KEENE, J., SEIDEL, C., BOHR, D. F.: Manganese on calcium flux and norepinephrine-induced tension in arterial smooth muscle. Proc. Soc. exp. Biol. (N. Y.) **139**, 1083 (1972).

KHAIRALLAH, P. A., DAVILA, D., PAPANICOLAOU, N., GLENDE, N. M., MEYER, P.: Effects of angiotensin infusion on catecholamine uptake and reactivity in blood vessels. Circulat. Res. 28 and 29 (Suppl. II), II—96 (1971).
KHAIRALLAH, P. A., PAGE, I. H.: Mechanism of action of angiotensin and bradykinin on smooth muscle in situ. Amer. J. Physiol. 200, 51 (1961).
KHAIRALLAH, P. A., PAGE, I. H., BUMPUS, F. M., TÜRKER, R. K.: Angiotensin tachyphylaxis and its reversal. Circulat. Res. 19, 247 (1966).
KIRAN, B. K., KHAIRALLAH, P. A.: Angiotensin and norepinephrine efflux. Europ. J. Pharmacol. 6, 102 (1969).
KORNER, P. I., STOKES, G. S., WHITE, S. W., CHALMERS, J. P.: Role of the autonomic nervous system in the renal vasoconstriction response to hemorrhage in the rabbit. Circulat. Res. 20, 676 (1967).
LIEBAU, H., DISTLER, A., WOLFF, H. P.: The noradrenalin releasing effect of angiotensin II in isolated blood vessels. Acta endocr. (Kbh.) 100 (Suppl.), 138 (1965).
LUMBERS, E. R., WHALEN, R. F.: Tachyphylaxis to angiotensin in man. Cardiovasc. Res. 4, 312 (1970).
MAZURKIEWICZ-KWILECKI, I. M.: Antagonistic effects of β-adrenergic blocking agents on responses to adrenaline in vascular smooth muscle. Arch. int. Pharmacodyn. 174, 199 (1968).
MCNEILL, J. R., STARK, R. D., GREENWAY, C. V.: Intestinal vasoconstriction after hemorrhage: roles of vasopressin and angiotensin. Amer. J. Physiol. 219, 1342 (1970).
MEYER, P., PAPADIMITRIOU, A., WORCEL, M.: Possible existence of different types of angiotensin II receptors. Brit. J. Pharmacol. 40, 541 P (1970).
NISSEN, O. I., GALSKOV, A.: Direct measurement of superficial and deep venous flow in the cat kidney. Circulat. Res. 30, 82 (1972).
PALAIC, D., LEMORVAN, P.: Angiotensin tachyphylaxis in guinea-pig aortic strips. J. Pharmacol. exp. Ther. 179, 522 (1971).
PALS, D. T., FULTON, R. W., MASUCCI, F. D.: Angiotensin, cocaine and desipramine: Comparison of effects on blood pressure responses to norepinephrine, tyramine and phenylephrine in the pithed rat. J. Pharmacol. exp. Ther. 162, 85 (1968).
PANISSET, J. C., BOURDOIS, P.: Effect of angiotensin on the response to noradrenaline and sympathetic nerve stimulation, and on ^{3}H-noradrenaline uptake in cat mesenteric blood vessels. Canad. J. Physiol. Pharmacol. 46, 125 (1968).
PEART, W. S.: The renin-angiotensin system. Pharmacol. Rev. 17, 143 (1965).
PERRY, H. M., Jr., SCHOEPFLE, E., BOURGOIGNIE, J.: In vitro production and inhibition of aortic vasoconstriction by mercuric, cadmium, and other metal ions. Proc. Soc. exp. Biol. (N. Y.) 124, 485 (1967).
POPOVIC, J., KOVILCIK, V., SMYK, L., BALSKOVA, I.: Folia. Fac. Med. Univ. Comenianae Bratislav. 6, 205 (1968).
SHEHADEH, Z., PRICE, W. E., JACOBSON, E. D.: Effects of vasoactive agents on intestinal blood flow and motility in the dog. Amer. J. Physiol. 216, 386 (1969).
SITRIN, M. D., BOHR, D. F.: Ca and Na interaction in vascular smooth muscle contraction. Amer. J. Physiol. 220, 1124 (1971).
SOMLYO, A. P., SOMLYO, A. V.: Vascular smooth muscle II. Pharmacology of normal and hypertensive vessels. Pharmacol. Rev. 22, 249 (1970).
SOMLYO, A. P., SOMLYO, A. V.: Electrophysiological correlates of the inequality of maximal vascular smooth muscle contraction elicited by drugs. Proc. Symp. Physiol. Pharmacol. Vascular Neuroeffector Systems, p. 216. Basel: S. Karger 1971.
SPARROW, M. P., MAXWELL, L. C., RUEGG, J. C., BOHR, D. F.: Preparation and properties of a calcium ion-sensitive actomyosin from arteries. Amer. J. Physiol. 219, 1366 (1970).
STOLC, S.: Vztah medzi tonusom mezenterialneho riecista a jeho citlivostou na niektore vazokonstrikcne latky u psa. (Relationship between the tonus of the canine mesenteric vascular bed and its sensitivity to some vasoconstrictor drugs.) Bratislavske lekarske listy 52, 303 (1969).
SULLIVAN, L. J., BRIGGS, A. H.: Effects of manganese on the response of aortic strips to angiotensin and norepinephrine contraction. J. Pharmacol. exp. Ther. 161, 205 (1968).
THIND, G. S., PETERSON, L. H.: Effects of autonomic nervous system blocking (ANSB) agents on angiotensin responses. J. clin. Invest. 47, 96 a (1968).
THIND, G. S., STEPHAN, K. F., BLAKEMORE, W. S.: Vascular responsiveness in cadmium-induced hypertension. Fed. Proc. 28, 329 (1969).
THIND, G. S., STEPHAN, K. F., BLAKEMORE, W. S.: Inhibition of vasopressor responses by cadmium. Amer. J. Physiol. 219, 577 (1970).
TÜRKER, R. K., PAGE, I. H., KHAIRALLAH, P. A.: Angiotensin alteration of sodium fluxes in smooth muscle. Arch. int. Pharmacodyn. 165, 394 (1967).

VAN BREEMEN, C., FARINAS, B. R., GERBA, P., MCNAUGHTON, E. D.: Excitation-contraction coupling in rabbit aorta studied by the lanthanum method for measuring cellular calcium influx. Circulat. Res. **30**, 44 (1972).
VILLAMIL, M. F., NACHEV, P., KLEEMAN, C. R.: Effect of prolonged infusion of angiotensin II on ionic composition of the arterial wall. Amer. J. Physiol. **218**, 1281 (1970).
VOTH, D., AGSTEN, M., SCHIPP, R., LÜBCKE, H.: Untersuchungen zur Wirkung von Angiotensin II auf einen autorhythmischen glatten Gefäßmuskel (Pfortader der Ratte). Arch. Kreisl.-Forsch. **65**, 41 (1971).
WALTER, P., BASSENGE, E.: Effect of angiotensin on vascular smooth muscle. Pflügers Arch. ges. Physiol. **307**, 70 (1969).
WARD, C. O., GAUTIERI, R. F.: Effect of certain drugs on perfused human placenta IX: Mode of action of angiotensin. J. Pharmac. Sci. **58**, 592 (1969).
WORCEL, M., MEYER, P., D'AURIAC, G. A., PAPANICOLAOU, N., MILLIEZ, P.: The role of angiotensin. Indirect studies with antiangiotensin plasma. Circulat. Res. **26** and **27** (Suppl. II), II—223 (1970).

Circulatory Effects of Angiotensin

Ruben D. Buñag

Studies on the cardiovascular effects of angiotensin became possible only after it was recognized that angiotensin, and not renin, was the active vasoconstrictor of the renal pressor system. This was discovered almost simultaneously in 1940 by Page and Helmer and by Braun-Menendez et al. From then on, everyone used partially purified natural products until 1957 when Bumpus, Schwyzer, and their respective co-workers made synthetic angiotensin available. Because most early studies have already been reviewed elsewhere (see Page and Bumpus, 1961; Peart, 1965; Page and McCubbin, 1968), the bulk of material presented here is limited to those reports published after 1960. However, some findings made earlier with the natural angiotensins deserve mention since they remain valid even now.

Selective arteriolar vasoconstriction produced by natural angiotensin was first described in 1942 by Abell and Page. They implanted transparent moat chambers to allow direct microscopic examination of vascular changes in the ears of unanesthetized rabbits. With moderate doses of angiotensin, only arterioles constricted while venules and capillaries were unaffected.

Cardiac effects of natural angiotensin were initially studied on perfused, isolated cat hearts by Hill and Andrus (1940); they found coronary blood flow reduced and amplitude of contraction markedly increased. Middleton and Wiggers (1944) later showed that in anesthetized dogs, cardiac output is always diminished by angiotensin because of reflex bradycardia. Similarly, in normotensive human subjects, cardiac output measured by ballistocardiography has been found consistently reduced by angiotensin (Bradley and Parker, 1941; Taylor and Page; 1943; Wilkins and Duncan, 1941).

I. Effects on the Heart

A. Myocardial Contractility

A positive inotropic effect of angiotensin has been consistently demonstrable on isolated papillary muscles from cat hearts but it is weaker than that of norepinephrine (Downing and Sonnenblick, 1963; Fowler and Holmes, 1964; Koch-Weser, 1964; Lefer, 1967). This effect has also been found in isolated atria and papillary muscles from guinea-pig hearts (Heeg and Meng, 1965). Analysis of high-speed recordings of isometric contractions led Koch-Weser (1964) to conclude that angiotensin's inotropic action is due almost entirely to an increase in rate of tension development. He later (Koch-Weser, 1965) showed that the inotropic response of isolated cat papillary muscle to angiotensin is not significantly altered by pretreatment with reserpine or β-adrenergic blocking agents. Because increase in calcium concentration inhibited responsiveness, he suggested that angiotensin increases contractility by facilitating entry of calcium ions into myocardial fibers.

Results from isolated hearts perfused following the Langendorff technique are conflicting. Positive (MEIER et al., 1958; STARKE et al., 1969) or negative (BIANCHI et al., 1960) inotropic responses have been produced in rabbit hearts by angiotensin. It has also been reported to increase (BIANCHI et al., 1960) or decrease (HEEG and MENG, 1965) the contractility of guinea-pig hearts. The discrepancy is probably due to differences not only in animal species but also in doses of angiotensin used since BIANCHI et al. (1960) found that in rabbit hearts, large doses initially inhibit and then increase force of contraction.

While positive inotropic responses to angiotensin are more reproducible in dog heart-lung preparations (ARESKOG, 1962; FOWLER and HOLMES, 1964; FARR and GRUPP, 1967), opinions differ as to the mechanisms involved. FOWLER and HOLMES (1964) observed that ventricular contractile force, measured with a strain-gage arch, is increased by angiotensin (40 μg) even in hearts from reserpine-pretreated dogs. They concluded that increased contractility is due to a direct cardiac action which does not depend on endogenous myocardial catecholamines. However, FARR and GRUPP (1967) subsequently found that inotropic stimulation in heart-lung preparations requires 60 times more angiotensin than that needed to produce the same effect in intact animals. Also, they showed that in anesthetized dogs the inotropic response to small doses of angiotensin (1 μg/kg) was markedly reduced by β-adrenergic blockade, reserpine pretreatment, or acute surgical decentralization of the heart. Prevention of the inotropic response by pronethalol has been confirmed by others (BERRY et al., 1964; KAKO et al., 1964; ROSS, 1967). More recently, FARR and GRUPP (1971) found that crushing the caudal cervical ganglia or cutting their postganglionic fibers also diminish the response. These findings all suggest that augmentation of myocardial contractility by angiotensin in intact animals is mediated indirectly via sympathetic nerves, but there are other explanations.

Inotropic responses are difficult to study in intact animals because cardiac activity *in situ* is strongly influenced by other cardiovascular changes. Many studies in man have shown that angiotensin increases left atrial and end-diastolic ventricular pressures (YU et al., 1961; ROSS and BRAUNWALD, 1964; KROVETZ et al., 1968). It has been argued (KRASNEY, 1968) that with elevation of systemic arterial pressure, heart rate is slowed reflexly and ventricular filling time, residual volume and end-diastolic pressure are all increased. These effects alone could then increase stroke volume through a Frank-Starling mechanism, even if angiotensin had no direct effects on the myocardium. To eliminate some of the variables involved, DOWNING and SONNENBLICK (1963) used cat preparations in which arterial pressure, cardiac output, and heart rate could be controlled independently. When ventricular work was kept constant, infusion of angiotensin transiently reduced coronary blood flow with concomittant myocardial depression. Negative inotropic responses have also been elicited in intact anesthetized dogs by others (KRASNEY, 1968; DRIMAL et al., 1969; FRANK et al., 1970). KRASNEY (1968) studied the effects of angiotensin on stroke volume by measuring cardiac output with electromagnetic flowmeters implanted on the base of the aorta. When arterial pressure was allowed to rise, aortic blood flow and stroke volume both increased while heart rate fell. But when the systemic pressor response was minimized by mechanical stabilization of arterial and venous pressures, stroke volume diminished, probably because of the reduction in coronary blood flow. KRASNEY (1968) therefore concluded that augmentation of stroke volume by angiotensin in intact animals is due mainly to a Frank-Starling effect secondary to the rise in systemic pressure.

B. Heart Rate

Cardio-acceleration induced by angiotensin went unnoticed in early studies because it was usually obscured by reflex bradycardia during the systemic pressor response. Studies on isolated hearts or heart-lung preparations yielded results varying from increases (BIANCHI et al., 1960), to decreases (ARESKOG, 1962; FARR and GRUPP, 1967), and to no consistent change (FOWLER and HOLMES, 1964; HEEG and MENG, 1965). In man, most investigators have found that angiotensin produces bradycardia (SEGEL et al., 1960; FINNERTY, 1962; DE BONO et al., 1963; SCROOP et al., 1965; NOLAN et al., 1967; BROD et al., 1969) that is blocked by atropine (SEGEL et al., 1960; FINNERTY, 1962; NOLAN et al., 1967).

The first clear demonstration of angiotensin-induced tachycardia was given by NISHITH et al. (1962), who used a mechanical compensator to buffer the pressor response in anesthetized dogs. When the compensator was not connected and systemic pressure was allowed to rise, angiotensin produced initial slowing of heart rate followed by acceleration. By contrast, when the compensator was used to prevent the pressor response, reflex bradycardia did not occur and the magnitude of cardio-acceleration was greater than that in unbuffered animals. Similarly, after sino-aortic denervation, the tachycardia was enhanced and was not preceded by an inhibitory phase. Because previous studies had shown that angiotensin does not accelerate isolated or denervated hearts, NISHITH et al. suggested that the chronotropic response *in vivo* is mediated via sympathetic nerves. Much evidence now supports this interpretation since the chronotropic response is abolished or markedly reduced by β-adrenergic blockade (BERRY et al., 1964; JAMES, 1965; KRASNEY et al., 1965; FARR and GRUPP, 1967; HUGHES, 1968), bretylium (KRASNEY et al., 1965; HUGHES, 1968), or reserpine (GROSS et al., 1965; FARR and GRUPP, 1967).

As angiotensin does not produce cardioacceleration by stimulating central sympathetic sites the response is unaffected by surgical sympathectomy or transection of the spinal cord (KRASNEY et al., 1965) or by pharmacologic ganglion blockade (KRASNEY et al., 1965; FARR and GRUPP, 1967; AIKEN and REIT, 1968; HUGHES, 1968). Bilateral adrenalectomy is also ineffective (KRASNEY et al., 1966; FARR and GRUPP, 1967), so that by a process of elimination it is clear that the site of action is peripheral. However, its exact localization remains uncertain.

JAMES (1965) infused angiotensin into the branch of the right coronary artery that supplies the sinus node in dogs and was unable to elicit significant cardio-acceleration. Upon finding that the chronotropic response to systemically administered angiotensin could be prevented by perfusing the sinus node with pronethalol, he surmised that the tachycardia was caused by catecholamines delivered to the heart from extracardiac sources. The results of KRASNEY et al. (1961) are in contrast to this; they showed that angiotensin causes cardio-acceleration within 1 to 2 sec after injection into the main right coronary artery. Since a similar latent period was required for injected norepinephrine, they concluded that angiotensin acts by releasing endogenous catecholamines from adrenergic nerve endings in the myocardium. This same conclusion was later reached by THOMPSON (1970) because the cardio-acceleration he produced by electrical stimulation of sympathetic nerves in isolated rabbit hearts was increased during infusion of angiotensin. On the other hand, AIKEN and REIT (1968) found no evidence for a direct effect of angiotensin on either the sino-atrial node or sympathetic nerve endings in the heart. They favor the stellate ganglion as the site of stimulation since cardio-acceleration produced in spinal cats by close intra-arterial injection of angiotensin towards the ganglion is abolished by removal of the ganglion. There may also be species differences. Recent studies by FARR and GRUPP (1971) show that in anesthetized dogs the cardiac effects of angiotensin are unaffected by destruction of the stellate ganglia but are reduced by crushing the caudal cervical ganglia or cutting their postganglionic fibers.

C. Cardiac Output

Despite angiotensin's proven ability to stimulate positive inotropic and chronotropic responses in certain experimental situations, it rarely increases cardiac output in intact animals. Variable effects have been obtained partly because of differences in animal species studied and in methods of measurement used. MANDEL and SAPIRSTEIN (1962) and GOMORI et al. (1962) used indicator-dilution techniques to measure cardiac output in anesthetized rats and found it unaffected by angiotensin. However, when thermodilution methods were later used in the same species by GROSS et al. (1965), they found it significantly reduced. BARER (1961) and ROSS and WHITE (1966) measured aortic flow with electromagnetic flowmeters in anesthetized cats, and found that angiotensin had no constant effects on cardiac output. Similarly, when measured with various techniques in anesthetized dogs, cardiac output has been reported to decrease (MCCAA et al., 1967; GILES et al., 1969), remain unaltered (CHIMOSKEY et al., 1962; KAKO et al., 1964; FRANK et al., 1970), or even increase (ROSS, 1967; KRASNEY, 1968).

Divergent results occur even when similar methods are used in the same species. Although electromagnetic flowmeters implanted on the ascending aorta were commonly used, MCCAA et al. (1967) found cardiac output decreased, while both ROSS (1967) and KRASNEY (1968) found it increased. Also, EMERSON (1966) has shown that venous return to the heart was reduced by angiotensin, which would in turn diminish cardiac output. Interpretation of these experiments is complicated because they were all made on open-chest, anesthetized dogs. In earlier studies on conscious dogs, PAGE and OLMSTED (1961) used chronically implanted electromagnetic flowmeters too but they always found cardiac output reduced by angiotensin. This observation is in keeping with those made recently by FORSYTH et al. (1971) in monkeys and also with most studies in man.

Early reports by SANCETTA (1960) and YU et al. (1961) indicated that cardiac output in man is unaffected by angiotensin but almost every investigation since then has shown that it is reduced (SEGEL et al., 1960; FINNERTY, 1962; JOHNSON and BRUCE, 1962; CHIANDUSSI et al., 1963; DE BONO et al., 1963; NOLAN et al., 1967; BROD et al., 1969). A possible explanation for this amazing uniformity is that most clinical investigators have used standard indicator-dilution techniques for measuring cardiac output. Lowering of cardiac output by angiotensin has also been found in children (KROVETZ et al., 1968) and in patients after open-heart surgery (MUELLER et al., 1970). The increase in cardiac output during exercise is also lessened by angiotensin (JOHNSON and BRUCE, 1962; SANNERSTEDT et al., 1963; SANNERSTEDT and VARNAUKASAS, 1968). Most investigators attribute reduction in cardiac output to reflex bradycardia (SEGEL et al., 1960; FINNERTY, 1962; DE BONO et al., 1963; NOLAN et al., 1967; BROD et al., 1969), but some believe it is due to reduced stroke volume (JOHNSON and BRUCE, 1962; SANNERSTEDT et al., 1963; MUELLER et al., 1970).

In summary, the positive inotropic and chronotropic effects produced by angiotensin on isolated heart preparations are probably mediated via sympathetic nerves. However, their possible contribution to the systemic pressor response in intact animals is doubtful since angiotensin has little or no effect on cardiac output. Its only prominent cardiac effect in intact animals is a reflex bradycardia that is secondary to the elevated arterial pressure.

II. Effects on Regional Blood Flow

A. Coronary Circulation

Blood flow in any organ is determined mainly by perfusion pressure and vascular resistance but the coronary vessels are unique in that their caliber is greatly influenced by mechanical compression during myocardial contraction. Consequently, coronary vascular resistance varies widely during the cardiac cycle and it is affected indirectly by changes in heart rate or blood pressure. Direct effects of angiotensin on the coronary vessels are therefore difficult to assess in intact animals because of its other effects on cardiac activity and arterial pressure. Limitations of methods used to measure flow probably also contribute to the difficulty; FORTE et al. (1960), using the nitrous oxide method in dogs, were unable to measure coronary blood flow accurately because of its great variance.

Coronary flow is most easily measured in isolated, perfused hearts and it is consistently reduced by angiotensin in hearts from guinea pigs (BIANCHI et al., 1960; HEEG and MENG, 1965), rabbits (MEIER et al., 1958; BIANCHI et al., 1960; STARKE et al., 1969), and cats (DOUGLAS et al., 1964). To keep cardiac work and its effects on coronary blood flow constant, DOWNING and SONNENBLICK (1963) used a cat right-heart bypass preparation in which heart rate, cardiac output and arterial pressure were controlled. Angiotensin had a biphasic effect on coronary blood flow, an initial transient reduction being followed by an increase. Using a similar preparation, MEIER et al. (1965) found that coronary blood flow increased during the systemic pressor response to angiotensin but decreased slightly when the pressor response was prevented. This finding has recently been confirmed by DRIMAL et al. (1969). In anesthetized, open-chest animals, coronary blood flow measured with a Shipley-Wilson rotameter (BIANCHI et al., 1960) or an electromagnetic flowmeter (BARER, 1961; ROSS, 1967) is always reduced upon injection of angiotensin into a coronary artery. The coronary response may be dose-dependent since MARCHETTI et al. (1965) showed that while flow is reduced by small doses of angiotensin, it is increased by large doses.

Determination of angiotensin's effects on coronary blood flow by means of indicator-dilution techniques indicates possible species differences in response. Many authors using tissue uptake of radioactive ^{86}Rb to indicate blood flow distribution have found coronary blood flow increased by angiotensin in anesthetized rats (GOMORI et al., 1962; MANDEL and SAPIRSTEIN, 1962; KAPITOLA et al., 1968). In contrast, when the same technique was used in dogs, LOVE et al. (1965) found that coronary blood flow was usually unaltered during the systemic pressor response to angiotensin. Absence of change in coronary flow of dogs was also observed by MAXWELL et al. (1959) using the nitrous oxide method, by DRIMAL et al. (1969) using thermodilution, and by FRANK et al. (1970) using krypton 85 as an indicator. It was reasonably assumed in all these studies that coronary vascular resistance had been increased by angiotensin since coronary flow did not change in spite of the increase in perfusion pressure. In patients after open-heart surgery MUELLER et al. (1970) recently found that both coronary blood flow (measured using ^{131}I iodoantipyrine as indicator) and calculated vascular resistance are increased by angiotensin.

B. Pulmonary Circulation

The pulmonary vessels in cats and dogs are relatively insensitive to angiotensin. Doses adequate for elevating systemic pressure in anesthetized animals increase pulmonary arterial pressure only slightly (YU et al., 1961; CHIMOSKEY et al., 1962; FOWLER and HOLMES, 1965; GILES et al., 1969) or not at all (CARLIER et al., 1958;

MAXWELL et al., 1959; BIANCHI et al., 1960; BARER, 1961). By substituting a pump for the left ventricle, ROSE et al. (1962) were able to distinguish between direct effects on pulmonary vessels and indirect effects caused by changes in left atrial or systemic arterial pressure. Since angiotensin had no direct effects they attributed the transient pulmonary hypertension to factors other than pulmonary vasoconstriction. This conclusion agrees with that of CHIMOSKEY et al. (1962) who found that both central blood volume and left atrial pressure were increased during infusion of angiotensin. A plausible interpretation is that pulmonary arterial pressure rises because systemic vasoconstriction forces blood into the pulmonary circuit.

Results in rats differ not only from those of other species but also from one report to another. Tissue clearance of radioactive Rb^{86} was first used as an indicator for blood flow distribution by MANDEL and SAPIRSTEIN (1962), and they found that angiotensin increased blood flow to the lungs while vascular resistance was essentially unaltered. GOMORI et al. (1962) used the same technique but with opposite results; flow was either reduced or unchanged but vascular resistance was increased. Still another study made later by KAPITOLA et al. (1968) using the same technique showed that following injection of large doses of angiotensin, the greatest increase in regional blood flow occurs in the lungs.

Increase in pulmonary arterial and wedge pressures by angiotensin has been a unanimous finding in man (NELSON et al., 1955; SANCETTA, 1960; YU et al., 1961; SEGEL et al., 1961; JOHNSON and BRUCE, 1962; DE BONO et al., 1963) but there is no agreement as to the mechanisms involved. YU et al. (1961) found no significant change in either central blood volume or in pressure gradient from the pulmonary artery to the left atrium. They therefore concluded that pulmonary arterial pressure increases passively because of elevation in left ventricular diastolic pressure. On the other hand, SEGEL et al. (1960) interpret the absence of change in pressure drop across the pulmonary circuit as an indication of active pulmonary vasoconstriction because pulmonary blood flow is reduced. Subsequent studies by DE BONO et al. (1963), in which pulmonary arterial and capillary pressures were measured simultaneously, showed that both pressures were increased before systemic arterial pressure, thus indicating a primary effect on the pulmonary vessels.

C. Splanchnic Circulation

Angiotensin reduces blood flow to most abdominal organs. BARER (1961) found blood flow in the main mesenteric vein of cats prominently diminished during the systemic pressor response. Decreased flow in the hepatic artery with increase in portal vein pressure was seen in dogs by SCHOLTHOLT and SHIRAISHI (1968). In isolated, perfused bovine liver preparations, angiotensin injected into either the portal vein or hepatic artery transiently increased pressure in both vessels (KELLY and NYHUS, 1966). Of the many vasoconstrictors studied by HADDY et al. (1962) in anesthetized dogs, angiotensin was the most potent in increasing resistance of the perfused superior mesenteric vascular bed. McCUBBIN et al. (1962) showed that intra-arterial injection of angiotensin into the mesenteric circulation caused constriction mainly of small arteries with slight effect on veins. KRASNEY (1968) found variable effects in intact dogs but when the systemic pressor response was minimized by means of a mechanical stabilizer, angiotensin always reduced superior mesenteric blood flow.

Some reports are contradictory. In anesthetized rats, intestinal blood flow has been found unaffected (MANDEL and SAPIRSTEIN, 1962) or reduced (GOMORI et al., 1962; KAPITOLA et al., 1968) while hepatic blood flow is either increased (GOMORI et al., 1962) or unchanged (MANDEL and SAPIRSTEIN, 1962; KAPITOLA et al., 1968).

While similar techniques of measurement were used and the authors seemed aware of each other's results, there has been no attempt to account for these conflicting results. Splenic blood flow is slightly increased by angiotensin in rats (MANDEL and SAPIRSTEIN, 1962) but decreased in cats (GREENWAY and STARK, 1970).

Recently FORSYTH et al. (1971) used the labeled-microsphere technique to measure blood-flow distribution. They found that in unanesthetized rhesus monkeys intravenously infused angiotensin reduced blood flow to liver and mesentery more than that to other abdominal organs. In man, estimations of splanchnic blood flow based on the Fick principle indicate that it is also diminished by angiotensin but the site of increased vascular resistance (mesenteric or hepatic vessels) is unknown (DE BONO et al., 1963). Infusions of angiotensin have been reported to decrease hepatic and splanchnic blood flow in normal subjects and cirrhotic patients (CHIANDUSSI et al., 1963; SEGEL et al., 1963; NOLAN et al., 1967).

D. Cerebral Circulation

Published reports on the cerebrovascular effects of angiotensin fall into two groups. At one extreme are those indicating that cerebral blood flow is increased by angiotensin, perhaps passively as a result of elevation in systemic arterial pressure. When angiotensin is injected intravenously into anesthetized cats, pial arterioles are markedly constricted (MEYER et al., 1960) but carotid blood flow is transiently increased (BARER, 1961). An interesting but unconfirmed finding is that of MANDEL and SAPIRSTEIN (1962) who observed that angiotensin increased cerebral blood flow in anesthetized rats even when only subpressor doses were infused.

On the other hand, most other reports indicate that angiotensin reduces cerebral blood flow. FUKIYAMA (1967) found that in dogs flow in the internal carotid increased during the systemic pressor response to angiotensin but that in the basilar artery was unaffected. He concluded that angiotensin increased vascular resistance in the area of the brain stem supplied by the basilar artery. In earlier studies, IKEDA et al. (1963) used photoelectric drop-counters to measure blood flow in the external and internal carotid arteries of unanesthetized rabbits. Angiotensin was presumed to constrict cerebral vessels selectively because it reduced flow in both internal and external carotids equally while norepinephrine affected only that in the external carotid. When KRASNEY (1968) used a mechanical stabilizer to prevent elevation of systemic pressure in dogs, he found that internal carotid vascular resistance was always increased and flow correspondingly lowered. In patients infused with angiotensin, GREENFIELD and TINDALL (1968) observed no significant effects on internal carotid flow but calculated vascular resistance was invariably increased. Interpretation of all these studies is complicated by the possibility that the changes observed may not be occurring solely in the cerebral vessels since the internal carotid also supplies extracranial structures. Reduction of blood flow to the brain by angiotensin has also been produced recently in conscious monkeys by FORSYTH et al. (1971).

E. Other Vascular Beds

Effects on the renal circulation are discussed elsewhere (see page 455).

Uterine blood flow was increased in pregnant dogs and sheep in the study by ASSALI and WESTERSTEN (1961) but they attributed it to the systemic pressor response to angiotensin rather than peripheral vasodilation. Subsequent studies in pregnant rabbits (BERGER and BOUCEK, 1964; CARTER and GOTHLIN, 1970) and sheep (GREISS and VAN WILKES, 1964) showed that angiotensin constricts uterine arteries and reduces blood flow.

Cutaneous vasoconstriction produced by angiotensin in man results in reduction of both temperature and blood flow in the skin (BOCK et al., 1958; PEART, 1959; IMHOFF et al., 1959; JOHNSON and BRUCE, 1962; DE BONO et al., 1963; BROD et al., 1969). A similar response in unanesthetized monkeys following infusion of angiotensin was described recently by FORSYTH et al. (1971). The slight increase in skin blood flow of anesthetized rats (GOMORI et al., 1962; MANDEL and SAPIRSTEIN, 1962) is probably secondary to increase in perfusion pressure. Intracutaneous injection of angiotensin in guinea pigs causes wheal formation (BISSET and LEWIS, 1962). A diagnostic aid for clinical hypertension based on cutaneous ischemia produced by intradermal injection of angiotensin has been proposed but has proven of no value.

Skeletal muscle blood flow is usually not measured directly. Effects of angiotensin on flow to various extremities (i.e. animal fore or hind limbs, or human digits, hands or arms) represent changes not only in skeletal muscles but also in bones and skin. Measurements made using indicator-dilution methods imply that angiotensin does not affect muscle blood flow in rats (KAPITOLA et al., 1968) or monkeys (FORSYTH et al., 1971). In man, BROD et al. (1969) calculated muscle blood flow from differences between total forearm and skin blood flow. They found muscle blood flow increased and vascular resistance reduced by angiotensin; this, together with marked renal vasoconstriction presumably causes redistribution of cardiac output, which is shifted from the kidneys to the muscles.

In summary, most vascular beds are constricted by angiotensin when it is injected intra-arterially or studied on isolated, perfused tissues. When angiotensin is administered intravenously in intact animals, it has two opposite effects on regional blood flow and the end-result depends on which one predominates. Elevation of perfusion pressure during the systemic pressor response tends to increase blood flow while local vasoconstriction tends to reduce it. Blood flow is markedly reduced in the splanchnic area, liver and skin because of predominant vasoconstriction. On the other hand, it may be increased passively in the skeletal muscles, brain, heart and uterus because of elevated perfusion pressure. The overall effect is an increase in total peripheral resistance which is primarily responsible for the elevation in systemic arterial pressure.

III. Effects on Systemic Circulation

A. Venous System

It is well established that angiotensin affects veins much less than arteries. FOLKOW et al. (1961) initially showed that venous or capacitance vessels in cats are constricted more strongly by norepinephrine than by angiotensin. On the other hand, precapillary or resistance vessels are more responsive to angiotensin than to norepinephrine. These differences were attributed to variations in receptor distribution, receptors for norepinephrine being present on both arterial and venous sides of the circulation while those for angiotensin are predominantly found only on the arterial side. Similar evidence attesting to angiotensin's weak venoconstrictor activity has since been obtained in dogs (GROSS and BOCK, 1962; HADDY et al., 1962; ROSE et al., 1962) and in man [MCQUEEN and MORRISON, 1961; DE PASQUALE and BURCH, 1963 (2); DOLLERY et al., 1963; SCROOP et al., 1965]. In sharp contrast are the results of EMERSON et al. (1965) who found that in all species they examined, on an equimolar basis angiotensin was a more potent small vein constrictor than norepinephrine.

Venous segments studied *in situ* are generally insensitive to angiotensin. While occluded segments of canine mesenteric or femoral veins constrict upon topical application of norepinephrine, they do not respond to angiotensin (Rose et al., 1962). To localize venous effects of angiotensin in man, De Pasquale and Burch [1963 (2)] studied isolated venous segments on the forearms of normal subjects. Direct injection of angiotensin into the venous segments was ineffective but intravenous injection caused a significant increase in segmental venous pressure. Since this venoconstriction was prevented by regional nerve block, they concluded that though angiotensin has no direct effect on forearm veins, it can influence venous tone through reflex neural mechanisms.

Central venous pressure invariably increases during the systemic pressor response to angiotensin [Gross and Bock, 1962; De Pasquale and Burch, 1963 (1); Scroop et al., 1965; Emerson, 1966]. Gross and Bock (1962) estimated in unanesthetized dogs that the potency ratio on a weight basis of angiotensin to norepinephrine is 10:1 for arterial pressure and 5:1 for venous pressure. They suggested that angiotensin's effect on venous pressure is of reflex origin, because it is reduced by atropine or thiopental anesthesia. In man, for any given elevation in systemic arterial pressure, norepinephrine produces a greater increase in central venous pressure than angiotensin (Scroop et al., 1965).

B. Arterial Pressure

Partly because elevation of systemic arterial pressure is the best known of its many diverse effects, angiotensin is generally acclaimed as the most potent pressor substance now available. De Bono et al. (1963) estimated that angiotensin was 6 to 8 times stronger on a weight basis and 40 to 50 times stronger on a molecular basis than norepinephrine when infused intravenously into normal human subjects. In all animal species including man, the characteristic response to a single intravenous injection is a sharp rise in arterial pressure which begins within 20 to 30 sec and reaches a peak in 1 to 2 min. Pressure then returns to its initial level in 3 to 5 min. Magnitude and duration of pressor responses are usually dose-dependent. Responses to small doses are fairly reproducible but large doses frequently cause tachyphylaxis.

Route of administration has a marked effect on response to angiotensin. When it is given by subcutaneous or intramuscular injection, doses 5 to 100 times larger than those used intravenously are required to elicit a pressor response (Gross and Turrian, 1960; Bock, 1966). Many have observed that intra-arterial infusion into liver (Chamberlain et al., 1964; Methot et al., 1964; Kokubu et al., 1967) or kidneys (Akinkugbe et al., 1966) causes a much smaller increase in systemic blood pressure than the same dose infused intravenously. Similarly, Scroop et al. (1965) found that in normal human subjects, intra-arterial infusions of angiotensin were only half as effective as those of norepinephrine in constricting hand vessels. By contrast, when infused intravenously, angiotensin had 8 times more constrictor effect than norepinephrine. The usual explanation for these findings is inactivation of angiotensin by various capillary beds but another possibility has recently been proposed.

Haas and his associates (1968) compared intra-arterial with intravenous infusions in unanesthetized dogs and they found pressor responses to angiotensin and norepinephrine reduced when these were infused into a femoral artery. Addition of a co-factor prepared from bovine or human serum restored response to angiotensin but did not affect that to norepinephrine. They later (1969) showed that this phenomenon is demonstrable only in conscious dogs because in dogs anesthetized with pentobarbital, angiotensin is equally effective when injected either intra-arterially or intravenously. HAAS et al. therefore postulated that loss of pressor activity during intra-arterial infusion in unanesthetized dogs is due to retention of angiotensin by its attachment to specific receptors in the femoral vascular bed. The co-factor, when present, then prevents loss of pressor activity by interfering with the interaction between angiotensin and its receptors.

Systemic arterial pressure can be kept elevated for hours or even days by intravenous infusion of angiotensin and when infusion is discontinued, pressure rapidly returns to, or falls below, the preinfusion level (PAGE and OLMSTED, 1961; BROWN et al., 1964). The type of response obtained is mainly determined by the dose of angiotensin infused. With very large doses, there is an initially prominent increase in arterial pressure but this then falls back to the preinfusion level despite continued infusion (BOCK and GROSS, 1961; BROWN et al., 1964; OLMSTED and PAGE, 1965). Inability to sustain pressure elevation with infusion of large doses is probably due to development of tachyphylaxis. An entirely different pressor response elicited during infusion of initially subpressor amounts of angiotensin was first described by McCUBBIN et al. (1965) and later confirmed by others (KEZDI and NOMURA, 1968; FORSYTH et al., 1971). In contrast to the direct cardiovascular effect of large doses, this response has been ascribed to stimulation of the sympathetic nervous system by angiotensin (see page 418).

In summary, the prominent systemic pressor response produced by angiotensin in intact animals is caused by constriction of resistance or precapillary vessels, while the veins or capacitance vessels, being relatively insensitive, remain unaltered. Dose and route of administration of angiotensin determine both the magnitude and the characteristics of the pressor response. Intra-arterial administration usually produces smaller responses than those elicited intravenously. With infusion of large doses, elevation of arterial pressure is not sustained because tachyphylaxis develops. Continuous infusion of doses that are initially subpressor results in hypertension mediated via stimulation of the sympathetic nervous system.

References

ABELL, R. G., PAGE, I. H.: The reaction of peripheral blood vessels to angiotonin, renin, and other pressor agents. J. exp. Med. **75**, 305 (1942).

AIKEN, J. W., REIT, E.: Stimulation of the cat stellate ganglion by angiotensin. J. Pharmacol. exp. Ther. **159**, 107 (1968).

AKINKUGBE, O. O., BROWN, W. C. B., CRANSTON, W. I.: Pressor effects of angiotensin infusions into different vascular beds in the rabbit. Clin. Sci. **30**, 409 (1966).

ARESKOG, N. H.: The effect of catecholamines, corticosteroids and angiotensin II on the heart-lung preparation of the dog. Acta Soc. Med. upsalien. **67**, 164 (1962).

ASSALI, N. S., WESTERSTEN, A.: Regional flow-pressure relationship in response to angiotensin in the intact dog and sheep. Circulat. Res. **9**, 189 (1961).

BARER, G. R.: A comparison of the circulatory effects of angiotensin, vasopressin and adrenaline in the anesthetized cat. J. Physiol. **156**, 49 (1961).

BERGER, M., BOUCEK, R. J.: Irreversible uterine and renal changes induced by placental ischemia (rabbit). Amer. J. Obstet. Gynec. **89**, 230 (1964).

BERRY, W. B., AUSTEN, W. G., CLARK, W. D.: Studies on the relative cardiac and peripheral actions of angiotensin. Ann. Surg. **159**, 520 (1964).

BIANCHI, A., DE SCHAEPDRYVER, A. F., DE VLEESCHHOUWER, G. R., PREZIOSI, P.: On the pharmacology of synthetic hypertensine. Arch. int. Pharmacodyn. **124**, 21 (1960).

BISSET, G. W., LEWIS, G. P.: A spectrum of pharmacological activity in some biologically active peptides. Brit. J. Pharmacol. **19**, 168 (1962).

BOCK, K. D.: Angiotensin, Pharmacologie und klinische Anwendung. Heidelberg: Hüthig 1966.

BOCK, K. D., GROSS, F.: Renin and angiotensin tachyphylaxis. Circulat. Res. **9**, 1044 (1961).

BOCK, K. D., KRECKE, H. J., KUHN, H. M.: Untersuchungen über die Wirkung von synthetischem Hypertensin II auf Blutdruck, Atmung und Extremitätendurchblutung des Menschen. Klin. Wschr. **36**, 254 (1958).

BRADLEY, S. E., PARKER, B.: Hemodynamic effect of angiotonin in normal man. J. clin. Invest. **20**, 715 (1941).

BRAUN-MENENDEZ, E., FASCIOLO, J. C., LELOIR, L. F., MUNOZ, J. M.: The substance causing renal hypertension. J. Physiol. **98**, 283 (1940).

BROD, J., HEJL, Z., HORNYCH, A., JIRKA, J., SLECHTA, V., BURIANOVA, B.: Comparison of haemodynamic effects on equipressor doses of intravenous angiotensin and noradrenaline in man. Clin. Sci. **36**, 161 (1969).

BUMPUS, F. M., SCHWARZ, H., PAGE, I. H.: Synthesis and pharmacology of the octapeptide angiotonin. Science **125**, 3253 (1957).

CARLIER, J., LEJEUNE-LEDANT, G., BARAC, G.: Angiotensine, 5-hydroxytryptamine et circulation pulmonaire chez le chien. C. R. Soc. Biol. (Paris) **152**, 1034 (1958).

CARTER, A. M., GOTHLIN, J.: Effects of angiotensin, oxytocin and vasopressin on placental circulation. Invest. Radiol. **5**, 86 (1970).

CHAMBERLAIN, M. J., BROUSE, N. L., GIBSON, D. G., GLEESON, J. A.: Angiotensin and renoportal anastomosis. Brit. Med. J. **1964 II**, 1507.

CHIANDUSSI, L., VACCARINO, A., GRECO, F., MURATORI, F., CESANO, L., INDOVINA, D.: Effect of drug infusion on the splanchnic circulation. I. Angiotensin infusion in normal and cirrhotic subjects. Proc. Soc. exp. Biol. **112**, 324 (1963).

CHIMOSKEY, J. E., BLAQUIER, P. C., TAQUINI, A. C., Jr., BOHR, D. F.: Effects of angiotensin on pulmonary and systemic hemodynamics. Amer. J. Physiol. **202**, 690 (1962).

DE BONO, E., LEE, G. DE J., MOTTRAM, F. R., PICKERING, G. W.: The action of angiotensin in man. Clin. Sci. **25**, 123 (1963).

DE PASQUALE, N. P., BURCH, G. E.: (1) Angiotensin II, digital blood flow, and the precapillary and postcapillary blood vessels of man. Ann. intern. Med. **58**, 278 (1963).

DE PASQUALE, N. P., BURCH, G. E.: (2) Effect of angiotensin II on the intact forearm veins of man. Circulat. Res. **13**, 239 (1963).

DOLLERY, C. T., HILL, D. W., HODGE, J. V.: The response of normal retinal blood vessels to angiotensin and noradrenaline. J. Physiol. **165**, 500 (1963).

DOUGLAS, C. R., PONCR-ZUMINE, A., RUIZ-PETRICH, E., PUIG, F., TALESNIK, J.: Effect of angiotensin upon coronary flow and oxygen consumption of the isolated heart of the cat. Acta physiol. lat.-amer. **14**, 161 (1964).

DOWNING, S. E., SONNENBLICK, E. H.: Effects of continuous administration of angiotensin II on ventricular performance. J. appl. Physiol. **18**, 585 (1963).

DRIMAL, J., PAVEK, K., SELECKY, F. V.: Primary and secondary effects of angiotensin on the coronary circulation. Cardiologia (Basel) **54**, 1 (1969).

EMERSON, T. E., Jr.: Effects of angiotensin, epinephrine, norepinephrine, and vasopressin on venous return. Amer. J. Physiol. **210**, 933 (1966).

EMERSON, T. E., Jr., HINSHAW, L. B., BRAKE, C. M.: Vascular effects of angiotensin and norepinephrine in the dog, cat, and monkey. Amer. J. Physiol. **208**, 260 (1965).

FARR, W. C., GRUPP, G.: Sympathetically mediated effects of angiotensin on the dog heart in situ. J. Pharmacol. exp. Ther. **156**, 528 (1967).

FARR, W. C., GRUPP, G.: Ganglionic stimulation. Mechanism of the positive inotropic and chronotropic effects of angiotensin. J. Pharmacol. exp. Ther. **177**, 48 (1971).

FINNERTY, F. A., Jr.: Hemodynamics of angiotensin in man. Circulation **25**, 255 (1962).

FOLKOW, B., JOHANSON, B., MELLANDER, S.: The comparative effects of angiotensin and noradrenalin on consecutive vascular sections. Acta physiol. scand. **53**, 99 (1961).

FORSYTH, R. P., HOFFBRAND, B. I., MELMON, K. L.: Hemodynamic effects of angiotensin in normal and environmentally stressed monkeys. Circulation **44**, 119 (1971).

FORTE, I. E., POTFIETER, L., SCHMITTHENNER, J. E.: Effects of hypertensin on arterial pressure, heart work, and cardiac oxygen utilization. Circulat. Res. **8**, 1235 (1960).

FOWLER, N. O., HOLMES, J. C.: Coronary and myocardial actions of angiotensin. Circulat. Res. **14**, 191 (1964).

FOWLER, N. O., HOLMES, J. C.: Pulmonary pressor action of 1-norepinephrine and angiotensin. Amer. Heart J. **70**, 66 (1965).

FRANK, M. J., NADIMI, M., CASANEGRA, P., STEIN, P., PEKAAR, R.: Effect of angiotensin on myocardial function. Amer. J. Physiol. **218**, 1267 (1970).

FUKIYAMA, K.: An experimental study on basilar artery flow in anesthetized dogs. Fukuoka Acta med. **58**, 345 (1967).

GILES, T. D., SHEN, Y., DHURANDHAR, R. W., BURCH, G. E., QUIROZ, A. C.: Influence of angiotensin II on the systemic and pulmonary circulations of intact anesthetized dogs. Proc. Soc. exp. Biol. Med. (N. Y.) **132**, 845 (1969).

GOMORI, P., TAKACS, L., KALLAY, K.: The effect of synthetic angiotensin II on the redistribution and shifting of blood. Arch. int. Pharmacodyn. **138**, 254 (1962).
GREENFIELD, J. C., Jr., TINDALL, G. T.: Effect of norepinephrine, epinephrine, and angiotensin on blood flow in the internal carotid artery of man. J. clin. Invest. **47**, 1672 (1968).
GREENWAY, C. V., STARK, R. D.: The vascular responses of the spleen to intravenous infusions of catecholamines, angiotensin and vasopressin in the anesthetized cat. Brit. J. Pharmacol. **38**, 583 (1970).
GREISS, F. C., VAN WILKES, D.: Effects of sympathomimetic drugs and angiotensin on the uterine vascular bed. Obstet. gynec. Surg. **23**, 925 (1964).
GROSS, F., BOCK, K. D.: Some contributions to the pharmacology of synthetic angiotensin. Circulation **25**, 193 (1962).
GROSS, F., TURRIAN, H.: Pharmacology of hypertensin and synthetic analogues. In: Polypeptides which affect smooth muscles and blood vessels (SCHACHTER, M., Ed.). Oxford: Pergamon Press 1960.
GROSS, M., MONTAGUE, D., ROSAS, R., BOHR, D. F.: Cardiac action of vasoactive polypeptides in the rat. I. Angiotensin. Circulat. Res. **16**, 151 (1965).
HAAS, E., GOLDBLATT, H., LEWIS, L., GIPSON, E. C.: Inhibition of angiotensin and its protection by a co-factor in blood. Amer. J. Physiol. **215**, 1420 (1968).
HAAS, E., GOLDBLATT, H., LEWIS, L., GIPSON, E. C.: Angiotensin-protective cofactor. Amer. J. Physiol. **217**, 981 (1969).
HADDY, F. J., MOLNAR, J. I., BORDEN, C. W., TEXTER, E. C., Jr.: Comparison of direct effects of angiotensin and other vasoactive agents on small and large blood vessels in several vascular beds. Circulation **25**, 239 (1962).
HEEG, E., MENG, K.: Die Wirkung des Bradykinins, Angiotensins und Vasopressins auf Vorhof, Papillarmuskel und isoliert durchströmte Herzpräparate des Meerschweinchens. Naunyn-Schmiedebergs Arch. Pharmak. exp. Path. **250**, 35 (1965).
HILL, W. H. P., ANDRUS, E. C.: Effects of renin and angiotonin upon isolated perfused heart. Proc. Soc. exp. Biol. (N. Y.) **44**, 213 (1940).
HUGHES, I. E.: Chronotropic and pressor responses to angiotensin in rats anesthetized with urethane. Europ. J. Pharmacol. **3**, 189 (1968).
IKEDA, M., FUJII, J., MURATA, K., TERASAWA, F., OZAWA, T., HOSODA, S., KURIHARA, H., KIMATA, S., OKINAKA, S.: Effect of angiotensin on cerebral circulation in unanesthetized rabbit. Jap. Circulat. J. (En.) **27**, 277 (1963).
IMHOFF, P., HURLIMANN, A., STEINMANN, B.: Periphere Kreislaufuntersuchungen mit synthetischen Hypertensin II. Cardiologia **3**, 120 (1959).
JAMES, T. N.: Absence of direct chronotropic action of angiotensin infused into the sinus node artery. Amer. J. Physiol. **209**, 571 (1965).
JOHNSON, W. P., BRUCE, R. A.: Hemodynamic and metabolic effects of angiotensin II during rest and exercise in normal healthy subjects. Amer. Heart J. **63**, 212 (1962).
KAKO, K., KRAYENBUHL, H. P., LUTHY, E., HEGGLIN, R.: Hemodynamic effects of angiotensin in intact dogs. Amer. J. Cardiol. **14**, 362 (1964).
KAPITOLA, J., KUCHEL, O., SCHREIBEROVA, O., JAHODA, I.: Blood flow through organs of the rat after an intravenous injection of angiotensin. Physiol. bohemoslov. **17**, 437 (1968).
KELLY, K. A., NYHUS, L. M.: Angiotensin and the liver. Amer. J. Physiol. **210**, 305 (1966).
KEZDI, P., NOMURA, G.: Potentiation of sympathetic output by chronic angiotensin infusion and the effect of altered carotid sinus mechanism. Hypertension **16**, 39 (1968).
KOCH-WESER, J.: Myocardial actions of angiotensin. Circulat. Res. **14**, 337 (1964).
KOCH-WESER, J.: Nature of the inotropic action of angiotensin on ventricular myocardium. Circulat. Res. **16**, 230 (1965).
KOKUBU, T., FUJIMOTO, S., HIWADA, K., AKUTSU, H., KATO, A., YAMAMURA, Y.: Inactivation of angiotensin II in liver. Jap. Circulat. J. (En.) **31**, 879 (1967).
KRASNEY, J. A.: Effects of angiotensin on stroke volume and regional blood flow and resistance. Amer. J. Physiol. **215**, 1454 (1968).
KRASNEY, J A., THOMPSON, J. L., LOWE, R. F.: Cardiac effects of angiotensin injections into perfused right coronary artery. Amer. J. Physiol. **213**, 134 (1967).
KRASNEY, J. A., PAUDLER, F. T., HOGAN, P. M., LOWE, R. F., YOUMANS, W. B.: Peripheral adrenergic basis for cardioaccelerator action of angiotensin. Amer. J. Physiol. **211**, 1447 (1966).
KRASNEY, J. A., PAUDLER, F. T., SMITH, D. C., DAVIS, L. D., YOUMANS, W. B.: Mechanisms of carioaccelerator action of angiotensin. Amer. J. Physiol. **209**, 539 (1965).
KROVETZ, L. J., MCLOUGHLIN, T. G., SCHIEBLER, G. L.: Left ventricular function in children studied by increasing peripheral resistance with angiotensin. Circulation **37**, 729 (1968).
LEFER, A. M.: Influence of mineralocorticoids and cations on the inotropic effect of angiotensin and norepinephrine in isolated cardiac muscle. Amer. Heart J. **73**, 674 (1967).

LOVE, W. D., MONFORD, R. S., ABRAHAM, R. E.: Comparison of the effects of l-norepinephrine angiotensin, dipyridamole, digitoxin, and reserpine on the regional distribution of coronary blood flow. J. Lab. clin. Med. **66**, 423 (1965).
MANDEL, M. J., SAPIRSTEIN, L. A.: Effect of angiotensin infusion on regional blood flow and regional vascular resistance in the rat. Circulat. Res. **10**, 807 (1962).
MARCHETTI, G. V., MERLO, L., NOSEDA, V.: Effects of angiotensin on coronary circulation. Arzneimittel-Forsch. **10**, 1244 (1965).
MAXWELL, G. M., CASTILLO, C. A., CRUMPTON, C. W., CLIFFORD, J. E., ROWE, G. G.: The effect of synthetic angiotensin upon the heart of the intact dog. J. Lab. clin. Med. **54**, 876 (1959).
MCCAA, R. E., RICHARDSON, T. Q., LANGFORD, H. G., DOUGLAS, B. H.: Circulatory changes following angiotensin administration. Amer. J. Physiol. **212**, 565 (1967)
MCCUBBIN, J. W., DE MOURA, R. S., PAGE, I. H., OLMSTED, F.: Arterial hypertension elicited by subpressor amounts of angiotensin. Science **149**, 1394 (1965).
MCCUBBIN, J. W., KANEKO, Y., PAGE, I. H.: Inhibition of neurogenic vasoconstriction by serotonin. Circulat. Res. **11**, 74 (1962).
MCQUEEN, E. G., MORRISON, R. B. I.: The effects of synthetic angiotensin and noradrenaline on blood pressure and renal function. Brit. Heart J. **23**, 1 (1961).
MEIER, M., WIRZ, E., BRUNNER, H., STAMM, W.: Effects of norepinephrine and angiotensin II amide on coronary flow and myocardial oxygen consumption in the cat. Cardiologia **47**, 127 (1965).
MEIER, R., TRIPOD, J., STUDER, A.: Comparison des proprietes vasculaires peripheriques de l'hypertensin synthetique et de divers vasoconstricteurs. Arch. int. Pharmacodyn. **117**, 185 (1958).
METHOT, A. L., MEYER, P., BIRON, B., LORAINE, M. F., LAGRUE, G., MILLIEZ, P.: Hepatic inactivation of angiotensin. Nature (Lond.) **203**, 531 (1964).
MEYER, J. S., WALTZ, A. G., GOTOH, F.: Pathogenesis of cerebral vasospasm in hypertensin encephalopathy. Neurology (Minneap.) **10**, 735 (1960).
MIDDLETON, S., WIGGERS, C. J.: The effects of renin and angiotonin on cardiac output and total peripheral resistance. Amer. J. Physiol. **141**, 128 (1944).
MUELLER, H. S., GREGORY, J. J., GIANNELLI, S., Jr., AYRES, S. M.: Systemic hemodynamic and myocardial metabolic effects of isoproterenol and angiotensin after open-heart surgery. Circulation **42**, 491 (1970).
NELSON, R. A., MAY, L. G., BENNETT, A., KOBAYASHI, M., GREGORY, R.: Comparison of the effects of pressor and depressor agents and influences on pulmonary and systemic pressures on normotensive and hypertensive subjects. Amer. Heart J. **50**, 172 (1955).
NISHITH, S. D., DAVIS, L. D., YOUMANS, W. B.: Cardioaccelerator action of angiotensin. Amer. J. Physiol. **202**, 237 (1962).
NOLAN, J. P., COBB, L. A., THOMPSON, J. I.: Circulatory responses to angiotensin in man. Clin. Pharmacol. Ther. 8, 235 (1967).
OLMSTED, F., PAGE, I. H.: Hemodynamic aspects of prolonged infusion of angiotensin into unanesthetized dogs. Circulat. Res. **16**, 140 (1965).
PAGE, I. H., BUMPUS, F. M.: Angiotensin. Physiol. Rev. **41**, 331 (1961).
PAGE, I. H., HELMER, O. M.: A crystalline pressor substance (angiotonin) resulting from the reaction between renin and renin-activator. J. exp. Med. **71**, 29 (1940).
PEART, W. S.: Hypertension and the kidney. II. Experimental basis of renal hypertension. Brit. Med. J. **1959 II**, 1421.
PEART, W. S.: The renin-angiotensin system. Pharmacol. Rev. **17**, 143 (1965).
ROSE, J. C., KOT, P. A., COHN, J. N., FRRIS, E. D., ECKERT, G. E.: Comparison of effects of angiotensin and norepinephrine on pulmonary circulation, systemic arteries and veins, and systemic vascular capacity in the dog. Circulation **25**, 247 (1962).
ROSS, J., Jr., BRAUNWALD, E.: The study of left ventricular function in man by increasing resistance to ventricular ejection with angiotensin. Circulation **29**, 739 (1964).
ROSS, G.: Effects of angiotensin on the heart and coronary circulation of the dog before and after beta-adrenergic blockade. Cardiovasc. Res. **1**, 255 (1967).
ROSS, G., WHITE, F. N.: Role of catecholamine release in cardiovascular responses to angiotensin. Amer. J. Physiol. **211**, 1419 (1966).
SANCETTA, S. M.: General and pulmonary hemodynamic effects of pure decapeptide angiotensin in normotensive man. Circulat. Res. **8**, 616 (1960).
SANNERSTEDT, R., BOJS, G., VARNAUSKAS, E.: Hemodynamic effect of angiotensin II in minute amounts: observations on normal subjects at rest and during exercise. Scand. J. clin. Lab. Invest. **15**, 159 (1963).
SANNERSTEDT, R., VARNAUSKAS, E.: Influence of angiotensin on the hemodynamic response to exercise in normotensive subjects. Circulation **38**, 1097 (1968).

SCHOLTHOLT, J., SHIRAISHI, T.: Die Wirkung von Acetylcholin, Bradykinin und Angiotensin auf die Durchblutung der Leber des narkotisierten Hundes und auf den endstandigen Druck im Ductus Choledochus. Pflügers Arch. ges. Physiol. **300**, 189 (1968).

SCHWYZER, R., ISELIN, B., KAPPELER, H., RINIKER, B., RITTAL, W., ZUBER, H.: Synthese von Hypertensin-Peptiden. Chemie **11**, 335 (1957).

SCROOP, G. C., WALSH, J. A., WHELAN, R. F.: A comparison of the effects of intra-arterial and intravenous infusions of angiotensin and noradrenaline on the circulation in man. Clin. Sci. **29**, 315 (1965).

SEGEL, N., BAYLEY, T. J., PATON, A., DYKES, P. W., BISHOP, J. M.: The effects of synthetic vasopressin and angiotensin on the circulation in cirrhosis of the liver. Clin. Sci. **25**, 43 (1963).

SEGEL, N., HARRIS, P., BISHOP, J. M.: The effects of synthetic hypertensin on the systemic and pulmonary circulations in man. Clin. Sci. **20**, 49 (1960).

STARKE, K., WERNER, U., SCHUMANN, H. J.: Wirkung von Angiotensin auf Funktion und Noradrenalinabgabe isolierter Kaninchenherzen in Ruhe und bei Sympathicusreizung. Naunyn-Schmiedebergs Arch. Pharmak. exp. Path. **265**, 1970 (1969).

TAYLOR, R. D., PAGE, I. H.: The effect of antipressor kidney extract, angiotonin, methylguanidine and tyramine on cardiac output as measured by the ballistocardiograph in hypertensive and normal persons. Amer. J. med. Sci. **205**, 66 (1943).

WILKINS, R. W., DUNCAN, C. N.: The nature of arterial hypertension produced in normal subjects by the administration of angiotonin. J. clin. Invest. **20**, 721 (1941).

YU, P. N., LURIA, M. N., FINLAYSON, J. K., STANFIELD, C. A., CONSTANTINE, H., FLATLEY, F. J.: The effects of angiotensin on pulmonary circulation and ventricular function. Circulation **24**, 1326 (1961).

Effects of Angiotensin on the Renal Circulation

LUIS G. NAVAR and HERBERT G. LANGFORD

With 2 Figures

I. General Effects of Angiotensin on Renal Hemodynamics

The intravenous injection or infusion of renin or angiotensin produces a marked decrease in renal blood flow, a lesser decrease in glomerular filtration, and, therefore, an increase in filtration fraction (CORCORAN and PAGE, 1939, 1940, 1941; HERRICK et al., 1942; HUGHES-JONES et al., 1949; WHITNEY et al., 1954). When the effects of bolus injections of renin and angiotensin were compared, it was found that renin in doses sufficient to cause a pressor response of approximately 60 mmHg decreased renal blood flow within 30 sec to 1 min, with the maximum effect occurring at about 2 min. This period of maximum vasoconstriction was short, and within 3 to 5 min renal blood flow returned to about one-half the control value and was maintained there for several minutes. The effects of angiotensin were more immediate and transient with the renal blood flow immediately decreasing to its minimum in less than 1 min and returning to the control value within 2 to 3 min (HERRICK et al., 1941, 1942).

The effects of renin and angiotensin on urine flow and sodium-excretion rate are dose dependent; both an antidiuretic and antinatriuretic effect and a diuretic and natriuretic effect have been reported (CROXATTO et al., 1952; MASSON et al., 1950, 1953; MERRILL et al., 1938; PICKERING and PRINZMETAL, 1940; SELLERS et al., 1951).

II. Effects of Small Doses on Renal Blood Flow, Glomerular Filtration Rate and Urine Flow

1. Effects of Intravenous Infusions

The renal response to low doses (1 to 50 ng/kg/min) of angiotensin has been consistent although there is some species variation. A moderate to marked decrease in renal blood flow, a lesser decrease in glomerular filtration rate, and a decrease in urine flow and sodium excretion occur when the blood pressure to the kidney is controlled or where the pressor response is not marked.

These findings were observed in man at 1 to 5 ng/kg/min, a dose which produced minimal pressor responses (AURELL, 1969; BARBOUR et al., 1965; TORRES et al., 1970); 20 to 40 ng/kg/min elicited pressor responses of 20 to 40 mmHg (AGNOLI et al., 1970; BIRON et al., 1962; DE BONO et al., 1962; FINNERTY et al., 1961; GILL et al., 1964; LOUIS and DOYLE, 1965), and doses of 100 ng/kg/min caused increases of 30 to 50 mmHg in arterial pressure (BOCK and KRECKE, 1958). The decrease in renal blood flow, glomerular filtration rate, urine flow, and sodium excretion were proportional to the log of the dose (BOCK et al., 1958). Fig. 1 shows the percentage decreases in renal blood flow or renal plasma flow, glomerular filtration rate, and urine flow plotted as a function of the dose of angiotensin infused. The points indicating the responses of the human subjects are shown as (X) and generally show relatively high sensitivity to the angiotensin. At these doses, sodium-excretion rates essentially parallel the fluid excretion rates (BOCK et al., 1958).

The effect of intravenous infusion in dogs is also plotted on Fig. 1. There have been several studies and the range of doses used is wide (AUKLAND, 1968; FOURCADE, 1972, personal communication, unpublished results; HEALY et al., 1965; LAMEIJER et al., 1966; LOUIS and DOYLE, 1965; MCGIFF et al., 1969; SCHMID, 1968). The vascular reactivity to the same dose of angiotensin appears to be lower in dogs than in man (Fig. 1). While the effects of the low doses have

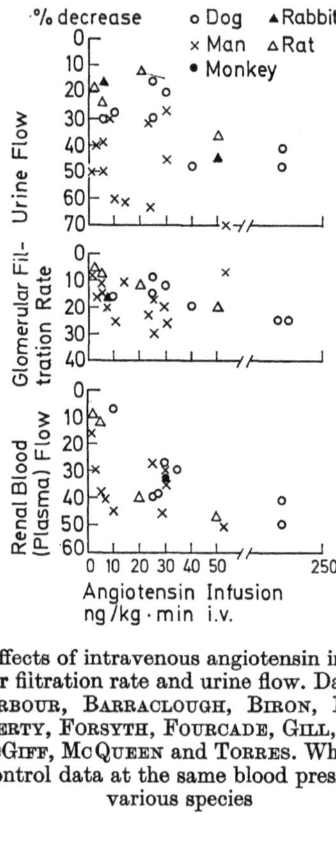

Fig. 1. Composite graph of effects of intravenous angiotensin infusions on renal blood flow or renal plasma flow, glomerular filtration rate and urine flow. Data were obtained from studies of AUKLAND, AURELL, BARBOUR, BARRACLOUGH, BIRON, BOCK, BONJOUR, COLLIGNON, DE BONO, DEL GRECO, FINNERTY, FORSYTH, FOURCADE, GILL, HEALY, ITSKOVITZ, LAMEIJER LARAGH, LOUIS, MALVIN, MCGIFF, MCQUEEN and TORRES. Where possible, the experimental, data was compared to the control data at the same blood pressure. The symbols indicate the various species

been studied most extensively in these two species, other investigations have indicated that comparable doses result in the same qualitative responses in rabbits (BARRACLOUGH, 1965), rats [BARRACLOUGH et al., 1967 (3); BONJOUR and MALVIN, 1969 (2); MALVIN and VANDER, 1967], and monkeys (FORSYTH et al., 1971).

Water diuresis has little effect on the response to angiotensin infusions at these low doses (BARBOUR et al., 1962; DEL GRECO, 1962; GILL et al., 1964). This survey supports the suggestion of BARRACLOUGH (1965) that equivalent doses of angiotensin cause essentially the same responses in the various species studied. It also demonstrates the relatively large variation in the urine-flow responses. On the other hand, the changes in glomerular filtration rate appear fairly uniform and are less dramatic than the changes in renal blood flow. Thus the filtration fraction increases substantially.

The decreased urine flow in response to low doses of angiotensin could be entirely due to the changes in renal hemodynamics or a consequence of an effect on the tubules as has been suggested by BARRACLOUGH et al. (1967). There is usually a significant correlation between the decrease in urine flow and either the decrease in glomerular filtration rate or that in renal plasma flow [AURELL, 1969; BOCK et al., 1958; BONJOUR and MALVIN, 1969 (2); SCHMID, 1968]. Studies involving effects of angiotensin on free water clearance have also generally indicated that the decrease in free water reabsorption is roughly proportional to the decrease in urine flow (BARBOUR et al., 1962; GILL et al., 1964). However DEL GRECO (1962) infused doses of 2.5 to 5 ng/kg/min, angiotensin into patients with diabetes insipidus and demonstrated that the decrease in free water clearance was greater than the decrease in urine flow; he suggested that angiotensin might have an additional tubular antidiuretic effect.

It is unnecessary to postulate a tubular effect to explain the decreases in urine flow and sodium excretion occurring with small doses of angiotensin. If a tubular effect increasing the fractional tubular reabsorption of sodium and water exists, the possibility of alteration in the peritubular capillary reabsorption forces must be considered (EARLEY and FRIEDLER, 1966). The observed decreases in intrarenal venous pressure (DI SALVO et al., 1971) indicate that changes in peritubular forces probably occur.

2. Effects of Intra-Arterial Infusion of Angiotensin I and II

Intra-arterial infusion of Ang. II elicits a local effect without producing genera circulatory changes such as follow intravenous infusion of angiotensin. Although large doses can reduce blood flow practically to zero (DI SALVO and FELL, 1970; FURUYAMA et al., 1967) the maximum sustained reduction is approximately 50% Approximately the same reduction is produced by 0.1 μg/min (FOURCADE et al., 1971; FURAYAMA, 1967) as by 1.0 to 1.4 μg/min (DEL GRECO and PAGE, 1961; KOVER et al., 1971). However, the data indicate that following doses of angiotensin given either intravenously or intra-arterially decreases of renal blood flow by much more than 50% are not sustained and the sustained response may be of lesser magnitude than that to smaller doses (DI SALVO and FELL, 1970; FURUYAMA et al., 1967 and HEALY et al., 1965).

The direct arterial infusion of Ang. I has been used to determine if it has a irect vasoconstrictor action. Results from some studies (FRANKLIN et al., 1970; TILDESLEY et al., 1971) showed approximately 25% as much response with Ang. I. DI SALVO et al. (1971) demonstrated that inhibition of the converting enzyme completely prevented the renal vasoconstrictor response. DI SALVO et al. (1971) found an intrarenal conversion rate of 4%. OPARIL et al. (1970) estimated a 7 to 10% conversion rate. Most of the doses used to obtain these disparate estimates have been high.

3. Effect of Angiotensin on Renal Autoregulation

Several investigators have performed studies in which renal autoregulatory efficiency was tested before and during infusions of angiotensin (BELLEAU and EARLY, 1967; GAGNON et al., 1970; KIIL et al., 1968). The doses used have varied widely but have all been sufficient to cause a 30 to 50% reduction in renal blood flow. The administration of renin or angiotensin to the intact dog kidney preparation does not impair the normal intrarenal vasodilatory response that occurs following acute decreases in renal arterial pressure within the range of 80 to 160 mmHg. The vascular response to angiotensin is actually less when angiotensin is infused at lower perfusion pressures than normal (McNAY and KISHIMOTO, 1969). The evidence suggests that autoregulatory adjustments in renal resistance are not mediated by angiotensin.

III. Factors Modifying Renal Response to Angiotensin

1. Effect of Anesthesia

Although some investigators have suggested that antidiuretic doses in unanesthetized animals either had no effect or tended to cause diuresis and natriuresis in animals anesthetized with pentobarbital [BARRACLOUGH et al., 1967 (2); CANNON et al., 1966; LEVITIN et al., 1963], the modifications were relatively slight.

2. Role of the Autonomic Nerves

Section of the carotid sinus and aortic depressor nerves in dogs caused increased urine flow when renin was injected, while dogs with intact buffer nerves responded with decreased urine flow (DEL GRECO et al., 1962). Intact renal nerves appeared to be essential for the renal effects of angiotensin to be manifested (McGIFF and ITSKOVITZ, 1964; McGIFF and FASY, 1965). McGIFF (1967) showed that in dogs pretreated with reserpine and guanethidine, the vasoconstrictor effect of angiotensin was blunted and natriuresis developed (McGIFF, 1967). Blood pressure was not monitored in most of these studies and may have contributed to the differences observed. More recent investigations have failed to support the previous suggestions and have indicated that the renal responses in chronically denervated kidneys are essentially the same as those in normal preparations (BONJOUR and MALVIN, 1969; DI SALVO and FELL, 1970; and GELLER and KENDRICK, 1967). Thus, barring the indirect effects that renal denervation or buffer-nerve sectioning might have on systemic arterial pressure and resting level of sympathetic tone to the kidney, it appears that an intact renal innervation is of little significance with respect to the direct renal responses to angiotensin. This does not exclude the possibility that intact renal innervation may be important in long-term responses to very low doses of angiotensin.

3. Effect of Dose on Sustained Vascular Response

As shown in Fig. 1, relatively small doses of angiotensin result in a sustained decrease in renal blood flow, glomerular filtration rate and urine flow. However, several investigators have demonstrated that the rather marked decreases in renal function following administration of renin or angiotensin in large doses are usually not well sustained. This decrease in continued response has been demonstrated in rabbits with doses greater than 250 ng/kg/min [BROWN et al., 1964 (1)] and in dogs with doses greater than 50 ng/kg/min (FURUYAMA et al., 1967; HEALY et al., 1966; LAMEIJER et al., 1966; LOUIS and DOYLE, 1965). The loss of the vascular response also occurs with intermittent injections of angiotensin into the renal artery every 5 min (VILLARREAL et al., 1964). While this type of response may not be exactly the same as the pressor tachyphylaxis which is known to occur, it is likely that saturation of vascular receptor sites due to the excessive doses may be responsible for this phenomenon (KHAIRALLAH et al., 1966). This diminished vascular reactivity in response to high doses may be of considerable significance, since it appears to be a prerequisite for the development of natriuretic and diuretic responses to high doses (HEALY et al., 1966; LAMEIJER et al., 1966; LOUIS and DOYLE, 1965; VILLARREAL et al., 1964). In general, the data indicate that following this decrease in vascular reactivity, the glomerular filtration rate may increase toward control levels while the renal blood flow recovery may not be so extensive (HEALY et al., 1966). The degree of diminished vascular reactivity is also influenced by the dose. It thus yields a relationship between dose and sustained effects which is complex and which shows a maximum effect at an intermediate dose (MALVIN and VANDER, 1967).

4. Interrelationships between Arterial Pressure, Pressor Responses to Angiotensin and Renal Responses to Angiotensin

There is a curvilinear relationship between arterial pressure and urine-flow or sodium-excretion rate even under conditions in which renal blood flow and glomerular filtration rate are well regulated (SELKURT et al., 1949; THURAU and

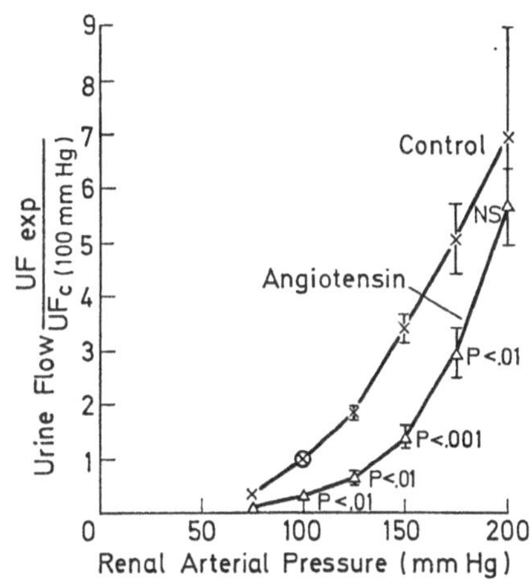

Fig. 2. Normalized graph showing a typical relationship between renal arterial pressure and urine flow and the same relationship as it is affected by angiotensin. Data was obtained from study by FOURCADE, NAVAR and GUYTON (1971)

DEETJEN, 1962). The cause of this phenomenon ("pressure diuresis") is not clear, but it is not due to medullary washout (NAVAR et al., 1971). The slope of the curve is influenced by the efficiency of autoregulation as altered by vasodilators (BAER et al., 1970).

The control curve presented in Fig. 2 was composed from data obtained by FOURCADE et al. (1971) and depicts a typical relationship between arterial pressure and urine flow. An increase of 25 mmHg in arterial pressure would result in approximately twice the increase in urine flow at a control arterial pressure of 150 mmHg compared to a normal control arterial pressure of about 100 mmHg. Small intra-arterial infusions of angiotensin of about 2.5 ng/kg/min (kidney weight), while causing a transient decrease in urine flow, did not alter the characteristics of the curve significantly. However, larger infusions which still caused sustained decreases in renal blood flow and glomerular filtration rate resulted in a change in the curve yielding a less steep relationship at the lower arterial pressures and a steeper slope than normal at higher arterial pressures. This curve is also shown in Fig. 2.

Infusions of angiotensin at normal arterial pressures could decrease urine flow even in the presence of a slight pressor response. The same infusions administered to a subject with much higher arterial pressure, in the order of 150 mmHg, could result in increased urine flow even with the same absolute pressor response. This type of analysis may help to explain the relatively consistent antidiuretic and antinatriuretic effects of angiotensin when given to normal subjects, while the responses obtained at higher arterial pressure have been somewhat variable. However, the pressure-diuresis phenomenon cannot explain all the observations reported in experimental preparations. At arterial pressures of more than 150 mmHg, the infusion of angiotensin at certain concentrations (approximately 250 ng/kg/min resulted in increased urine flow and sodium excretion even when the rise in arterial pressure was prevented (COLLIGNON and KULBERTUS, 1966; FOURCADE et al., 1971). These experiments indicate that the natriuretic and diuretic response to angiotensin cannot be completely explained by pressure diuresis.

IV. Influence of the Level of Salt Intake on Renal Responses to Angiotensin

Salt loading increases the vasoconstrictor effect of angiotensin (AURELL, 1969), and allows the influence of sub-pressor doses to become apparent [BARRACLOUGH, 1967 (1)]. Sodium depletion is accompanied by a diminished vascular sensitivity to low doses of angiotensin, substantial blunting of the antidiuretic response normally observed, and a greater probability of a diuretic and natriuretic effect [BARRACLOUGH et al., 1967 (2); LOUIS and DOYLE, 1966]. When diuresis occurs, the changes are relatively small and not of the magnitude observed when larger doses are given.

It is not clear why kidneys in salt-depleted people or animals have a decreased vascular response to angiotensin. Blood angiotensin levels are increased by salt depletion (AURELL, 1969; CATT et al., 1970; GOCKE et al., 1969), so the kidney may be responding to the sum of the endogenous and exogenous angiotensin. Further discussion of this subject will be found in Section VIII, 1.

V. Natriuretic Effects of High Doses of Angiotensin

PICKERING and PRINTZMETAL (1940) noted the diuretic effect of large doses of renin. Small doses were usually antidiuretic. Angiotensin was also antidiuretic when given in small amounts, such as 200 ng/kg/min, but natriuretic in doses of 1000 ng/kg/min (LANGFORD and PICKERING, 1965).

Glomerular filtration rate, markedly reduced during the first 10 to 40 min of infusion, approaches the control value at the time diuresis begins (AKINKUGBE et al., 1967; CANNON et al., 1966; HEALY et al., 1965; HUGHES-JONES et al., 1949; KLEIN et al., 1971; LANGFORD and PICKERING, 1965; PETERS, 1963). The filtration fraction is elevated during the natriuretic period (BONJOUR and MALVIN, 1969) ,and the kidneys are enlarged (MERRILL et al., 1938).

1. Time Related Nature of Diuretic Response

Infusions of large doses of angiotensin, 250 ng/μkg/min in rats [BONJOUR and MALVIN, 1969 (2)] and 1000 ng/kg/min in rabbits (LANGFORD and PICKERING, 1965), elicits a complex series of responses. The first response is marked renal vascular constriction and a sharp drop in urine flow [BARER, 1963; BARRACLOUGH, 1965; BARRACLOUGH et al., 1967 (3); FURUYAMA et al., 1967; HEALY et al., 1965; KLEIN et al., 1971; LAMEIJER et al., 1966; LOUIS and DOYLE, 1965]. There is marked blanching of the kidney with a decrease in size (FINBERG and PEART, 1970). This response is similar to that reported to occur in frog kidneys following topical application of angiotensin (WAKIN et al., 1941). In 10 to 40 min the urinary responses are reversed and a diuretic and natriuretic response occurs. It is postulated that the reversal time is related inversely to the magnitude of the dose (HEALY et al., 1965).

The marked natriuretic response is usually due to both an increase in urine flow and increased sodium and chloride concentration in the urine, some studies indicating an 8- to 30-fold increase in sodium excretion (FINBERG and PEART, 1970; LAMEIJER et al., 1966). This is important because it distinguishes the diuresis of high doses from the diuresis that may occasionally occur with low doses in preparations with uncontrolled blood pressure.

Marked proteinuria has frequently been observed, especially following renin injections (BRANDT and GRUHN, 1948; DEODHAR et al., 1964; MASSON et al., 1950, 1953; MERRILL et al., 1938; ROSENFELD et al., 1965) and it has been suggested that it is of glomerular origin (PESSINA et al., 1971).

The diuretic and natriuretic responses do not appear to be related to the pressor response, and the maximum natriuretic response usually occurs after blood pressure has fallen some way toward control levels (LOUIS and DOYLE, 1965; MASSON et al., 1950; MERRILL et al., 1938; VILLARREAL et al., 1964). Nor was any significant correlation found between the blood-pressure changes and the changes in urine flow or sodium excretion [BONJOUR and MALVIN, 1969 (2); PETERS, 1963].

Direct infusion of angiotensin into the renal artery has demonstrated that diuresis can be elicited. The kidney into which angiotensin has been infused shows a much greater diuretic and natriuretic response than the contralateral kidney (AKINKUGBE et al., 1966; BRICKER and COE, 1966). Also, HEALY and ELLIOTT (1971) have shown that when the blood pressure is controlled by bleeding during the infusion of angiotensin, the natriuretic response is still observed. No correlations can be established between the diuretic response and the changes in renal plasma flow or glomerular filtration rate (BONJOUR and MALVIN, 1969).

These observations and the finding that there are obvious increases in the tubular rejection fraction of sodium (BONJOUR et al., 1968; FURUYAMA et al., 1967), has led to the conclusion that high doses of angiotensin are capable of causing a decrease in the tubular reabsorption of sodium which is not accounted for by hemodynamic alterations.

2. Factors Influencing Diuretic Responses to Angiotensin

The same doses of angiotensin in the same species are sometimes associated with diuresis and sometimes with an antidiuretic response. Dehydrated rats do not usually exhibit any natriuretic response to intermediate doses of angiotensin (of about 200 ng/kg/min) (BONJOUR et al., 1968). However, expansion of the extracellular fluid with isotonic saline greatly facilitates the response which can then be elicited at doses which previously had an antidiuretic effect (CANNON et al., 1966). BONJOUR et al. (1968) found a direct correlation between the relative change in the tubular fraction in response to angiotensin and the control tubular rejection fraction. REGOLI (1969) reported that blood-volume expansion with iso-oncotic solutions of bovine albumin and Ringer's solution did not facilitate diuresis.

Diuretic responses to intermediate doses (100 to 500 ng/kg/min) can be explained on the basis of changes in blood pressure or changes in the glomerular filtration rate, especially when acute volume expansion has been imposed. The situation is complex because of the number of variables responsible for the changes in urine flow and sodium excretion. A true tubular natriuretic response should not be expected unless the decrease in the fractional reabsorption of sodium is greater than can be explained by hemodynamic changes. Changes in glomerular filtration rate and intrarenal pressure and the possible changes in the level of autoregulatory efficiency should all be considered. This problem is probably responsible for the contention by some investigators that all the diuretic effects of angiotensin can be explained by hemodynamic alterations and loss of vascular reactivity (EARLEY and FRIEDLER, 1966; SCHMID, 1968). Probably in most conditions, changes in sodium excretion result from renal vascular effects while in other conditions, especially with high doses, a tubular action is primarily responsible for the natriuresis.

3. Direct Evidence of the Tubular Effect of Angiotensin

While many experiments find circumstantial evidence favoring a tubular effect of angiotensin, few have given the matter direct consideration. VANDER (1963) performed stop-flow experiments in dogs and demonstrated that angiotensin infusion elevated the distal tubular sodium minimum. A nonspecific effect due to the pressor effects of angiotensin was ruled out since equipressor doses of norepinephrine did not reproduce these results. This finding suggested that angiotensin might act on the distal tubule sodium transport mechanisms. PETERS (1964) and BONJOUR et al. (1967) also suggested a distal effect in water-loaded rats since the relative increase in free-water clearance accompanying the increase in urine flow was not as great as would be expected from the increased distal load. LEYSSAC (1964), on the basis of tubular occlusion studies, suggested that angiotensin inhibited sodium transport in the proximal tubule. These studies, however, were not confirmed by other investigators (VON NAGEL et al., 1966).

A different approach took advantage of the separate glomerular and peritubular capillary blood supply of the chicken, and angiotensin was infused into the renal portal vein (CUYPERS, 1965; LANGFORD and FALLIS, 1963; LANGFORD, 1964). Angiotensin infusions into the portal vein of the chicken resulted in prompt diuresis, which was substantially more pronounced on the infused side than on the contralateral side. This suggests that angiotensin could have a direct effect on the tubules, most probably at distal sites. The micropuncture and microperfusion studies of HORSTER et al. (1966), however, showed no effect of angiotensin on tubular reabsorption. These studies were criticized because the experimental conditions were such that a diuresis would not be expected (BONJOUR et al., 1968). More recent micropuncture experiments of LOWITZ et al. (1969) have strengthened the hypothesis of a direct tubular effect by showing that peritubular capillary perfusion with angiotensin-containing solutions resulted in inhibition of sodium transport in the distal tubule. HEALY and ELLIOTT (1970) demonstrated that large doses of angiotensin resulted in decreased medullary concentration of sodium, chloride, and urea, and increased water content, suggesting an effect of angiotensin on the ascending limb of Henle. This agrees with the findings of LOWITZ et al. (1969), and is in accord with free water-clearance studies. Experiments in dogs prepared with thoracic caval occlusion (PORUSH et al., 1967), and those on patients with cirrhosis (LARAGH et al., 1963) indicate that a diuretic response in these conditions decreases the sodium reabsorption of the diluting segment of the distal nephron.

VI. Angiotensin Effects on Isolated Tissues

The hypothesis concerning a direct tubular effect of angiotensin would not be questioned to such an extent were it not for the negative results obtained from most studies of the effect of angiotensin on isolated tissues. Studies on toad skin

(BONJOUR et al., 1969), toad bladder (COVIELLO and CRABBE, 1965), isolated rabbit proximal tubules (BURG and ORLOFF, 1968; HEALY et al., 1969), and cortex slices (BONTING et al., 1964; HEALY and DOUGLAS, 1968) have generally failed to show an inhibitory action of angiotensin on short circuit current, sodium flux, or tubular enzymatic activity.

Angiotensin in low doses (10^{-12} g/ml) increases the rate of active sodium extrusion by rat kidney-cortex slices and inhibits potassium uptake (MUNDAY et al., 1971). This effect is not affected by conditions which would be expected to increase intracellular cyclic AMP levels, and is blocked by inhibitors of the translation stage of protein synthesis (MUNDAY et al., 1972).

The above studies of MUNDAY would explain the anti-natriuresis of low doses of angiotensin. Only BARTHA and SZOCS [1970 (1, 2)] and LEYSSAC et al. (1961) have obtained results which are compatible with either a direct or a permissive effect of angiotensin to decrease the net transport of sodium across the tubules. The work of DAVIES et al. (1970), using the rat colon, showed stimulation of Na transport by 10^{-12} g/ml of angiotensin and depression of transport by 10^{-7} g/ml of angiotensin.

Besides a direct effect on the tubular epithelium to inhibit the rate of sodium transport, other possibilities include a) a selective vasoconstriction of the renal medullary structures (LEVER, 1965), b) a possible redistribution of intrarenal blood flow, or c) changes in the vascular permeability of the glomerular or peritubular capillaries, perhaps changing the interstitial fluid pressure or interstitial protein concentration. The proteinuria which accompanies the diuresis of high doses and the finding that thoracic lymph flow increases after high doses of angiotensin (WENZE et al., 1965) lend credence to the possibility that changes in the permeability of the peritubular capillaries could play some role.

VII. Alterations in Intrarenal Hemodynamics with Angiotensin

1. Comparative Effects of Angiotensin on Renal and Other Vascular Beds

When angiotensin is given systemically, there is strong evidence that vascular resistance in the kidney increases more or at least as much as that in any other part of the body (ASSALI and WESTERSTEN, 1961; ASTOIN, 1965; FORSYTH et al., 1971; HERRICK et al., 1942; MANDEL and SAPIRSTEIN, 1962; MCGIFF and AVIADO, 1961). FORSYTH et al. (1971) showed that angiotensin infusions given to monkeys at rates varying from 15 to 210 ng/kg/min resulted in substantial decreases in renal, cutaneous, hepatic, and mesenteric blood flow (see Fig. 1). Of the major vascular beds, the kidney showed the greatest decrease. Skeletal muscle blood flow remained relatively constant.

Arteriographic studies have shown enlargement of the main renal artery during intravenous infusion of angiotensin, presumably reflecting constriction of the resistance arteries and passive hypertension-induced dilatation of the larger vessel (ELKIN and MENG, 1966).

The *in-vitro* studies of BOHR and UCHIDA (1967) are in conflict with the above results. Angiotensin completely failed to cause constriction of renal resistance arteries with outer diameters of 250 to 500 micra., though the vessel responded to epinephrine or norepinephrine, and resistance vessels from other beds responded to angiotensin.

The effects of equipressor doses of norepinephrine are more generalized (ASTOIN, 1965) and do not cause as pronounced a decrease in renal blood flow (MC QUEEN and MORRISON, 1961). Both angiotensin and norepinephrine cause a greater decrease in renal plasma flow than in glomerular filtration rate (BARCLAY et al., 1947; LARAGH et al., 1963), though the diuretic effect of an equipressor dose of norepinephrine is much less than that of angiotensin (FINBERG and PEART, 1970; LANGFORD and PICKERING, 1963; LARAGH, 1962).

2. Changes in Segmental Renal Vascular Resistance

The findings that both renin and angiotensin usually result in increased filtration fraction have been cited as evidence for a predominant role of angiotensin on the postglomerular arterioles. However, this conclusion is not completely justified. As early as 1942, LAMPORT attempted to evaluate the relative changes in the pre- and post-glomerular resistances following administration of renin and angiotensin. As he pointed out, the increase in filtration fraction of itself does not indicate a predominant effect on the efferent resistance but only that there is an effect on it. He calculated that angiotensin elicited increased glomerular capillary pressure and that there was no distinct indication that efferent resistance was the predominant site of increased resistance. More recently KIIL et al. (1969) have also evaluated the segmental changes in resistance with vasoconstrictors including angiotensin. The decreased G.F.R. with angiotensin does not necessarily indicate that glomerular pressure is reduced since the filtration fraction is elevated and the mean glomerular colloid osmotic pressure would thus be increased. If glomerular filtration rate was maintained, this would indicate increased glomerular pressure (LAMPORT, 1942).

Angiotensin infusions thus affect both the afferent and efferent arterioles, but the sustained effect is greater on the efferent resistance segments. The effects on the afferent segments are not directly associated with the autoregulating segments; autoregulatory capability in response to manipulations of the renal arterial pressure is well maintained during infusions of angiotensin. Studies using isolated perfused rabbit kidneys [REGOLI and GAUTHIER, 1971 (1, 2)] suggested that there is a distinct difference between angiotensin and epinephrine; angiotensin increased G.F.R. and urine flow while epinephrine decreased them. The G.F.R. changes are opposite to those found *in vivo* and are difficult to explain.

Changes in the resistance of the venous segments in response to angiotensin have not been studied in great detail. Only a slight increase in venous resistance (ZIMMERMAN et al., 1964) or no effect (DISALVO et al., 1971) is caused by either Ang. II or Ang. I.

3. Changes in Regional Intrarenal Vascular Resistance and Intrarenal Distribution of Renal Blood Flow

BARGER (1966) suggested that subtle alterations in the regional resistances to blood flow through the kidneys could be responsible for relative changes in sodium reabsorption to an extent greater than could be accounted for on the basis of renal blood flow and glomerular filtration rate of the whole kidney. The problem is complicated by the fact that there are several techniques used to estimate regional renal blood flow. DANIEL et al. (1954) suggested on the basis of angiographic studies that renin could cause relatively prolonged periods of cortical ischemia with constriction of the smaller intrarenal arteries. Presumably very high doses of renin were used.

Later, other investigators suggested that there was little evidence for redistribution between the outer cortical and juxta-medullary nephrons since angiotensin failed to affect the *tubular maximums* for P.A.H. and glucose (HEALY et al., 1965) and also failed to alter the P.A.H.-extraction ratio [AURELL, 1969; BONJOUR and MALVIN, 1969 (2); SCHROEDER et al., 1967]. Studies using the inert gas-washout technique support the concept that both Ang. I and Ang. II are capable of causing preferential decrease in cortical blood flow and either a maintained, or increased, relative blood flow through the deep juxtamedullary nephrons (CARRIERE and FRIBORG, 1969; CARRIERE and BIRON, 1970). These investigators used this interpretation to explain the antidiuretic effect of angiotensin as a result of a greater proportion of filtrate traversing longer nephrons where more sodium is reabsorbed. The diuretic effect has also been explained in this manner since FINBERG and PEART [1970 (1)], using a carbon-particle distribution technique, suggested that it may be due to relative redistribution of flow and G.F.R. toward the cortical nephrons.

Another relatively popular technique of measuring local blood-flow rates involves measurement of local clearance of a substance by the use of some probe. AUKLAND (1968) using the hydrogen gas-washout technique and GRANGSJO and PERSSON (1971) using the heated thermocouple method have both failed to obtain evidence that angiotensin in a wide range of doses causes a singificant redistribution of renal blood flow. Results obtained from experiments using the microsphere technique (RECTOR et al., 1971) are in agreement. Intra-arterial infusion of angiotensin (100 ng/min) to dogs resulted in a 40% decrease in renal blood flow, but no difference in microsphere distribution was observed.

It appears that the bulk of the evidence is not in favor of any marked redistribution effects of Ang. II on regional blood flow. The situation may be quite different for endogenously produced angiotensin, since most renin is found in the outer cortical glomeruli (BROWN et al., 1966).

VIII. Effect of Sodium Balance, Renin Content of the Kidneys, Pregnancy, Hypertension, and Cirrhosis on the Renal Response to Angiotensin

1. Sodium Balance

AUREL (1969) showed that there was a direct correlation between Na^+ excretion in the control periods and the percentage decrease in G.F.R. and P.A.H. clearance following angiotensin infusion in human beings. Patients infused with 1.1 to 1.5 ng/kg/min of angiotensin did not show any change in G.F.R. and P.A.H. clearance when the basal Na^+ excretion was 100 μE/min or less, but with increasing basal Na^+ excretion progressively greater vasoconstriction was produced. This important study may explain the findings in the studies of LOUIS and DOYLE (1966) and of LARAGH (1962), in which low doses of angiotensin were antidiuretic and antinatriuretic in the sodium-replete state but induced diuresis and natriuresis in saltdepleted subjects. If angiotensin fails to produce vasoconstriction in the kidney of the Na-depleted subject, the tubular diuretic effect may be unmasked, or the diuretic effects of increased arterial pressure may predominate.

2. Renal Artery Stenosis

If the increased plasma and renal angiotensin of Na-depletion are responsible for the decreased vasoreactivity and thus allow angiotensin-induced diuresis, several findings should follow. As the renin content of a kidney with a partially occluded artery is increased and that of the contralateral kidney reduced, angiotensin infusion might cause less vasoconstriction in the stenosed kidney and diuresis from it. The studies of MCGIFF and ITSKOVITZ (1964) fulfill these expectations. Acute ischemia markedly reduced the renal vasoconstrictor response to angiotensin but not to norepinephrine. The studies of PETERS (1965) in rats several weeks after unilateral narrowing of the renal artery were compatible to an extent. Diuresis and natriuresis occurred from the ischemic kidney but not from the intact kidney. The failure of the intact kidney to show diuresis could not be explained on the basis of a more pronounced decline in G.F.R., which actually rose. Similar results were found by BORKOWSKI (1965) in rats that became hypertensive after unilateral renal artery narrowing; but in similarly treated rats which did not become hypertensive, angiotensin was non-diuretic in both kidneys (G.F·R. was not measured).

JONES and BARRACLOUGH (1962) and PAUSESCU et al. (1970) noted diuresis from the normal but not the ischemic kidney when angiotensin was infused intravenously into hypertensive patients with unilateral renovascular disease, but BROWN (1964) and ITSKOVITZ et al. (1967) found no consistent difference in the response of the ischemic compared to the non-ischemic kidney. Most of the patients in the latter two studies showed the same findings as the majority of severe essential hypertensive subjects; diuresis from both kidneys at an angiotensin dose which would not produce diuresis in a normotensive patient.

The discrepancy between the above studies cannot be resolved at present. If further studies are performed, it would be of interest to determine the renin-secretion rate from both kidneys. The kidney which is ischemic, as shown by increased secretion of renin compared to the other may react in a different manner from a kidney with non-significant stenosis.

3. Hypertensive Patients

Two types of patients, cirrhotics and severe essential hypertensives, respond to angiotensin with diuresis at doses which normally produce antidiuresis. In patients with hypertension, angiotensin infusions may produce a natriuretic and diuretic response, while the P.A.H. and inulin clearance may be no lower than control levels. (BIRON et al., 1962; ITSKOVITZ et al., 1967; JAHN et al., 1967; NIJENSOHN, 1957; PEART and BROWN, 1961; VAGNUCCI et al., 1964; VILLARREAL et al., 1967). Similar doses of angiotensin (1 to 3 μg/min) given to normotensive patients lead to antidiuresis and depression of clearances (see Section II).

While the diuretic response has been reported to occur even without an increase in blood pressure (BROWN and PEART, 1962), this response occurs predominantly in severely hypertensive patients, disappears after control of their blood pressure, and is more marked in patients with positive sodium balance (DEL GRECO, 1961). It should be emphasized that not all the hypertensives studied have exhibited a diuretic and natriuretic response Approximately 30 to 50% of patients respond with a decreased urine flow (DUSTAN et al., 1955; VAGNUCCI et al., 1964; VILLARREAL et al., 1967). In the latter study patients were classified according to whether or not a natriuretic response was obtained. Table 1 present the mean data from this study. The most obvious difference between the two groups was in the mean arterial pressure, which was substantially lower in the patients who responded with antidiuresis than in those who responded with natriuresis. While differences in the G.F.R. responses were noted, no significant correlation was established in this study. In an experimental study on dogs, however, SCHMID (1968) demonstrated that the natriuretic effect of angiotensin infusions in dogs with chronic renal hypertension could be associated with an increased G.F.R. and thus supported the original contention of NIJENSOHN (1957). On the other hand, VAGNUCCI et al. (1964) showed that infusion of angiotensin in doses of 0.11 μg/kg/min into hypertensive patients caused a diuretic response in two-thirds of the patients, but seven of the nine had a decreased G.F.R. in response to the angiotensin. It is not certain that all of the facets of the diuretic response of hypertensives can be explained on the basis of hemodynamic alterations. Nevertheless, it is possible that a tubular effect may be contributing to the response since the natriuretic effect is usually quantitatively much greater than the diuretic effect.

Table 1. *Mean data of results reported in study of* Villarreal *et al., 1967. Angiotensin infusion of 4 μg/min or 50 to 70 ng/kg/min*

	I			II		
	C	A	P	C	A	P
Number of patients	11			16		
Sodium excretion μEq/min	224	149	<0.01	256	957	<0.001
Arterial blood pressure mmHg	125	157	<0.001	150	180	<0.001
G.F.R. ml/min	110	99	>0.05 N.S.	96	106	>0.05 N.S.
R.P.F. ml/min	396	288	<0.01	368	298	<0.01
Urine flow ml/min	4.56	1.85	<0.05	4.9	9.07	<0.01
EF Na (%)	1.51	1.26	<0.05	1.96	6.74	<0.001
EF H_2O (%)	4.16	2.21	<0.05	4.93	8.74	<0.01

Patients given 7 g NaCl supplement daily.
I responded with antidiuresis, II responded with diuresis, C control, A during angiotensin infusion, P probability values.

4. Hepatic Cirrhosis

After 3.8 μg/min angiotensin cirrhotic patients with ascites (Laragh et al., 1963) exhibited diuresis, unchanged G.F.R., and a decrease of about 25% in P.A.H. clearance. It was also shown that these patients required about three times as much angiotensin as normal for the same pressor response. Normal patients studied at this dosage retained Na^+ and water and their P.A.H. clearance decreased by 51% with unaltered G.F.R. Patients on a low Na diet, unlike those in the study of Louis and Doyle (1966), responded similarly to angiotensin infusion as those on a normal diet. In the latter study, diuresis was achieved with angiotensin, and the sodium depletion was probably more pronounced as diuretics were given early in the course of the sodium depletion.

Kuntzman et al. (1967) observed diuresis in only ten of forty-five edematous cirrhotic patients in response to angiotensin. Decreased G.F.R. was not more frequent in the patients who did not undergo diuresis, and diuresis occurred in some patients despite decreased G.F.R.; others retained Na^+ and water even though G.F.R. increased. The amount of angiotensin given was less than that used by Laragh (1962). There were no clinical characteristics found to predict whether the response to angiotensin would be natriuretic or antinatriuretic.

Ajzen et al. (1968) also studied cirrhotic patients with ascites. They pretreated the patients with aldosterone. Infusion of subpressor doses (0.2 μg/min) of angiotensin produced a significant fall in G.F.R., P.A.H. clearance, and sodium excretion. Pressor doses averaging 9.5 μg/min produced greater decreases in G.F.R. but approximately the same decreases in sodium excretion. As the authors pointed out, their studies are at variance with the results of Laragh. However,

LOUIS and DOYLE (1964) had earlier reported that pretreatment of cirrhotic patients with aldosterone reversed the natriuretic effect of angiotensin given in doses of 10 to 20 ng/kg/min. Thus it appears that administration of aldosterone prevents the natriuretic effect in cirrhotic subjects.

Therapy with spironolactone for varying periods of time did not change the effect of creatinine clearance but had a dramatic effect on sodium excretion (JAHN et al., 1967). Following prolonged treatment, the same dose of angiotensin which formerly caused natriuresis now caused sodium retention. Pretreatment with chlorthalidone had a similar effect to spironolactone pretreatment.

There is no ready explanation for the discrepancy between the study by LOUIS and DOYLE (1961), where exogenous aldosterone blunted the angiotensin-induced diuresis, and that of JAHN et al. (1967), where pre-treatment with an aldosterone antagonist or chlorthalidone also abolished angiotensin-induced natriuresis. Spironolactone and chlorthalidone should elicit a further increase in aldosterone secretion, but there is no apparent reason why increased aldosterone should reverse the response to angiotensin in patients who must have been producing it in large amounts before the additional administration.

When angiotensin-induced natriuresis is observed in both cirrhotic patients (LARAGH et al., 1963) and thoracic-caval dogs (PORUSH et al., 1967) under conditions of water diuresis, free-water clearance is depressed to an extent greater than can be accounted for an increased distal load. Norepinephrine infusions may also produce diuresis in cirrhotics, but the free-water clearance is not equally depressed. As the reduced free-water clearance with increase of total water excreted shows reduced fractional sodium reabsorption by the diluting segment of the distal nephron, angiotensin apparently depresses sodium reabsorption at this site.

5. Pregnancy

Pregnancy with elevated plasma renin is also accompanied by blunting of the renal response to angiotensin. CHESLEY et al. (1963) found that 0.5 μg/min produced much less depression of Na^+ and water excretion in pregnant women than in non-pregnant patients, and inulin clearance was less reduced in patients 26 to 35 weeks pregnant than in the control patients. There was no significant difference in inulin clearance response between the pregnant patients at full term and the controls.

MANGIONI and MORANDINI (1967) studied the effects of angiotensin on urine flow and electrolyte excretion in normal pregnancy. Angiotensin produced less antidiuresis in pregnant patients than in non-pregnant controls. Toxemic patients had even less reduction of Na^+ and water excretion than normal pregnant women.

IX. Resume

Low doses of angiotensin (1 to 50 ng/kg/min) in rat, dog, rabbit, and man cause renal vasoconstriction, the decrease in G.F.R. being slightly less than the decrease in blood flow. The decreased urine flow and sodium excretion appear to be due to vasoconstriction. When a diuretic response occurs at these doses, it is usually due to the increased arterial pressure resulting in pressure diuresis. At higher control arterial pressures, either in severe essential hypertension or high renal perfusion pressures and under conditions of sodium depletion, the above doses of angiotensin may lead to a slight diuretic effect. The diuresis may be related to the finding that vasoconstriction is less marked in sodium-depleted and other 'high-renin' states.

High doses of angiotensin cause much greater initial vasoconstriction, but the responses are less sustained. A marked natriuretic effect occurs under these conditions. There is strong evidence of a tubular effect of angiotensin to inhibit sodium reabsorption, probably in the ascending loop of Henle and the distal tubule. Manifestation of a tubular effect occurs with high angiotensin doses or in diseases in which plasma angiotensin may be elevated.

There is insufficient evidence to conclude that exogenous angiotensin administration leads to substantial redistribution of intrarenal blood flow or glomerular filtration rate. Analyses of segmental vascular resistance changes indicate that angiotensin affects both the pre- and the post-glomerular resistance elements but not the venous resistance segment. The autoregulatory ability of the kidney in response to decreases in arterial pressure is not perceptibily affected by angiotensin infusions although the blood-flow level at which autoregulation takes place is decreased.

Angiotensin infusions at doses which are normally antidiuretic may lead to natriuresis and diuresis in hypertension and hepatic cirrhosis with ascites, and in the presence of sodium depletion. Both a tubular effect of angiotensin and pressure diuresis appear to be responsible for the responses observed. Renal vascular reactivity to the infused angiotensin is probably diminished in these conditions. The latter phenomenon may represent tachyphylaxis produced by elevated endogenous angiotensin.

References

AGNOLI, G. C., BERNARDI, P., CARIANI, A., MONTINI, F. F. e T.: Sul controllo del filtrato glomerulare e deil'effecienza dei riassorbimenti tubulari durante l'infusione di angiotensina II. Bolletino soc. ital. **45**, 1515 (1970).

AJZEN, H. U. A., CIPULLO, J. P., SUSTOVICH, D. R., RAMOS, O. L.: Effect of angiotensin II on urinary sodium excretion in normal subject and cirrhotic patients. Amer. J. med. Sci. **256**, 373 (1968).

AKINKUGBE, O. O., BROWN, W. C. B., CRANSTON, W. I.: Response to angiotensin infusion before and after adrenalectomy in the rabbit. Amer. J. Physiol. **212**, 1147 (1967).

AKINKUGBE, O. O., BROWN, W. C., CRANSTON, W. I.: The direct renal action of angiotensin in the rabbit. Clin. Sci. **30**, 259 (1966).

ASSALI, N. S., WESTERSTEN, A.: Regional flow-pressure relationship in response to angiotensin in the intact dog and sheep. Circulat. Res. **9**, 189 (1961).

ASTOIN, M.: Effects compares de la noradrenaline et de l'angiotensine sur les resistances vasculaires renales et femorales. J. Physiol. **57**, 541 (1965).

AUKLAND, K.: Effect of adrenaline, noradrenaline, angiotensin and renal nerve stimulation on intrarenal distribution of blood flow in dogs. Acta physiol. scand. **72**, 498 (1968).

AURELL, M.: Renal response in man to plasma volume expansion and angiotensin: Scand. J. clin. Lab. Invest. **24** (Suppl. 112), (1969).

BAER, P. G., NAVAR, L. G., GUYTON, A. C.: Renal autoregulation filtration rate, and electrolyte excretion during vasodilatation. Amer. J. Physiol. **219**, 619 (1970).

BARBOUR, B. H., GILL, J. R., SLATER, J. D. H., BARTTER, F. C.: An explanation for the antidiuresis produced by angiotensin II in man. Clin. Res. **10**, 245 (1962).

BARCLAY, J., COOKE, W. T., KENNEY, R. A.: Observations on the effects of adrenalin on renal function and circulation in man. Amer. J. Physiol. **151**, 621 (1947).

BARER, G. R.: The action of vasopressin, a vasopressin analogue (PLV_2), oxytocin, angiotensin, bradykinin and theophylline ethylene diamine on renal blood flow in the anaesthetized cat. J. Physiol. **169**, 62 (1963).

BARGER, A.: Renal hemodynamic factor in congestive heart failure. Annals of N. Y. Acad. Sci. **139**, 276 (1966).

BARRACLOUGH, M. A.: Dose-dependent opposite effects of angiotensin on renal sodium excretion. Lancet **1965 II**, 987.

BARRACLOUGH, M. A., JONES, N. F., MARSDEN, C. D.: (3) Effect of angiotensin on renal function in the rat. Amer. J. Physiol. **212**, 1153 (1967).

BARRACLOUGH, M. A., JONES, N. F., MARSDEN, C. D., BRADFORD, B. C.: (1) Renal and pressor actions of angiotensin in salt loaded and depleted rabbits. Experientia (Basel) **23**, 553 (1967).

Barraclough, M. A., Perriello, V. A., Marsden, C. D., Jones, N. F.: (2) The inffuence of the experimental conditions on the renal response to angiotensin in the rat. Experientia (Basel) **23**, 140 (1967).

Bartha, J., Szocs, E.: (1) ^{24}Na uptake by renal cortical slices in the presence of angiotensin. Acta Physiol. Acad. Sci. Hung. **37**, 396 (1970).

Bartha, J., Szocs, E.: (2) ^{24}Na uptake and PAH accumulation of renal cortical lsices in the presence of angiotensin. Acta Physiol. Acad. Sci. Hung. **39**, 151 (1970).

Belleau, L. J., Earley, L. E.: Autoregulation of renal blood flow in the presence of angiotensin infusion. Amer. J. Physiol. **213**, 1590 (1967).

Biron, P., Chretien, M., Koiw, E., Genest, J.: Effect of angiotensin infusions on aldosterone and electrolyte excretion in normal subjects and patients with hypertension and adrenocortical disorders. Brit. Ned. J. **1962 I**, 1569.

Bock, K. D., Dengler, H., Krecke, H. J., Reichel, G.: Untersuchungen über die Wirkung von synthetischem Hypertensin II auf Elrktrolythaushalt, Nierenfunktion und Kreislauf beim Menschen. Klin. Wschr. **36**, 808 (1958).

Bock, K. D., Krecke, H. J.: Die Wirkung von synthetischem Hypertensin II auf die PAH und Inuiin-clearance, die renale Hamodynamik und die Diurese beim Menschen. Klin. Wschr. **36**, 69 (1958).

Bohr, D. F., Uchida, E.: Individualities of vascular smooth muscles in response to angiotensin. Circulat. Res. **21** (Suppl. II), 135 (1967).

Bonjour, J. P., Malvin, R. L.: (1) Effect of angiotensin on the denervated kidney in the dog. Proc. Soc. Exp. Biol. (N.Y.) **131**, 469 (1969).

Bonjour, J. P., Malvin, R. L.: (2) Renal extraction of PAH, GFR and U_{Na}-V in the rat during infusion of angiotensin. Amer. J. Physiol. **216**, 554 (1969).

Bonjour, J. P., Peters, G., Chomety, F., Regoli, D.: Renal effects of Val-5-angiotensin II-amide, vasopressin and iuretics in the rat, as influenced by water diuresis and by ethanol anesthesia. Europ. J. Pharmacol. **2**, 88 (1967).

Bonjour, J. P., Regoli, D., Roch-Ramel, F., Peters, G.: Prerequisites for the natriuretic effect of Val-5-angiotensin II amide in the rat. Amer. J. Physiol. **215**, 1133 (1968).

Bonting, S. L., Canady, M. R., Hawkins, N. M.: Angiotensin and renal Na-K activated adenosine triphosphates (Studies on Na-K activated ATPase, VIII). Biochim. biophys. Acta (Amst.) **82**, 427 (1964).

Borkowski, A. J., Howards, S. S., Laragh, J. H.: Angiotensin and electrolyte excretion in renovascular hypertension. Amer. J. Physiol. **208**, 1087 (1965).

Brandt, J. L., Gruhn, J. G.: Effect of renin on proteinuria and PAH clearance at low plasma levels. Amer. J. Physiol. **153**, 458 (1948).

Bricker, L. A., Coe, F. L.: Unilateral natriuresis from selective intrarenal infusion of angiotensin. Clin. Res. **14**, 489 (1966).

Brown, J. J., Peart, W. S.: The effect of angiotensin on urine flow and electrolyte excretion in hypertensive patients. Clin. Sci. **22**, 1 (1962).

Brown, J. J., Chapius, G., Robertson, J. I. S.: (1) The effect of prolonged intravenous infusion of angiotensin in the rabbit. Clin. Sci. **26**, 165 (1964).

Brown, J. J., Davies, D. L., Lever, A. F., Robertson, J. I. S.: Renin and angiotensin — A survey of some aspects. Postgrad. med. Journ. **42**, 153 (1966).

Brown, J. J., Matthew, G. K., Robertson, J. I. S.: (2) The effect of angiotensin on the function of the separate kidneys in patients with unilateral renal artery stenosis. Clin. Sci. **26**, 381 (1964).

Burg, M., Orloff, J.: Control of fluid absorption in the renal proximal tubule. J. clin. Invest. **47**, 2016 (1968).

Cannon, P. J., Ames, R. P., Laragh, J. H.: Indirect action of angiotensin infusion to inhibit renal tubular sodium reabsorption in dogs. Amer. J. Physiol. **211**, 1021 (1966).

Carriere, S., Biron, P.: Effect of angiotensin I on intrarenal blood flow distribution. Amer. J. Physiol. **219**, 1642 (1970).

Carriere, S., Friborg, J.: Intrarenal blood flow and PAH extraction during angiotensin infusion. Amer. J. Physiol. **217**, 1708 (1969).

Catt, K. J., Cain, M. D., Coghlan, J. P., Zimmet, P. Z., Cran, E., Best, J. B.: Metabolism and blood levels of angiotensin II in normal subjects, renal disease, and essential hypertension. Circulat. Res. **27** (Suppl.), 177 (1970).

Chesley, L. G., Wynn, R. M., Silverman, N. C.: Renal effects of angiotensin II infusions in normotensive pregnant and nonpregnant women. Circulat. Res. **13**, 232 (1963).

Collignon, P., Kulbertus, H.: Influence de lapression de perfusion sur la reponse a l'angiotensin du rein de chien transplante au cou. Arch. Int. Physiol. Biochim. **74**, 565 (1966).

Corcoran, A. C., Page, I. H.: The effects of renin, pitressin, and pitressin and atrophine on renal blood flow and clearance. Amer. J. Physiol. **126**, 354 (1939).

COVIELLO, A., CRABBE, J.: Effect of angiotensin II onanctive transport of sodium by toad bladder and skin. Biochem. Pharmacol. **14**, 1739 (1965).

CROXATTO, H., BARNAFI, L., PASSI, J.: Effect of renin on diuresis in rats. Science **116**, 507 (1952).

CUYPERS, Y.: L'Action tubulaire renale de 17-angiotensine II-amide chez le coq. Arch. Int. Pharmacodyn. **155**, 495 (1965).

DANIEL, P. M., PRICHARD, M. M. L., WARD-McQUAID: An angiographic study of the effect of renin upon the renal circulation. J. Physiol. **124**, 106 (1954).

DAVIES, N. T., MUNDAY, K. A., PARSONS, B. J.: The effect of angiotensin on the rat intestinal fluid transfer. J. Endocr. **48**, 391 (1970).

DEBONO, E., LEE, G. D. J., MOTTRAM, F. R., PICKERING, G. W.: The action of angiotensin in man. Clin. Sci. **25**, 123 (1963).

DEL GRECO, F.: Effects of valine-5 angiotensin II on excretion of water and salt in primary and secondary hypertension. Proc. Soc. Exp. Biol. (N.Y.) **107**, 943 (1961).

DEL GRECO, F.: Comparative effects of valine-5 angiotensin II amide and pitressin on renal excretory function in diabetes insipidus. Proc. Soc. Exp. Biol. (N.Y.) **109**, 105 (1962).

DEL GRECO, F., CORCORAN, A. C., PAGE, I. H.: Renal effects of renin in normal and buffer-nerve sectioned dogs. Proc. Soc. Exp. Biol. (N.Y.) **111**, 3 (1962).

DEL GRECO, F., PAGE, I. H.: Effects of intrarenal infusion of angiotensin in the dog. Circulation **24**, 917 (1961).

DEODHAR, S. D., CUPPAGE, F. E., GABLEMAN, E.: Studies on the mechanisms of experimental proteinuria induced by renin. J. exp. Med. **120**, 677 (1964).

DISALVO, J. and FELL, C.: Effects of angiotensin on canine renal blood flow. Proc. Soc. Exp. Biol. (N.Y.) **133**, 1432 (1970).

DISALVO, J., PETERSON, A., MONTEFUSCO, C., MENTA, M.: Intrarenal conversion of angiotensin I to angiotensin II in the dog. Circulat. Res. **29**, 398 (1971).

DUSTAN, H., NIJENSOHN, C., CORCORAN, A. C.: Natriuretic-diuretic effect of angiotensin in essential hypertension. J. clin. Invest. **34**, 931 (1955).

EARLEY, L. E., FRIEDLER, R. M.: The effects of combined renal vasodilation and pressor agents on renal hemodynamics and the tubular reabsorption of sodium. J. ciin. Res. **45**, 542 (1966).

ELKIN, M., MENG, C. H.: The effects of angiotensin on renal vascularity in dogs. Amer. J. Roentgenol. **98**, 927 (1966).

FINBERG, J. P. M., PEART, W. S.: Intrarenal blood flow distribution in the rat and the effect of angiotensin, noradrenaline and vasopressin. J. Physiol. **209**, 21P (1970).

FINNERTY, F. A., MASSARO, G. D., CHUPKOVICH, V., TUCKMAN, J.: Evaluation of the pressor, cardiac, and renal hemodynamic properties of angiotensin II in man. Circulat. Res. **9**, 256 (1961).

FORSYTH, R. P., HOFFBRAND, B. I., MELMON, K. L.: Hemodynamic effects of angiotensin in normal and environmentally stressed monkeys. Circulation **44**, 119 (1971).

FOURCADE, J. C., NAVAR, L. G., GUYTON, A. C.: Possibility that angiotensin resulting from unilateral kidney disease affects contralateral renal function. Nephron **8**, 81 (1971).

FRANKLIN, N. G., PEACH, M. J., GILMORE, J. P.: Evidence for the renal conversion of angiotensin I in the dog. Circulat Res. **27**, 321 (1970).

FURUAYAMA, C., SUZUKI, C., SHIOJI, R., SAITO, H., MAEBASHI, M., AIDA, M.: Effect of angiotensin on renal function of the dog. Tohoku J. exp. Med. **92**, 73 (1967).

GAGNON, J. A., KELLER, H. I., KOKOTIS, W., SCHRIER, R. W.: Analysis of role of renin-angiotensin system in autoregulation of glomerular filtration. Amer. J. Physiol. **219**, 491 (1970).

GELLER, R. G., KENDRICK, J. E.: Reduction in renal vascular responses to angiotensin and norepinephrine during coratid sinus stimulation. Circulat. Res. **20**, 321 (1967).

GILL, J. R., BARBOUR, B. H., SLATER, J. D. H., BARTTER, F. C.: Effect of angiotensin II on urinary dilution in normal man. Amer. J. Physiol. **206**, 750, 1964.

GOCKE, D. J., GERTEN, J., SHERWOOD, L. M., LARAGH, J. H.: Physiological and pathological variations of plasma angiotensin II in man. Circulat. Res. **24**, 131 (1969).

GRANGSJO, G., PERSSON, E.: Influence of some vaso-active substances on regional blood flow in the dog kidney. Acta anaesth. scand. **15**, 71 (1971).

HEALY, J. K., BARCENA, C., O'CONNELL, J. M. B., SCHREINER, G. E.: Renal and pressor action of angiotensin in the normal dog. Amer. J. Physiol. **208**, 1093 (1965).

HEALY, J. K., BARCENA, C., SCHREINER, G. E.: Effect of angiotensin on maximal tubular transport of PAH and glucose in dogs. Amer. J. Physiol. **209**, 651 (1965).

HEALY, J. K., DOUGLAS, J. B.: The effect of angiotensin on renal carbonic anhydrase.Biochim. biophys. Acta (Amst.) **151**, 520 (1968).

HEALY, J. K., DOUGLAS, J. B., ARNOLD, J. E.: The effect of angiotensin on isolated rabbit renal tubules. Clib. Sci. **37**, 583 (1969).

HEALY, J. K., ELLIOTT, A. J.: The effect of a natriuretic dose of angiotensin on rabbit kidney composition. Clin. Sci. **38**, 727 (1970).
HEALY, J. K., ELLIOTT, A. J.: Angiotensin-induced renal changes without pressor response. Clin. Res. **19**, 532 (1971).
HEALY, J. K., SUSZKIW, J. B., DENNIS, V. W., SCHREINER, G. E.: Effect of aldosterone and salt intake on renal and pressor actions of angiotensin. Nephron **3**, 329 (1966).
HERRICK, J. F., CORCORAN, A. C., ESSEX, H. E.: The effects of renin and of angiotonin on the renal blood flow and blood pressure of the dog. Amer. J. Physiol. **135**, 88 (1941—42).
HORSTER, M., NAGEL, W., v. SCHNERMANN, J., THURAU, K.: Zur Frage einer direkten Angiotensinwirkung auf die Natriumresorption im proximalen Tubulus und in der Henleschen Schleife der Rattenniere. Pflügers Archiv ges. Physiol. **292**, 118 (1966).
HUGHES-JONES, N. C., PICKERING, G. W., SANDERSON, P. H., SCARBOROUGH, H., VANDENBROUCKE, J.: The nature of the action of renin and hypertension on renal function in the rabbit. J. Physiol. **109**, 228 (1949).
ITSKOVITZ, H. D., MURPHY, J. J., SKHOENBERG, H. W.: Differential renal function studies on the effects of angiotensin in normotensive and hypertensive patients. Amer. J. med. Sci. **253**, 163 (1967).
JAHN, H., REVILLE, P., KURTZ, T., KUNTZMANN, F., STAHL, J.: Quelques aspects de l'action de l'angiotensine sur le rein. Path. et Biol. **15**, 641 (1967).
JONES, N. F., BARRACLOUGH, M. A., PERRIELLO, VA. A., MARSDEN, C. D.: Effect of angiotensin on urea reabsorption in man. Clin. Sci. **32**, 257 (1967).
KHAIRALLAH, P. A., PAGE, I. H., BUMPUS, F. M., TURKER, R. K.: Angiotensin tachyphylaxis and its reversal. Circulat. Res. **19**, 247 (1966).
KIIL, F., KJEKSHUS, J., LYNING, E.: Renal autoregulation during infusion of noradrenaline, angiotensin and acetylcholine. Acta physiol. scand. **76**, 10 (1969).
KLEIN, G. L., MILLS, I. H., WILSON, R. J.: Changes in renal function associated with the development of resistance of the renal vasculature to the arterial infusion of angiotensin. J. Physiol. **215**, 43P (1971).
KOVER, G., TOST, H., BALINT, T.: The effect of angiotensin on renal tubular function. Acta physiol. Acad. Sci. hung. **39**, 136 (1971).
KUNTZMAN, F., REVILLE, P., KURTZ, M. T., VASSAUX, C., JAHN, H., STAHL, J.: Effects de l'angiotensine sur le rein dans la cirrhose. Path. et Biol. **15**, 1133 (1967).
LAMEIJER, L. D. F., SOGHIKIAN, K., DE GRAEFF, J.: The effect of angiotensin on renal sodium excretion. Studies in normal dogs and in dogs with experimental renal artery stenosis. Clin. Sci. **30**, 529 (1966).
LAMPORT, H.: The effects on renal resistance to blood flow of renin angiotonin, pitressin and atropine, hypertension, and toxemia of pregnancy. J. clin. Invest. **21**, 685 (1942).
LANGFORD, H. G.: Tubular action of angiotensin. Canad. med. Ass. J. **90**, 332 (1964).
LANGFORD, H. G., FALLIS, N. E.: Tubular effect of angiotensin. Circulation **28**, 754 (1963).
LANGFORD, H. G., PICKERING, G. W.: The action of synthetic angiotensin on renal function in the unanaesthetized rabbit. J. Physiol. **177**, 161 (1965).
LARAGH, J. H.: Interrelationships between angiotensin, norepinephrine, epinephrine, aldosterone secretion, and electrolyte metabolism in man. Circulation **25**, 203 (1962).
LARAGH, J. H., CANNON, P. J., BENTZEL, C. H., SICINSKI, A. M., MELTZER, J. I.: Angiotensin II, norepinephrine, and renal transport of electrolytes and water in normal man and in cirrhosis with ascites. J. clin. Invest. **42**, 1179 (1963).
LEVER, A. F.: The vasa recta and countercurrent multiplication. Acta med. Scand. **434** (Suppl. V), 178 (1965).
LEVITIN, H., LEHMANN, W. B., PIGEON, G., WARREN, Y., GOLDENBERG, I. S.: The effect of anesthesia and adrenalectomy oh the renal response to angiotensin. J. clin. Invest. **42**, 951 (1963).
LEYSSAC, P. P.: The in vivo effect of angiotension on the proximal tubular reabsorption of salt in rat kidneys. Acta physiol. Scand. **62**, 436 (1964).
LEYSSAC, P. P., LASSEN, U. V., THAYSEN, J. H.: Inhibition of sodium transport in isolated renal tissue by angiotensin. Biochim. biophys. Acta (Amst.) **48**, 602 (1961).
LOUIS, W. J., DOYLE, A. E.: The effects of varying doses of angiotensin on renal function and blood pressure in man and dogs. Clin. Sci. **29**, 489 (1965).
LOUIS, W. J., DOYLE, A. E.: The renal action of angiotensin II. Austral. Ann. Med. **14**, 87 (1965).
LOUIS, W. J., DOYLE, A. E.: The effects of aldosterone and angiotensin on renal function. Clin. Sci. **30**, 179 (1966).
LOWITZ, H. D., STUMPE, K. O., OCHWADT, B.: Micropuncture study of the action of angiotensin II on tubular sodium and water reabsorption in the rat. Nephron. **6**, 173 (1969).
MALVIN, R. L., VANDER, A. J.: Effects of angiotensin infusion on renal function in the unanesthetized rat. Amer. J. Physiol. **213**, 1205 (1967).

MANDEL, M. J., SAPIRSTEIN, L. A.: Effect of angiotensin infusion on regional blood flow and regional vascular resistance in the rat. Circulat. Res. **10**, 807 (1962).

MANGIONI, C., MORANDINI, G.: Effect of angiotensin on urine flow and electrolyte excretion in normal and toxemic pregnancy. Mal. cardiovasc. 8, 515 (1967).

MASSON, G. M. C., CORCORAN, A. C., PAGE, I. H.: Some effects of chronic treatment of rats with renin. Amer. J. Physiol. **162**, 379 (1950).

MASSON, G. M. C., DEL GRECO, F., CORCORAN, A. C., PAGE, I. H.: Factors influencing renin diuresis and proteinuria. Proc. Soc. Exp. Biol. (N.Y.) **83**, 631 (1953).

MCGIFF, J. C.: Natriuretic effect of angiotensin in dogs revealed after administration of reserpine and guanethidine. Circulat. Res. **20**, 664 (1967).

MCGIFF, J. C., AVIADO: Differential response of renal femoral blood flows and vascular esistances — Hypotensive and hypertensive procedures. Circulat. Res. **9**, 1327 (1961).

MCGIFF, J. C., FASY, T. M.: The relationship of the renal vascular activity of angiotensin II to the autonomic nervous system. J. clin. Invest. **44**, 1911 (1965).

MCGIFF, J. C., ITSKOVITZ, H. D.: Loss of the renal vasoconstrictor activity of angiotensin II during renal ischemia. J. clin. Invest. **43**, 2359 (1964).

MCGIFF, J. C., LYNCH, J. R., LRINICKE, J. A., STRAND, J. C., ABOOSI, A.: Some determinants of the effects of Val-5-angiotensin II amide on glomerular filtration rate and sodium excretion in dogs. J. clin. Invest. **48**, 146 (1969).

MCNAY, J. L., KISHIMOTO, T.: Association between autoregulation and pressure dependency of renal vascular responsiveness in dogs. Circulat. Res. **24**, 599 (1969).

MCQUEEN, E. G., MORRISON, R. B. D.: The effects of synthetic angiotensin and nor-adrenaline on blood pressure and renal function. Brit. Heart J. **23**, 1(1961).

MERRILL, A., WILLIAMS, R. H., HARRISON, T. R.: The effects of a pressor substance obtained from the kidneys on the renal circulation of rats and dogs. Amer. J. med. Sci. **196**, 240 (1938).

MULROW, P. J., GOFFINET, J. A.: The renin-angiotensin system. In: Physiology of the Human Kidney, p. 465—520 (WESSON, G., Ed.). New York: Grune and Stratton 1969.

MUNDAY, K. A., PARSONS, B. J., POAT, J. A.: The effect of angiotensin on cation transport by rat kidney cortex slices. J. Physiol. **215**, 269 (1971).

MUNDAY, K. A., PARSONS, B. J., POAT, J. A.: Studies on the mechanism of action of angiotensin on ion transport by kidney cortex slices. J. Physiol. **224**, 195 (1972).

NAVAR, L. G., UTHER, J. B., BAER, P. G.: Pressure diuresis in dogs with diabetes insipidus. Nephron 8, 97 (1971).

NIJENSOHN, C. M.: Accion de la hipertensina angiotonina en la hipertension arterial humana. Sem. méd. (B. Aires) **111**, 205 (1957).

OPARIL, S., SANDERS, C. A., HABER, E.: In vivo and in vitro conversion of angiotensin I to angiotensin II in dog blood. Circulat. Res. **26**, 591 (1970).

PAUSESCU, E., BERONIADE, V., RADULESCU, C., CARNARU, S., LUGOJAN, R., OSIESCU, J.: Effects of angiotensin on the function and metabolism of the ischemic kidney. Arch. int. Pharmacodyn. **186**, 28 (1970).

PEART, W. S., BROWN, J. J.: Effect of angiotensin (hypertensin or angiotonin) on urine flow and electrolyte excretion in hypertensive patients. Lancet **1961 I**, 28.

PESSINA, A. C., HULME, B., PEART, W. S.: The effect of renin, angiotensin II and adrenalectomy on glomerular capillary permeability in the rat. Clin. Sci. **40**, 12p (1971).

PETERS, G.: Renal tubular effect of val-5-angiotensin II amide in rats. Proc. Soc. Exp. Biol. (N.Y.) **112**, 771 (1963).

PETERS, G.: Etude de l'effect natriuretique de l'angiotensinechez le rat. Helv. physiol. pharmacol. Acta **22**, C34 (1964).

PETERS, G.: Effect of val-angiotensin II amide and of hydrochlorothiazide on the kidneys of renal hypertensive rats. Nephron **2**, 94 (1965).

PICKERING, G. W., PRINZMETAL, M.: The effect of renin on urine formation. J. Physiol. **98**, (314 (1940).

PORUSH, J. G., KALOVANIDES, G. J., CACCIAGUIDA, R. J., ROSEN, S. M.: The effects of angiotensin II on renal water and electrolyte excretion in normal and caval dogs. J. clin. Invest. **46**, 2109 (1967).

RECTOR, J. B., BAY, W. H., STEIN, J. H., FERRIS, T. F.: Comparison of the effect of hemorrhagic hypotension and vasopressor administration on the distribution of renal cortical blood flow in the dog. Amer. Soc. Nephrol. **5**, 62 (1971).

REGOLI, D.: The renal action of angiotensin in rats after expansion of plasma volume or of extracellular fluid. Canad. J. Physiol. Pharmacol. **47**, 969 (1969).

REGOLI, D., GAUTHIER, R.: (1) (FR) studies on intrarenal role of renineffects of vasoconstrictors on an isolated rabbit kidney preparation. Union Medicale du Canad. **100**, 733 (1971).

REGOLI, D., GAUTHIER, R.: Site of action of angiotensin and other vasoconstrictors on the kidney. Canad. J. Physiol. **49**, 608 (1971).

ROSENFELD, S., KRAUS, R., MCCULLEN, A.: Effect of renin, ischemia and plasma protein loading on the isolated perfused kidney. Amer. J. Physiol. **209**, 835 (1965).
SCHMID, H. E.: Action of angiotensin in normal, adrenalectomized and renal hypertensive trained dogs. Nephron **5**, 265 (1968).
SCHROEDER, E. T., SHEAR, L., SANCETTA, S. M., GABUZDA, G. J.: Renal failure in patients with cirrhosis of the liver. III. Evaluation of intrarenal blood flow by para-aminohippurate extraction and response to angiotensin. Amer. J. Med. **43**, 887 (1967).
SELKURT, E. E., HALL, P. W., SPENCER, M. P.: Influence of graded arterial pressure decrement on renal clearance of creatinine, P-aminohippurate and sodium. Amer. J. Physiol. **159**, 369 (1949).
SELLERS, A. L., SMITH, S., III., GOODMAN, H. C., MARMORSTON, J.: Effects of renin on excretion of sodium chloride and water in the rat. Amer. J. Physiol. **166**, 619 (1951).
THURAU, K., DEETJEN, P.: Die Diurese bei arteriellen Drucksteigerungen. Pflügers Arch. ges. Physiol. **274**, 567 (1962).
TILDESLEY, G., OSBORN, E. C., WILLICOMBE, P. R., MAHLER, R. F.: The effect of angiotensin I on renal blood flow in sheep. J. Pharm. Pharmacol. **23**, 547 (1971).
TORRES, C., LOZANO, R., WHITTEMBURY, J., MONGE, C.: Effect of angiotensin on the kidney of the high altitude native. Nephron **7**, 489 (1970).
VAGNUCCI, A. I., LAULER, D. P., HICKLER, R. B., THORN, G. W.: Acute infusion of synthetic angiotensin II in patients with essential hypertension — Its effect on renal hemodynamics and on electrolyte and water excretion. Circulation **29**, 523 (1964).
VANDER, A. J.: Inhibition of distal tubular sodium reabsorption by angiotensin II. Amer. J. Physiol. **205**, 133 (1963).
VILLARREAL, H., ARCILA, H., DIAZ, J., SIERRA, P.: Effect of angiotensin on the renal transport of sodium in essential hypertension. Circulation **35**, 889 (1967).
VILLARREAL, H., DE PASCUAL, J. N., ARCILA, H., LOPEY-VINAS, C., SIERRA, P.: The action of angiotensin on renal transport of sodium in the dog. Nephron **1**, 338 (1964).
VON NAGEL, W., HORSTER, M., WAHL, M., THURAU, K., SCHNERMANN, J.: Die tubulare resorptionskapazität für Isotone NaCl-Lösung bei unterschiedlichrn Glomerulumfiltraten und unter Angiotensineinwirkung. Pflügers Arch. ges. Physcol. **291**, 1260 (1966).
WAKIM, K. G., ROOT, G. T., ESSEX, H. E.: Effect of angiotonin and renin on glomerular circulation in frog kidney. Proc. Exp. Biol. (N.Y.) **47**, 72 (1941).
WERNZE, H., FUJII, J., SEMBACH, B.: Der LymphfulB in ductus thoracicus unter Angiotensin und Noradrenalin. Z. ges. exp. Med. **139**, 70 (1965).
WHITNEY, J., SMITH, S., III., MARMORSTON, J., GOODMAN, H. C., SELLERS, A. L.: Antidiuretic effect of renin in the dog. Amer. J. Physiol. **176**, 419 (1954).
ZIMMERMAN, B. G., ABBOUD, F. M., ECKSTEIN, J. W.: Effects of norepinephrine and angiotensin on total venous resistance in the kidney. Amer. J. Physiol. **206**, 701 (1964).

Intrarenal Action of Angiotensin

Klaus Thurau

With 5 Figures

This chapter is concerned with the intrarenal action of angiotensin. The treatment of this subject has become extremely difficult during the last few years, as many observations indicate that angiotensin II is formed intrarenally in the vicinity of the juxtaglomerular apparatus (JGA). Here, specialized cells produce the enzyme renin, which is essential for the formation of Ang. II. Because the activity of this enzyme, like that of angiotensinase, is not homogeneously distributed among all JGAs in the kidney but varies according to the position of the JGA in different layers of the renal cortex (Brown et al., 1965, 1966; Cook et al., 1956; Granger et al., 1972; Peart, 1959), it is clear that any study must take this intrarenal pattern of enzyme activity into account. These aspects exclude the possibility of simulating the action associated with naturally occurring angiotensin by injecting this substance into the blood perfusing the kidney. The injection of synthetic angiotensin would be expected not only to have a uniform distribution within the entire kidney, but also to act upon vascular and tubular segments, which may not normally be exposed to intrarenally formed angiotensin. Therefore, the events following the exogenous administration of synthetic angiotensin may have little relation to *in-vivo* mechanisms.

With this in mind, the discussion in this chapter will be restricted primarily to those reports in the literature which are concerned with the analysis of intrarenally occurring angiotensin. This restriction is somewhat arbitrary since it excludes important material, e.g. extrarenal factors which stimulate intrarenal renin activity and influence renin release (for reference see Davis, 1971; Tobian, 1967; Page and McCubbin, 1968; Vander, 1967).

Location of the Enzymes of the Renin-Angiotensin System in the Kidney

During the last 15 years a number of observations have been made permitting the localization of the intrarenal formation of renin. Two main methods have been used for this purpose: a) immunological techniques in combination with fluorescence microscopy (Nairn et al., 1959; Edelman and Hartroft, 1961; Hartroft et al., 1964; Warren et al., 1966) and b) microdissection of renal tissue and its quantitative analysis for renin activity (Bing and Wiberg, 1958; Cook et al., 1956; Cook and Pickering, 1959; Bing and Kazimierczak, 1959, 1960, 1962; Peart et al., 1956; Cook, 1970, 1971; Faarup, 1967, 1971; Brown et al., 1963, 1965, 1966; Thurau et al., 1970; Dahlheim et al., 1970; Gavras et al., 1970; Granger et al., 1972).

There is general agreement that the enzyme renin is located almost exclusively at the vascular pole of the glomerulus in the epitheloid cells situated in the afferent arteriolar vessel wall (Fig. 1). Renin has not been found in aglomerular tissue, i.e. in the most superficial layer of the kidney (cortex corticis) and in the renal medulla (COOK et al., 1956). BING and KAZIMIERCZAK (1962) obtained some evidence that renin might be localized in the macula densa cells rather than in the epitheloid cells. However, in a subsequent study, FAARUP (1967), using a selective staining technique for the identification of juxtaglomerular granules in the epitheloid cells, found that the macula-densa cells were practically free of renin while the epitheloid cells contained almost all the renin present in the entire JGA (Fig. 2).

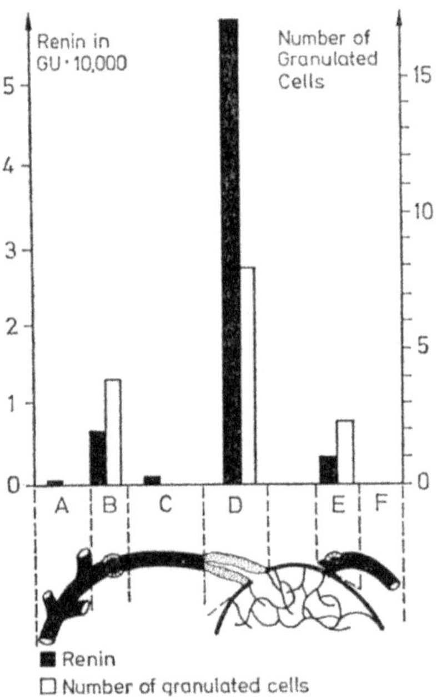

Fig. 1

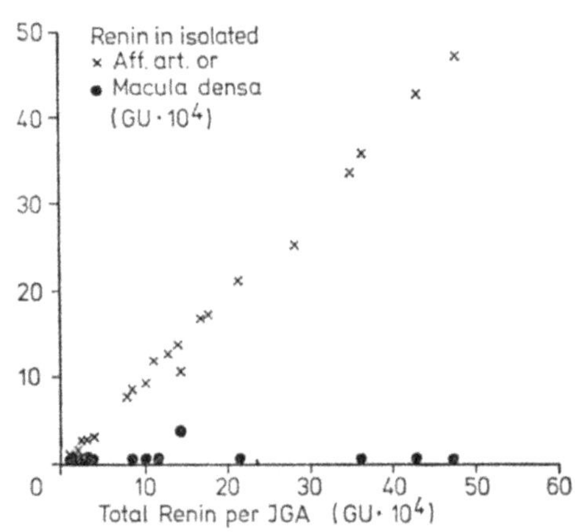

Fig. 2

Fig. 1. Renin content of different fractions of the vascular system of the nephron correlated to the occurrence of epitheloid cells containing juxtaglomerular granules. The renin content and the number of granulated cells are given as mean values per 100 microns length of the vascular fraction. (From FAARUP, 1971)

Fig. 2.: The renin content of the afferent arteriole and of the macula densa in freeze-dried tissue. Abscissa: The total renin content in both the afferent arteriole and the macula densa. Ordinate: Renin content of single fractions. (From FAARUP, 1972)

Direct evidence for the presence of renin in the epitheloid cells was furnished by COOKE (1970, 1971), who punctured these cells with glass pipettes and sampled a mixture of cytoplasm and granules in which renin activity was demonstrated. Samples taken from surrounding tubular cells contained no renin activity. It is not clear to date whether the granules are formed from renin molecules in an active or an inactive state. Ultrastructural studies have revealed different types of granules in the epitheloid cells. The identity of a specific type of granule which is the site of renin storage remains still to be established. Furthermore, there is some evidence that the renin activity, which can be measured in a homogenized single JGA, reflects only the number of physiologically active renin molecules rather than the total number of both active and inactive molecules (see p. 484). If so, this may explain the observation that in some conditions the number of granules in JGA cells does not correlate with the renin activity measured (ROBERTSON et al., 1966, GRANGER et al., 1971).

COOK et al. (1957) and BROWN et al. (1965, 1966) observed in the rabbit kidney that the more superficial the location of the JGA in the renal cortex, the higher the renin activity was. This is consistent with data obtained by PEART (1959), working with dog-kidney slices in which he showed a higher renin content per JGA in superficial than in deeper tissue layers. Such a renin gradient from superficial to juxtamedullary JGAs, however, probably does not exist in all species. In rats, GRANGER et al. (1972) found the renin activity of superficial and juxtamedullary microdissected JGAs to be essentially the same. The angiotensinase activity, however, showed a gradient such that its activity was lower in superficial than in deeper JGAs. This observation emphasizes the fact that the intrarenal cortico-juxtamedullary distribution of renin is not necessarily identical to the distribution of Ang. II, since renin is not the sole determinant for the local Ang.-II concentration. Other factors which also influence the rate of Ang. II formation and destruction (i.e. renin substrate, converting enzyme, angiotensinase) may exhibit a cortico-juxtamedullary gradient, thus effecting the intrarenal distribution pattern of Ang. II.

Intrarenal Formation of Angiotensin II

Ang. II can only be formed intrarenally if converting enzyme activity is present in addition to renin and renin substrate. In fact, converting-enzyme activity appears to be available in the kidney so that intrarenal formation of angiotensin can occur. THURAU et al. (1970) and GRANGER et al. (1972) found converting activity in single microdissected JGAs of the rat kidney.

Analysis of renal lymph furnishes indirect evidence for the presence of converting enzyme activity in the interstitial fluid of the kidney. BAILIE et al. (1971) found Ang.-II concentration in renal lymph of dogs to be higher than in renal arterial or venous blood. This difference became more pronounced during hemorrhagic hypotension, a procedure known to activate the renin-angiotensin system. Since the concentration of Ang. II in renal lymph may be as much as 60 times higher than that in renal venous blood, this difference in concentration cannot be explained by diffusion of Ang. II from the blood into the interstitial space. On the contrary, these data indicate that Ang. II is formed primarily in an interstitial compartment of the kidney, which presumes the availability of converting enzyme in this compartment. ITSKOVITZ and ODYA (1971) analyzed renal arterial and venous blood for Ang. I and II. They found that the concentration of Ang. I in the renal venous blood was higher than that in renal arterial blood and up to 45 times higher than that of Ang. II. They concluded that the enzymatic reaction is rapid enough to produce Ang. I in the renal vasculature, but that converting-enzyme activity in renal blood is too low to account for a significant formation of Ang. II in blood during passage through the kidney. These data are in keeping with the hypothesis that the primary site of action of converting enzyme is located somewhere in the renal tissue remote from the renal vasculature.

The existence of converting-enzyme activity of renal origin is also suggested by the results of HORKY et al. (1971). In the abdominal lymph of rats they found converting-enzyme activity which increased following the stimulation of the renin angiotensin system by the i.v. injection of the natriuretic substance furosemide and decreased after bilateral nephrectomy.

The existence of an *extravascular* site of angiotensin formation in the area of the JGA would render the assessment of the activity of the renal renin-angiotensin system difficult. The value of measuring renin and angiotensin in the renal venous blood is lost if these substances are not primarily released into the blood but into the interstitium. On the basis of the above arguments this appears to be a valid objection since renin activity and Ang. II concentrations are considerably higher in renal lymph than in renal venous blood. However, for two reasons, it is probably not feasible to calculate the effective angiotensin concentration of the JGA *in vivo* from the renal lymph values. Firstly, the total mass of the JGAs is only approximately 1/10,000 of the total kidney mass (MEYER, 1971), from which the entire renal lymph is drained. Secondly, Ang. II formation may continue to occur in the lymphatic fluid during its passage from the area of the JGA to the hilar lymph vessels where it can be collected.

There are data which indicate that the site of Ang. II formation in the area of the JGA may be within the epitheloid cells. In a fluorescent antibody study on pig juxtaglomerular cells, SUTHERLAND (1970) found evidence for the presence of α_2-globulin within the JGA cells. Since renin substrate is an α_2-globulin it may be assumed that the membranes of the juxtaglomerular cells are permeable to the renin substrate. BING (1964), in an earlier study, had already suggested that substrate may pass into the juxtaglomerular cells, this process being a prerequisite for an intracellular formation of angiotensin.

If Ang. II is formed intracellularly, it could act on cellular contractile elements, since the renin-producing cells do have myofilaments.

Several authors have investigated the possible existence of converting-enzyme activity in the kidney by adding Ang. I to the renal arterial blood and estimating its conversion to Ang. II from the change in renal resistance. This technique, however, has several inherent limitations which excludes its use as a quantitative assay: Pharmacologically induced changes in renal resistance occur primarily in the arterioles, i.e. in a vascular segment which is proximal to the capillaries. If these changes in resistance are taken as a quantitative measure for the conversion of Ang. I to Ang. II, all converted molecules must have access to the smooth-muscle receptor sites in the arterioles. This fundamental prerequisite, however, appears not to be met. If converting-enzyme activity is bound to intrarenal cellular structures, Ang. I molecules which have been added to the blood can be exposed to this enzyme only after diffusion across the capillary membranes into the interstitium, i.e. beyond the arteriolar segment. Only a small undefinable fraction of Ang. II formed in this way will reach the smooth muscle receptor sites, because most of the renal interstitial fluid is not in contact with the arterioles. These objections are equally valid if converting activity is restricted to specialized cell complexes in the kidney such as the JGA: In this case the fraction of infused Ang. I which reaches the site of converting activity is also unpredictable.

Thus it must be concluded that the method of addition of Ang. I to the renal arterial blood is unsuitable for the quantitative assay of intrarenal converting-enzyme activity. NG and VANE (1967) found practically no increase in renal resistance following the injection of Ang. I into the renal artery, whereas FRANKLIN et al. (1970) reported that 19% of the Ang. I was converted into Ang. II. REGOLI and GAUTHIER (1971), using an isolated rabbit kidney preparation, found that 10 to 20% of Ang. I was converted into Ang. II. Injection of high doses of Ang. I into the renal artery resulted in a 7 to 10% conversion as measured by radioimmunoassay (OPARIL et al., 1970).

The Action of Angiotensin on Tubular Resorption of Sodium

Numerous clearance studies have been performed to elucidate the effect of angiotensin on tubular Na reabsorption and both natriuretic and antinatriuretic response reported (for reference see THURAU et al., 1968). Two fundamental difficulties inherent in the clearance method prevent this technique from yielding detailed information about tubular Na transport. Clearance studies can only measure net changes in Na handling; neither the factors responsible nor the site of action can be pinpointed. Furthermore, it is not possible to distinguish between a direct influence of the peptide on the tubular epithelium and an indirect effect brought about by its vasoactive action. For these reasons the following discussion will be limited to those results which permit the evaluation of a possible direct effect of angiotensin on the reabsorptive capacity of the tubular epithelium.

The concept of an inhibitory action of angiotensin on tubular sodium reabsorption was favoured by LEYSSAC (1967). Following the i.v. injection of 5 to 25 ng angiotensin amide, he found proximal tubular reabsorption capacity was decreased, as measured by the occlusion time. These results, however, could not be confirmed by WAHL et al. (1967) who found that the occlusion time was independent of glomerular filtration rate and of intravenously injected angiotensin (12.5 to 50 ng) THURAU et al. (1967). Also in disagreement with the existence of an inhibitory effect of angiotensin upon tubular sodium reabsorption are the results of HORSTER et al. (1966). Using the splitdroplet technique they were not able to detect a change in the reabsorption capacity after either intratubular (25 to 250 μg/100 ml) or peritubular (0.18 μg/kg/min BW, i.v.) application of angiotensin. Similar conclusions were drawn by BURG and ORLOFF (1968) after perfusion of isolated rabbit renal proximal tubules. The reabsorption rate without angiotensin was 0.95 nl/mm/min, and in the presence of angiotensin in the bath medium (2.5 ng/ml) it was 0.90 nl/mm/min. This difference was not statistically significant. At very high intratubular concentrations of angiotensin (10 mg/100 ml) GERTZ (1962) reported a 30% prolongation of reabsorption half-time in split-droplet experiments on rat proximal tubules. This inhibition of reabsorption rate was confirmed by HORSTER et al. (1966). However, since at this unphysiologically high concentration of angiotensin the tubular epithelium changed its visual appearance, they considered this effect to be a pharmacological artefact.

The results obtained from studies on the loop of Henle and distal tubule are even less conclusive. In microperfusion experiments on the loop of Henle of the rat kidney, HORSTER et al. (1966) could not detect any effect on net reabsorption when angiotensin was included in the perfusion fluid at concentrations of 0.5 and 5 μg/100 ml.

On the basis of stop-flow analysis VANDER (1963) postulated a distal tubular inhibitory effect of angiotensin. However, it must be noted that this conclusion was based on an increase of only 4 mEq/l in sodium concentration in the distal tubular stop-flow sample. More evidence for an inhibitory effect of angiotensin on distal reabsorption capacity is obtained by OCHWADT's micropuncture experiments (LOWITZ et al., 1969). When the peritubular capillaries were perfused with Krebs-Henseleit solution containing angiotensin at a concentration of 2.5 μg/ml, reabsorption capacity, as measured by the split oil droplet, decreased (reabsorption half-time increased from 35.6 to 67.7 sec). Accordingly, distal intratubular free-flow sodium concentration increased by some 15 mEq/l during i.v. infusion of 1.5 μg/min/kg BW. The application of angiotensin to the *luminal* membrane of the distal convolution did not change reabsorptive capacity, a finding consistent with the results obtained by HORSTER et al. (1966) on the proximal convolution and on the loop of Henle.

Because of the difficulties inherent in the experimental evaluation of a direct effect of angiotensin on tubular reabsorption processes, several laboratories have investigated the effect of this peptide on the sodium transport in the frog skin, toad skin and toad bladder (BARBOUR et al., 1964; COVIELLO and CRABBE, 1965; MCAFFEE and LOCKE, 1967). They all deny an inhibitory effect of angiotensin on sodium transport. MCAFEE and LOCKE (1967) reported sodium transport of the frog skin to be enhanced by angiotensin. Finally, BONTING et al. (1964) were unable to demonstrate any effect of angiotensin upon the Na-K activated ATPase of kidney homogenates.

Before a clear conclusion about a primary effect on tubular function can be achieved, a good deal more quantitative investigations are required. The preceding data may allow one temporary conclusion, namely, that if Ang. II has any direct effect upon net tubular sodium reabsorption, this is restricted to the distal part of the nephron.

Angiotensin: Its Role in the Tubulo-Glomerular Feedback Mechanism

The juxtaglomerular apparatus, with its renin-producing granular cells, forms part of each afferent arteriole and establishes a point of close contact between the tubular epithelium at the end of Henle's loop (macula densa cells) and the vascular pole of the glomerulus belonging to the same nephron. This tubulo-vascular intimacy suggested to GOORMAGHTIGH (1937, 1944, 1945) that the composition of the tubular fluid flowing past the JGA might be sensed by the macula densa cells, thereby influencing the function of the granular cells and thus regulating the rate of blood flow through the glomerulus. There is now much evidence that the function of this juxtaglomerular structure may be directly involved in the adjustment of blood flow through the glomerulus by its ability to form vasoactive angiotensin locally. Since one intrarenal stimulus for the varying formation rate of angiotensin is thought to be the composition of the tubular fluid at the macula densa cells, this functional connection is referred to as a juxtaglomerular or tubulo-vascular feedback mechanism. Such a feedback system may serve to adjust glomerular filtration rate to the reabsorption capacity of the tubular epithelium. Hence, the adjustment of renal blood flow under many conditions, including autoregulation, may be merely a by-product of a system which regulates filtration rate by changes in vascular resistance (THURAU, 1967).

In 1963, THURAU suggested that intrarenally formed angiotensin might be involved in the autoregulation of renal blood flow and filtration rate. This theory, which is centered on this tubulo-vascular feed-back mechanism, proposes that some tubular fluid characteristics, which vary with filtration rate and are detected at the macula densa cells, influence the local formation rate of Ang. II in the JGA, thereby regulating glomerular blood flow and filtration rate.

Several investigators have tried to elucidate the nature of the macula densa signal. Using an analog computer simulation of hypothetical feedback mechanisms, GUYTON et al. (1964) concluded that the afferent arteriolar resistance might be controlled by the tubular fluid osmolarity at the macula densa site. In a theoretical paper, BRITTON (1968) attempted to unify various views of a number of different investigators into a renin renal autoregulation hypothesis in which the feedback control of glomerular filtration rate plays the central role.

From micropuncture experiments by THURAU and SCHNERMANN (1965) it was concluded that the intratubular NaCl, which can vary in concentration and load in the macula densa segment, provides the stimulus for the local formation of angiotensin. When the sodium concentration in the macula densa segment is increased to isotonicity by microinjection, the proximal convolution belonging to the same nephron unit collapses. This was interpreted as an indication of the interruption of filtrate formation in this nephron. Because cessation of filtration as a response to increased sodium concentration at the macula densa is restricted to the individual nephron under study and the JGA is the only contact between macula densa segment and glomerulus, it was suggested that this reaction is mediated by an increase in local formation of vasoactive angiotensin in the area of the vascular pole. This leads to increased vascular resistance, thereby decreasing blood flow

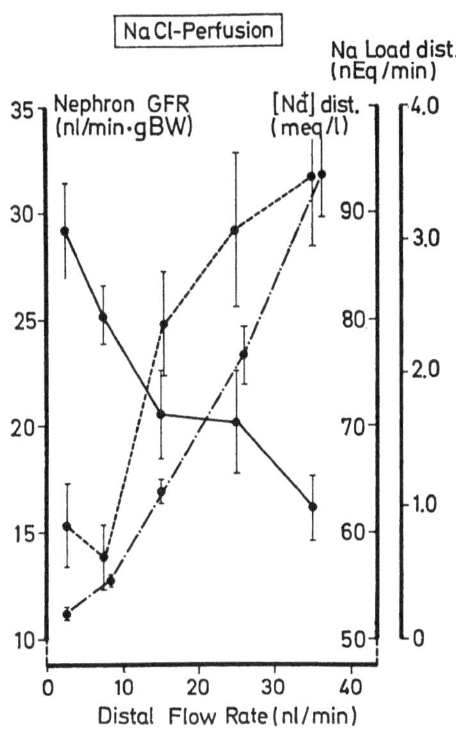

Fig. 3. Correlation between distal flow rate and single nephron glomerular filtration rate (left coordinate), and distal sodium concentration and distal sodium load respectively (right coordinate) during sodium chloride perfusion of the loop of Henle. (From SCHNERMANN et al., 1970)

and filtration rate. SCHNERMANN et al. (1970) used an elegant refinement of the micropuncture technique to give a quantitative demonstration of the operation of a feedback mechanism between Na at the macula densa cells and single nephron filtration rate. Using changes in loop of Henle perfusion rate to mimic changes in filtration rate, they observed a direct correlation between flow rate through the loop and early distal Na load or Na concentration. This, in turn, was inversely related to filtration rate simultaneously measured in the same nephron as shown in Fig. 3. Pressure control in the proximal tubule excluded the possibility that this response was mediated by a primary change in proximal tubular pressure, a mechanism suggested by LEYSSAC (1967). He proposed that changes in filtration rate are achieved by primary alterations in proximal tubular pressure. These were to result from changes in tubular volume reabsorption brought about by variations in the rate of angiotensin formation.

MORGAN (1971), applying a similar technique to that used by SCHNERMANN et al. (1970), was not able to demonstrate feedback control of single-nephron filtration rate. However, this may be explained by the fact that early distal Na concentration and load were not measured and constancy of proximal tubular pressure was not verified, a prerequisite for undisturbed function of the filtration mechanism. In addition, MORGAN (1971) did not measure loop perfusion rate directly but relied on a precalibrated perfusion pump. This may explain the wide scatter in MORGAN's results which, when averaged, fail to demonstrate the operation of a feedback mechanism.

The question of whether an increase or a decrease in Na concentration or load at the macula densa cells stimulates angiotensin formation (or renin release) has been a matter of controversy over the last few years. NASH et al. (1968) found evidence for a sodium chloride-sensitive tubular mechanism affecting renin release. They suggested that renin release was independent of renal blood flow, blood pressure and total body salt and water content. On the other hand, renin release appeared to be dependent on some tubular parameter varying directly with filtered sodium load. VANDER and MILLER (1969) concluded that renin secretion, when elevated by aortic constriction, was inhibited following the administration of natriuretic agents which almost certainly increase Na load in the macula densa segment. An increase in early distal sodium load achieved by natriuretic agents raises additional aspects which must be considered in the interpretation of such results (see p. 484). In this series of experiments VANDER and MILLER (1969) noted an inhibition of renin release during osmotic diuresis. In this situation early distal sodium *load* may well be increased but sodium *concentration* has been found to be decreased (ULLRICH et al., 1963; MALNIC et al., 1966). Thus, these data are consistent with the assumption that the sodium concentration in the tubular fluid at the macula densa cells is a stimulus for renin activation.

The results of experiments in which early distal Na concentration was increased by the use of natriuretic agents and its effect on renin secretion observed are in keeping with a direct correlation between Na concentration at the macula densa cells and renin activity. An increase in early distal Na concentration caused by the administration of ethacrynic acid or furosemide is followed within minutes by an increase in renal venous renin activity, as observed by COOKE et al. (1970) and IMBS et al. (1970). This activation does not occur when the natriuretic agent is administered after cessation of fluid flow past the macula densa achieved by ureteral occlusion. Following release of the occlusion and flow restoration in the tubules, a prompt rise in renal venous renin was again observed within 5 min. These data are in agreement with the assumption that the presence of tubular urine flow with a high NaCl concentration is a prerequisite for prompt stimulation of renin. Similar conclusions were drawn in an earlier study by MEYER et al. (1968), who studied the effect of furosemide on renin release in rabbits. When urinary loss was prevented by shunting urine into the femoral vein, the furosemide-induced increase in plasma-renin activity occurred despite the constancy of blood pressure, plasma-sodium concentration and plasma volume.

Recent observations by THURAU et al. (1971, 1972) have delivered more direct information about the interrelationship between renin activity in the JGA and sodium concentration or load in the macula densa. These investigators varied tubular fluid composition in the macula densa segment of single nephrons and analyzed the renin activity of the attached JGA. When NaCl concentration in the macula densa segment of the nephron was elevated from its naturally low value of 40 mM to 140 mM for 4 to 20 min, the attached JGA showed a highly significant increase in renin activity when compared to control JGAs. Fig. 4a u. b summarizes the changes in renin activity of single JGAs after perfusion of their macula densa region with different test solutions. In each group the juxtaglomerular renin activity of the artificially perfused nephron, shown by the

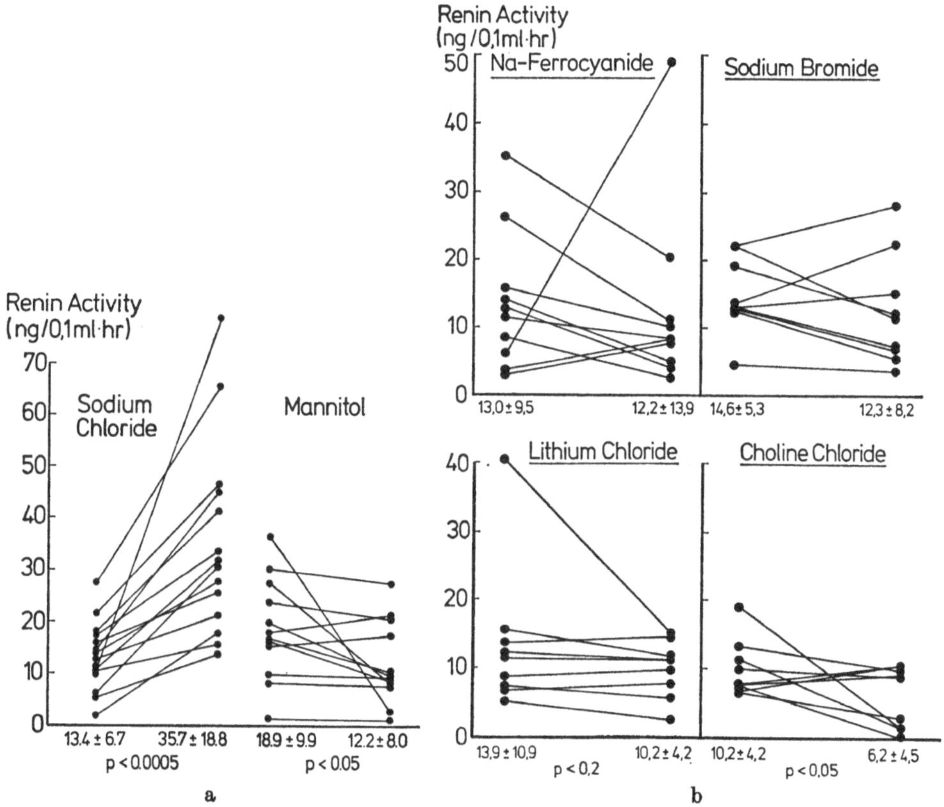

Fig. 4. Dependence of renin activity of single juxtaglomerular apparatuses upon fluid composition at the macula densa segment. The values on the left of each group are mean values of 2 to 4 control juxtaglomerular apparatuses, whose macula densa segments were not artificially perfused. The values on the right of each group represent values of single juxtaglomerular apparatuses following perfusion. The lines connect values obtained from one kidney. At the bottom mean values with S.D. a) Perfusion of the macula densa segment with sodium chloride 140 mM/l and with mannitol 300 mM/l. b) Perfusion of the macula densa segment with sodium ferrocyanide, sodium bromide, lithium chloride and choline chloride respectively. All solutions were isomotic to plasma. (From THURAU, DAHLHEIM, GRÜNER, MASON and GRANGER, unpublished)

symbols on the right, is compared with the mean renin activity of several juxtaglomerular regions from spontaneously perfused nephrons of the same kidney, shown on the left. At an elevated NaCl concentration of 140 mM, renin activity increased from the control value of 13.4 ± 6.7 to 35.7 ng/0.1 ml/h ± 18.8 S.D. This threefold increase is highly significant. Thus, increasing the NaCl concentration at the macula densa cells above its normal hypotonic value of approximately 40 mM raises the renin activity of the JGA. Following Na-free or Cl-free perfusion of the macula densa segment, renin activity of the attached JGA is not increased. The fact that renin activity is not significantly reduced during Na^+ and Cl^- free perfusion is not surprising. The NaCl concentration at the macula densa cells is normally already low and can be made only slightly lower because transepithelial influx of NaCl into the perfusate precludes the possibility of achieving a totally NaCl-free solution in this tubular segment.

These data suggest that both ions, Na^+ and Cl^-, are essential to the activation of renin in the JGA when stimulated from the site of the macula densa cells. This is at variance with results obtained *in vitro* on kidney slices and isolated glomeruli. Renin release from these preparations increases when the Na^+ concentration is elevated in the incubation medium without a concomitant increase in Cl^- concentration (HAMMERSEN et al., 1971; OELKERS et al., 1970; FORGACS et al., 1971).

The observation of an increase in JGA renin activity even after only 4 min of perfusion of the macula densa with 140 mM NaCl raises some doubts about the possibility that this increase in renin activity reflects *de-novo* synthesis. It rather suggests the activation of preformed but physiologically inactive enzyme molecules, an assumption consistent with the experiments of DE VITO et al. (1970), performed on kidney slices, in which they found evidence for the existence of inactive renin molecules (prerenin). Whether these inactive molecules are bound to or are identical to the granules in the epitheloid cells remains to be established.

There is experimental evidence (THURAU, 1972) that it is the NaCl which can move across the luminal membrane into the macula densa cells, and not the intratubular NaCl *per se*, which acts upon the function of the JGA. Studies on the frog skin (BENTLEY, 1969; EIGLER and CRABBE, 1969; NAGEL and DÖRGE, 1970) have shown that the diuretic substance amiloride acts upon net sodium movement by primarily reducing the passive entry of NaCl into the cell. Assuming a similar action upon tubular cells, and this assumption is supported by the results of DUARTE et al. (1971), amiloride would lower the permeability of the luminal membrane of the macula densa cells thus reducing the inflow of NaCl from the tubular fluid. When the macula densa segment is perfused with 140 mM NaCl, which itself increases the JGA renin activity, the addition of amiloride (10^{-4} M) to the perfusate prevents the activation (Fig. 5). Thus, it appears that the NaCl must move across the luminal membrane of the macula densa cells to initiate the reaction which activates renin.

The data obtained by microperfusion of the macula densa segment, together with analysis of renin activity in the JGA, furnish direct evidence for a modifying influence of NaCl in the tubular fluid at the macula densa cells on JGA renin activity. The juxtaglomerular cell complex is positioned between the end of Henle's loop and the vascular pole of the glomerulus belonging to the same nephron unit. In terms of renal function, this cellular complex ties together the tubular system, whose function is energetically bound to the metabolism of the kidney, with the glomerular system whose function is hemodynamic and which is energetically bound to the heart metabolism. It is generally appreciated that the kidney can perform its normal function only when these two partial functions of each nephron unit are in balance with each other. The data presented here strongly suggest that the enzymatic vasoactive principle of the JGA contributes to the balance of the two energetically independent processes by adjusting glomerular blood flow, and hence filtration rate, to the reabsorption capacity of the nephron. It therefore appears that the JGA, with its ability to form angiotensin locally, exercises its physiological role in the phenomenon of tubulo-glomerular balance.

Two groups of investigators (BELLEAU and EARLEY, 1967; GAGNON et al., 1970) have tried to evaluate the contribution of the intrarenal renin-angiotensin system to autoregulation by minimizing the intrarenal renin activity. They did this by maintaining animals on a high-salt diet, supplemented in some cases by DOCA administration. This procedure has been found to lower the JGA renin activity (GAVRAS et al., 1970; GRANGER et al., 1972). If the intrarenal formation of angiotensin is essential for autoregulation and if renin is the limiting factor in the formation of vasoactive Ang. II, then, one would except the efficiency of autoregulation to be diminished in the above conditions. However, in these studies both autoregulation of GFR as well as RBF remained practically unchanged. Unfortunately, the intrarenal renin activity was not determined simultaneously, nor is it possible to deduce whether or not the low renin activity is maintained during the course of an acute experiment and whether renin is the limiting factor in the formation of

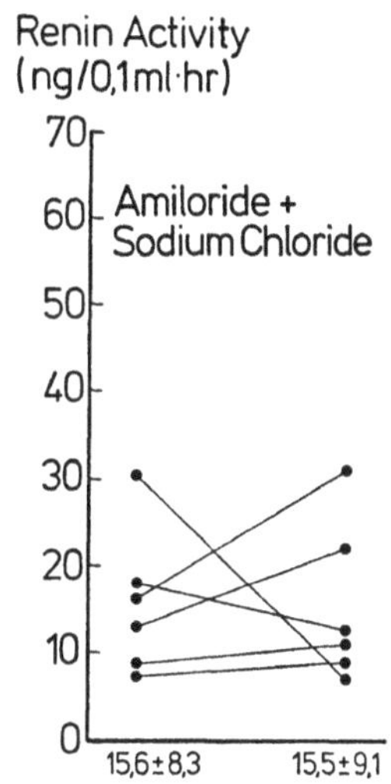

Fig. 5. Perfusion of the macula densa segment with 140 mM/l sodium chloride solution containing amiloride (10^{-4}). For details see legend Fig. 4. (From THURAU, DAHLHEIM, GRÜNER, MASON and GRANGER, unpublished)

Ang. II. Therefore, these data neither prove nor disprove participation of intra renally formed Ang. II in autoregulatory changes in renal resistance.

Several laboratories have tried to assess the contribution of the renin-angiotensin system to renal autoregulation by calculating renal secretion of renin from RBF and arterio-venous difference for renin during changes in arterial pressure. The results of these experiments are not only contradictory but also difficult to interpret. VANDER (1967) and NASH et al. (1968) observed that the changes in renal renin secretion induced by altering renal arterial pressure can be dissociated from hemodynamic parameters by changing the tubular handling of sodium chloride. It therefore appears that factors other than renal arterial pressure play a role. It is also evident that any change in arterial blood pressure or renal blood flow induces changes in glomerular and tubular functions which themselves have been shown to affect juxtaglomerular renin activity.

From the literature it appears that when arterial blood pressure is reduced, renal renin secretion (RBF × a.v. difference) increases (IMBS et al., 1970). However, few reports are available in which glomerular filtration rate and renal blood flow have been measured simultaneously with changes in blood pressure to verify the existence of autoregulation. FOJAS and SCHMID (1970) found the renal renin secretion decreased from 7.2 ± 2.3 S.E. to 3.1 ± 2.2 ng/g kidney/min when blood pressure was lowered in the autoregulatory range from 130 to 103 mmHg and both GFR and RBF remained constant. The simultaneous renal vasodilation may well be the result of this decrease in renin secretion. When blood pressure was further reduced below the autoregulatory range, renal renin secretion (RBF × a.v. diffe-ence) increased.

The different behaviour in renin secretion, which depends on the level of arterial pressure at which the pressure is reduced, is at variance with the results of SKINNER et al. (1964), who reported an inverse relationship between blood pressure and renin "secretion" even in the autoregulatory range.

There is a fundamental problem in attempting to relate these data to the autoregulatory phenomenon insofar as only one component for the formation of vaso-active Ang. II is analyzed when renin secretion rate is measured. Furthermore this procedure does not take into account the amount of renin which leaves the kidney via the lymphatics. Since renin concentration in renal lymph is much higher than in renal venous blood, this *lymphatic* fraction of renin may represent a considerable part of renal renin production. In addition, since changes in lymphatic hydrodynamics during blood pressure alterations may be quite massive whereas blood flow remains relatively constant, it is quite possible that renin outflow through these two routes does not change in parallel. Therefore, the change in renal venous renin secretion cannot be expected to parallel a change in intrarenal renin production. Furthermore, according to the laws of enzymatic reactions, it is not the amount of the renin released by the kidney but rather the local activity at the site of reaction which determines the intrarenal formation rate of angiotensin.

References

BAILIE, M. D., RECTOR, F. C., SELDIN, D. W.: Angiotensin II in arterial and renal venous plasma and renal lymph in the dog. J. clin. Invest. **50**, 119—126 (1971).

BARBOUR, B. H., GILL, J. R., BARTTER, F. C.: Effects of angiotensin on the toad skin. Proc. Soc. exp. Biol. (N. Y.) **116**, 806—809 (1964).

BELLEAU, L. J., EARLEY, L. E.: Autoregulation of renal blood flow in the presence of angiotensin infusion. Amer. J. Physiol. **213**, 1590—1595 (1967).

BENTLEY, P. J.: Amiloride: a potent inhibitor of sodium transport across the toad bladder. J. Physiol. (Lond.) **195**, 317—330 (1969).

BING, J.: Morphological aspects of the renin-angiotensin system. Dan. med. Bull. **11**, 24—32 (1964).

BING, J., KAZIMIERCZAK, J.: Location of renin in the kidney, II. Acta path. microbiol. scand. **47**, 105—112 (1959).

BING, J., KAZIMIERCZAK, J.: Renin content of the different parts of the periglomerular circumference. Localization of renin in the kidney, III. Acta path. microbiol. scand. **50**, 1—11 (1960).

BING, J., KAZIMIERCZAK, J.: Renin content of the different parts of the juxtaglomerular apparatus. 4. Localization of renin in the kidney. Acta path. microbiol. scand. **54**, 80—84 (1962).

BING, J., WIBERG, B.: Localization of renin in the kidney. Acta path. microbiol. scand. **44**, 138—145 (1958).

BONTING, S. L., CANADY, M. R., HAWKINS, N. M.: Angiotensin and renal Na-K activated adenosine triphosphatase. Biochim. biophys. Acta (Amst.) **82**, 427—429 (1964).

BRITTON, K. E.: Renin and renal autoregulation. Lancet **1968 II**, 329—333.

BROWN, J. J., DAVIES, D. L., LEVER, A. F., PARKER, R., ROBERTSON, J. I. S.: Assay of renin in single glomeruli. Renin distribution in the normal rabbit kidney. Lancet **1963 II**, 668—670.

BROWN, J. J., DAVIES, D. L., LEVER, A. F., PARKER, R., ROBERTSON, J. I. S.: The assay of renin in single glomeruli in the normal rabbit and the appearance of the juxtaglomerular apparatus. J. Physiol. (Lond.) **176**, 418—428 (1965).

BROWN, J. J., DAVIES, D. L., LEVER, A. F., PARKER, R. A., ROBERTSON, J. I. S.: The assay of renin in single glomeruli and the appearance of the juxtaglomerular apparatus in the rabbit following renal artery constriction. Clin. Sci. **30**, 223—235 (1966).

BURG, M. B., ORLOFF, J.: Control of fluid absorption in the renal proximal tubule. J. clin. Invest. **47**, 2016—2024 (1968).

COOK, W. F.: Juxtaglomerular cells, the storage site of kidney renin. In: Proc. IV Internat. Congr. of Nephrol., Stockholm, Vol. 2, p. 12—13 (ALWALL, N., BERGLUND, F., JOSEPHSON, B., Eds.). Basel-Munich-New York: S. Karger 1970.

COOK, W. F.: Cellular localization of renin. In: Kidney hormones, p. 117—128 (FISHER, J. W., Ed.). London-New York: Academic Press 1971.

COOK, W. F., GORDON, D. B., PEART, W. S.: The location of renin in the rabbit kidney. J. Physiol. (Lond.) **135**, 46 P (1956).

COOK, W. F., PICKERING, G. W.: The location of renin in the rabbit kidney. J. Physiol. (Lond.) **149**, 526—536 (1959).

COOKE, C. R., BROWN, T. C., ZACHERLE, B. J., WALKER, W. G.: The effect of altered sodium concentration in the distal nephron segment on renin release. J. clin. Invest. **49**, 1630—1638 (1970).

COVIELLO, A., CRABBE, J.: Effect of angiotensin II on active transport of sodium by toad bladder and skin. Biochem. Pharmacol. **14**, 1739—1744 (1965).

DAHLHEIM, H., GRANGER, P., THURAU, K.: A sensitive method for determination of renin activity in the single juxtaglomerular apparatus of the rat kidney. Pflügers Arch. ges. Physiol. **321**, 303—315 (1970).

DAVIS, J. O.: What signals the kidney to release renin. Circulat. Res. **28**, 301—306 (1971).

DE VITO. E.. CABRERA, R. R., FASCIOLO, J. C.: Renin production and release by rat kidney slices. Amer. J. Physiol. **219**, 1042—1045 (1970).

DUARTE, C. G., CHOMETY, F., GIEBISCH, G.: Effect of amiloride, ouabain and furosemide on distal tubular function in the rat. Amer. J. Physiol. **221**, 632—640 (1971).

EDELMAN, R., HARTROFT, P. M.: Localization of renin in juxtaglomerular cells of rabbit and dog through the use of the fluorescent antibody technique. Circulat. Res. **9**, 1069—1077 (1961).

EIGLER, J., CRABBE, J.: Effect of diuretics on active Na-transport in amphibian membranes. In: Renal transport and diuretics, p. 195—208 (THURAU, K., JAHRMÄRKER, J., Eds.). Berlin-Heidelberg-New York: Springer 1969.

FAARUP, P.: Renin location in the different part of the juxtaglomerular apparatus. I. The afferent arteriole and the macula densa. Acta path. microbiol. scand. **71**, 509—521 (1967).

FAARUP, P.: Renin location in the different parts of the juxtaglomerular apparatus in the cat kidney. 2. Fractions of the afferent arteriole, the cell group of Goormaghtigh, the efferent arteriole and the glomerulus. Acta path. microbiol. scand. **72**, 109—117 (1968).

FAARUP, P.: Morphological aspects of the renin-angiotensin system. Copenhagen Bogtrykkeriet Forum 1971.

FOJAS, J. E., SCHMID, H. E.: Renin release, renal autoregulation and sodium excretion in the dog. Amer. J. Physiol. **219**, 464—468 (1970).

FORGÁCS, I., GAÁL, K.: Effect of sodium and osmotic concentration on renin release by renal cortical slices in vitro. Acta physiol. Acad. Sci. hung. **40**, 139—144 (1971).

FRANKLIN, W. G., PEACH, M. J., GILMORE, J. P.: Evidence for the renal conversion of angiotensin I in the dog. Circulat. Res. **27**, 321—324 (1970).

GAGNON, J. A., KELLER, H. I., KOKOTIS, W., SCHRIER, R. W.: Analysis of role of renin-angiotensin system in autoregulation of glomerular filtration. Amer. J. Physiol. **219**, 491—496 (1970).

GAVRAS, H., BROWN, J. J., LEVER, A. F., ROBERTSON, J. I. S.: Changes of renin in individual glomeruli in response to variations of sodium intake in the rabbit. Clin. Sci. **38**, 409—414 (1970).

GERTZ, K. H.: Direct measurement of the transtubular flux of electrolytes and nonelectrolytes in the intact rat kidney. In: Proc. XXII Intern. Congr. Physiol. Sciences, Leiden 1962, p. 370.

GOORMAGHTIGH, N.: L'appareil neuromyoartériel juxtaglomérulaire du rein: ses reactions en pathologie et ses rapports avec le tube urinefère. C. R. Soc. Biol. (Paris) **124**, 293 (1937).

GOORMAGHTIGH, N.: La fonction endocrine des artérioles rénales. Louvain: Fonteyn 1944.

GOORMAGHTIGH, N.: Facts in favour of an endocrine function of the renal arterioles. J. Path. Bact. **57**, 392 (1945).

GRANGER, P., DAHLHEIM, H., THURAU, K.: Enzyme activities of single juxtaglomerular apparatuses in the rat kidney. Kidney International **1**, 78—88 (1972).

GRANGER, P., ROJO-ORTEGA, J. M., CASADO PEREX, S., BOUCHER, R., GENEST, J.: The renin-angiotensin system in newborn dogs. Canad. J. Physiol. Pharmacol. **49**, 134—138 (1971).

GUYTON, A. C., LANGSTONE, J. B., NAVAR, G.: Theory for renal autoregulation by feedback of the juxtaglomerular apparatus. Circulat. Res. **14/15** (Suppl. I), 187—196 (1964).

Hammersen, G., Karsunky, K.-P., Fischinger, J., Rosenthal, J., Taugner, R.: Einfluß der Natriumkonzentration auf die Reninabgabe aus Nierenrindenschnitten und isolierten Glomerula. Pflügers Arch. ges. Physiol. **328**, 344—355 (1971).

Hartroft, P. M., Sutherland, L. E., Hartroft, W. S.: Juxtaglomerular cells as the source of renin. Further studies with the fluorescent antibody technique and the effect of passive transfer of antirenin. Canad. med. Ass. J. **90**, 163—166 (1964).

Horky, K., Rojo-Ortega, J. M., Rodriguez, J., Boucher, R., Genest, J.: Renin, renin substrate and angiotensin I-converting enzyme in the lymph of rats. Amer. J. Physiol. **220**, 307—311 (1971).

Horster, M., Nagel, W., Schnermann, J., Thurau, K.: Zur Frage einer direkten Angiotensinwirkung auf die Natriumresorption im proximalen Tubulus und in der Henle'schen Schleife der Rattenniere. Pflügers Arch. ges. Physiol. **292**, 118—128 (1966).

Imbs, J. L., Velly, J., Fontaine, J. L., Schwartz, J.: Controle de la sécrétion de rénine. Nephron **7**, 499—511 (1970).

Itskovits, H. D., Odya, C.: Intrarenal formation of angiotensin I. Science **174**, 58 (1971).

Leyssac, P. P.: Intrarenal function of angiotensin. Fed. Proc. **26**, 55—59 (1967).

Lowitz, H.-D., Stumpe, K. O., Ochwadt, B.: Micropuncture study of the action of angiotensin-II on tubular sodium and water reabsorption in the rat. Nephron **6**, 173—187 (1969).

Malnic, G., Klose, R. M., Giebisch, G.: Microperfusion study of distal tubular potassium and sodium transfer in rat kidney. Amer. J. Physiol. **211**, 548—559 (1966).

McAfee, R., Locke, W.: Effect of angiotensin amide on sodium isotope flux and short-circuit current of isolated frog skin. Endocrinology **81**, 1301—1305 (1967).

Meyer, D.: Normale und pathologische Morphologie des juxtaglomerulären Apparates. In: Fortschritte der Nephrologie, p. 443—444 (Bohle, A., Schubert, G. E., Eds.). Stuttgart-New York: F. K. Schattauer 1971.

Meyer, P., Menard, J., Papanicolaou, N., Alexandre, J. M., Deveaux, C., Milliez, P.: Mechanism of renin release following furosemide diuresis in rabbit. Amer. J. Physiol. **215**, 908—915 (1968).

Morgan, T.: A microperfusion study of influence of macula densa on glomerular filtration rate. Amer. J. Physiol. **220**, 186—190 (1971).

Nagel, W., Dörge, A.: Effect of amiloride on sodium transport of frog skin. I. Action on intracellular sodium content. Pflügers Arch. ges. Physiol. **317**, 84—92 (1970).

Nairn, R., Fraser, K. B., Chadwick, C. S.: The histological localization of renin with fluorescent antibody. Brit. J. exp. Path. **40**, 155—163 (1959).

Nash, F. D., Rostorfer, H. H., Bailie, M. D., Wathen, R. L., Schneider, E. G.: Renin release. Relation to renal sodium load and dissociation from hemodynamic changes. Circulat. Res. **22**, 473—487 (1968).

Ng, K. K. F., Vane, J. R.: Conversion of angiotensin I to angiotensin II. Nature (Lond.) **216**, 762—766 (1967).

Oelkers, W., Molzahn, M., Samwer, K. F., Kreiser, H., Kutschke, H.: Reninabgabe aus Nierenschnitten in Abhängigkeit von der Elektrolytzusammensetzung des Mediums. Pflügers Arch. ges. Physiol. **321**, 67—82 (1970).

Oparil, S., Sanders, C. A., Haber, E.: In-vivo and in-vitro conversion of angiotensin I to angiotensin II in dog blood. Circulat. Res. **26**, 591 (1970).

Peart, W. S., Gordon, D., Cook, W., Pickering, C.: Distribution of renin in the rabbit kidney. Circulation **14**, 981—982 (1956).

Peart, W. S.: Renin and hypertension. Ergebn. Physiol. **50**, 409—432 (1959).

Regoli, D., Gauthier, R.: Studies on the intrarenal role of renin: effects of vasoconstrictors on an isolated rabbit kidney preparation. Un. méd. Can. **100**, 733—739 (1971).

Schnermann, J., Wright, F. S., Davis, J. M., Stackelberg, W., von, Grill, G.: Regulation of superficial nephron filtration rate by tubulo-glomerular feedback. Pflügers Arch. ges. Physiol. **318**, 147—175 (1970).

Skinner, S. L., McCubbin, J. W., Page, I. H.: Control of renin secretion. Circulat. Res. **15**, 64—76 (1964).

Sutherland, L. E.: A fluorescent antibody study of juxtaglomerular cells using the freeze-substitution technique. Nephron **7**, 512—523 (1970).

Thurau, K.: Fundamentals of renal circulation. In: Proc. 2nd Intern. Congr. Nephrol., Prague 1963, p. 51—61. Amsterdam: Excerpta Med. Found. 1964.

Thurau, K.: The nature of autoregulation of renal blood flow. In: Proc. III Intern. Congr. Nephrology, Vol. I, p. 162—173 (Handler, J. S., Ed.). Basel-New York: Hans Huber 1967.

Thurau, K., Schnermann, J.: Die Natriumkonzentration an den Macula densa-Zellen als regulierender Faktor für das Glomerulumfiltrat. Klin. Wschr. **43**, 410—413 (1965).

Thurau, K., Schnermann, J., Nagel, W., Horster, M., Wahl, M.: Composition of tubular fluid in the macula densa segment as a factor regulating the function of the juxtaglomerular apparatus. Circulat. Res. **20/21** (Suppl. 2), 79—89 (1967).

THURAU, K.: Juxtaglomerular apparatus: Its role in the function of the single nephron unit. In: Modern diuretic therapy in the treatment of cardiovascular and renal disease. Excerpta Medica Amsterdam 1973, p. 84—92 (A. F. LANT and G. M. WILSON, Eds.).

THURAU, K., DAHLHEIM, H., GRANGER, P.: On the local formation of angiotensin at the site of the juxtaglomerular apparatus. In: Proc. Intern. Congr. Nephrol. Stockholm 1969, Vol. 1, p. 24—30 (HEPTINSTALL, R. H., Ed.). Basel-New York: S. Karger 1970.

THURAU, K., DAHLHEIM, H., GRÜNER, A., MASON, J., GRANGER, P.: The dependence of renin activity in the single juxtaglomerular apparatus of the rat nephron upon NaCl in the fluid of the macula densa segment. In: Proc. XXV Intern. Congr. Physiol. Sciences Munich, 1971, p. 564.

THURAU, K., DAHLHEIM, H., GRÜNER, A., MASON, J., GRANGER, P.: Functional and enzymatic analyses of single juxtaglomerular apparatus. In: Hypertension — 1972, p. 63—72 (GENEST, J., KOIW, E., Eds.). Berlin-Heidelberg-New York: Springer 1972.

THURAU, K., VALTIN, H., SCHNERMANN, J.: Kidney. Ann. Rev. Physiol. **30**, 441—524 (1968).

TOBIAN, L.: Renin release and its role in renal function and control of salt balance and arterial pressure. Fed. Proc. **26**, 48—54 (1967).

ULLRICH, K. J., SCHMIDT-NIELSEN, B., O'DELL, R., PEHLING, G., GOTTSCHALK, C. W., LASSITER, W. E., MYLLE, M.: Micropuncture study of composition of proximal and distal tubular fluid in rat kidney. Amer. J. Physiol. **204**, 527—531 (1963).

VANDER, A. J.: Inhibition of distal tubular sodium reabsorption by angiotensin II. Amer. J. Physiol. **205**, 133—138 (1963).

VANDER, A. J.: Control of renin release. Physiol. Rev. **47**, 359—382 (1967).

VANDER, A. J., MILLER, R.: Control of renin secretion in the unanesthetized dog. Amer. J. Physiol. **207**, 537—546 (1969).

WAHL, M., NAGEL, W., THURAU, K.: On the application of the occlusion time method for measurements of lateral net fluxes in the proximal convolution of the rat kidney. Pflügers Arch. ges. Physiol. **298**, 141—153 (1967).

WARREN, B., JOHNSON, A. G., HOOBLER, S. W.: Characterisation of the renin-antirenin system. J. exp. Med. **123**, 1109—1120 (1966).

Morphological Effects of Angiotensin in Arteries

PRISCILLA KINCAID-SMITH, A. FRIEDMAN, and J. B. HOBBS

This review will consider the morphological effects of angiotensin on vessels, compare these with the findings in other types of acute vascular injury and discuss the possible role of angiotensin in the pathogenesis of hypertensive vascular injury.

Vessel Changes

The direct action of angiotensin on vascular smooth muscle preparations is always contraction (ZUBERBUHLER and BOHR, 1964; WALTER and BASSENGE, 1969; BOHR and UCHIDA, 1967; KIPROV et al., 1968) or in the case of small renal artery preparations, no effect at all (BOHR and UCHIDA, 1967). The effect on intact vessels is more complex and both central (BICKERTON and BUCKLEY, 1961) and peripheral sympathetic mechanisms (MCCUBBIN and PAGE, 1963; BENELLI et al., 1964) have been demonstrated. A direct vasoconstrictor effect was long ago demonstrated on the vascular smooth muscle.

In the intact anesthetized rat, infusion with varying doses of angiotensin over periods of 5 to 25 min has resulted in an increase in blood pressure and total peripheral resistance without increasing cardiac output (MANDEL and SAPIRSTEIN, 1962). Simultaneous measurement of the regional blood flow and regional vascular resistance was shown to be reduced or unchanged, whereas renal vascular resistance was increased by 100 to 200%. Vascular resistance of the coronary and pulmonary circulation was unchanged, that of the spleen and adrenal slightly increased, and a larger increase was found in resistance of the skin vessels.

A. Aorta and Major Branches

A large amount of Angiotensin II (66 μg) injected as a bolus into the common iliac artery of rats and fixed within 20 to 30 sec by perfusion with 5% buffered glutaraldehyde resulted in separation of interendothelial cell junctions without any other change visible by electron microscopy (CONSTANTINIDES and ROBINSON, 1969). In some cases a large area of subendothelial collagen was exposed to the circulating blood. The authors believe that the presence of endothelial pseudopods in some areas, and pronounced flattening of the endothelium, suggested that separation of the junction was due to angiotensin-induced contraction of the endothelial cells.

ROBERTSON and KHAIRALLAH (1971) studied endothelial-cell contraction induced in adult rats by intracardiac injections of much smaller doses of several vasoactive agents. Temporary widening of intercellular spaces or junctions with appearance of tortuous interendothelial channels or gaps (IEGs) were demonstrated by rapid (12 to 15 sec) injections of Ang. II (total dose 0.1 to 10 ng) and simultaneous administration of electron markers (colloidal carbon, ferritin, horseradish peroxidase) or labeled serum lipoprotein fractions. Injections were followed by immediate *in-vivo* perfusion-fixation and processing for light and electron microscopy-radioautography.

In similar studies using tritiated Ang. II (ROBERTSON and KHAIRALLAH, in press) radioactivity was found in the nuclear zone of vascular and cardiac muscle cells as well as in mitochondria but not in other intracellular organelles. Control injections of either tritiated L-tyrosine or isoleucine failed to show passage of these amino acids in the short time of the injections beyond the endothelial layers of the aorta or coronary arteries. These findings were interpreted as suggesting that either Ang. II or some of its rapidly generated metabolic fragments may have an action on vascular muscle cell nuclei.

B. Small Arteries

1. Mesentery and Intestine

An important contribution to pathogenesis of acute hypertensive vascular disease was made by GIESE (1964) who observed the *in-vivo* pattern of reactivity of small arteries to angiotensin through an abdominal-window technique developed by PALMER and WILKINS (1960). Infusion of angiotensin (about 1.7 μg/kg/min) produced an immediate response of the vessels which coincided with a rise in blood pressure. Pronounced dilatations appeared in the proximal parts of the mesenteric arteries; sometimes separated by a short segment of constriction. Distally many arteries showed a pattern of alternating dilatation and constriction. Some vessels were uniformly constricted and others showed mild dilatation. As the infusion was continued this pattern persisted in some animals and disappeared in others. With repeated angiotensin infusions the areas of dilatation and constriction tended to reappear in the same areas.

GIESE (1961) also demonstrated deposits of serum (conjugated with lissamine rhodamine B 200) in the walls of small arteries and arterioles of pancreas, intestine and mesentery following angiotensin infusion. These deposits sometimes involved the whole circumference of the vessel though often discrete sections were affected. These areas of fluorescence were noted to correspond with the site of PAS-positive deposits. In this experiment 10 μg doses of angiotensin had been injected every 2 to 5 min for between 2 and $4^1/_2$ h before the animal was killed. This time lapse may have been long enough to permit medial necrosis to occur and thus did not help to resolve the question as to whether extrusion of plasma precedes and causes medial necrosis (SCHURMANN and MACMAHON, 1933) or muscle degeneration precedes regional necrosis (MONTGOMERY and MUIRHEAD, 1954). GIESE (1964) subsequently combined vital microscopy with colloidal carbon infusion, and observed the time sequence of permeability changes. Carbon deposits in the walls of arteries formed very rapidly within as little as 50 sec after the appearance of dilatations and constrictions in the vessels. Thus increased permeability was shown to account for the PAS-positive deposits which could not have been due to degenerative changes in the medial smooth muscle in this short time.

A distinctive pattern of carbon labeling of the vessels was observed. The constricted arterial segments never showed labeling and this was predominantly seen in widely dilated areas, although not all dilated segments became labeled. The proximal dilated parts of the intestinal arteries were most commonly involved. Diffuse labeling, suggesting capillary leakage, also occurred, often in relation to labeled arterioles. The arteriolar labeling was arranged in parallel streaks in the media of the vessels, perpendicular to the long axis of the artery and included discrete collections of carbon in the intercellular areas between smooth muscle cells of the media. Carbon particles were found on either side of the internal elastic membrane.

OLSEN (1968) has confirmed these findings and shown fluorescence in the walls of arteries 60 to 100 micron in diameter in the same distribution as the carbon labeling observed by GIESE. Only dilated parts showed marked labeling but in occasional constricted areas single grains of fluorescent protein could be seen. About 20% of dilated areas showed evidence of permeability and in such areas the vessel wall appeared thicker. The deposition of plasma proteins in the vessel wall had a hyaline appearance on hematoxylin and eosin stain and the nuclei of the smooth muscle cells appeared normal.

When hydralazine was added to the continuing infusion of angiotensin in the experiments of GIESE (1964) the blood pressure returned to normal over about 10 min during which time all the constrictions and most of the dilatations also returned to normal. Some of the areas of dilatation persisted, however, and when colloidal carbon was injected after the blood pressure had returned to normal, labeling was confined to these areas. If a rise in blood pressure was prevented by prior administration of dihydralazine fewer areas of dilatation and constriction were seen and no labeling was noted.

Hence, in response to angiotensin-induced acute hypertension there are focal changes in the caliber of the walls of arteries. The constrictions and some of the dilatations promptly revert to normal on reduction of blood pressure, whereas some areas of dilatation persist and permit continued entry of colloidal carbon into the wall.

Our experiments with angiotensin infusions into rats confirm the changes which GIESE described in the mesentery and intestinal arteries. We examined ultramicroscopic changes in vessels fixed within 3 min of the development of areas of dilatation and constriction in vessels. The most obvious ultrastructural abnormalities were observed in dilated areas of the vessel wall. The minimal changes observed were vacuolation and swelling of the endothelial cells, without separation of the endothelial junctions. More marked changes occurred when noradrenaline was used together with angiotensin (KINCAID-SMITH et al., 1972). On occasions platelet aggregation was seen in relation to these areas. Gaps in the endothelium packed with platelet thrombi were also seen and some arteries showed very thin rregular walls.

2. *Renal Vessels*

Injection of angiotensin into normal rats causes blanching of the kidney (BYROM, 1964). The renal artery becomes markedly dilated as far as or slightly beyond the origins of its primary branches. More distally the vessels show marked narrowing. Within about 5 min the blood pressure returns to normal and kidneys examined at this time showed no frank necrosis in the hilar arteries, but in a number of rats these arteries were dilated and thin-walled with irregularities in outline. A few showed patchy loss of medial staining, suggesting rupture of muscle fibers. Since the vaso-activity was present for only about 5 min these changes could not be due to ischemic damage, which takes at least 60 min to cause arterial necrosis (SHEEHAN and DAVIS, 1959). When the other kidney was removed the next day, necroses of larger arteries in the hilum and, occasionally, of smaller vessels were seen. The necroses were medial and involved part or all of the circumference. Intermittent subcutaneous doses of angiotensin (2 μg three times daily) producing mild transient increases in blood pressure, resulted in loss of nuclear staining in muscle cells of the media of medium sized arteries within 24 h (KATZ et al., 1962). PAS-positive material was seen in the groundsubstance of the media.

After 7 days of intermittent subcutaneous injections of angiotensin the degenerative changes were much worse than those observed after 24 h. Marked proliferation of both cellular and fibrous elements of the intima were seen, the internal elastic lamina was fragmented and vacuoles seen throughout the vessel wall. Vessels of brain, heart, aorta, liver and spleen were also examined after 2 weeks of intermittent angiotensin injections and showed no degenerative lesions.

Degenerative changes in the media of renal vessels were not seen by KOLETSKY et al. (1966) nor by KAMURA et al. (1966). The former authors gave angiotensin infusions lasting 8 to 10 h on each of 5 days. This caused a moderate elevation of blood pressure (150 to 180 mmHg systolic) during the infusion. Diffuse thickening of arterioles with narrowing of lumen were seen in vessels of 30 to 100 u external diameter in the kidney, gastrointestinal tract, adrenal and pancreas. Endothelial cells were enlarged and projected into the lumen. The internal elastic lamina was prominently scalloped and areas of fibrinoid necrosis were also seen. KAMURA et al. (1966) gave a constant infusion of Ang. II for 1 h. The dose is not specified, but it was sufficient to maintain the blood pressure at over 180 mmHg systolic and 150 mmHg diastolic. The small arcuate and interlobular arteries were contracted showing marked wrinkling of the internal elastic lamina and thickened media, and slight vacuolation of the media was noted.

Renovascular hypertensive rats, with a clip on the artery of the solitary kidney showed more severe and extensive damage following angiotensin than that seen in normal rats (BYROM, 1964). Arterial necrosis was found at 1 day in the solitary kidney in 9 of 10 animals studied. This involved arteries of all sizes and in 3 animals included numerous aneurysms and necroses in the glomerular capillaries. In 5 hypertensive rats with one clipped and one untouched kidney the clipped kidney showed extensive arterial necrosis. When the clip was removed, just before the angiotensin injection, the damage to the previously clipped kidney was massive, almost every artery between the afferent arterioles being necrotic (BYROM, 1969). It is possible that exposure of the vessels in the untouched kidney to the high blood pressure may render them more resistant to the further acute rise in blood pressure. By comparison the vessels in the clipped kidney had been partially protected by the clip from hypertensive effects and thus seemed to be more susceptible to acute hypertensive damage.

The glomerular lesions were of two types (BYROM, 1964), aneurysms and focal necroses. The necrotic areas contained fibrin and the demonstration of a basement membrane encircling the periphery of each necrotic area confirmed their aneurysmal nature.

3. *Rabbit Ear Chamber*

Vascular changes were also observed by us *in vivo* in renal vessels grafted as fetal allografts into a modified Sandison-Clark transparent ear chamber by a method previously described by HOBBS and CLIFF (1971). Injections of 1 μg/kg of angiotensin were given into the contralateral ear vein and there was an acute rise in systolic blood pressure from 85 to 90 mmHg to 120 mmHg within 20 sec. Within 30 sec the observed interlobular renal arteries, and more particularly the afferent arterioles, developed constrictions separated by areas of relative dilatation. The effect increased over 3 to 4 min and finally all the glomeruli stopped flowing as these vessels became intensely constricted. The circulation appeared to cease for 30 sec. Then, from $5^1/_2$ min after injection, the vessels rapidly resumed their original diameter and a brisk blood flow resulted. A second injection given within the next 2 h produced a similar result but the intensity of the vasoconstriction was reduced by about half.

When these vessels showed a primary response the whole graft was flooded with Karnovsky fixative *in situ* so that the constrictions could be observed until fixation was complete. After trimming to section the observed constrictions, light microscopic and ultrastructural evidence of damage appeared to be limited to the endothelial cells which showed marked vacuolation especially in regions where the endothelial cells bulged into the vessel lumen, suggesting this was the point of constriction. There appeared to be an increase in distance between these cells and the underlying muscle, with some derangement of the microtubules connecting the two. The endothelial junctions were very well preserved and the intracellular vacuolation appeared quite remote from the intercellular borders.

At the time of the experiment the grafted tissue had differentiated to a stage of maturity about 2 weeks post-partum, judging from the glomerular and tubular maturity. The graft retains local nervous responses to stimuli, such as direct pressure, adrenaline, noradrenaline and serotonin, but whether the vascular nerves are anastomosed to those of the recipient is unconfirmed.

C. Afferent Arterioles and Juxtaglomerular Apparatus

RUYTER (1925) first described the cytoplasmic granules in specific cells (epithelioid-like cells) within the media of the distal portion of the afferent arteriole to the glomerulus. The epithelioid cells are larger than smooth muscle cells, and contain a large round or oval nucleus with a delicate chromatin structure. In most stains the cytoplasm of the cell is larger and paler than the cytoplasm of smooth muscle cells (FAARUP, 1971).

The pressor activity of renal extracts was described in 1898 (TIGERSTEDT and BERGMAN) and the epithelioid cells and granules were described by RUYTER (1925). However, it was not until GOORMAGHTIGH (1939, 1940) observed epithelioid-cell hyperplasia and hypergranulation in the afferent arterioles in the clipped kidney in unilateral renovascular hypertension that he suggested that these cells were the site of renin production. In some cases of hypertension, epithelioid cells and granular cytoplasmic deposits may be found in much more proximal sites along the afferent arteriole, well separated from the juxtaglomerular apparatus (FAARUP et al., 1970).

Rats given 2 μg angiotensin subcutaneously three times daily for up to 14 days were studied by KATZ et al. (1962). This regime caused intermittent blood pressure elevations of about 30 mmHg lasting about $1^1/_2$ h. On the first day after angiotensin injections there was an increase in the number of epithelioid cells and in their granularity, as calculated by the method of HARTROFT and HARTROFT (1953). The number of granules increased up to day 7 of angiotensin injections, but in those examined at 14 days the granularity had returned towards control values. The epithelioid cells retained their swollen appearance. A group of rats given 20 μg epinephrine three times daily, which gave a similar blood pressure response, showed no obvious changes in the epithelioid cell, or the degree of granularity. When aldosterone was given at the same time as the angiotensin, the increase in granularity did not occur.

Pathogenesis of Hypertensive Vascular Damage

A. Role of Angiotensin

Angiotensin may be an important initiating event leading to the structural lesions that are characteristic of malignant or accelerated hypertension. Angiotensin causes endothelial damage to the aorta (ROBERTSON and KHAIRALLAH,

1971), the large arteries (CONSTANTINIDES and ROBINSON, 1969), and the small arteries (KINCAID-SMITH et al., 1972). The damage is apparent as swelling and vacuolation of the endothelium, and in the larger vessels endothelial cell separation has been observed. This exposes the underlying collagen to the circulating blood. Collagen is a powerful cause of platelet aggregation (MUSTARD, 1967) and this is probably augmented by the enhancing effect of angiotensin on adrenaline and ADP-induced platelet aggregation (POPLAWSKI, 1970). Increased platelet adhesion has been shown by the glass bead-column method in human hypertensive cardiovascular disease (POPLAWSKI et al., 1968). In some of our preparations platelet aggregations in relation to intact though abnormal endothelium have been observed. With platelet aggregation ADP is released, which in turn induces the release of platelet serotonin (PACKHAM et al., 1967) and a factor or factors increasing vessel permeability (MUSTARD, 1967). In human hypertensive biopsy material BIAVA et al. (1964) have shown quite substantial deposits of hyaline material in arteriolar walls with no apparent ultramicroscopic changes in the smooth muscle or endothelium. LENDRUM (1963) observed fibrin under the internal elastic membrane and considered this deposit important in causing the subsequent degeneration of the internal elastic lamina and the media. BYROM (1969) believes that the endothelial proliferation seen in acute hypertensive lesions may be an attempt to plug a leak in an overstretched or necrotic media.

It is still widely believed that the renin-angiotensin system is involved in causing renovascular malignant hypertension (CATT et al., 1971) although LOUIS et al. (1970) were able to produce experimental renovascular hypertension in the presence of apparently successful immunization against Ang. II. CARRETERO and BUJAK (1972) found that in acute malignant hypertension antibodies against Ang. II produced a striking fall in the blood pressure and increase in survival. No such effect was noted in benign hypertension. The vascular pattern of dilatation and constriction in experimental renovascular hypertension is very similar to that seen with angiotensin infusions. These changes have been seen during hypertensive crises and also in experimental malignant hypertension in the mesenteric vessels (BYROM, 1954) and in the cerebral vessels of the hypertensive rat. Retinal arteries also showed definite constrictions and dilatations (ABT and BRUCKNER, 1950; BYROM, 1963). These variations in caliber disappear and reappear in the same sites with variations in the blood pressure. For many years it had been believed that the clinical and pathological manifestations of malignant hypertension were caused by intense vasoconstriction with resultant focal ischemia (VOLHARD, 1948; BYROM, 1954). Accordingly ABT and BRUCKNER (1950) looked for degenerative changes in the constricted areas and found none. There is no mention of dilated aıeas being examined. BYROM (1963) found that after a few weeks of hypertension, lowering of the blood pressure did not abolish the changes in the caliber of the vessel wall, suggesting that a structural lesion had developed. However, if the clip was removed from the renal artery many constrictions and dilatations of the arteries disappeared. Gross focal dilatations rarely returned to normal. These findings are analogous to those of GIESE (1964) with angiotensin infusions. While the renal artery clips were in place and angiotensin levels presumably high, the vascular reactive pattern persisted, in spite of reduction of the blood pressure to normal. When the clips were removed and the kidneys were no longer ischemic, the blood pressure, and probably the angiotensin levels, returned to normal, as did the functional variations in caliber. However, some dilatations show increased permeability and vascular damage, and these would not be expected to return to normal.

Areas of vessels which have undergone dilatation with angiotensin are capable of constriction under appropriate conditions, if for example pressure is lowered by venesection. As the blood volume is restored the variations in caliber reappear (GIESE, 1964).

By the use of a combined microangiographic and histologic technique in steroid-induced hypertension in the rat, HILL and HEPTINSTALL (1968) were able to confirm the presence of dilatations and constrictions in the kidney. The interlobular arteries were most affected and some of the dilated vessels had fibrinoid accumulation in the wall and lumen, with some adventitial and interstitial cellular reaction and often a necrotic or hyalinized muscularis. By contrast the constricted vessels were usually normal in appearance.

B. Mechanical Factors

1. Distension

As has been mentioned above, prevention of the rise in blood pressure by prior administration of dihydralazine (GIESE, 1964) resulted in a lessening of the vascular reactive pattern of segmental dilatation and constriction and in absence of the increased permeability of the vessels usually produced by angiotensin infusion. Acute distension of the arterial system by forcible injection of sufficient Ringer's solution, to raise the blood pressure acutely by some 100 mmHg in the rat resulted in focal necrosis of arterial walls at 3 days (BYROM and DODSON, 1948). Renal vessels appeared to be especially vulnerable as the renal arcuate, interlobular and afferent arterioles were all affected though arteries in other areas were not. MASSON et al. (1951), in a similar experiment, witnessed intimal edema, distension and fibrinoid necrosis of small arteries. The lesions did not appear until the third day and were limited to the kidneys. Vessels of the pancreas and mesentery were also involved in the experiments of WOLFGARTEN and MARGAREY (1959). They measured accurately the blood pressure responses to acute distension of the vasculature and were also able to demonstrate a positive statistical correlation between the blood-pressure changes and the development of microscopic lesions. They examined the tissues earlier than the other groups, and found fibrinoid necrosis present as early as 12 h. In 2 of 9 animals killed between 14 and 21 days there was intimal proliferation in the small arteries, which in some cases almost occluded the lumen. Thus vascular lesions can be caused by an increase in blood pressure caused by a sudden increase in vascular volume. Whether the vessels undergo localized dilatations and constrictions, and whether the pathogenetic mechanisms are the same as with angiotensin-induced hypertension, is not known.

2. Vascular Dynamics

The flow of blood under pulsatile pressure through a constricted vessel into a dilated channel results in low pressure turbulent flow. Two further phenomena occur at the most proximal part of the dilated segments. One of these is relative stasis within eddy currents, which would favor the formation of platelet microthrombi. ROBB and JACOBSON (1963) have used vital microphotography in the rat mesentery, and observed the formation of platelet microthrombi in relation to the endothelium just distal to segmental constrictions. These rapidly dislodged and were seen to float away to embolize smaller vessels more distally. By their release of enzymes, including permeability factors, these platelet aggregates could contribute to the increased permeability seen at the dilated areas, and within the microcirculation supplied by the affected vessels as noted by GIESE (1964).

Another factor which could possibly contribute is the Ventury effect causing a sucking action on the endothelium. The magnitude of this effect would be dependent on the blood pressure as well as the extent of the segmental dilatations and constrictions induced by angiotensin.

3. Hypertension

The persistence of some areas of dilatation after the blood pressure has been lowered by use of hydralazine (GIESE, 1964) suggests that angiotensin has effects on the blood vessel wall which are unrelated to its effects on blood pressure. The areas of dilatation are the areas of increased permeability and damage, and yet not all the dilated areas show this increased permeability. Both GIESE (1966) and OLSEN (1968) suggest that factors other than angiotensin must be involved. As well as the effect of angiotensin on the vessel wall and its effect on platelets (POPLAWSKI, 1970) the other major factor may be the actual blood pressure elevation. Both of these often interrelated factors appear to be important. Without a rise in blood pressure, angiotensin causes only mild changes in vessel caliber and no evidence of increased permeability. Vascular damage is not as severe when hypertension is due to pressor agents other than angiotensin (GIESE, 1962, 1964). Extremely high elevations of the blood pressure are required to produce vessel lesions using methoxamine, for example (GIESE, 1962). Similarly, mechanical distension will only cause vessel lesions when the blood pressure is raised to very high levels (BYROM and DODSON, 1948; WOLFGARTEN and MARGAREY, 1959).

Other pressor agents can also cause vascular injury. GIESE (1964) infused norepinephrine and methoxamine into nephrectomized rats and observed mainly vasoconstriction, but occasionally moderate distension of the intestinal arteries. Colloidal carbon deposits were seen to form early in dilated areas. HERBERTSON and KELLAWAY (1960) noted with methoxamine-induced lesions that vessels with extensive medial necrosis were usually dilated, and when a segment of vessel wall was affected a local dilatation was often found. It was not possible to tell in this study whether injury was the cause of the dilatation or whether dilatation preceded the observable damage.

Summary

Infusion of angiotensin produces areas of constriction and dilatation in arteries and arterioles. Damage consisting of hyaline deposits in the walls of these vessels is limited to dilated areas. This may be due to mechanical stretching with separation of endothelial desmosomes and leakage of plasma constituents into the vessel wall.

The constrictions and dilatations are more marked when the blood pressure is elevated but may persist after the blood pressure is lowered to normal levels. Damage in dilated areas may also continue when the blood pressure is normal provided that dilatations and constrictions persist. Although hypertension is undoubtedly one of the factors contributing to the vessel damage it appears that angiotensin may cause vascular damage in other ways. It may have a direct effect on the endothelium. Additional damage could be due to local turbulence in dilated areas and to the formation of platelet aggregates in the proximal portion of dilated areas. Angiotensin also enhances platelet aggregation produced by adrenalin and ADP and platelet thrombi may themselves further damage vessel walls by release of enzymes and permeability factors.

References

ABT, K., BRUCKNER, R.: Netzhautgefäßspasmen bei artifiziell hypertonischen Ratten. Ophthalmologica (Basel) **119**, 17 (1950).

ALTURA, B. M.: Evaluation of neurohumeral substances in local regulation of blood flow. Amer. J. Physiol. **212**, 1447 (1967).

BENELLI, G., DELLA BELLA, D., GANDINI, A.: Angiotensin and peripheral sympathetic nerve activity. Brit. J. Pharmacol. **22**, 211 (1964).

BIAVA, C. G., DYRDA, I., GENEST, J., BENCOSANE, S. A.: Renal hyaline arteriosclerosis. An electron microscope study. Amer. J. Path. **44**, 349 (1964).

BICKERTON, R. K., BUCKLEY, J. P.: Evidence for a central mechanism in angiotensin induced hypertension. Proc. Soc. exp. Biol. (N. Y.) **106**, 834 (1961).

BOHR, D. F., UCHIDA, E.: Individualities of vascular smooth muscles in response to angiotensin. Circulat. Res. **21** (Suppl. II), 135 (1967).

BYROM, F. B.: The nature of malignancy in hypertensive disease. Evidence from the retina of the rat. Lancet **1963 I**, 516.

BYROM, F. B.: Angiotensin and renal vascular damage. Brit. J. exp. Path. **45**, 7 (1964).

BYROM, F. B.: The hypertensive vascular crisis. An experimental study. London: William Heinemann 1969.

BYROM, F. B.: The pathogenesis of hypertensive encephalopathy and its relation to the malignant phase of hypertension. Lancet **1954 II**, 201.

CARRETERO, O. A., BUJAK, B.: The role of angiotensin in benign and malignant experimental hypertension. An immunological approach. In: Hypertension — 1972. 2nd International Symposium on the Renin-Angiotensin-Aldosterone-Sodium System, p. 473 (GENEST, J., KOIW, E., Eds.). Berlin-Heidelberg-New York: Springer 1972.

CATT, K. J., ZIMMET, P. Z., CAIN, M. D., CRAN, E., BEST, J. B., COGHLAN, J. P.: Angiotensin II blood levels in human hypertension. Lancet **1971 I**, 459.

CONSTANTINIDES, P., ROBINSON, M.: Ultrastructural injury of arterial endothelium. II. Effects of vasoactive amines. Arch. Path. **88**, 106 (1969).

DAY, M. D., OWEN, D. A. A.: The interaction between angiotensin and sympathetic vasoconstriction in the isolated artery of the rabbit ear. Brit. J. Pharmacol. **34**, 499 (1968).

FAARUP, P.: Morphological aspects of the renin-angiotensin system. Kopenhagen: Bogtrykkeriet Forum 1971.

FAARUP, P., NIELSEN, I., JENSEN, G., CLAUSEN, E., KEMP, E.: Renin location in human contracted kidneys. Acta path. microbiol. scand. **78**, 674 (1970).

GIESE, J.: Deposition of serum proteins in vascular walls during acute hypertension. Acta path. microbiol. scand. **53**, 167 (1961).

GIESE, J.: Acute vascular disease caused by severe renal ischaemia. Acta path. microbiol. scand. **56**, 399 (1962).

GIESE, J.: Acute hypertensive vascular disease. 2. Studies on vascular reaction patterns and permeability changes by means of vital microscopy and colloidal tracer technique. Acta path. microbiol. scand. **62**, 497 (1964).

GIESE, J.: The pathogenesis of hypertensive vascular disease. Kopenhagen: Munksgaard 1966.

GOORMAGHTIGH, N.: Existence of an endocrine gland in the media of the renal arterioles. Proc. Soc. exp. Biol. (N. Y.) **42**, 688 (1939).

GOORMAGHTIGH, N.: Histological changes in the ischaemic kidney with special reference to the juxtaglomerular apparatus. Amer. J. Path. **16** (2), 409 (1940).

HARTROFT, P. M., HARTROFT, W. S.: Studies on renal juxtaglomerular cells. 1. Variations produced by sodium chloride and desoxycorticosterone acetate. J. exp. Med. **97**, 415 (1953).

HERBERTSON, B. M., KELLAWAY, T. D.: Arterial necrosis in the rat produced by methoxamine. J. Path. Bact. **80**, 87 (1960).

HILL, G. S., HEPTINSTALL, R. H.: Steroid-induced hypertension in the rat. A microangiographic and histologic study on the pathogenesis of hypertensive vascular and glomerular lesions. Amer. J. Path. **52**, 1 (1968).

HOBBS, J. B., CLIFF, W. J.: Observations on tissue grafts established in rabbit ear chambers. A combined light and electron microscopic study. J. exp. Med. **134**, 963 (1971).

KAMURA, S., NIWA, T., SKELTON, F. R., BERNARDIS, L. L.: Effects of angiotensin II and epinephrine infusion on juxtaglomerular cell granularity and arterioles of the rat kidney. Experientia (Basel) **22**, 547 (1966).

KATZ, V. J., PATEK, P. R., BERNICK, S.: Effect of angiotensin on juxtaglomerular cells and vessels of the kidney. Circulat. Res. **11**, 955 (1962).

KINCAID-SMITH, P., HOBBS, J. B., FRIEDMAN, A.: Structural and ultrastructural alterations in mesenteric and renal arterioles following infusion of vaso-active agents. In: Hypertension — 1972. 2nd International Symposium on the Renin-Angiotensin-Aldosterone-Sodium System, p. 97 (GENEST, G., KOIW, E., Eds.). Berlin-Heidelberg-New York: Springer 1972.

KIPROV, D. I., PUKHLEV, A. R., SOMOVA, L. M.: The role of vessel wall reactivity in experimental hypertension. Cor et vase (Praha) **10**, 228 (1968).

KOLETSKY, S., RIVERA-VEL z, J. M., PRITCHARD, W. H.: Production of hypertension and vascular disease by angiotensin. Arch. Path. **82**, 99 (1966).
LENDRUM, A. C.: The hypertensive diabetic kidney as a model of the so-called collagen diseases. Canad. med. Ass. J. **88**, 442 (1963).
LOUIS, W. J., RENGINI, V., MACDONALD, G. J., BOYD, G. W., PEART, W. S.: Renal clip hypertension in rabbits immunized against angiotensin II. Lancet **1970 I**, 333.
MANDEL, M. J., SAPIRSTEIN, L. A.: Effect of angiotensin infusion on regional blood flow and regional vascular resistance in rat. Circulat. Res. **10**, 807 (1962).
MASSON, G. M. C., CORCORAN, A. C., PAGE, I. H.: Role du rein dans l'hypertension experimentale chez le rat. Rev. canad. Biol. **10**, 309 (1951).
MCCUBBIN, J. W., PAGE, I. H.: Renal pressar system and neurogenic control of arterial pressure. Circulat. Res. **12**, 553 (1963).
MONTGOMERY, P. O'B., MUIRHEAD, E. E.: A microspectroscopic study of arterioles in benign and malignant hypertension. Amer. J. Path. **30**, 1181 (1954).
MUSTARD, J. F.: Recent advances in molecular pathology; A review. Platelet aggregation, vascular injury and atherosclerosis. Exp. molec. Path. **7**, 366 (1967).
OLSEN, F.: Penetration of circulating fluorescent proteins into walls of arterioles and venules in rats with intermittent acute angiotensin-hypertension. Acta path. microbiol. scand. **74**, 325 (1968).
PACKHAM, M. A., NISHIZAWA, E. E., MUSTARD, J. F.: The response of platelets to tissue injury. Biochem. Pharmacol. (Suppl.) (1967).
PALMER, A. A., WILKINS, A. G.: A closed method for the microscopic study of the living rat pancreas in situ. Aust. J. exp. Biol. med. Sci. **38**, 467 (1960).
POPLAWSKI, A.: The effect of angiotensin II on the platelet aggregation induced by adenosinediphosphate, epinephrine and thrombin. Experientia (Basel) **26**, 86 (1970).
POPLAWSKI, A., SKORULSKE, M., NIEWIAROWSKI, S.: Increased platelet adhesiveness in hypertensive cardiovascular disease. J. Atheroscler. Res. **8**, 721 (1968).
ROBB, H. J., JACOBSON, L. F.: Microvascular responses to trauma. J. Trauma **3**, 407 (1963).
ROBERTSON, A. L., KHAIRALLAH, P. A.: Angiotensin II: Rapid localization in nuclei of smooth and cardiac muscle. Science **172**, 1138 (1971).
RUYTER, J. H. C.: Über einen merkwürdigen Abschnitt der Vasa Afferentia in der Mäuseniere. Z. Zellforsch. **2**, 242 (1925).
SCHURMANN, P., MACMAHON, H. E.: Die maligne Nephrosklerose, zugleich ein Beitrag zur Frage der Bedeutung der Blutgewebsschranke. Virchows Arch. path. Anat. **291**, 47 (1933).
SHEEHAN, H. L., DAVIS, J. C.: Renal ischaemia with good reflow. J. Path. Bact. **78**, 351 (1959).
TIGERSTEDT, R., BERGMAN, P.: Niere und Kreislauf. Scand. Arch. Pysiol. **8**, 223 (1898).
VOLHARD, F.: Über die Pathogenese des roten (essentielien) arteriellen Hochdrucks unter der malignen Sklerose. Schweiz. med. Wschr. **78**, 1189 und 1224 (1948).
WALTER, P., BASSENGE, E.: Effect of angiotensin on vascular smooth muscles. Pflügers Arch. ges. Physiol. **307**, 70 (1969).
WOLFGARTEN, M., MARGAREY, F. R.: Vascular fibrinoid necrosis in hypertension. J. Path. Bact. **77**, 597 (1959).
ZUBERBUHLER, R. C., BOHR, D. F.: Responses of coronary smooth muscle to catecholamines. Circulat. Res. **16**, 431 (1965).

Effects of Angiotensin II on the Permeability of the Vascular Wall

A. LAZZARINI ROBERTSON and P. A. KHAIRALLAH

With 6 Figures

Endothelial cells have long been considered selective functional barriers for the transport of blood components across the wall of large blood vessels with a "continuous" endothelial lining because of their intimate contact with circulating blood. Two major routes have been described for blood macromolecules escaping from the vascular lumen: one by intracellular incorporation and transport across the endothelial cell cytoplasm, the other through interendothelial spaces or "tight" junctions. The latter is considered to be morphologically, if not functionally, equivalent to the "small pore" system (less than 90 Å in diameter) found in peripheral capillaries (FLOREY and SHEPPARD, 1970).

Experimental data has suggested the presence of extremely rapid transport of water, salts and even plasma macromolecules across some types of endothelium. Recent morphological studies in search of functional pathways to explain this phenomenon have attempted to correlate function with ultrastructural findings (FRENCH, 1966). Because of the relative organizational simplicity of the capillary wall, earlier studies were directed at evaluation of capillary endothelium rather than that of larger blood vessels. More recently, electron markers of known particle size, such as colloidal carbon (250 to 500 Å), horse spleen ferritin (80 to 110 Å) or horseradish peroxidase (40 to 50 Å), have been used for this purpose [ROBERTSON and KHAIRALLAH, 1973).

Larger particles such as lipoproteins and chylomicrons normally found in the circulation and measuring up to 5,000 to 10,000 Å in diameter, were considered too large to be able to travel across normal endothelial lining (CASLEY-SMITH, 1962; FRENCH, 1963). The distribution, size and number of intercellular junctions anchoring endothelial cells in different vessels is relatively uniform in spite of occasional local variations such as those found in the fenestrated endothelia of adipose tissue capillaries and in liver sinusoids.

In man, one of the major ultrastructural differences between large and small arteries with continuous endothelium occurs in the subendothelial space or intima which varies greatly both in thickness and in number of cellular components with age. In the arteries of the newborn, endothelial cells are directly in contact with the underlying internal elastic membrane. In the adult human aorta, however, the intimal layer containing abundant cells and extracellular components becomes progressively thicker in contrast with other mammals in which the intimal lining of major arteries remains inconspicuous throughout life.

SCHWARTZ and BENDITT have recently described (1972) four categories of arterial interendothelial junctions in Wistar Firth/Mai rats based on the degree of complexity and surface contact between two adjacent endothelial cells. In Sprague-Dawley rats, the so-called "mortice" type of endothelial junction is by far the most common both in the aorta and main coronary arteries (ROBERTSON and KHAIRALLAH, 1973).

The substance filling vascular interendothelial junctions, best shown following surface staining with silver salts, was described by early anatomists as "intercellular cement" (FLOREY, 1964). Its staining characteristics are likely due, at least in part, to the condensation of mucopolysaccharide coats covering the surfaces of contiguous endothelial cells overlapping one another (FRENCH, 1966).

Following routine chemical fixation, evaluation of the functional significance of the intercellular junctions of arterial endothelium is subject to those difficulties inherent in reviewing ultrastructural characteristics of other highly elastic organs. It is possible to avoid some of these shortcomings by *in-vivo* fixation with *low* concentrations of buffered aldehydes in isotonic solutions injected within physiological pressure ranges. When this method was used, combined with serial sections perpendicular as well as parallel to the interendothelial junction, it was possible to identify, following injection of angiotensin II and other vasoactive agents, the presence of tortuous and *temporary* intercellular spaces. They have been named "interendothelial gaps" or IEGs [ROBERTSON and KHAIRALLAH, 1973).

Endothelial Cell Contraction

Studies by MAJNO et al. (1969) and by CONSTANTINIDES and ROBINSON (1969) have suggested that arterial endothelial cells may respond by contraction to

Table 1. *Acute ultrastructural effects of circulating vasoactive agents on arterial cells*

	Total injection ($\times 10^{-9}$ g)[a]	Av. time (sec)	Endothelium			Medical smooth muscle cells	
			Pino-cytosis	I.E.G.[b]	Cont.[c]	Pino cytosis	Cont.[a]
Angiotensin II	0.1—10	38	±	+ + +	+ + +	+	+ + +
Prostaglandin E_1	10—20	46	+	+ +	+ + +	+	+ + +
Serotonin	10—200	44	+ +	±(+ + +)	+ +	+	+ +
Bradykinin	10—20	51	+	±	+	+	+ +
Norepinephrine	100—200	48	+ +	±	+ +	+	+ +
Control L-isoleucine or L-tyrosine	2400—3800	78	–	–	–	–	–
Control Ringer's solution	2 ml	240	±	–	–	–	–

[a] In 1 ml Ringer's solution injected in left ventricle of a 200 g Sprague-Dawley rat.
[b] Formation of interendothelial gaps demonstrated by colloidal C, Fe, HRP or ^{3}H lipids.
[c] Estimated by nuclear membrane pinching after MAJNO et al. (J. Cell Biol. 42, 647, 1969).

stimuli induced by high blood levels of several vasoactive agents. In the latter study, although increased vascular permeability resulted, the effects of such substances on interendothelial junctions, short of irreversible cell injury, was not clear. For this reason, other experimental designs have been recently used combined with the *in-vivo* fixation technique mentioned above (ROBERTSON and KHAIRALLAH, 1973). In one set of experiments, rapid left intraventricular injections of Ang. I or II, norepinephrine, serotonin, prostaglandins E_1, $F_{2\alpha}$, or bradykinin were used in anesthetized pathogen-free fasting adult female Sprague-Dawley rats

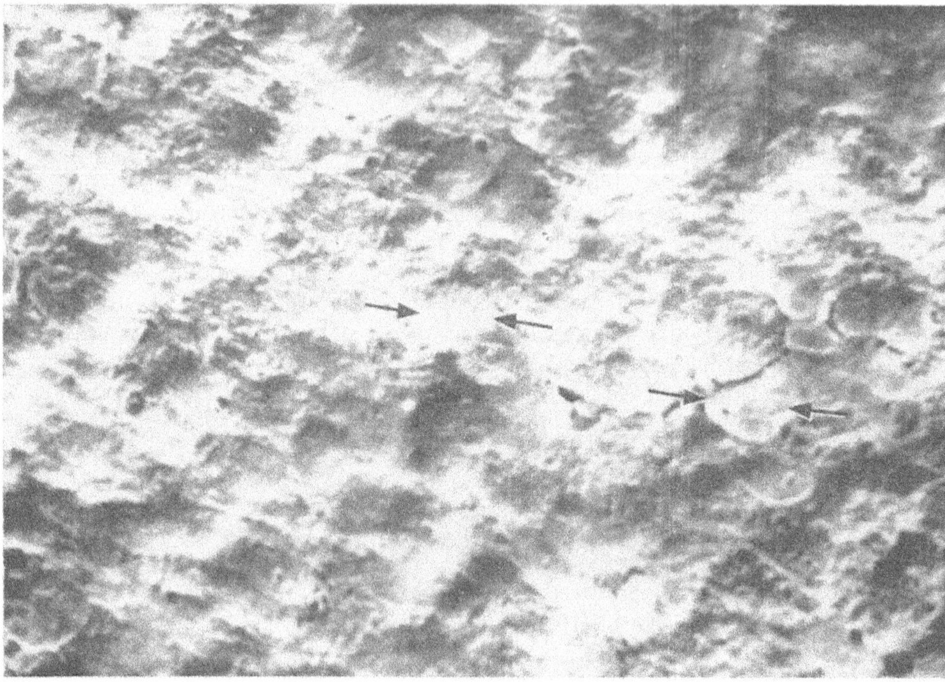

a

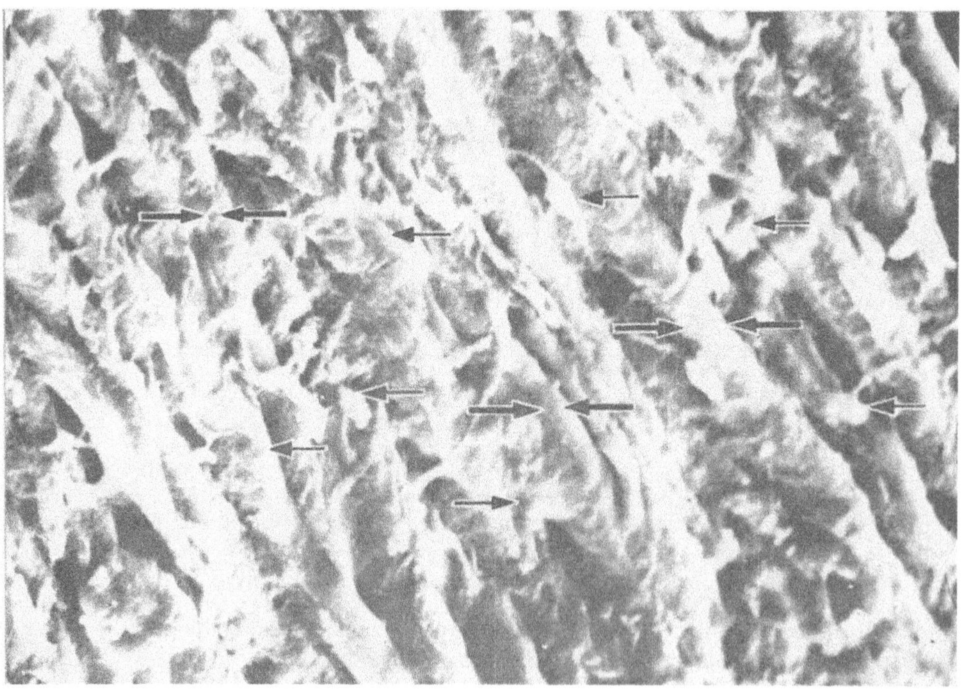

b

Fig. 1. Scanning electronmicrographs of the response of the endothelial lining of the rat thoracic aorta after intraventricular injection of 0.1 nanograms of Ang. II. a) control preparation. Note individual flat endothelial cells (arrows) (× 1200), b) similar to a), but 40 sec after injection of the octapeptide. Note irregularities of the vascular surface with projection of contracted endotheiial cells into the lumen (large arrows). Scattered blood cells are attached to the endothelium (small arrows) (× 1200)

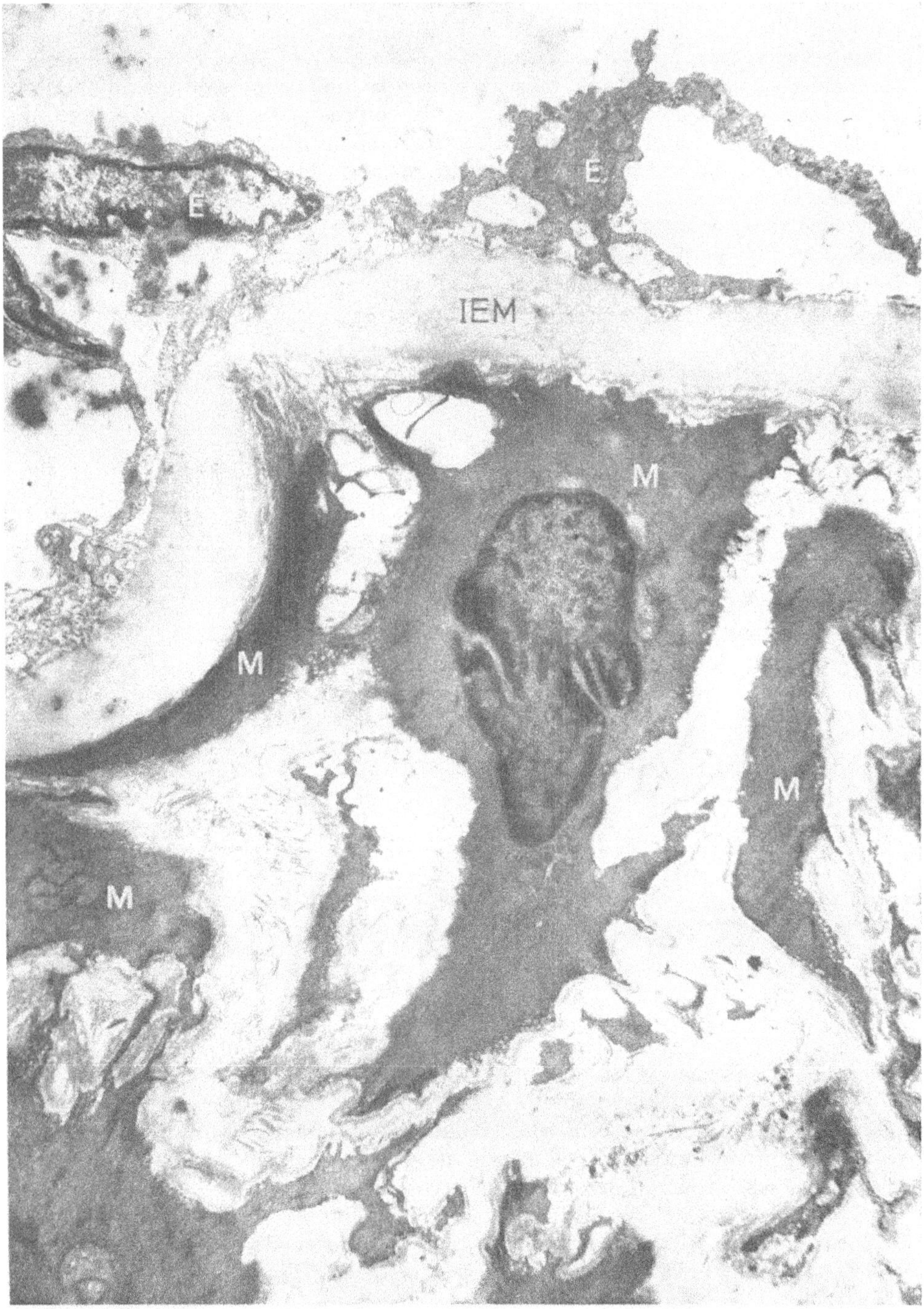

Fig. 2. Transmission electronmicrograph of rat superior mesenteric artery under experimental conditions similar to those of 1 b). Note projection of endothelial cells (E) with large intracellular vacuoles resting directly over irregular internal elastic membrane (IEM), separating them from underlying and partially contracted medial smooth muscle cells (M). Uranyl acetate — lead citrate staining (× 9800)

followed by immediate *in-vivo* fixation with ascending concentrations of buffered aldehyde solutions.

Injections of up to 100 nanograms of the decapeptide, Ang. I, did not induce endothelial or vascular smooth muscle cell contraction or increase the number of pinocytotic cytoplasmic vesicles (Table 1). In contrast, intracardiac injections of 0.1 to 10 nanograms of the octapeptide, Ang. II, in less than 40 sec produced striking endothelial and muscle cell changes in the aorta, coronary and peripheral arteries (Figs. 1 and 2). Morphological changes found in the mesenteric artery, resembled those described by Kincaid-Smith et al. (1972) (see also Chap. "Morphological Effects of Angiotensin on Arteries" in this book). As a result of contraction of individual endothelial cells, widening of interendothelial spaces

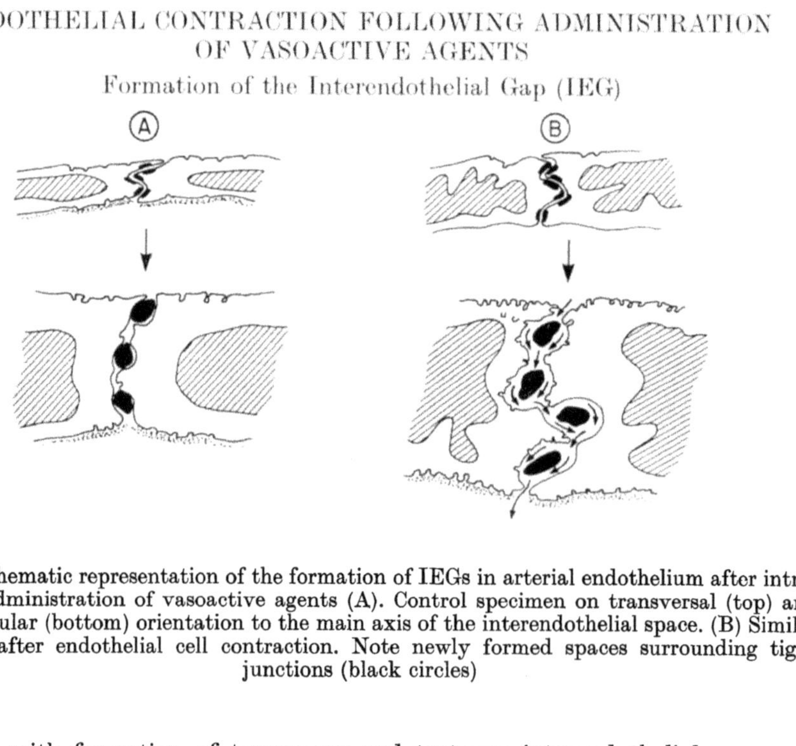

Fig. 3. Schematic representation of the formation of IEGs in arterial endothelium after intracardiac administration of vasoactive agents (A). Control specimen on transversal (top) and perpendicular (bottom) orientation to the main axis of the interendothelial space. (B) Similar junction after endothelial cell contraction. Note newly formed spaces surrounding tight junctions (black circles)

occurred with formation of temporary and tortuous interendothelial spaces or gaps (IEGs). They varied considerably in width, measuring 750 Å at their widest points. Following three dimensional reconstruction of serial sections, IEGs seem to occur by separation of the cell membrane or plasmalemma of two contiguous endothelial cells around desmosomes, or tight junctions rather than by morphological changes in these intercellular connections (Fig. 3).

Serotonin also induced temporary widening of interendothelial junctions but its effects seemed to be more limited than those of Ang. II. Although many endothelial cells appeared to contract, this was not a universal phenomenon. Bradykinin at concentrations ten times higher than those needed for Ang. II was found to have intermediate effects between those of the octapeptide and serotonin. Prostaglandin E_1, on the other hand, produced severe endothelial contraction. Further evidence for the temporary formation of interendothelial gaps was obtained using electron markers. Acute transendothelial passage, particularly of colloidal carbon, ferritin, or horseradish peroxidase (Fig. 4) was most evident if injected simultaneously with Ang. II. If the injection of the marker was delayed more than 480 sec after the injection of the octapeptide, morphological evidence for IEGs was not found and only the smaller electron markers, particularly horseradish peroxidase, could be demonstrated in the subendothelial space as previously shown in other blood vessels (KARNOVSKY, 1967). The ultrastructural characteristics of the vascular wall of those animals receiving delayed injections were similar

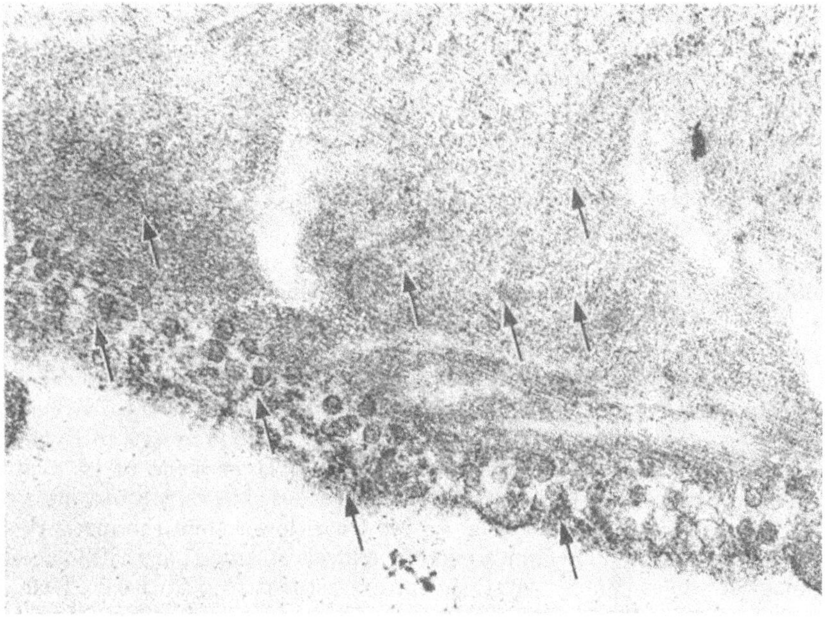

Fig. 4. Aortic rat endothelium 45 sec after simultaneous intraventricular injection of 0.1 nanograms of Ang. II and horseradish peroxidase. Note the reaction product appearing not only in endothelial pinocytotic vesicles (arrows) but also in considerable amounts in the subendothelial space (s) shown here in oblique projection due to specimen orientation (× 38,000)

to those of controls injected with Ringer's solution alone. When labeled hyperlipemic sera or lipoprotein fractions were injected simultaneously with Ang. II, lipid retention was highest in the intima-medial arterial layers, but diminished rapidly if intervals of 60 sec or longer occurred between injections. In the coronary vessels, retention of low density lipoprotein fractions after simultaneous injection with Ang. II in the left ventricle seemed to be localized primarily in the subendothelial space.

When ^{3}H angiotensin was used under similar experimental conditions, the isotope was found by light and electron microscopy-autoradiography in the endothelial cell nucleus as well as in the mitochondria and nuclei of the underlying medial smooth muscle cells. If labeled amino acids were injected simultaneously with "cold" Ang. II, they were very rapidly distributed across the full thickness of the arterial wall without selective intracellular localizations (ROBERTSON and KHAIRALLAH, 1971). To evaluate further the distribution of areas of increased aortic endothelial permeability following local injection of Ang. II, studies were carried out in normolipemic rabbits [ROBERTSON and KHAIRALLAH, 1973). They were based on a method originally suggested by PACKHAM et al. (1967) using the azo-dye Evans blue, known to be carried in the blood bound to serum albumin. SOMER and SCHWARTZ have used this technique and have recently shown (1971) that Evans blue-stained areas of the arch of the aorta of young pigs were also characterized by increased permeability to ^{3}H cholesterol. They correspond anatomically to areas where spontaneous arterial lesions are often found in older animals.

In our studies, 0.1 nanograms of Ang. II was injected through a fine needle into a temporarily isolated segment of the abdominal aorta of a rabbit that had 15 min earlier received intravenously 60 mg/kg of Evans blue dye in Ringer's solution. Sixty sec after injection of the octapeptide, a dramatic increase in endothelial permeability occurred only in areas of the aorta exposed to the vasoactive agent. Endothelial surfaces, proximal and distal to the isolated site of injection, showed no changes. Control experiments using injections of Ringer's solution alone showed no increased endothelial permeability.

These experimental results suggest that sudden changes in aortic endothelial permeability may indeed occur following temporary and shortlived increases in circulating Ang. II. Acute increases in endothelial permeability may elicit self-perpetuating metabolic alterations resulting in an abnormal "trapping" of circulating macromolecules such as lipoproteins, globulins and fibrogens in the arterial wall. These changes in turn may lead to arterial cell proliferation, degeneration and eventual development of overt vascular disease. As part of the above studies, we also investigated the permeability of skin dermal blood vessels to Evans blue dye following intradermal administration of Ang. II or some of its synthetic analogs. The experimental results showed that rabbit skin vessels become permeable to the dye after doses of Ang. II 100 times lower than those reported by BISSET and LEWIS (1962) in guinea pigs. Such levels of Ang. II are within accepted physiological ranges (VANE, 1969). Qualitative estimation of its local effects were made by measuring the blueing area surrounding the site of injection of the octapeptide. Similar to the findings of BISSET and LEWIS (1962) in the guinea pig, these effects of Ang. II on peripheral vascular permeability were found not to be histamine-mediated in the rabbit; local or systemic administration of antihistaminics did not prevent the vascular response. These results seem to suggest that the primary local action of the peptide on skin vascular permeability may be caused by contraction of endothelial cells and the temporary development of interendothelial gaps in dermal arteries and venules similar to those described above for arterial endothelium.

Effects of Angiotensin II in Other Vascular Cells

Studies on the effects of sustained perfusion of Ang. II in Ringer's solution were performed utilizing an intra-aortic catheter in unanesthetized rats (ROBERTSON et al., 1972). It was found that individual myocardial cells of both the left and the right ventricle adjacent to the subendocardium rapidly developed ultrastructural and histochemical changes compatible with acute hypoxia and early myocardial infarction. Although the distribution of these cellular changes was focal, they did not occur in the epicardial myocardium containing intraparenchymal coronary artery branches. Control injections of Ringer's solution under identical laboratory conditions produced no myocardial changes. These observations suggest that the focal effects of Ang. II on individual cardiac muscle cells may result in severe and possibly irreversible myocardial damage leading eventually to myocardial infarction.

Role of Platelets

It is well known that circulating platelets carry a number of intracellular hormones which are rapidly released after cell contraction and degranulation (MUSTARD et al., 1970). Intravascular injections of Ang. II, as previously described, induced temporary platelet aggregation, contraction, and degranulation (Fig. 5). Local release of platelet granules containing vasoactive agents resulted, in turn, in prolongation of endothelial cell contraction and maintenance of IEGs. Circulating macromolecules or electron markers were trapped by the arterial wall [ROBERTSON and KHAIRALLAH, 1973).

The proposed role of platelets in prolonging abnormal endothelial permeability and, indirectly, in induction of vascular disease is shown schematically in Table 2.

Table 2. *Proposed role of Ang. II and other vasoactive agents on platelet aggregation and vascular permeability*

↓ 1) *Circulating vasoactive agent*, acting independently or combined with hypoxia, immunological insults or hemodynamic changes produce
↓ 2) Short-lived *endothelial contraction* with exposure of subendothelial basement membrane collagen and
↓ 3) Local aggregation of *circulating platelets* followed by *contraction* and *degranulation* inducing
↓ 4) *Focal release* of platelet serotonin, histamine, and other vasoactive agents resulting in
↓ 5) Prolonged *endothelial contraction* with increased permeability of the vascular wall to plasma macromolecules.

After appearance of interendothelial gaps following endothelial cell contraction under the stimuli of circulating vasoactive agents, short-lived platelet aggregation could be initiated by temporary exposure of endothelial basement membrane. It has recently been reported (MAJNO, 1970) that such membrane is rich in hydroxyproline and is digested by collagenase. It is known, on the other hand (MUSTARD et al., 1970), that collagen fibers are strong inducers of platelet aggregation. Exposure of endothelial basement membrane following cell contraction may thus initiate platelet aggregation at sites of IEGs. This phenomenon can then be followed by the release of serotonin and other vasoactive agents carried by platelets. It would be of considerable interest to determine if reserpine and other serotonin depleters could partially or totally inhibit such a phenomenon.

It should be emphasized that experimental data from our laboratory suggest that the microscopic demonstration of these platelet aggregates is a very transitory phenomenon. This is in contrast to the usual finding of platelet aggregates containing cells at different stages of degranulation and lysis encountered in the early stages of intravascular thrombosis.

The multiple effects of Ang. II in endothelial and vascular smooth muscle cells reviewed here are illustrated schematically in Fig. 6. Like other powerful hormones, this agent may have several related intracellular actions involving both the metabolism and the function of the target cells.

Besides the cell surface effects of Ang. II involving Ca-dependent specific receptor sites, metabolic cell changes involving protein and nucleotide synthesis may occur (see GOODFRIEND, in this book). The above phenomena could explain

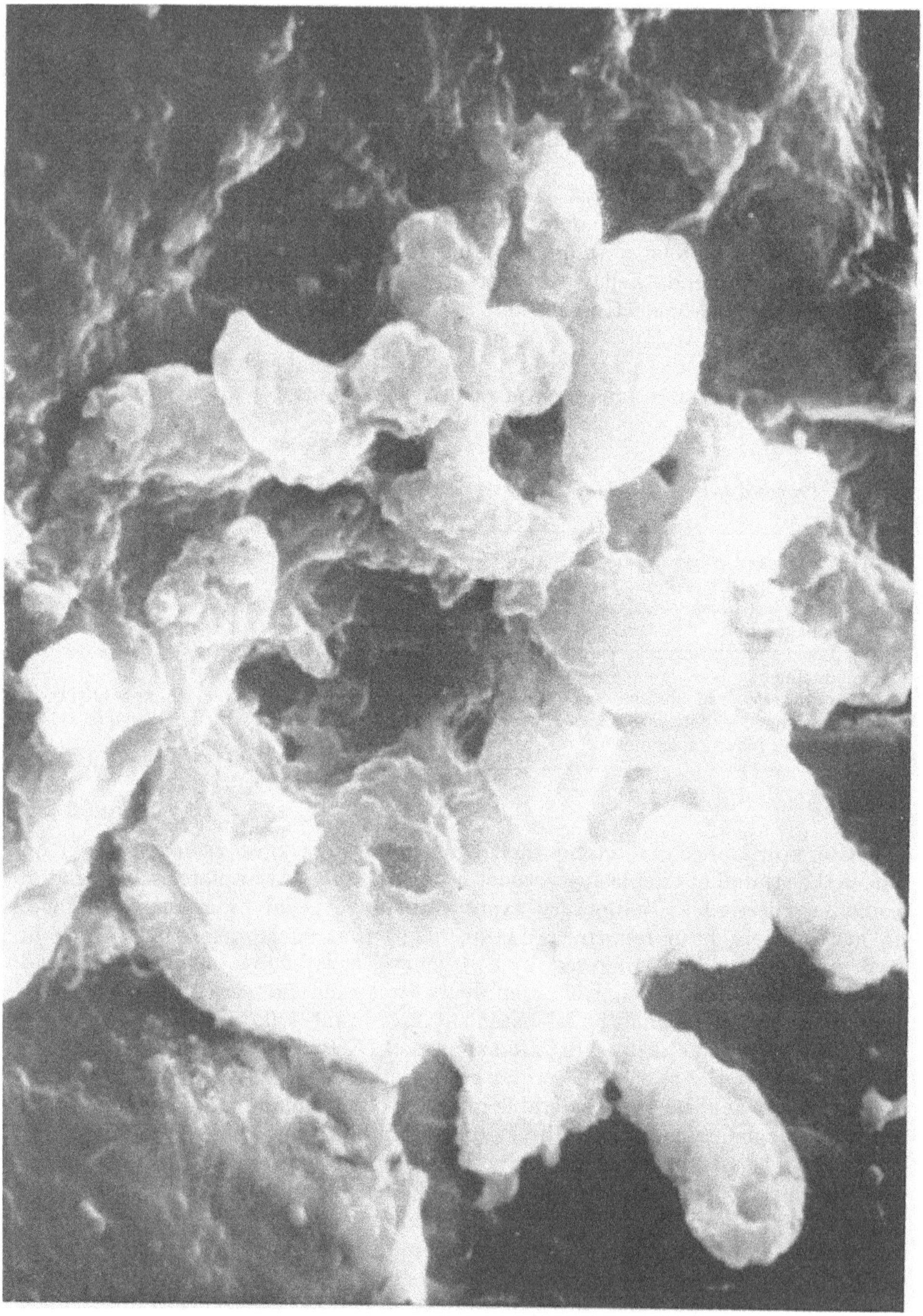

Fig. 5. Scanning electronmicrograph showing platelets and other blood cells attached to the endothelial surface at IEGs ($\times$ 2100)

the rapid intracellular localization of the octapeptide or some of its molecular fragments found in previous studies (KHAIRALLAH et al., 1972). It is not yet known whether these are simultaneous or successive phenomena and to what extent they are associated with the ability of all vascular cells to contract.

The sudden increases in vascular permeability described above are assumed from these findings to be associated with endothelial cell contraction. If they occur simultaneously with increases in protein biosynthesis by myocardial and vascular

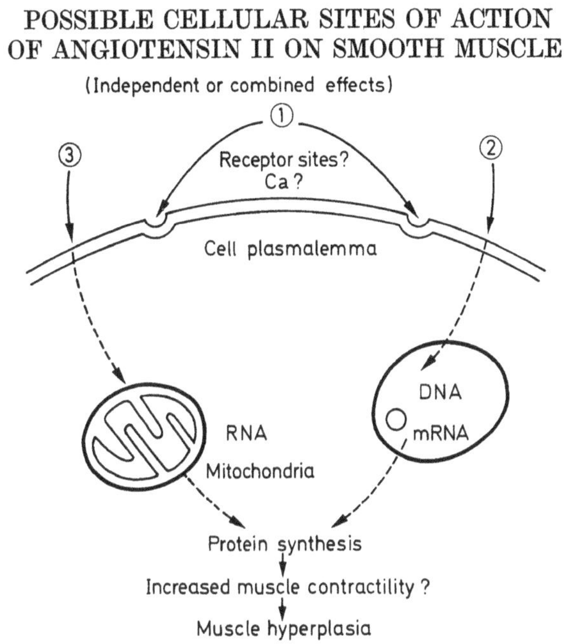

Fig. 6. Schematic representation of the proposed multiple effects of Ang. II in the target vascular cell

smooth muscle cells, it is tempting to speculate that arterial and cardiac muscle hypertrophy found in hypertensives may be the cause rather than the result of sustained increases in blood pressure.

References

BISSET, G. W., LEWIS, G. P.: A spectrum of pharmacological activity in some biologically active peptides. Brit. J. Pharmacol. **19**, 168 (1962).

CASLEY-SMITH, J. R.: The identification of chylomicra and lipoproteins in tissue sections and their passage into jejunal lacteals. J. Cell Biol. **15**, 259 (1962).

CONSTANTINIDES, P., ROBINSON, M.: Ultrastructural injury of arterial endothelium. I. Effects of pH, osmolarity, anoxia, and temperature. II. Effects of vasoactive amines. Arch. Path. **88**, 99 (1969).

FLOREY, H. W.: The transport of materials across the capillary wall. Quart. J. exp. Physiol. **49**, 117 (1964).

FLOREY, L., SHEPPARD, B. L.: The permeability of arterial endothelium to horseradish peroxidase. Proc. roy. Soc. **174**, 435 (1970).

FRENCH, J. E.: The behavior of chylomicra in the circulation; observations with the electron microscope. In: Proc. VIth Intern. Conf. Biochemical Problems Lipids. Amsterdam: Elsevier 1963.

FRENCH, J. E.: Atherosclerosis in relation to the structure and function of arterial intima, with special reference to the endothelium. In: International Review of Experimental Pathology, Vol. 5. New York: Academic Press 1966.

KARNOVSKY, J.: The ultrastructural basis of capillary permeability studied with peroxidase as a tracer. J. Cell Biol. **35**, 213 (1967).

KHAIRALLAH, P. A., ROBERTSON, A. L., DAVILA, D.: Effects of angiotensin II on DNA, RNA and protein synthesis. In: Hypertension — 1972, p. 212 (GENEST, J., KOIW, E., Eds.). Berlin-Heidelberg-New York: Springer 1972.

KINCAID-SMITH, P., HOBBS, J. B., FRIEDMAN, A., MATHEWS, D. C.: Structural and ultrastructural alterations in mesenteric and renal arterioles following infusion of vaso-active agents. In: Hypertension — 1972, p. 97 (GENEST, J., KOIW, E., Eds.). Berlin-Heidelberg-New York: Springer 1972.

MAJNO, G., SHEA, S. M., LEVENTHAL, M.: Endothelial contraction induced by histamine-type mediators. An electron microscopic study. J. Cell Biol. **42**, 647 (1969).

MAJNO, G.: Endothelial contraction, collagenase digestion of the basement membrane. In: Vascular Factors and Thrombosis. Stuttgart: F. K. Schattauer 1970.

MUSTARD, J. F., JORGENSEN, L., PACKHAM, M. A.: Formed elements as a source of vascular injury. In: Vascular Factors and Thrombosis (BRINKHOUS, K. M., Ed.). Stuttgart: F. K. Schattauer 1970.

PACKHAM, M. A., ROWSELL, H. C., JORGENSEN, L., MUSTARD, J. G.: Localized protein accumulation in the wall of the aorta. Exp. molec. Path. **7**, 214 (1967).

ROBERTSON, A. L., KHAIRALLAH, P. A.: Angiotensin II: Rapid localization in nuclei of smooth and cardiac muscle. Science **172**, 1138 (1971).

ROBERTSON, A. L., KHAIRALLAH, P. A., KYNCL, J.: Role of endothelial contraction and platelets in atherogenesis. Circulation **65—66** (abstract), II—252 (1972).

ROBERTSON, A. L., KHAIRALLAH, P. A.: Effects of angiotensin II and some analogs on vascular permeability in the rabbit. Circ. Res. **31**, 923 (1972).

ROBERTSON, A. L., KHAIRALLAH, P. A.: Arterial endothelial permeability and vascular disease. The "trap door" effect. Exp. molec. Path. **18**, 241 (1973).

SCHWARTZ, S. M., BENDITT, E. P.: Studies on aortic intima. I. Structure and permeability of rat thoracic aortic intima. Amer. J. Path. **66**, 241 (1972).

SOMER, J. B., SCHWARTZ, C. J.: Focal ^{3}H-cholesterol uptake in the pig aorta. Atherosclerosis **13**, 293 (1971).

VANE, J. R.: Release and fate of vasoactive hormones in tke circulation. Br. J. Pharmacol. **35**, 209 (1969).

Biochemical Effects of Angiotensin

THEODORE L. GOODFRIEND, FREJ FYHRQUIST, and DAVID ALLMANN

Two kinds of biochemical effects of angiotensin will be described in this section: effects on chemical aspects measured in intact organisms, and direct effects on target cells or cell fractions.

I. Effects on Intact Organisms

In the case of the hormone epinephrine and the chemical effect hyperglycemia, the change measured in blood is a direct manifestation of a chemical event induced by the hormone at the target cell. Epinephrine activates glycogen phosphorylase by way of an effect on adenyl cyclase (ROBISON et al., 1971). The product of the reaction eventually appears in the blood as glucose. An even more direct chemical effect of hormone action can be observed after administration of parathormone, when cyclic AMP itself appears in the urine (CHASE and AURBACH, 1967). By contrast, the chemical events observed after angiotensin administration are probably not intimately related to the cellular mechanism of action of the hormone. In fact, there is little evidence of the nature of the primary event. Instead, the biochemical changes reflect the potency of angiotensin as a vasoconstrictor, a stimulant to adrenal cortical and medullary hormone release, and a participant in autonomic nervous function.

Elevations of plasma lactate observed after angiotensin infusion probably result from tissue ischemia or catecholamine release (HEIDENREICH et al., 1964). Angiotensin causes a transient rise in blood glucose, which may be attributable in part to a direct effect on kidney or liver, to catecholamine release, and to reduced plasma insulin (HEIDENREICH et al., 1964; AKINKUGBE, 1965). Decreased plasma insulin probably results from a normal islet cell response to diminished flow of blood and glucose through the pancreas and to sympathetic nerves or mediators (MINTZ et al., 1967). Infused angiotensin lowers plasma fatty acids, and this change can be blocked by atropine (ROTHLIN et al., 1962; HEIDENREICH et al., 1964; NAKANO and KUSAKARI, 1966; IIZUKA et al., 1970).

In addition to the well-known effect of angiotensin on aldosterone, there is stimulation of glucocorticoid release at high doses of angiotensin in the dog (KAPLAN and BARTTER, 1962; SLATER et al., 1963), and inhibition of glucocorticoid release at low doses in man (RAYYIS and HORTON, 1971). The work of RAYYIS and HORTON (1971) also demonstrated a rise in ACTH during angiotensin infusion. These endocrine alterations inevitably affect blood constituents, such as glucose.

Angiotensin has a variety of effects on the kidney, and these, in turn, alter the chemical and cellular components of the blood (LANGFORD, this volume). Angiotensin is reported to release erythropoietin from the kidney, and long-standing renal hypertension is accompanied by elevated hemoglobin concentration (FISHER and ROH, 1971; WERNING et al., 1971). Renin infusion increases albumin catabolism by the isolated perfused kidney, but there is no evidence of a change in albumin concentration after angiotensin infusion or during renal hypertension in intact animals (ROSENFELD et al., 1967). There is evidence that angiotensin causes the release of prostaglandins from the kidneys, but there is no data supporting a change in these chemicals in the general circulation (MCGIFF et al., 1970).

It is apparent from the preceding paragraphs that angiotensin affects the chemistry of the blood and body fluids in a variety of ways. There is data to support effects on the absorption, excretion, and metabolism of many compounds. There are effects of angiotensin on the classical endocrine modulators of metabolism and excretion. However, none of the changes reported in intact animals appears to reflect the intimate molecular events begun by angiotensin at its target.

Although "sub-pressor" doses of angiotensin are frequently administered in an attempt to avoid the effects of vasoconstriction on various facets, most of these experiments do not include measurement of regional blood flow, that may change before blood pressure rises. However, newer analogues of angiotensin that exert profound effects virtually devoid of pressure or flow changes offer another approach to the dissection of this hormone's manifold properties (PEACH et al., 1969; KHAIRALLAH, 1970).

Patients with Bartter's syndrome, in whom the pressor response to angiotensin is absent despite high levels of endogenous angiotensin, present a clinical avenue to elucidation of non-pressor effects of the hormone (BARTTER et al., 1962). The high plasma lipid and low magnesium levels reported by BARTTER may be examples of direct biochemical effects of angiotensin (BARTTER, 1969). These patients are "complicated" by hyperaldosteronism and hypokalemia, however, and would represent ideal subjects for study only in the rare instances in which they undergo therapeutic adrenalectomy.

II. Effects in Vitro

The remainder of this chapter reports experiments with isolated tissues and subcellular fractions *in vitro*. Such experiments permit a clear statement of causal relationships between hormone and observation.

A. Effects on Intact Tissues

Human platelets suspended in plasma aggregate in the presence of epinephrine or adenosine diphosphate. This aggregation is accelerated by the addition of nanogram quantitites of [Asp^1, Val^5] angiotensin II (POPLAWSKI, 1969). The common mechanism for many platelet agglutinations is release of ADP, but this effect has not been proven for the acceleration induced by angiotensin.

Altered ion fluxes in cells of isolated uteri, vessels, intestinal smooth muscle, adrenal cortex, kidney, frog skin, and cardiac tissue have been observed after exposure to angiotensin. The most dramatic experimental effect was an increased efflux of radioactive sodium from rat uterus and dog carotid artery (TÜRKER et al., 1967). At high hormone levels, angiotensin increased the rate of influx of radioactive calcium into rat uterus and guinea-pig taenia coli (SHIBATA et al., 1968; KHAIRALLAH, 1971). The effect on colonic smooth muscle is distinct from an effect on fluid transfer across the entire thickness of the colon, observed at physiologic levels of the hormone added *in vitro* (DAVIES et al., 1969). In guinea-pig atria, angiotensin accelerated the rate of efflux of radioactive rubidium, a potassium analogue (VAN ZWIETEN, 1968). In porcine adrenal slices, high doses of angiotensin inhibited potassium uptake (SZALAY, 1969). In rat kidney cortex slices, angiotensin at very low concentrations inhibited potassium accumulation and accelerated sodium extrusion (MUNDAY et al., 1971). The renal effect was not inhibited by ouabain, but was inhibited by inhibitors of protein synthesis (MUNDAY et al., 1972).

Of these effects on ion fluxes only the effect on kidney slices has been correlated convincingly with effects of angiotensin *in vivo*.

Levels of 3', 5' cyclic adenosine monophosphate in both rat uterus and arteries have been reduced by application of angiotensin (Volicer and Hynie, 1971; Angles d'Auriac et al., 1972). The effect in uterus was blocked by theophylline suggesting that angiotensin affected the phosphodiesterase that destroys cyclic AMP. In addition, angiotensin decreased the activity of uterine adenyl cyclase in the presence of epinephrine (Angles d'Auriac et al., 1972). These effects are consistent with the postulated role of the cyclic AMP system in smooth muscle-decreasing levels accompanying contraction and increasing levels accompanying relaxation. Causal relationships are not proven, however.

Khairallah and Robertson (1972) measured incorporation of labeled nucleotides and amino acids into DNA, RNA, and protein in isolated rat atria incubated for 120 min. Ang. II at 3 ng/ml increased the rate of incorporation of the precursors into all three macromolecules. This study was prompted by the observation that infused tritiated Ang. II localized over myocardial nuclei and mitochondria (Robertson and Khairallah, 1971). The observed stimulation was not caused by changes in precursor specific activity, making it unlikely that it was a result of permeability changes. The observations of macromolecular synthesis were repeated in intact rats. Infused angiotensin stimulated DNA synthesis by heart and kidney, RNA synthesis by heart, kidney, spleen, brain, and liver, and protein synthesis by heart and kidney. The work of Hyde (1968), showing an increased rate of liver regeneration after renal ischemia, or injections of kidney homogenate may now be interpreted as secondary to angiotensin actions on hepatic protein synthesis.

Other experiments suggesting an action of angiotensin on macromolecular biosynthesis are the observation that inhibitors of protein synthesis blocked the effects of angiotensin on fluid transfer by isolated rat colon (Davies et al., 1969), and rat kidney (Munday et al., 1972), and the observation that one inhibitor of protein synthesis, puromycin, blocked the effect of angiotensin on steroid release by rabbit adrenal slices (Cosby et al., 1971).

B. Effects on Subcellular Fractions

1. *Receptors*

Angiotensin presumably initiates chemical and physiologic events in cells by combining with receptors. Evidence that specialized binding sites exist has been presented (Lin and Goodfriend, 1970; Baudouin et al., 1972), but proof is lacking that these sites are responsible for subsequent events triggered by the hormone.

Many of the experiments on subcellular fractions attempt to answer two questions at the same time, i.e., the nature of the primary event triggered by angiotensin, and the locus of the initial binding site or receptor. When the first is answered, the second will follow easily. For example, proof that angiotensin exerted one or more of its effects by stimulating oxidative phosphorylation would be strong evidence that the receptors for the hormone were located in mitochondria. Until the mechanism(s) of action are defined, studies on binding to subcellular particles or extracts of tissues offer only clues to new angiotensin targets, possible subcellular sites of action, and possible potent hormone derivatives (Goodfriend et al., 1972).

2. *Microsomes*

BAUDOUIN et al. (1972) demonstrated an effect of Ang. II on calcium translocation by microsome vesicles from homogenized rabbit aorta. The vesicles appeared to be formed from membranes, but the original location of the membranes in the aorta before homogenization is not known. The effect of angiotensin was to decrease binding of calcium by these vesicles and to increase the rate at which trapped calcium was released. This may affect overall calcium distribution *in vivo* (DANIELS et al., 1967). Thus these results are appealing as evidence for angiotensin's mechanism of action at the subcellular level in vascular tissue, and the membrane locus of one of its receptors.

LEVIN (1970) has observed that angiotensin stimulates the Na^+, K^+-activated ATPase in microsomes from rat kidney and heart. The effect was slight, strictly dependent on pH, and transient. These requirements may explain the fact that BONTING et al. (1964) failed to observe stimulation in rabbit kidney homogenates. LEVIN's effect required 1 μg of Ang. II amide per ml of incubation medium. This concentration is at least 10,000 times higher than circulating levels of the hormone. The observation may reflect a non-specific effect of angiotensin, or may indicate that a congener of the octapeptide, such as the heptapeptide, is the true effector. This possibility would be easy to study.

C. Mitochondria

Angiotensin has multiple effects on the metabolism of mitochondria, *in vitro* (GOODFRIEND et al., 1972). The most responsive organelles are those from bovine or feline heart and bovine adrenal cortex. The rate, efficiency (P/O ratio), and "coupling" (respiratory control index) of oxidative phosphorylation are increased, especially in mitochondria that have been "aged" to reduce their baseline phosphorylation efficiency (ALLMANN and GOODFRIEND, 1971). The effects on P/O ratio require high concentrations of angiotensin, in the range of 1 μg/ml. Since they are not observed unless the mitochondria have undergone some deterioration *in vitro*, they may not be representative of effects *in vivo*.

The ATPase of heart mitochondria is inhibited by angiotensin. This effect is also seen in submitochondrial fragments, the "electron-transport-particles", which are everted sacs of inner mitochondrial membrane. Inhibition of this ATPase is consistent with improved coupling of respiration and ATP synthesis in intact mitochondria. It is not related to the ATPase described above.

The phosphorylation of exogenous and endogenous protein ("protein kinase activity") by bovine and rat heart mitochondria is increased by angiotensin. Protein kinase activity is stimulated by cyclic AMP in many tissues, but the stimulation by angiotensin is observed under conditions in which cyclic AMP is inactive. As mentioned above, angiotensin's effect on adenyl cyclase is either absent or inhibitory. The relationship of stimulated protein kinase activity to the other mitochondrial effects of angiotensin, or to physiologic responses, is unknown. It is observed, however, at low hormone concentrations, and is not observed with hexapeptide (amino acids, 3-8) or heptapeptide (amino acids, 1-7) both of which are physiologically inactive.

Mitochondrial effects of angiotensin have not been proven in living tissues. There is indirect evidence that they occur. The hormone was observed to localize at the site of mitochondria, when labeled hormone was infused into intact heart (ROBERTSON and KHAIRALLAH, 1971). Intact adrenal cells exposed to radioactive angiotensin bind the label to mitochondria. Finally, the effectiveness of the Ang. II heptapeptide (2-8) as a positive inotropic agent in cat papillary muscles is greater at low levels of oxygen when mitochondrial function may be more critical to the heart muscle (KENT et al., 1972). However, direct measurement of mitochondrial function in intact tissues exposed to angiotensin has not been performed.

D. Effects on Miscellaneous Chemicals

Angiotensin has been known to form complexes with the divalent cations of zinc, copper, iron and cobalt (SCHWYZER, 1963). The relevance of this observation to living systems is unknown.

Lecithin, other phospholipids, and some fatty acids interact with angiotensins *in vitro* (FYHRQUIST and GOODFRIEND, 1971). This was demonstrated by the ability of the lipids to inhibit binding of labeled angiotensin to antibody and to receptors isolated from adrenal cortex, and their ability to carry labeled angiotensin from aqueous buffer into chloroform.

The ability of various lipids to carry labeled polypeptide into chloroform varied from lipid to lipid, in a way that was not related to charge or to any obvious physical property. The lipids also varied in their individual abilities to carry various analogues of angiotensin into chloroform. In general, the biologically active polypeptides were better carried than inactive labeled analogues. Two exceptions to this rule were hexapeptide 3-8 of Ang. II, and the phenylalanine^6 analogue, both of which were more soluble in chloroform and more readily solubilized by lipids. The significance of this interaction of angiotensins and lipids is not clear.

Discussion

Angiotensin is similar to other vasoactive hormones in that it exerts effects on intact organisms that can be measured chemically as well as physiologically. Also, like other hormones, it exerts effects on isolated organs, cell organelles, and chemicals *in vitro*. However, the relationships of these several effects to each other and to the basic cellular event stimulated by angiotensin are obscure. It seems reasonable to expect many biochemical phenomena to be modified by angiotensin, all of which will hopefully make a constellation of responses easy to understand as "valuable" to an animal.

Angiotensin appears to share with other complex hormones the property that its "precursor" and "product" (decapeptide and heptapeptide 2-8) are potent hormones in their own right (PEACH et al., 1971). These additional polypeptides in the angiotensin sequence have not been extensively investigated for biochemical effects.

References

AKINKUGBE, O. O.: Glycosuria and raised blood glucose during intravenous infusion of angiotensin in the unanaesthetized rabbit. J. Physiol. **178**, 16 P—17 P (1965).

ALLMANN, D. W., GOODFRIEND, T.: The role of endogenous free fatty acids in regulating mitochondrial function. In: Proc. First Europ. Biophys. Congr. Berlin-Heidelberg-New York: Springer-Lederer 1971.

ANGLES D'AURIAC, G., BAUDOUIN, M., MEYER, P.: Mechanisms of action of angiotensin in smooth muscle cell; biochemical changes following the interaction of the hormone with its membrane receptors. Circulat. Res. **XXXI**, II-151—II-157 (1912).

BARTTER, F. C.: So-called Bartter's Syndrome. New Engl. J. Med. **281**, 1483—1484 (1969).

BAUDOUIN, M., MEYER, P., FERMANDJIAN, S., MORGAT, J. L.: Calcium release induced by interaction of angiotensin with its receptors in smooth muscle microsomes. Nature (Lond.) **235**, 336 (1972).

CHASE, L. R., AURBACH, G. D.: Parathyroid function and the renal excretion of 3'5'-adenylic acid. Proc. nat. Acad. Sci. (Wash.) **58**, 518—525 (1967).

COSBY, L. A., SARTORELLI, A. C., ROTH, R. H.: Studies on angiotensin-induced synthesis of aldosterone in rabbit adrenal slices. Pharmacologist **13**, 214 (1971).

DANIELS, A. E., SEVERS, W. B., BUCKLEY, J. P.: The effects of angiotensin II on the ^{45}Ca distribution of the rat. Life Sci. **6**, 545—549 (1967).

DAVIES, N. T., MUNDAY, K. A., PARSONS, B. J.: Dose-dependent biphasic effects of angiotensin on fluid transfer by rat colon. J. Physiol. (Lond.) **204**, 142 P—143 P (1969).

DAVIES, N. T., MUNDAY, K. A., PARSONS, B. J.: The effects of protein synthesis inhibitors on angiotensin stimulated colonic fluid transfer. J. Physiol. (Lond.) **205** (abstract), 17 P—19 P (1969).

FISHER, J. W., ROH, B. L.: Factors influencing renal and extrarenal erythropoietin production. In: Renal Pharmacology. New York: Appleton-Centry-Crofts 1971.

FYHRQUIST, F., GOODFRIEND, T.: Angiotensin interactions with cholesterol and steroids. Clin. Res. **20**, 312 (1972).

GOODFRIEND, T. L., FYHRQUIST, F., GUTMANN, F., KNYCH, E., HOLLEMANS, H., ALLMANN, D., KENT, K. M., COOPER, T.: Clinical and conceptual uses of angiotensin receptors. In: Hypertension — 1972. International Symposium on the Renin-Angiotensin-Aldosterone-Sodium System in Hypertension, p. 549 (GENEST, J., KOIW, E., Eds.). Berlin-Heidelberg-New York: Springer 1972.

HEIDENREICH, O., KOOK, Y., BAUMEISTER, L., REUS, E.: Stoffwechselwirkungen von synthetischem Angiotensin II. Arch. int. Pharmacodyn. **148**, 309—319 (1964).

HYDE, T. A.: The effect of nephrectomy and renal ischaemia on liver regeneration. J. Path. Bact. **96**, 131—136 (1968).

IIZUKA, T., ECKSTEIN, J. W., ABBOUD, F. M.: Effects of angiotensin and atropine on plasma free fatty acids. Amer. J. Physiol. **219**, 528—533 (1970).

KAPLAN, N., BARTTER, F. C.: The effect of ACTH, renin, angiotensin II, and various precursors on biosynthesis of aldosterone by adrenal slices. J. clin. Invest. **41**, 715—724 (196?).

KENT, K. M., GOODFRIEND, T. L., MCCALLUM, Z. T., DEMPSEY, P. J., COOPER, T.: Inotropic agents in hypoxic cat myocardium — depression and potentiation. Circulat. Res. **30**, 196—204 (1972).

KHAIRALLAH, P. A.: Discussion. Supplement I to Circulat. Res. **26** and **27**, I—170 and I—174 (1970).

KHAIRALLAH, P. A.: Pharmacology of angiotensin. In: Kidney hormones. London-New York: Academic Press 1971.

KHAIRALLAH, P. A., ROBERTSON, A. L., Jr., DAVILA, D.: Effects of angiotensin II on DNA, RNA and protein synthesis. In: Hypertension — 1972. International Symposium on the Renin-Angiotensin-Aldosterone-Sodium System in Hypertension, p. 212 (GENEST, J., KOIW, E., Eds.). Berlin-Heidelberg-New York: Springer 1972.

LEVIN, K.: The stimulating effect of angiotensin and vasopressin on adenosine triphosphatase activity *in vitro*. Acta physiol. scand. **79**, 37—49 (1970).

LIN, S. Y., GOODFRIEND, T. L.: Angiotensin receptors. Amer. J. Physiol. **218**, 1319—1328 (1970).

MCGIFF, J. C., CROWSHAW, K., TERRAGNO, N. A., LONIGRO, A. J.: Release of a prostaglandin-like substance into renal venous blood in response to angiotensin II. In: Hypertension, Vol. XVIII — Mechanisms of Hypertension. New York: The American Heart Association 1970.

MINTZ, D. H., FINSTER, J., STEPT, M.: Effect of angiotensin II on immunoreactive insulin. J. clin. Endocr. **27**, 671—678 (1967).

MUNDAY, K. A., PARSONS, B. J., POAT, J. A.: The effect of angiotensin on cation-transport by rat kidney cortex slices. J. Physiol. (Lond.) **215**, 269—282 (1971).

MUNDAY, K. A., PARSONS, B. J., POAT, J. A.: Studies on the mechanism of action of angiotensin on ion transport by kidney cortex slices. J. Physiol. (Lond.) **224**, 195—206 (1972).

NAKANO, J., KUSAKARI, T.: Effects of synthetic angiotensin on plasma free fatty acid and blood glucose-levels. Nature (Lond.) **209**, 922—923 (1966).

PEACH, M. J., BUMPUS, F. M., KHAIRALLAH, P. A.: Inhibition of norepinephrine uptake in hearts by angiotensin II and analogs. J. Pharmacol. exp. Ther. **167**, 291—299 (1969).

PEACH, M. J., BUMPUS, F. M., KHAIRALLAH, P. A.: Release of adrenal catecholamines by angiotensin I. J. Pharmacol. exp. Ther. **176**, 366—376 (1971).

POPLAWSKI, A.: The effect of angiotensin II on the platelet aggregation induced by adenosine-diphosphate, epinephrine and thrombin. Experientia (Basel) **26**, 86 (1969).

RAYYIS, S. S., HORTON, R.: Effect of angiotensin II on adrenal and pituitary function in man. J. clin. Endocr. **32**, 539—546 (1971).

ROBERTSON, A. L., Jr., KHAIRALLAH, P. A.: Angiotensin II: Rapid localization in nuclei of smooth and cardiac muscle. Science **172**, 1138—1139 (1971).

ROBISON, G. A., BUTCHER, R. W., SUTHERLAND, E. W.: Cyclic AMP. New York, London: Academic Press 1971.

ROSENFELD, S., BONORRIS, G., KRAUS, L. R., MCCULLEN, A.: Effect of renin and plasma protein loading on albumin catabolism in the isolated perfused kidney. Proc. Soc. exp. Biol. (N. Y.) **125**, 1118—1122 (1967).

ROTHLIN, M. E., ROTHLIN, C. B., WENDT, V. E.: Free fatty acid concentration and composition in arterial blood. Amer. J. Physiol. **203**, 306—310 (1962).

SCHWYZER, R.: Chemical structure and biological activity in the field of polypeptide hormones. Pure Appl. Chem. **6**, 265—295 (1963).

SHIBATA, S., CARRIER, O., Jr., FRANKENHEIM, J., DARNELL, J. R.: Effect of chlorpromazine, dibenamine and phenoxybenzamine on the contractile response of *taenia coli* to potassium, acetylcholine, angiotensin and barium. J. Pharmacol. exp. Ther. **160**, 106—111 (1968).

SLATER, J. D. H., BARBOUR, B. H., HENDERSON, H. H., CASPER, A. G. T., BARTTER, F. C.: Influence of the pituitary and the renin-angiotensin system on the secretion of aldosterone cortisol, and corticosterone. J. clin. Invest. **42**, 1504—1520 (1963).

SZALAY, K. S.: Inhibiting effect of angiotensin on potassium accumulation of adrenal cortex. Biochem. Pharmacol. 18, 962—964 (1969).

TÜRKER, R. K., PAGE, I. H., KHAIRALLAH, P. A.: Angiotensin alteration of sodium fluxes in smooth muscle. Arch. int. Pharmacodyn. **165**, 394—404 (1967).

VOLICER, L., HYNIE, S.: Effect of catecholamines and angiotensin on cyclic AMP in rat aorta and tail artery. Europ. J. Pharmacol. **15**, 214—220 (1971).

WERNING, V. C., STIEL, W., SCHWEIKERT, H. U., STIEL, D., VETTER, W., SIEGENTHALER, W.: Korrelationen zwischen Plasmareninaktivität und Blutdruck, Erythrocytenzahl, Hämoglobin, Hämatokrit sowie Natrium, Kalium, Harnstoff und Kreatinin im Serum bei Hypertonikern. Z. klin. Chem. **9**, 13—17 (1971).

ZWIETEN, P. A., VAN: Der Einfluß von adrenergen Pharmaka und von Val^5-Hypertensin II-amid auf die mittels ^{86}Rb gemessene Membranpermeabilität am isolierten Herzvorhof von Meerschweinchen. Naunyn-Schmiedeberg Arch. Pharmak. exp. Path. **261**, 441—457 (1968).

Some Possible Functions of Angiotensin

I. H. PAGE

Nothing is more treacherous than engaging in uninhibited soothsaying; more popularly known as "futurism", a guessing game widely practiced by the news media and all-season prophets. The regular occurrence of constant amounts of a substance in the body is seldom without purpose. The organism also exhibits an inner economy and prudence by using one substance for several functions. Epinephrine immediately comes to mind as such a substance. This is a warning that widely distributed single-function substances are rare.

The relative importance of a substance is an almost unanswerable question because the counter-question arises, "importance relative to what?" The question has merit usually only in comparing of the interrelationships of one substance with others performing the same, or similar functions. Thus, aldosterone secretion is stimulated by angiotensin and ACTH but the former usually seems the more important. But if the source of angiotensin is abolished, as in anephric patients, then ACTH or other substances may become the chief stimulants. It is this interplay of regulatory mechanisms, this ability of the body to use alternative regulatory systems, that makes the hemodynamic problems of the perfusion of tissue, and hence arterial pressure, so complicated. This is essential in the example of aldosterone, since aldosterone is so important in the organization of electrolyte homeostasis. Thus, angiotensin is an integral part of the mechanism of salt and water metabolism.

Angiotensin has *a* function and probably *multiple* ones. The two currently most discussed are the regulation of blood pressure and that of sodium metabolism. Its participation in both is scarcely to be doubted. It has both direct and complicated indirect mechanisms to achieve these two purposes. But it is nonsense to say that it is the only humoral regulatory system.

For years the problem of the participation of angiotensin in the mechanism of hypertension has been studied. Even today about the best that can be said is that most evidence strongly suggests active participation in the acute phase of renal hypertension. But there is still the uncertain evidence that anti-renin as shown by WAKERLIN and GOLDBLATT lowers the pressure in a few dogs with long-standing chronic experimental renal hypertension. Some believe that anti-renin is effective in the acute phase as well. Immunization with synthetic angiotensin in rabbits does not prevent the occurrence of hypertension in rabbits with perinephric compression or renal artery clip. Nor does it lower pressure in hypertension. The numbers of animals in these experiments are small but the conclusion drawn is firm that renin and angiotensin play no part in the development or maintenance of experimental renal hypertension. On the other hand, the results are all mutually contradictory, so that prudence requires that no firm conclusions be drawn from this group of experiments.

The recent advent of synthetic analogs of angiotensin, which compete with angiotensin for receptor sites, further strengthens the belief in participation during the acute phase. Here again the evidence is not definitive. There are those who believe that some analogs sharply reduce blood pressure during the acute phase but not to normal while having little or a slight pressor effect in chronic hypertension.

Angiotensin seems to be involved in the mechanism of malignant hypertension and of primary hyperaldosteronism. How and to what degree it participates in the mechanisms of renal and essential hypertension is still not clear. One by one many of the false pathways of men's minds are being recognized. Thus, it may be that renin and angiotensin within the blood vessel walls and brain are more involved than those deriving from the kidneys. Few deny the direct action of angiotensin on smooth muscle but this may not be its prime action in hypertension, rather its action on the sympathetic nervous system tending to be paramount. It is only recently being recognized that as methodology improves in specificity and sensitivity, it is becoming possible to deal with the amounts of such powerful pressor substances as angiotensin such as might occur in chronic, rather than acute, changes in arterial blood pressure and also to measure the angiotensin itself rather than the levels of plasma renin activity. Further, turnover rates are in some circumstances measurable, instead of levels.

Over the years I have become increasingly impressed by the possibility that angiotensin is the so-called "angiotoxic substance" responsible indirectly for the hemorrhagic necrotizing arteriolitis seen in malignant hypertension and hypertensive encephalopathy. I would even go so far as to suggest that it has a hand in the production of the miliary aneurysms probably responsible for many cerebral hemorrhages and possibly some myocardial infarctions (PAGE, 1972). This surely is far enough for a conservative to look into the future without a better pair of glasses for my mind's eye!

I strongly suspect that there are a number of other functions that will be uncovered by some lonely investigator who is not on any committee that tells him how and what to look for. Only recently FITZSIMONS has found good evidence that angiotensin might have been called "the thirst hormone" if its role in the body's water balance had first been studied.

Still another late development is the possibility that angiotensin is concerned in the control of renal blood flow and urine formation working in association with renal prostaglandins. Only weak evidence for this hypothesis exists.

Perhaps we have too long considered the kidneys as the only source of renin. Recent evidence suggests it is widespread. Whether it is produced outside the kidneys or is produced within the kidneys but stored elsewhere is unknown. Since SKEGGS' analyses show that there are various renins, the question arises as to the nature of renin in organs other than the kidneys or indeed, whether "renin-activity" is merely a proteolytic activity produced by a variety of enzymes. The observation of the occurrence of an angiotensin-like substance in brain suggests that renin-like activity is of local origin within the brain, which could cast quite a different light on the central action of angiotensin.

Author Index

Page numbers in *italics* refer to the bibliography

Subject Index

Handbuch der experimentellen Pharmakologie /

Handbook of Experimental Pharmacology

Heffter—Heubner, New Series

Vol. IV: **General Pharmacology**
ISBN 3-540-04845-6 DM 76,00; US $34.30

Vol. X: **Die Pharmakologie anorganischer Anionen**
ISBN 3-540-01465-9 DM 205,00; US $92.40

Vol. XI: **Lobelin und Lobeliaalkaloide**
ISBN 3-540-01910-3 DM 16,00; US $7.30

Vol. XII: **Morphin und morphinähnlich wirkende Verbindungen**
ISBN 3-540-02158-2 DM 79,00; US $35.60

Vol. XIII: **The Alkali Metal Ions in Biology.** In preparation

Vol. XIV:

Part 1 **The Adrenocortical Hormones I**
ISBN 3-540-02830-7 DM 260,00; US $117.10

Part 2 **The Adrenocortical Hormones II**
ISBN 3-540-03146-4 DM 75,00; US $33.80

Part 3 **The Adrenocortical Hormones III**
ISBN 3-540-04147-8 DM 152,00; US $68.50

Vol. XV: **Cholinesterases and Anticholinesterase Agents**
ISBN 3-540-02988-5 DM 328,00; US $147.80

Vol. XVI: **Erzeugung von Krankheitszuständen durch das Experiment**

Part 1 **Blut/Blood.** In preparation

Part 2 **Atemwege**
ISBN 3-540-04517-1 DM 124,00; US $55.90

Part 3 **Herz und Kreislauf / Heart and Circulation.** In preparation

Part 4 **Niere, Nierenbecken, Blase**
ISBN 3-540-03305-X DM 152,00; US $68.50

Part 5 **Leber.** In preparation

Part 6 **Schilddrüse.** In preparation

Part 7 **Zentralnervensystem**
ISBN 3-540-02831-5 DM 123,00; US $55.40

Part 8 **Stütz- und Hartgewebe**
ISBN 3-540-04518-X DM 98,00; US $44.20

Part 9 **Infektionen I**
ISBN 3-540-03147-2 DM 152,00; US $68.50

Part 10 **Infektionen II**
ISBN 3-540-03531-1 DM 169,00; US $76.20

Part 11A **Infektionen III**
ISBN 3-540-03840-X DM 150,00; US $67.60

Part 11B **Infektionen IV.** In preparation
ISBN 3-540-06290-4

Part 12 **Tumoren I**
ISBN 3-540-03532-X DM 150,00; US $67.60

Part 13 **Tumoren II**
ISBN 3-540-03533-8 DM 90,00; US $40.60

Part 14 **Tumoren III.** In preparation

Part 15 **Kohlenhydratstoffwechsel, Fieber / Carbohydrate Metabolism, Fever**
ISBN 3-540-03534-6 DM 150,00; US $67.60

Vol. XVII:

Part 1 **Ions, alcalino-terreux I. Systèmes isolés**
ISBN 3-540-02989-3 DM 162,00; US $73.00

Part 2 **Ions alcalino-terreux II. Organismes entiers**
ISBN 3-540-03148-0 DM 218,00; US $98.20

Vol. XVIII:

Part 1 **Histamine**
ISBN 3-540-03535-4 DM 202,00; US $91.00

Part 2 **Anti-Histaminics.** In preparation

Vol. XIX: **5-Hydroxytryptamine and Related Indolealkylamines**
ISBN 3-540-03536-2 DM 202,00; US $91.00

Vol. XX:
Part 1 **Pharmacology of Fluorides I**
ISBN 3-540-03537-0 DM 158,00; US $71.20
Part 2 **Pharmacology of Fluorides II**
ISBN 3-540-04846-4 DM 146,00; US $65.80

Vol. XXI: **Beryllium**
ISBN 3-540-03538-9 DM 40,00; US $18.10

Vol. XXII:
Part 1 **Die Gestagene I**
ISBN 3-540-04148-6 DM 320,00; US $144.20
Part 2 **Die Gestagene II**
ISBN 3-540-04519-8 DM 320,00; US $144.20

Vol. XXIII: **Neurohypophysial Hormones and Similar Polypeptides**
ISBN 3-540-04149-4 DM 192,00; US $86.50

Vol. XXIV: **Diuretica**
ISBN 3-540-04520-1 DM 248,00; US $111.70

Vol. XXV: **Bradykinin, Kallidin and Kallikrein**
ISBN 3-540-04847-2 DM 248,00; US $111.70

Vol. XXVI: **Vergleichende Pharmakologie von Überträgersubstanzen in tiersystematischer Darstellung**
ISBN 3-540-05132-5 DM 148,00; US $66.70

Vol. XXVII: **Anticoagulantien**
ISBN 3-540-05133-3 DM 198,00; US $89.20

Vol. XXVIII:
Part 1 **Concepts in Biochemical Pharmacology I**
ISBN 3-540-05134-1 DM 174,00; US $78.40
Part 2 **Concepts in Biochemical Pharmacology II**
ISBN 3-540-05389-1 DM 248,00; US $111.70
Part 3 **Concepts in Biochemical Pharmacology III.** In preparation

Vol. XXIX: **Oral wirksame Antidiabetika**
ISBN 3-540-05554-1 DM 296,00; US $133.40

Vol. XXX: **Modern Inhalation Anesthetics**
ISBN 3-540-05135-X DM 198,00; US $89.20

Vol. XXXI: **Antianginal Drugs**
ISBN 3-540-05365-4 DM 168,00; US $75.70

Vol. XXXII:
Part 1 **Insulin I**
ISBN 3-540-05470-7 DM 248,00; US $111.70
Part 2 **Insulin II.** In preparation

Vol. XXXIII: **Catecholamines**
ISBN 3-540-05517-7 DM 396,00; US $178.40

Vol. XXXIV: **Secretin, Cholecystokinin-Pancreozymin and Gastrin**
ISBN 3-540-05952-0 DM 165,00; US $74.40

Vol. XXXV:
Part 1 **Androgene I**
ISBN 3-540-05706-4 DM 298,00; US $134.30
Part 2 **Androgene II und Antiandrogene.** In preparation

Vol. XXXVI: **Uranium-Plutonium-Transplutonic Elements**
ISBN 3-540-06168-1 DM 374,00; US $168.50

Vol. XXXVII: **Angiotensin**
ISBN 3-540-06276-9 DM 224,00; US $100.90

Vol. XXXVIII: **Antineoplastic and Immunosuppressive Agents.**
ISBN 3-540-06402-8. In preparation

Preisänderungen vorbehalten / Prices are subject to change without notice

Reprint from

Handbuch der experimentellen Pharmakologie
Handbook of Experimental Pharmacology

New Series

Edited by: **O. Eichler, A. Farah, H. Herken, A. D. Welch**

Volume XXXVII

Editors: **I. H. Page and F. M. Bumpus**

Springer Verlag · Berlin · Heidelberg · New York 1973
Printed in Germany

The Biological Production of Angiotensin

L. T. Skeggs, F. E. Dorer, J. R. Kahn,
K. E. Lentz, and M. Levine

Reprint from

Handbuch der experimentellen Pharmakologie
Handbook of Experimental Pharmacology

New Series

Edited by: **O. Eichler, A. Farah, H. Herken, A. D. Welch**

Volume XXXVII

Editors: **I. H. Page and F. M. Bumpus**

Springer Verlag · Berlin · Heidelberg · New York 1973
Printed in Germany

The Fate of Angiotensin I

J. R. Vane

(Not in Circulation)

Reprint from

Handbuch der experimentellen Pharmakologie
Handbook of Experimental Pharmacology

New Series

Edited by: **O. Eichler, A. Farah, H. Herken, A. D. Welch**

Volume XXXVII

Editors: **I. H. Page and F. M. Bumpus**

Springer Verlag · Berlin · Heidelberg · New York 1973
Printed in Germany

Converting Enzyme in Vitro Measurement and Properties

Y. S. Bakhle

(Not in Circulation)

Reprint from

Handbuch der experimentellen Pharmakologie
Handbook of Experimental Pharmacology
New Series

Edited by: **O. Eichler, A. Farah, H. Herken, A. D. Welch**

Volume XXXVII
Editors: **I. H. Page and F. M. Bumpus**

Springer Verlag · Berlin · Heidelberg · New York 1973
Printed in Germany

The Fate of Angiotensin II

J. W. Ryan

(Not in Circulation)

Reprint from

Handbuch der experimentellen Pharmakologie
Handbook of Experimental Pharmacology

New Series

Edited by: **O. Eichler, A. Farah, H. Herken, A. D. Welch**

Volume XXXVII

Editors: **I. H. Page and F. M. Bumpus**

Springer Verlag · Berlin · Heidelberg · New York 1973
Printed in Germany

Catabolism of Angiotensin II

J. G. Ledingham and W. P. Leary

(Not in Circulation)

Reprint from
Handbuch der experimentellen Pharmakologie
Handbook of Experimental Pharmacology
New Series
Edited by: **O. Eichler, A. Farah, H. Herken, A. D. Welch**
Volume XXXVII
Editors: **I. H. Page and F. M. Bumpus**
Springer Verlag · Berlin · Heidelberg · New York 1973
Printed in Germany

Structure-Activity Relationship in Angiotensin II Analogs

M. C. Khosla, R. R. Smeby, and F. M. Bumpus

Reprint from

Handbuch der experimentellen Pharmakologie
Handbook of Experimental Pharmacology

New Series

Edited by: **O. Eichler, A. Farah, H. Herken, A. D. Welch**

Volume XXXVII

Editors: **I. H. Page and F. M. Bumpus**

Springer Verlag · Berlin · Heidelberg · New York 1973
Printed in Germany

Antagonists of Angiotensin II

R. K. Türker, I. H. Page, and F. M. Bumpus

(Not in Circulation)

Reprint from

Handbuch der experimentellen Pharmakologie
Handbook of Experimental Pharmacology

New Series

Edited by: **O. Eichler, A. Farah, H. Herken, A. D. Welch**

Volume XXXVII

Editors: **I. H. Page and F. M. Bumpus**

Springer Verlag · Berlin · Heidelberg · New York 1973
Printed in Germany

Tachyphylaxis to Angiotensin

J. M. Stewart

(Not in Circulation)

Reprint from

Handbuch der experimentellen Pharmakologie
Handbook of Experimental Pharmacology

New Series

Edited by: **O. Eichler, A. Farah, H. Herken, A. D. Welch**

Volume XXXVII

Editors: **I. H. Page and F. M. Bumpus**

Springer Verlag · Berlin · Heidelberg · New York 1973
Printed in Germany

Immunogenicity and Antigenicity of Angiotensin I and II

M. B. Vallotton

(Not in Circulation)

Reprint from

Handbuch der experimentellen Pharmakologie
Handbook of Experimental Pharmacology

New Series

Edited by: **O. Eichler, A. Farah, H. Herken, A. D. Welch**

Volume XXXVII

Editors: **I. H. Page and F. M. Bumpus**

Springer Verlag · Berlin · Heidelberg · New York 1973
Printed in Germany

Measurement of Renin and of Angiotensin (Extraction and Bioassay)

R. Boucher and J. Genest

(Not in Circulation)

Reprint from

Handbuch der experimentellen Pharmakologie
Handbook of Experimental Pharmacology
New Series

Edited by: **O. Eichler, A. Farah, H. Herken, A. D. Welch**

Volume XXXVII
Editors: **I. H. Page and F. M. Bumpus**

Springer Verlag · Berlin · Heidelberg · New York 1973
Printed in Germany

Angiotensin Immunoassay

G. W. Boyd and W. S. Peart

(Not in Circulation)

Reprint from

Handbuch der experimentellen Pharmakologie
Handbook of Experimental Pharmacology

New Series

Edited by: **O. Eichler, A. Farah, H. Herken, A. D. Welch**

Volume XXXVII

Editors: **I. H. Page and F. M. Bumpus**

Springer Verlag · Berlin · Heidelberg · New York 1973
Printed in Germany

Bioassay of Angiotensin

P. A. Khairallah and R. R. Smeby

(Not in Circulation)

Reprint from

Handbuch der experimentellen Pharmakologie
Handbook of Experimental Pharmacology

New Series

Edited by: **O. Eichler, A. Farah, H. Herken, A. D. Welch**

Volume XXXVII

Editors: **I. H. Page and F. M. Bumpus**

Springer Verlag · Berlin · Heidelberg · New York 1973
Printed in Germany

Plasma of Serum Vasopressor Peptides Other than Angiotensins

H. R. Croxatto

(Not in Circulation)

Reprint from

Handbuch der experimentellen Pharmakologie
Handbook of Experimental Pharmacology

New Series

Edited by: **O. Eichler, A. Farah, H. Herken, A. D. Welch**

Volume XXXVII

Editors: **I. H. Page and F. M. Bumpus**

Springer Verlag · Berlin · Heidelberg · New York 1973
Printed in Germany

Primary Aldosteronism: Importance of the Level of Plasma Renin as an Adjunct in Diagnosis

J. W. Conn and E. L. Cohen

(Not in Circulation)

Reprint from

Handbuch der experimentellen Pharmakologie
Handbook of Experimental Pharmacology

New Series

Edited by: **O. Eichler, A. Farah, H. Herken, A. D. Welch**

Volume XXXVII

Editors: **I. H. Page and F. M. Bumpus**

Springer Verlag · Berlin · Heidelberg · New York 1973
Printed in Germany

Secondary Hyperaldosteronism

E. G. Biglieri, J. R. Stockigt, M. Schambelan, and R. D. Collins

(Not in Circulation)

Reprint from

Handbuch der experimentellen Pharmakologie
Handbook of Experimental Pharmacology
New Series

Edited by: **O. Eichler, A. Farah, H. Herken, A. D. Welch**

Volume XXXVII
Editors: **I. H. Page and F. M. Bumpus**

Springer Verlag · Berlin · Heidelberg · New York 1973
Printed in Germany

Intermediary Metabolism of Aldosterone

J. C. Melby

(Not in Circulation)

Reprint from

Handbuch der experimentellen Pharmakologie
Handbook of Experimental Pharmacology

New Series

Edited by: **O. Eichler, A. Farah, H. Herken, A. D. Welch**

Volume XXXVII

Editors: **I. H. Page and F. M. Bumpus**

Springer Verlag · Berlin · Heidelberg · New York 1973
Printed in Germany

The Renin-Angiotensin System in the Control of Aldosterone Secretion

J. O. Davis

(Not in Circulation)

Reprint from

Handbuch der experimentellen Pharmakologie
Handbook of Experimental Pharmacology

New Series

Edited by: **O. Eichler, A. Farah, H. Herken, A. D. Welch**

Volume XXXVII

Editors: **I. H. Page and F. M. Bumpus**

Springer Verlag · Berlin · Heidelberg · New York 1973
Printed in Germany

Aldosterone Regulation in Sodium Deficiency: Role of Ionic Factors and Angiotensin II

J. R. Blair-West, J. P. Coghlan, D. A. Denton, and B. A. Scoggins

Reprint from

Handbuch der experimentellen Pharmakologie
Handbook of Experimental Pharmacology

New Series

Edited by: **O. Eichler, A. Farah, H. Herken, A. D. Welch**

Volume XXXVII

Editors: **I. H. Page and F. M. Bumpus**

Springer Verlag · Berlin · Heidelberg · New York 1973
Printed in Germany

Effects of Aldosterone on Blood Pressure, Water, and Electrolytes

F. Gross

(Not in Circulation)

Reprint from

Handbuch der experimentellen Pharmakologie
Handbook of Experimental Pharmacology

New Series

Edited by: **O. Eichler, A. Farah, H. Herken, A. D. Welch**

Volume XXXVII

Editors: **I. H. Page and F. M. Bumpus**

Springer Verlag · Berlin · Heidelberg · New York 1973
Printed in Germany

Adrenal Medulla

M. J. Peach

(Not in Circulation)

Reprint from

Handbuch der experimentellen Pharmakologie
Handbook of Experimental Pharmacology

New Series

Edited by: **O. Eichler, A. Farah, H. Herken, A. D. Welch**

Volume XXXVII

Editors: **I. H. Page and F. M. Bumpus**

Springer Verlag · Berlin · Heidelberg · New York 1973
Printed in Germany

Central Neurogenic Effects of Angiotensin

C. J. Dickinson and C. M. Ferrario

(Not in Circulation)

Reprint from

Handbuch der experimentellen Pharmakologie
Handbook of Experimental Pharmacology

New Series

Edited by: **O. Eichler, A. Farah, H. Herken, A. D. Welch**

Volume XXXVII

Editors: **I. H. Page and F. M. Bumpus**

Springer Verlag · Berlin · Heidelberg · New York 1973
Printed in Germany

Peripheral Effects of Angiotensin on the Autonomic Nervous System

J. W. McCubbin

(Not in Circulation)

Reprint from

Handbuch der experimentellen Pharmakologie
Handbook of Experimental Pharmacology

New Series

Edited by: **O. Eichler, A. Farah, H. Herken, A. D. Welch**

Volume XXXVII

Editors: **I. H. Page and F. M. Bumpus**

Springer Verlag · Berlin · Heidelberg · New York 1973
Printed in Germany

Angiotensin on Vascular Smooth Muscle

D. F. Bohr

(Not in Circulation)

Reprint from

Handbuch der experimentellen Pharmakologie
Handbook of Experimental Pharmacology

New Series

Edited by: **O. Eichler, A. Farah, H. Herken, A. D. Welch**

Volume XXXVII

Editors: **I. H. Page and F. M. Bumpus**

Springer Verlag · Berlin · Heidelberg · New York 1973
Printed in Germany

Circulatory Effects of Angiotensin

R. D. Buñag

(Not in Circulation)

Reprint from

Handbuch der experimentellen Pharmakologie
Handbook of Experimental Pharmacology

New Series

Edited by: **O. Eichler, A. Farah, H. Herken, A. D. Welch**

Volume XXXVII

Editors: **I. H. Page and F. M. Bumpus**

Springer Verlag · Berlin · Heidelberg · New York 1973
Printed in Germany

Effects of Angiotensin on the Renal Circulation

L. G. Navar and H. G. Langford

(Not in Circulation)

Reprint from

Handbuch der experimentellen Pharmakologie
Handbook of Experimental Pharmacology

New Series

Edited by: **O. Eichler, A. Farah, H. Herken, A. D. Welch**

Volume XXXVII

Editors: **I. H. Page and F. M. Bumpus**

Springer Verlag · Berlin · Heidelberg · New York 1973
Printed in Germany

Intrarenal Action of Angiotensin

K. Thurau

(Not in Circulation)

Reprint from

Handbuch der experimentellen Pharmakologie
Handbook of Experimental Pharmacology

New Series

Edited by: **O. Eichler, A. Farah, H. Herken, A. D. Welch**

Volume XXXVII

Editors: **I. H. Page and F. M. Bumpus**

Springer Verlag · Berlin · Heidelberg · New York 1973
Printed in Germany

Morphological Effects of Angiotensin on Arteries

P. Kincaid-Smith, A. Friedman, and J. B. Hobbs

Reprint from

Handbuch der experimentellen Pharmakologie
Handbook of Experimental Pharmacology

New Series

Edited by: **O. Eichler, A. Farah, H. Herken, A. D. Welch**

Volume XXXVII

Editors: **I. H. Page and F. M. Bumpus**

Springer Verlag · Berlin · Heidelberg · New York 1973
Printed in Germany

Effects of Angiotensin II on the Permeability of the Vascular Wall

A. Lazzarini Robertson and P. A. Khairallah

(Not in Circulation)

Reprint from

Handbuch der experimentellen Pharmakologie
Handbook of Experimental Pharmacology

New Series

Edited by: **O. Eichler, A. Farah, H. Herken, A. D. Welch**

Volume XXXVII

Editors: **I. H. Page and F. M. Bumpus**

Springer Verlag · Berlin · Heidelberg · New York 1973
Printed in Germany

Biochemical Effects of Angiotensin

T. L. Goodfriend, F. Fyhrquist, and D. Allman

(Not in Circulation)

Reprint from

Handbuch der experimentellen Pharmakologie
Handbook of Experimental Pharmacology

New Series

Edited by: **O. Eichler, A. Farah, H. Herken, A. D. Welch**

Volume XXXVII

Editors: **I. H. Page and F. M. Bumpus**

Springer Verlag · Berlin · Heidelberg · New York 1973
Printed in Germany

Some Possible Functions of Angiotensin

I. H. Page

(Not in Circulation)

www.ingramcontent.com/pod-product-compliance
Lightning Source LLC
Chambersburg PA
CBHW080535250926
51846CB00016B/964
* 9 7 8 3 6 4 2 6 5 6 0 2 6 *